Neuroepidemiology

Neuroepidemiology

From Principles to Practice

Edited by
Lorene M. Nelson
Caroline M. Tanner
Stephen K. Van Den Eeden
Valerie M. McGuire

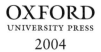

OXFORD
UNIVERSITY PRESS
2004

OXFORD

UNIVERSITY PRESS

Oxford New York
Auckland Bangkok Buenos Aires Cape Town Chennai
Dar es Salaam Delhi Hong Kong Istanbul Karachi Kolkata
Kuala Lumpur Madrid Melbourne Mexico City Mumbai
Nairobi São Paulo Shanghai Singapore Taipei Tokyo Toronto

Copyright © 2004 by Oxford University Press, Inc.

Published by Oxford University Press, Inc.
198 Madison Avenue, New York, New York, 10016
http://www.oup.com

Oxford is a registered trademark of Oxford University Press

Library of Congress Cataloging-in-Publication Data
Neuroepidemiology : from principles to practice /
edited by Lorene M. Nelson, Caroline M. Tanner, Stephen K. Van Den Eeden,
and Valerie M. McGuire.
p. ; cm. Includes bibliographical references and index.
ISBN 0-19-513379-X
1. Nervous system—Diseases—Epidemiology.
I. Nelson, Lorene M. II. Tanner, Caroline M.
III. Van Den Eeden, Stephen K., IV. McGuire, Valerie M.
[DNLM: 1. Nervous System Diseases—epidemiology.
2. Epidemiologic Methods.
WL 140 N4912 2004] RA645.N48N47 2004 614.5′98—dc21 2003042959

2 4 6 8 9 7 5 3 1

Printed in the United States of America
on acid-free paper

For Dave, Colin, and Adrienne
—L.M.N.

For Ana, Pam, Dorothy, and Richard
—C.M.T.

For Assia and Stella
—S.K.V.

Preface

Neurologic disorders are major contributors to death and disability. Disorders that begin in early or midlife, such as seizure disorders, brain injury, repetitive trauma disorders, and multiple sclerosis, are responsible for a considerable lifetime burden of chronic disability and lost productivity. Disorders that affect the elderly, such as stroke, dementia, and Parkinson's disease will be of increasingly greater importance as the population ages. Although the field of neuroepidemiology is young compared with other epidemiologic specialties such as cancer and cardiovascular disease epidemiology, the number and quality of neuroepidemiologic studies have rapidly increased in the last two decades.

The aim of this book is to provide new researchers with a comprehensive overview of basic epidemiologic research methods and to provide experienced researchers with strategies for adapting traditional research methods for the study of neurologic conditions. We begin with the basic principles of study design and end with the final application of these methods in translational research including clinical trials, health services research, and evidence-based medicine in neurology. The book is intended for practicing neurologists, epidemiologists, biostatisticians, health services researchers, and public health professionals, as well as students of these disciplines.

Several excellent texts already provide epidemiologic reviews of neurologic disorders. In this volume, we have a different goal. We have chosen to emphasize the methodologic aspects of epidemiologic research especially relevant to investigating neurologic disease. The book has three parts. In the first section, we focus on classic principles of epidemiologic and clinical research, including study design, sources of study bias, and methods for assessing the role of environmental and genetic factors in neurologic disorders. In the second part, we provide a critical summary of epidemiologic research on the major neurologic disorders, describe the methodologic challenges of studying each disorder, and identify research questions that merit further study. The third section is devoted to clinical and translational research methods, including the design and conduct of clinical trials and prognostic studies, as well as the principles of health services research and evidence-based medicine. Each chapter includes expanded examples illustrating important concepts, making this volume appropriate as a classroom text and as a research handbook for those who already have training in the field.

Early neuroepidemiologic studies emphasized the descriptive aspects of neurologic disease, such as patterns of incidence, prevalence, and mortality. These studies laid the groundwork for more recent analytic studies that identified factors associated with the occurrence of neurologic disorders. Some noteworthy examples are studies that have discovered the apolipoprotein $\epsilon4$ allele as a susceptibility gene for Alzheimer's disease, studies identifying the use of oral contraceptives as a risk factor for thromboembolic stroke, and studies determining that folate supplementation is a protective factor for neural tube defects. Study populations have also changed, so that investigations in smaller populations are being supplanted by large-scale population-based studies. In recent years, the use of genetic and biological markers, coupled with improved methods for risk-factor assessment, have improved the quality of neuroepidemiologic studies. We hope that the book will spur interest and growth in the evolving field of neuroepidemiology.

Stanford, California   L.M.N.
Sunnyvale, California   C.M.T.
Oakland, California   S.K.V.D.E.
Stanford, California   V.M.M.

Acknowledgments

This book is the sum of the contributions of many who have inspired, advised, and supported the editors throughout our careers. Among them are teachers, students, colleagues, and friends. Only a few of these individuals can be named here.

Our first debt of gratitude is to the colleagues who contributed to this volume. Without their dedicated work, our dream of a methodologically oriented textbook of neuroepidemiology would not have been possible. We are particularly grateful to them for their willingness to adopt the concept for this text and to participate in the many revisions needed to make this work a uniform whole. We are also indebted to Dr. Kristin Cobb, who added tremendously to this work through her in-depth understanding of epidemiology and biostatistics, her crisp prose, and her energy and good humor despite tight deadlines and late hours.

The vision and leadership of those epidemiologists who established the field of neuroepidemiology have inspired us to follow in their footsteps. We particularly acknowledge the recent loss of two of these dear colleagues—Drs. Leonard Kurland and John Annegers. Dr. Kurland had a lifelong commitment to neuroepidemiology, contributing immensely to the theoretical and practical developments of this field and training countless neuroepidemiologists worldwide. Among Dr. Kurland's most important contributions was the use of the Mayo Clinic medical records linkage system for neuroepidemiologic research. Dr. Kurland also championed the investigation of an unusual neurodegenerative disease clustered in the Western Pacific, the syndrome of amyotrophic lateral sclerosis, parkinsonism, and dementia. Dr. Kurland passed away in December of 2002. We also mourn the loss of Dr. John (Fred) Annegers, Professor of Epidemiology at the University of Texas School of Public Health. He made many contributions to our understanding of the neuroepidemiology of epilepsy and amyotrophic lateral sclerosis, especially as they affect minority populations. In February of 2000, Dr. Annegers passed away at the young age of 55. We are extremely grateful to him for his conscientious work on Chapter 12 (Epilepsy). Both Dr. Kurland and Dr. Annegers are greatly missed by their friends and colleagues, and their tremendous contributions to the field of neuroepidemiology will not be forgotten.

We have been fortunate to have many inspiring and generous teachers. Our love of epidemiology can be traced to many distinguished faculty, in particular, University of Washington Professors Tom Koepsell, Noel Weiss, Will Longstreth, Gary Franklin, Harvey Checkoway, and Gerald Van Belle, and University of California-Berkeley Professors Martyn Smith, William Satariano, and Robert Spear. Dr. Tanner is equally indebted to many teachers of neurology, notably Harold Klawans, Frank Morell, and Christopher Goetz.

The critical comments of our colleagues and students, many of whom read early drafts of chapters in this book, have been invaluable. Among these are David Thom, Rita Popat, Annette Langer-Gould, Diana Aston, Monica Korell, and Kathleen Comyns. Sarah Larson provided expert administrative support for every aspect of the book, from its inception to its finish. The editors are also grateful to others who worked on the many aspects of book production, including Michael Shino, Amethyst Leimpeter, Susan Sanborn, Robert Field, and Liv Trondsen.

Perhaps our deepest debt is to those patients with neurologic disorders who have volunteered as participants in epidemiologic and clinical studies. Without their selflessness in the face of personal misfortune, research to understand and combat diseases of the nervous system would not be possible. We hope that this book will return the favor of their contribution by improving the rigor of neuroepidemiologic research and by attracting new investigators to join this important field; such developments will in turn improve the treatment and prevention of neurologic disorders.

Finally, we offer our thanks to our family members, without whose love and support this book would not have been possible. We are grateful for their many years of encouragement, as well as their enduring patience while we toiled away on the manuscript.

Contents

Clinical Epidemiology

Contributors

J. FRED ANNEGERS, PhD*
University of Texas School of Public Health
Houston, Texas

CARMEL ARMON, MD, MHS
Department of Neurology
Loma Linda University School of Medicine
Loma Linda, California

ALBERTO ASCHERIO, MD, DrPH
Departments of Nutrition and Epidemiology
Harvard School of Public Health
Boston, Massachusetts

BERNADETTE BODEN-ALBALA, DrPH, MPH
Neurological Institute, Columbia University
New York, New York

MELISSA BONDY, PhD
Department of Epidemiology
The University of Texas M. D. Anderson Cancer Center
University of Texas
Houston, Texas

*Deceased

AMY BORENSTEIN GRAVES, PhD, MPH
Department of Epidemiology and Biostatistics
College of Public Health
University of South Florida
Tampa, Florida

COLEEN A. BOYLE, PhD
National Center on Birth Defects and Developmental Disabilities
Centers for Disease Control and Prevention
Atlanta, Georgia

TERRI CHEW, MPH
Department of Epidemiology and Biostatistics
University of California
San Francisco, California

KRISTIN COBB, PhD, MS
Division of Epidemiology, Department of Health Research & Policy
Stanford University School of Medicine
Stanford, California

MARIEKE C.J. DEKKER, PhD
Department of Epidemiology & Biostatistics
Erasmus Medical Center
Rotterdam, The Netherlands

GARY M. FRANKLIN, MD, MPH
Department of Environmental Health
University of Washington
Seattle, Washington

SANDRA W. HAMELSKY, PhD, MPH
New Jersey School of Public Health
University of Medicine and Dentistry of New Jersey
Piscataway, New Jersey
Bristol-Myers Squibb
Hillside, New Jersey

ROBERT G. HOLLOWAY, MD, MPH
Department of Neurology
University of Rochester
Rochester, New York

KARL KIEBURTZ, MD, MPH
Department of Neurology
University of Rochester
Rochester, New York

JESS F. KRAUS, PhD, MPH
Southern California Injury Prevention Research Center
Department of Epidemiology
UCLA School of Public Health
Los Angeles, California

RICHARD B. LIPTON, MD
Departments of Neurology, Epidemiology, and Social Medicine
Albert Einstein College of Medicine
Headache Unit, Montefiore Medical Center
Bronx, New York
Innovative Medical Research
Stamford, Connecticut

W.T. LONGSTRETH JR., MD, MPH
Department of Neurology
University of Washington
Seattle, Washington

KAREN MARDER, MD, MS
Gertrude H. Sergievsky Center and
Department of Neurology College of Physicians and Surgeons
Columbia University
New York, New York

CONNIE MARRAS, MD
The Parkinson's Institute
Sunnyvale, California

DAVID L. MCARTHUR, PHD, MPH
UCLA Brain Injury Research Center
Division of Neurosurgery
The Geffen School of Medicine at UCLA
Los Angeles, California

VALERIE MCGUIRE, PHD, MPH
Division of Epidemiology, Department of Health Research & Policy
Stanford University School of Medicine
Stanford, California

YURIKO MINN, MS
Department of Neurology
Stanford University School of Medicine
Stanford, California

KASSANDRA MUNGER, MSc
Department of Nutrition
Harvard School of Public Health
Boston, Massachusetts

CATHERINE C. MURPHY, PHD
National Center on Birth Defects and Developmental Disabilities
Centers for Disease Control and Prevention
Atlanta, Georgia

LORENE M. NELSON, PHD, MS
Division of Epidemiology, Department of Health Research & Policy
Stanford University School of Medicine
Stanford, California

BEATE RITZ, MD, PhD
School of Public Health
University of California Los Angeles
Los Angeles, California

G. WEBSTER ROSS, MD
Honolulu Department of Veteran Affairs
Pacific Health Research Institute
Honolulu, Hawaii

RALPH L. SACCO, MD, MS
Neurological Institute, Columbia University
New York, New York

STEVEN R. SCHWID MD
Department of Neurology
University of Rochester
Rochester, New York

WALTER F. STEWART, PhD, MPH
Geisinger Health Systems
Danville, Pennsylvania

CAROLINE M. TANNER, MD, PhD
Parkinson's Institute
Sunnyvale, California

DAVID H. THOM, MD, PhD
UCSF Department of Family Medicine
San Francisco, California

STEPHEN K. VAN DEN EEDEN, PhD
Division of Research
Kaiser Permanente
Oakland, California

CORNELIA M. VAN DUIJN, PhD
Department of Epidemiology & Biostatistics
Erasmus Medical Center
Rotterdam, The Netherlands

BARBARA G. VICKREY, MD, MPH
UCLA Department of Neurology
Los Angeles, California

MARGARET WRENSCH, PhD
Department of Epidemiology and Biostatistics
University of California
San Francisco, California

Neuroepidemiology

1

Neuroepidemiology: Fundamental Considerations

CAROLINE M. TANNER AND G. WEBSTER ROSS

Neuroepidemiology addresses the distribution and determinants of neurologic diseases in populations with the ultimate aim of preventing disease. Our goal in this book is to provide the basic information necessary for planning and implementing public health research in diseases of the nervous system. We hope to be equally useful to epidemiologists who are not familiar with neurologic disease and neurologists who are not familiar with epidemiologic approaches. Knowledge of the unique characteristics of the nervous system is essential to the design and conduct of studies of neurologic diseases. This first chapter briefly presents essential concepts for the reader not trained in neuroscience. The chapter also provides an overview of epidemiologic study design, emphasizing aspects relevant to the investigation of neurologic disease. Basic methodologic topics important to all neuroepidemiologic studies are covered here and in Chapters 2 and 3. Then individual chapters address major categories of neurologic disease and specific types of study (genetic epidemiology, clinical trials, prognosis, health services and utilization). Because these chapters emphasize the design, conduct, and interpretation of neuroepidemiologic studies, many details about particular neurologic disorders have been omitted. For more in-depth discussion, the reader is referred to several excellent textbooks on epidemiology and clinical research (Kelsey et al. 1996; Rothman and Greenland 1998; Gordis 2000; Portney and Watkins 2000) and on neurology and neuroscience (Rowland 1995; Bradley et al. 1999; Kandel et al. 2000; Victor and Ropper 2001; Goetz 2003; Koepsell and Weiss 2003; Squire et al. 2003).

The Nervous System

The nervous system is comprised of the brain, spinal cord, and peripheral nerves. The brain and spinal cord are complex assemblages of functionally specific individual nerve cell populations and supportive tissues. The brain and spinal cord are encased in a bony skull and vertebrae. This enclosed space protects nervous system tissue but may contribute to injury in pathologic states causing an increase in the volume of the contents (such as hemorrhage, masses). The brain and spinal cord have central cavities, the ventricles and spinal canal. The external surfaces are covered by a thick protective membrane (the dura). The cerebrospinal fluid (CSF) is produced within the ventricles by the choroid plexus and circulates out to bathe the external surfaces within the subdural space before being absorbed by the blood stream.

An awareness of the unique characteristics of the nervous system is important in understanding the diseases affecting these tissues. First, essentially all body functions are controlled or regulated by the nervous system. These include consciousness, thought in all of its complexities, learning and memory, sleep, voluntary and involuntary behaviors, emotion, sensory perception, and control or modulation of visceral function. Second, nervous system tissue, on the whole, does not repair itself or regenerate after injury. Third, the nervous system is relatively protected from exogenous exposures by the blood–brain barrier and the blood–nerve barrier. Fourth, the brain has high metabolic requirements and is vulnerable to injury within minutes after interruption of its metabolic needs. Fifth, within the brain and spinal cord, the old real estate adage "location, location, location" is particularly relevant. Cell populations separated by only millimeters can control dramatically different functions and can exist in very different biochemical and physiological milieu. Sixth, the brain and spinal cord are on the whole not easily accessible tissues. Each of these features adds to the complexity of investigations of the nervous system in health and disease. Failure to consider the unique characteristics of the nervous system can lead to mistaken inferences.

Diagnosing Neurologic Disease

Because direct examination of the brain (for example, by inspection or biopsy) is difficult and carries the risk of injury, indirect methods for evaluating nervous system function are central to the assessment of the nervous system in the living human. Each method, however, provides an incomplete picture, based on only some aspects of brain function, and interpreting results requires highly trained experts. Even with the expertise of specialists, in some cases a definite diagnosis may not be possible until the brain is examined at postmortem. The need to examine the brain postmortem presents a tremendous challenge in designing epidemiologic studies of some disorders, as follow-up to death can be costly. Moreover, even with high rates of follow-up, few subjects may consent to postmortem evaluation of the brain. In such situations, well-studied diagnostic criteria, with known sensitivity and specificity, will provide insight into the potential for diagnostic misclassification (see below).

The basic tool in neurologic diagnosis is expert examination. The clinical neurologist, trained in neuroanatomy, obtains the neurologic history from the patient including onset date and symptoms, conducts a neurologic exam to elicit clinical signs of neurologic dysfunction, and identifies the specific area of brain injury to predict the likely causes of injury. Neuroimaging techniques that reveal the structures of the brain and spinal cord tissue, such as computerized axial tomography (CAT) and magnetic resonance imaging (MRI), can supplement the clinical exam. Neuroimaging studies show changes in the gross anatomy of nervous system structures but miss smaller anatomic changes, microscopic changes, or changes in function without clear-cut anatomic changes. Many neurologic illnesses are characterized by these less obvious changes. In many cases, even when an anatomic change is identified, neither the cause nor the pathologic or clinical effect of the change can be determined from the image. Some imaging approaches take advantage of unique metabolic or neurotransmitter characteristics of tissues to identify areas of injury (positron emission tomography [PET], single photon emission computerized tomography [SPECT], functional MRI [fMRI]).

Communication from neuron to neuron occurs electrochemically, and diagnostic tests based on measuring the electrical activity of the nervous system (e.g., the electroencephalogram [EEG], electromyogram [EMG], and evoked responses [ERs]) can be useful diagnostic adjuncts to neuroimaging techniques. CSF evaluation can be helpful in diagnosing some diseases such as meningitis and multiple sclerosis. Other tests, such as blood or urine analyses, are less often useful in the identification of primary neurologic illnesses, although in some genetic disorders DNA evaluation can be diagnostic.

Disease-specific Challenges in the Conduct of Neuroepidemiologic Research

The specific characteristics of a disorder as well as the special features of the nervous system can pose challenges in the investigation of neurologic disease (Table 1–1). First, many neurologic diseases are relatively rare. This makes it difficult to assemble a large population-based sample of patients with the disease. One consequence of having a small number of subjects with a condition is that the statistical precision of estimates of disease

Table 1–1 Challenges in Neuroepidemiology

1. Diagnostic criteria may vary across studies and/or over time.
2. Definite diagnosis may require postmortem examination.
3. Diagnosis during life may require an expert.
4. Many neurologic diseases are relatively rare.
5. Precise time of disease onset may be uncertain.
6. There is a long latent period before diagnosis in some diseases.
7. Intermittent symptoms and signs occur in some diseases.
8. Most neurologic diseases not reportable in the United States, and there are few disease registries.

frequency or association measures such as the relative risk and the odds ratio will be lower. Also, rare disorders may be unfamiliar to many generalist physicians, resulting in greater diagnostic misclassification. Expert examination can often improve diagnostic accuracy, but these are costly and often unfeasible. Diagnostic criteria may vary tremendously across studies, or over time, making it difficult to compare studies. The potential for missing cases is greatest for disorders without a good diagnostic test. If cases of disease are not identified, disease frequency will be underestimated. Reporting is not required for most neurologic diseases in the United States. As a consequence, disease registries are not available for many neurologic disorders. For some disorders, voluntary registries exist, but registry cases may not be representative of all cases in the population.

Because it is essential to life, the nervous system has tremendous reserve capacity. For many chronic neurologic diseases, the pathophysiologic mechanisms causing the illness may be active, but clinical signs or symptoms may be absent for months or years (Fig. 1–1). If symptom onset is insidious, the diseased person may not seek medical care at first onset. For uncommon diseases, diagnosis may be delayed further if the physician is unfamiliar with the disorder. Consequently, the actual time of disease onset often may not be easily determined. This can affect retrospective risk factor identification, since the exposure time of greatest interest would be before the onset of the pathogenetic process, not the time of diagnosis. Finally, many neurologic diseases have intermittent symptoms and signs, so that population surveys based on a single contact with the subject may miss affected persons.

The Research Question

The first and most essential step in any research study is to clearly articulate the research question (Table 1–2). A clear state-

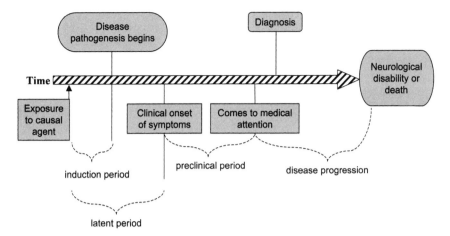

Figure 1–1 Schematic relationship between exposure, disease pathogenesis, and symptom onset. During the period from exposure to disease manifestations, the *latent period,* clinical signs and symptoms are absent. The patient experiences symptoms when neuronal injury is sufficient to cause disease manifestations. Even after patient experiences symptoms, a preclinical interval of several months or even years can occur before the patient seeks medical care and receives a correct diagnosis. Identification of causative factors is challenging in this situation.

ment of the study aims and the specific hypotheses to be addressed will guide selection of the study design, the outcome measures, the population, and the analysis plan. Common epidemiologic questions include the following:

1. How many cases of the disease are there in a population?
2. What are the demographic features of the disease?
3. What is the natural history of the disease?
4. What factors determine a good or poor prognosis of the disease?
5. What are the determinants of the disease—both genetic and environmental?
6. What are the economic characteristics of the disease?
7. What are the best treatments for the disease?
8. How can the disease be prevented?

These broad questions typically are addressed by answering a logical series of more focused questions, ideally refined through a dialogue of clinicians, epidemiologists and basic scientists.

The research question may address a novel hypothesis, provide better quality data to address an existing hypothesis, or reformulate an existing hypothesis to gain a better understanding of the underlying mechanism. Often, iteration of the question among epidemiologists, clinicians, and basic researchers results in heightened understanding of the disease and a more focused direction of the inquiry (Fig. 1–2).

Example 1–1 Early in the twentieth century, Parkinson's disease was popularly held to be the result of genetic predisposition or exposure to influenza virus (Tanner and Goldman, 1996). Investigation of a cluster of young narcotic addicts with rapid-onset parkinsonism in the early 1980s led to identification of the neurotoxin MPTP (1-methyl 4-phenyl tetrahydropyridine) as the cause of the parkinsonism (Langston et al., 1983). MPTP, a contaminant in a locally manufactured "designer" narcotic, was injected intravenously by those affected. It has provided a useful animal model for Parkinson's disease. Because MPTP resembles compounds such as the pesticide paraquat and blocks mitochondrial respiration, it fanned interest in the environmental causes of Parkinson's disease. Several case–control studies have demonstrated a role for pesticides in risk for Parkinson's disease. In recent years, knowledge about the etiology of Parkinson's disease has taken great steps forward through the active collaboration of epidemiologists, neurologists, neuroscientists, geneticists, and toxicologists.

In formulating a hypothesis, it is important to critically review the clinical, epidemiologic, and basic science literature. Some caveats are also important. First, there is often a publication bias, so that more "positive" studies than negative studies are published Overconfidence in published studies can also influence the results of subsequent studies. Investigators may make false assumptions or limit the scope of their study designs on the basis of previously published conclusions. Specific published results may also influence those affected with disease and result in a form of information bias (i.e., "recall" bias) in which the case has spent more time considering exposure to a risk factor than has a control (see Chapter 2).

Articulation of a clear set of hypotheses will direct the choice of study outcome measures (see Chapters 3 and 18) and of the appropriate design, study population, and study methods (Table 1–2).

Table 1–2 Steps Involved in Epidemiologic Research, Chapter Coverage of Concepts

Step	Activity	Coverage of concept
1	Develop research question to address etiology, diagnosis, prognosis, or treatment	Chapters 1, 4
2	Determine outcome measures	Chapters 1 (overview), 3 (detail)
3	Choose optimal study design to address the research question	Chapters 1 (overview), 2 (detail)
4	Define source population in which to conduct study	Chapter 1
5	Decide on sampling method for selecting subjects from source population (i.e., identify "study base")	Chapters 1, 2
6	Use thorough methods for identifying neurologic patients for study	Chapter 1
7	Apply disease definition according to strict criteria (i.e, case definition), define inclusion and exclusion criteria	Chapter 1
8	Determine sample size needs and statistical power to detect associations of interest	Chapter 3
9	Design study to avoid common biases such as selection bias, confounding, and measurement error	Chapters 2, 3
10	Collect data regarding health predictors or risk factors for neurologic condition	Chapters 2, 3
11	Apply quality control methods to ensure data integrity, examine reliability and validity	Chapter 3
12	Analyze association between predictors or risk factors and neurological outcome	Chapter 3
13	Control for biases in conduct of the study and in data analysis	Chapters 2, 3
14	Make inferences about the nature of associations (i.e., causal or only associated?)	Chapter 2
15	Determine public health impact of associations, identify preventive health practices to reduce frequency and severity of disease	Chapters 2, 3
16	Determine how study findings will affect the practice of medicine, develop evidence-based practice guidelines	Chapter 19
17	Use information about disease frequency and severity to plan delivery of health care, emphasizing quality and cost-effectiveness	Chapter 18

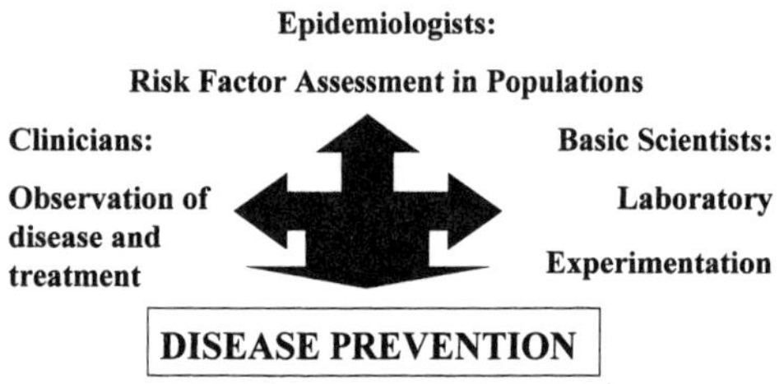

Epidemiologists:

Risk Factor Assessment in Populations

Clinicians: Basic Scientists:

Observation of   Laboratory
disease and
treatment   Experimentation

DISEASE PREVENTION

Figure 1–2 The ultimate goal of neuroepidemiology is to identify the causes of disease, to allow prevention, or to cure disease. This is most efficiently achieved via the dynamic collaboration of clinical, laboratory, and epidemiologic investigators.

Study Design

The first step in designing a study is to identify the ideal scientific approach to address the research question at hand. This optimal design may later be tempered by ethical concerns or practical considerations. However, the effect of these compromises on the scientific integrity of the study must always be considered. If a study design poses significant ethical concerns, it should be abandoned.

Epidemiologic studies can be classified in several broad ways (Table 1–3, Fig. 1–3). Studies can be grouped by purpose (descriptive or analytical). Descriptive studies identify patterns of disease in populations. Analytic studies address the determinants or risk factors of disease. Studies can also be classified according to the study design used, such as experimental and observational (nonexperimental) studies. Finally, epidemiologic studies can be classified temporally, as prospective or retrospective studies. Both disease ascertainment and exposure assessment can be performed prospectively or retrospectively. By definition, experimental studies (randomized trials) are prospective. The exposure is introduced by the researcher as part of the study, and subjects are followed to determine the outcome.

Descriptive studies describe the pattern of disease in the population. All descriptive studies employ observational designs. These can be cross-sectional, retrospective, or prospective. Cross-sectional descriptive studies can report on the incidence of disease among different populations defined geographically or demographically. Retrospective descriptive studies can examine changes in disease prevalence over time, while prospective descriptive studies can look at the incident of new cases and the natural history of disease, including mortality rates. Observing disease patterns within a population and comparing disease patterns across populations can lead to hypotheses regarding the causes of or treatments for a disease.

Analytic studies investigate the cause, treatment, or prevention of a disease. Analytic studies may have experimental or observational designs. In experimental stud-

Table 1–3 Types of Epidemiologic Studies

Experimental Studies

Types

Clinical trials
Field trials
Community interventions

Limitations

Resource intensive
Practical constraints preclude some questions
Ethical constraints preclude some questions

Strengths

Scientifically sound
Controlled, randomized design possible
Can determine cause and effect

Nonexperimental (Observational) Studies

Types

Cohort studies
Case–control studies
Cross-sectional studies
Ecological studies

Limitations

Measure association only
Not controlled or randomized

Strengths

Less resource intensive
Fewer practical constraints
Fewer ethical constraints

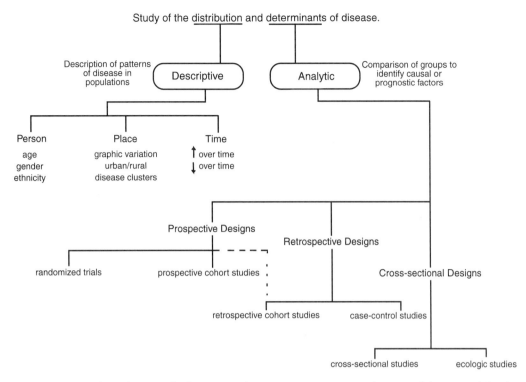

Study of the <u>distribution</u> and <u>determinants</u> of disease.

Description of patterns of disease in populations — **Descriptive**

Analytic — Comparison of groups to identify causal or prognostic factors

Person
age
gender
ethnicity

Place
graphic variation
urban/rural
disease clusters

Time
↑ over time
↓ over time

Prospective Designs

Retrospective Designs

randomized trials

prospective cohort studies

Cross-sectional Designs

retrospective cohort studies

case-control studies

cross-sectional studies

ecologic studies

Figure 1–3 Epidemiologic study designs can be classified by study purpose, as descriptive or analytic. Further classification describes population, outcome, and temporal features of the design (see text for detailed discussion).

ies, a specific action is performed to obtain the answer to a research question—that is, an experiment is carried out. The prototypic experimental study is a randomized controlled clinical trial in which a proposed treatment and identical placebo are compared to determine whether the proposed treatment is safe and effective (Fig. 1–4, see also Chapter 17). Other studies in this category are variations applied to nonclinical settings, such as field trials and community interventions. Such trials may also focus on primary prevention of disease. In experimental studies, conditions can be carefully controlled so that only the factor in question is altered between comparison groups. A well-designed experimental study is the ideal investigational approach to hypothesis testing. While this approach is easily applied in the laboratory, in clinical settings, in which research subjects are usually involved as volunteers, experimentation must

be tempered by ethical and practical considerations. For example, investigating whether or not a particular risk factor causes disease would not be an appropriate question for a controlled trial, as this would require causing disease in previously

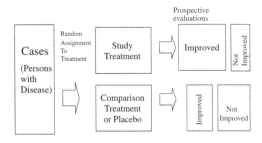

Figure 1–4 Schematic representation of randomized trials. First a representative sample of cases is identified. The study and comparison treatments are then introduced. Subjects are followed prospectively to assess outcome.

nondiseased persons. Similarly, it would be impractical to design a controlled trial to investigate whether a specific diet during infancy could prevent Alzheimer's disease, since the expense involved in life-long follow-up of individuals in each treatment arm would be prohibitive.

Observational analytic studies include cross-sectional studies as well as cohort and case–control studies. In some cross-sectional studies, risk factor exposure is assessed in addition to the disease distribution (Fig. 1–5). However, cross-sectional designs have limited value for analytical purposes, because the timing of exposure relative to disease onset cannot be determined. In ecological studies, the frequencies of disease and exposure are compared among populations without individual enumeration of persons with disease or exposure (Fig. 1–6). Because exposure and disease are correlated on an ecological (group) basis rather than within individuals, it is not possible to be certain that the risk factor and the disease are actually associated, further limiting any conclusions derived from this type of cross-sectional study. Other observational studies address the determinants of disease risk by comparing putative risk factors for disease between a group of cases and a group of controls. The

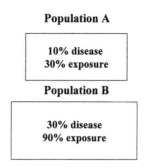

Population A

10% disease
30% exposure

Population B

30% disease
90% exposure

Figure 1–6 Schematic representation of ecological studies. Populations are identified in aggregate; individuals are not enumerated. The frequencies of exposure and disease are identified for each population at the same time point.

risk factor information can be obtained prospectively or retrospectively. Ideally, information is collected independent of awareness of disease status. In prospective cohort studies (Fig. 1–7), exposure information is collected on a population, or *cohort*, before the onset of disease. The cohort is followed into the future to identify new cases of disease. In some cases, exposure information may be collected retrospectively in an established cohort. In case–control studies (Fig. 1–8), risk factor exposure is determined for persons with disease (cases) and a comparison group (controls), and exposure information is collected retrospectively.

Observational studies share one critical limitation: cause and effect cannot be tested

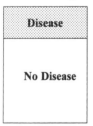

Persons with disease are
ascertained at a single time

Disease

No Disease

Figure 1–5 Schematic representation of cross-sectional studies. First a study population sample is identified. Cases with disease are then ascertained at a single time point. Exposure or other factors may also be identified at the same time.

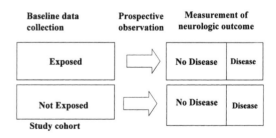

Baseline data collection	Prospective observation	Measurement of neurologic outcome	
Exposed	⇨	No Disease	Disease
Not Exposed	⇨	No Disease	Disease

Study cohort

Figure 1–7 Schematic representation of cohort studies. A representative population sample is identified. Exposure information is collected at baseline. Subjects are followed for development of disease.

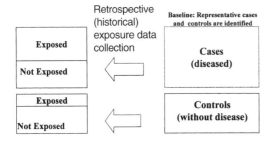

Figure 1–8 Schematic representation of case–control studies. A study population sample is first identified. Cases with disease are ascertained, and controls are selected. Exposure information is collected retrospectively.

directly; only the *association* of outcome and exposure can be determined. Inferences regarding the study hypothesis must include an awareness of this limitation (see Chapters 2, 3). Examples of erroneous conclusions due to inappropriate inference based on observational studies are legion. Observational studies are also more prone to study biases, such as selection bias and confounding, than are randomized trials. Randomized trials are not altogether exempt from study biases, however (see Chapters 2, 17).

Choosing the Study Population

A critical step in the design of an epidemiologic study is the selection of the study population. A meticulously conducted study can be rendered useless if the population investigated is inappropriate for the research question. Choice of the correct study population is guided by the research question and tempered by practical considerations. The goal is to investigate the research question in a study population that most represents the entire population of interest (sometimes called the "target" population). Ideally, all members of a population would be assessed in an epidemiologic study, although such an approach is rarely possible. An alternative is to take a sample of subjects from the study population (sometimes referred to as a "source" pop-

ulation) similar to the entire population of interest (also called the "base" population), and with the appropriate characteristics to allow investigation of the study hypothesis. Study populations may be established or assembled specifically to address the research question of interest (Table 1–4). For many research questions, it is essential that the base population is enumerated or can be numerated using a list or census. For example, the number of persons in the base population must be known to estimate incidence or prevalence. Because many neurologic disorders are relatively uncommon, identifying or assembling populations of adequate size can be challenging. Use of populations assembled for other purposes can sometimes provide a useful alternative. Other study designs, such as clinical trials or case–control studies, do not require a fully enumerated base population. However, the more closely the study population represents the "target" population (to whom the results will be extrapolated) the more valid the study will be.

Table 1–4 Source Populations for Epidemiologic Studies

A. Base Population Enumerated

Existing Populations

Birth and death records
Public records (census, voting records, automobile licensees)
Health-care utilization records (National Health Insurance, HCFA, HMOs)
Disease registries (mandatory reporting)

Study-specific Populations

Exposure/risk factor cohorts
Demographic cohorts (birth, gender, race/ethnicity)
Surveys with household enumeration
Family studies with complete enumeration

B. Base Population Not Enumerated

Hospital/private medical practice
Members of voluntary organizations
Respondents to advertisements, some surveys
Industry or occupational workers
Disease registries (voluntary)
Disease clusters (familial, geographic, temporal)

HCFA, Health Care Financing Administration; HMO, health maintenance organization.

Populations for Experimental Studies

Experimental epidemiologic studies typically address the value of an intervention with respect to a disease outcome. In a clinical trial, persons with the disease who receive the treatment of interest are compared to others with the disease who do not receive the treatment. Persons in each comparison group should be similar except for the intervention that will be assigned. This correspondence is achieved if a population of persons with the disease of interest is assembled, and each person is randomly assigned to the intervention being studied or a comparison intervention (usually either a placebo or standard therapy). If treatment assignment is not random, the group receiving the treatment is likely to differ from the untreated group. Persons participating in the study would ideally be representative of all persons with the disease who might ultimately receive the therapy being tested. Representativeness may not be easily achieved, however, as persons volunteering for clinical trials typically differ from those not participating in important ways (such as age, gender, race/ethnicity, socioeconomic status, disease severity), and the application of inclusion and exclusion criteria may further limit the representative nature of the group. Investigators must include in their design specific plans to identify and include the most representative sample possible. When this cannot be achieved, conclusions drawn from a study must be tempered by the lack of representativeness of the study population. The same principles apply to other experimental studies, although the "unit" of comparison may differ.

Populations for Observational Studies

Populations for Descriptive Studies. When the goal is to describe the pattern and frequency of disease, it is essential that the descriptive characteristics of the base population and the study population are well known. For example, determining the age-, gender-, and race-specific distribution of disease requires that the age, gender, and racial characteristics of the base population be known. The base population should closely resemble the target population for the descriptive characteristics assessed in the study. If the base population and target population differ, extrapolation may not be appropriate. For example, it may not be valid to apply disease incidence rates obtained from investigating an urban county to the population in a rural region. The relationship between the study population and the base population must also be clear. For example, age, gender, race, and disease status may be well known for the participants in a physician's private practice. However, the relationship of the participants in the practice and the entire community in which that practice occurs is unknown. Therefore, the practice would not be an appropriate study population for an estimate of disease frequency in that community. A second important feature in choosing a population for descriptive studies is the quality of information available regarding the disease (see below). For example, death records provide complete enumeration of deaths for a population, but would not be a useful source for a descriptive study of headache, as disease status would not be coded on the death certificate.

Populations for Analytic Studies. A characteristic of all analytic observational studies is that the study question assesses an association between a risk factor and disease. Because the conclusion is determined by this comparison, it is critical that the study population be representative of the target population with respect to the risk factors of interest. For example, a study conducted in a predominantly male population may not allow similar reasoning about risk factors for women. Or, a study conducted in an industrialized country may not be valid for a primarily agrarian country. Representativeness is best achieved if the study population is systematically assembled from the base population. Established databases such as cancer registries or death records can sometimes serve this purpose, although at other times it may be necessary to assemble a population to address certain questions. Ideally, the diseased and nondiseased populations will have similar opportunities for exposure to the risk factors of interest. This is most easily achieved through the investigation of a cohort assembled to allow measurement of the risk factors. Few large cohorts have been established to study risk factors for neurologic disease; however, many cohorts originally established to investigate risk factors for other common diseases, such as cardiovascular disease, may be useful in the investigation of risk factors for neurologic disease.

Example 1–2 The Honolulu Heart Program was established in 1965 to investigate risk factors for cardiovascular disease. Men of Japanese and Okinawan descent born between 1900 and 1919 and living in Honolulu were enrolled (Kagan et al. 1974; White et al. 1996). Risk factor information was collected in 1965–67, 1967–70, 1971–74, 1991–93, 1994–96, and 1996–98. Beginning in 1990, Parkinson's disease was ascertained in the cohort. Risk factor analyses have identified strong inverse associations between cigarette smoking and coffee drinking and risk of Parkinson's disease (Grandinetti et al. 1994; Ross et al. 2000). Because exposure information was collected prospectively, long before disease was diagnosed, recall bias and respondent bias are minimized. A single cohort study can thus provide more conclusive evidence about an association than can several case–control studies of the same association.

Assembling and maintaining a cohort for decades is costly, and size must be limited by practical concerns. For this reason, cohort studies are not practical for investigating rare diseases. However, increasingly the data from large cohorts are being pooled. This strategy may in the future provide opportunity to study less common diseases (or risk factors) using a cohort method.

Case–control studies provide a less resource-intensive alternative to cohort studies. The study population is identified by the presence (cases) or absence (controls) of disease. Ideally, cases enrolled will be representative of the target population. Both cases and controls should be selected from the same base population, with the same opportunity for exposure to the risk factor. This is most easily accomplished if cases and controls are recruited from a defined population (such as the residents of a defined geographic area or members of a health maintenance organization) using the same ascertainment strategies. When a suitable defined population is not available, ensuring that cases and controls are selected in a similar fashion presents a methodologic challenge. Cases commonly are identified through medical care facilities. Identification of controls from the same facility is appropriate only if the same selection forces determined the use of that facility by the control. For example, a specialty clinic may attract a greater proportion of cases with a high socioeconomic status. In contrast, those seeking routine care at the same medical center may have primarily moderate or low socioeconomic status. Comparing cases and controls will show an association of disease and higher socioeconomic status, as well as many commonly studied factors that are associated with socioeconomic status (e.g., occupational exposures, smoking, dietary intake). However, these associations would be the result of the selection process, and not necessarily identify true risk factors for disease.

Cognitive impairment can be a feature of many neurologic disorders. If a case is cognitively impaired, an additional source of information about risk factors will be needed. This may be a proxy informant or an existing data source (such as a medical record). For control selection, proxy informants may need to be recruited to ensure the integrity of the comparison when case information is collected via proxies. In addition, some population controls who have cognitive impairment may be selected, especially in studying late-life diseases (since dementia is more common in older populations). Control inclusion criteria should include a plan for handling cognitively impaired subjects (see Chapter 2).

For some diseases, most notably cancer, population-based disease registries exist, and reporting cancer is mandatory in the United States. Because the symptoms of brain tumors are severe, persons with brain tumors almost always seek medical attention. Therefore most cases of malignant cancer affecting the brain will be reported. Cancer registries generally do not collect risk factor information, however. Cases or their surviving family members will be needed to provide these data. Control selection also poses a problem, as persons without cancer will not be registered. Since brain tumors and other cancers may have shared risk factors, use of registered persons without brain cancer (but with other cancers) as controls could cause invalid results.

Health professionals are not required to report most neurologic diseases, however. Voluntary groups, recognizing the potential scientific value of a registry, often establish registries among their membership. Such registries are subject to many biases, particularly nonrepresentativeness. Cases voluntarily registering likely differ from those not registering in many ways, including in age, gender, socioeconomic status, race/ethnicity, and disease severity.

Case Finding and Diagnostic Accuracy

The foundation for diagnosis of most neurologic conditions is clinical information obtained from the medical history and physical examination. Unlike many other disciplines, confirmatory diagnostic tests for neurologic conditions usually do not exist and tissue diagnosis is rarely possible during life. Thus, for clinical research in neurology, the best diagnosis often depends on the use of standardized diagnostic criteria applied by experienced physicians who have undergone special training. Clearly,

this type of diagnostic process can be time consuming and expensive. Ideally, epidemiologic studies of neurologic disorders include funds for clinical examination of subjects by study neurologists. Unfortunately, this is often not feasible for large-scale investigations such as large case–control studies or health-services research that utilizes large health-care databases.

The goal of case identification in epidemiologic research is to obtain a standardized diagnosis that is the most accurate possible considering the study design and available resources. Misclassification of disease status dilutes the true association between exposure and disease when misclassification is random and may falsely elevate the degree of association between an exposure and disease risk when there are systematic case identification errors (bias).

In addition to an accurate diagnosis, it is essential to measure characteristics of the disease that may be useful for determining etiology and prognosis and that may provide outcome measures for intervention studies. These characteristics include age at onset, disease symptoms and signs that may be quantifiable by the use of rating scales, as well as disease effects on functioning ability and quality of life.

Unique characteristics of the brain, including lack of neuronal regeneration capacity, absence of functional redundancy, and inaccessibility of the brain and spinal cord, make tissue diagnosis relatively impractical and unsafe. An exception is nervous system neoplasms. Here, tissue diagnosis by biopsy or complete removal is the standard of care.

As with cancer research in other disciplines, population-based nervous system tumor registries exist. A registry includes all cases of the disease reported in a defined population and can be used to calculate disease rates. Generally, patients participating in the registry are followed up to determine case status. In this way, registries support research on risk factors, prognosis, treatment effects, and survival. Additionally, patterns of disease distribution in the community become evident, which promotes community awareness and helps to focus public health efforts on controlling the disease (Valanis 1999). For example, the German Childhood Cancer Registry is a population-based registry. Information from this registry accumulated over 10 years indicates that the incidence rate for brain tumors in children less than 15 years of age was 2.6 per 100,000. The 5-year survival rate for all brain tumors combined was 64% (Kaatsch et al. 2001).

When tissue diagnosis is not feasible for the neurologic disease being studied, a limited number of other diagnostic tests can increase the accuracy of case definition if study design and resources allow. When combined with the appropriate clinical presentation, for example, neuroimaging can confirm the diagnosis of stroke and can provide support for the diagnosis of multiple sclerosis. Likewise, electroencephalography may confirm the diagnosis of epilepsy and electromyography and nerve conduction studies can support or confirm the diagnosis of neuromuscular disorders. Cerebrospinal fluid analysis is critical for diagnosing infections of the central nervous system and can also support the diagnosis of multiple sclerosis.

For most studies of neurologic diseases, routine clinical diagnosis by neurologists (often in conjunction with standardized published diagnostic criteria) is the most practical method for case identification. However, routine clinical diagnosis depends on the expertise of the clinician and can be affected by variations in disease presentation and in the attitudes of physicians toward the diagnosis in different cultures. Standardized diagnostic criteria are also imperfect but can help to ensure that various groups involved in research are in fact studying the same entity. For this reason, standardized criteria are often incorporated into diagnostic methods designed by researchers who plan to compare their findings with those of other published studies. In multicenter studies, this strategy can be strengthened by having centralized training for diagnosticians. Levels of certainty can also be assigned for the diagnosis, such as definite, probable, or possible. Researchers can then select cases in any of these categories, depending on requirements of the study design. Often more than one set of diagnostic criteria has been developed by different groups for a single disease. Decisions about which criteria to use for a particular study depend on community acceptance and study design, goals, and budget.

Example 1–3 There are several sets of published criteria for diagnosis of multiple sclerosis (MS) (see Chapter 8). Most of the early criteria required clinical evidence of neurologic lesions separated in time and neuroanatomical space (Schumacher et al. 1965; Poser et al. 1983). A more recently developed set of criteria allows for the diagnosis after clinical evidence of one lesion if there is imaging or electrodiagnostic evidence of a second lesion (McDonald et al. 2001). These criteria are complex and may be feasible for use in clinical trials of MS, but more difficult to apply in epidemiologic studies because the investigators have less control over whether or not the subject has neurodiagnostic tests that are needed for full application of the criteria. Thus the use of criteria allowing laboratory evidence of lesions is not practical for survey research involving large populations but may be very useful for identification of early cases that are the most suitable subjects for clinical trials (Nelson and Anderson 1995).

For most sets of clinical criteria, diagnostic accuracy can be determined by eventual evaluation of the diagnosed cases by postmortem pathologic examination. Some neurologic disease categories, however, have no accepted standard pathological criteria. A recent clinicopathologic study revealed that 76% of 100 patients with Parkinson's disease (PD) clinically diagnosed by neurologists actually had pathological evidence of the disease. Diagnostic accuracy improved to 82% when the neurologists used standardized criteria

(Hughes et al. 1992). This demonstrates that while the use of standardized criteria improves diagnostic accuracy, they are not perfect. The misclassification rate of PD in the best of circumstances still allows the inclusion of approximately 18% without true PD. Furthermore, it has been demonstrated that rates of PD can vary depending on the specific criteria used, making it essential to specify the use of criteria that are best suited for the study design and then to stick to these criteria for the duration of the study (Bower et al. 2000).

Example 1–4 No universal agreement exists regarding the type, size, number, and location of cerebrovascular lesions necessary for the pathologic diagnosis of vascular dementia. Consequently, clinical diagnoses cannot be tested against a pathologic "gold standard." A recent analysis comparing five different sets of criteria for vascular dementia applied all of these criteria to an unselected group of 167 patients. Concordance between the criteria was low. There were only five patients that met the criteria for vascular dementia for every set of criteria (Wetterling et al. 1996).

Accuracy of clinical diagnosis usually improves with longer follow-up of patients. For Alzheimer's disease, research centers that followed patients for the duration of their illness found diagnostic accuracy of greater than 80% using National Institute of Neurological Disorders and Stroke (NINCDS) criteria. Studies that used a diagnosis made on the first appointment and that failed to observe participants over time had lower diagnostic accuracy (Petrovitch et al. 2001). Similar results have been reported for Parkinson's disease. In one study, the accuracy of the initial clinical diagnosis improved from 65% to 76% after 12 years of follow-up (Rajput et al. 1991), prompting the authors to recommend that studies of Parkinson's disease restrict enrollment to subjects who have had the disease for 5 or more years. This suggestion, however, is impractical for studies that require subjects to be early in their disease course, such as case–control studies that ideally would select newly diagnosed (incident) cases for study. Similarly, clinical trials aimed at altering disease progression must enroll subjects who are in the earliest stages of disease, when intervention is likely to be the most beneficial. Additionally, longitudinal observational studies of disease incidence usually use less stringent diagnostic criteria that do not require long duration of disease as a diagnostic factor.

In some types of study design, the use of any standardized diagnostic technique is impractical. Large medical databases with cases identified by diagnostic codes assigned by physicians are very useful for evaluating the economic impact of disease and for studying other health services–related questions. For example, in a recently published study of incidence and mortality of status epilepticus, investigators used a statewide hospital discharge database to identify all hospitalizations for status epilepticus by International Diagnostic Codes, Ninth Revision–Clinical Modification (ICD-9-CM) code (Wu et al. 2002).

For studies attempting to identify risk factors with smaller numbers of subjects, the accuracy of diagnosis becomes more critical. Accuracy can be improved by medical record review after case finding by ICD code. This allows the use of standardized definitions of cases and can provide information on date of disease onset. Medical abstractors can be helpful in this process, as they can obtain specific information from the medical record and make decisions about additional items that are needed to secure the diagnosis. However, because final pathologic diagnoses are not usually available for neurologic diseases, a neurologist is often required to review this information and arrive at a diagnosis.

Surveys designed to determine prevalence and cohort studies designed to determine incidence rates and risk factors often screen large populations to identify persons with the disease of interest. Consideration of disease demographics will enable investigators to determine the most efficient population to be screened. Diseases such a migraine and epilepsy may affect persons of all ages, while developmental diseases affect infants and children. Multiple sclerosis occurs in early adulthood, and neurodegenerative diseases such as Alzheimer's disease, amyotrophic lateral sclerosis, and Parkinson's disease usually occur later in life.

Once the population to be screened is determined, a screening tool can be created. Ideally, the instrument should be designed without bias related to age, educational, and cultural differences within the chosen population. If bias is unavoidable, the factors that introduce bias and the degree to which the instrument is affected must be clearly identified and quantified so that statistical adjustments can be made. For example, the Mini-Mental Status Exam (MMSE) is commonly used as a screening instrument for dementia, but age and education influence the score. If the effects of age and education on test score are precisely known, these factors can be accounted for by adjusting the screening cut point based on a participant's age and level of education. The primary determinants of the screening cut point are the sensitivity and specificity of the screening tool, which must be determined for the population under study (Tables 1–5 and 1–6). Sensitivity and specificity measurements for a test with a continuous result, such as the MMSE, allows for the construction of receiver operator characteristic (ROC) curves (Henderson 1993) that determine the specificity for any given value of sensitivity. The most use-

Table 1–5 Sensitivity and Specificity for Correct Classification of a Neurologic Disorder

Definitions

Sensitivity = $[a/(a + c)]$

Definition: proportion of those who truly have the disease that are correctly classified as having it by the diagnostic test or case definition criteria

Specificity = $[d/(b + d)]$

Definition: proportion of those who truly do not have the characteristic that are correctly classified as not having it by the diagnostic test or case definition criteria.

False-negative rate = $c/(a + c)$
(or false negative = $1 - $ sensitivity)

False-positive rate = $b/(b + d)$
(or false positive = $1 - $ specificity)

ful cut point can then be established. An estimate of missed cases in the population can also be calculated using these measures.

Once positively screened subjects or potential cases are identified, a thorough examination is usually required to confirm case status. Often, only specially trained neurologists are qualified to perform such examinations, and they are time consuming and costly. If neurologists are unavailable or the cost is too high, a consensus panel composed of experts may be used to review all clinical information and arrive at a final diagnosis.

For example, large epidemiologic studies of dementia perform mental status testing and elementary neurologic examinations on hundreds of subjects. Consensus committees composed of neuropsychologists, neurologists, and geriatricians are able to

Table 1–6 Example of Classification of Neurologic Disorder

| Imperfect classification[†] | TRUE CLASSIFICATION OF NEUROLOGIC DISORDER* | |
	Present	Absent
Present	a (true positive)	b (false positive)
Absent	c (false negative)	d (true negative)
	a + c	b + d

*Ascertained by autopsy confirmation or best "consensus" among neurologist panel.

†As indicated by a diagnostic test, or epidemiologic case definition.

review all the clinical information and combine expertise to arrive at the best possible diagnosis (Graves et al. 1996; White et al. 1996). Studies that require examinations of subjects over wide geographic distributions, such as the WWII veterans twins study of Parkinson's disease, employ multiple examiners (Tanner et al. 1999). A consensus panel composed of experts in movement disorders reviews the examination results and can both apply their expertise to the diagnosis of Parkinson's disease and help to reduce errors related to interrater variation.

A highly accurate method of diagnosis is critical in selecting participants for clinical trials. Investigators in clinical trials must calculate sample sizes with little margin for error because of the large expense involved in conducting these studies and the need for definitive results. The effect of enrolling misclassified non-cases may under- or overestimate the efficacy of the study drug, depending on whether the misclassified case is randomized to the active treatment or control group. Potential cases recruited from clinics, advertisements, or other health care–related facilities are usually confirmed as cases in face-to-face interviews and examinations. Several screening visits may be required to determine final eligibility based on accurate diagnosis, clinical stage or severity, treatment status, and other characteristics.

Defining Study Outcomes

The appropriate selection and accurate measurement of disease outcome are vital to generating interpretable study results and generalizable findings. Possible clinical outcomes include disease diagnosis and stage; measurement of disease symptoms and signs; assessment of level of functioning, disability, or quality of life; and mortality. An ideal outcome for clinical research is one that (1) measures what it is intended to measure (referred to as "validity" or "accuracy"); (2) is inexpensive and easy to use; and (3) does not vary with repeated meas-

ures, across time, with different observers, or with different populations.

Objective measurement of the outcome should be possible without using overly invasive or risky procedures. For example, modern stereotactic techniques have made biopsy of cortical tumors a relatively safe and accurate diagnostic procedure for cerebral neoplasms. Since tissue diagnosis is unavailable for most neurologic diseases and outcomes, most research relies on clinical measures. The accuracy of such clinical measures can be estimated. Criterion-related validity refers to the extent to which a clinical measure agrees with an external criterion ("gold standard") (Herndon 1997).

Example 1–5 The Schumacher diagnostic criteria for multiple sclerosis were developed to standardize the criteria used to diagnose multiple sclerosis in clinical trials (Schumacher 1965; Herndon and Goodkin 1997). Diagnoses of multiple sclerosis made using these criteria have been compared to the gold standard pathological diagnosis. In one study, 518 consecutive patients with definite multiple sclerosis by clinical criteria were examined postmortem and 485 (94%) were found to have multiple sclerosis by neuropathological examination (Engell 1988).

Sensitivity and specificity evaluate how well an outcome or test predicts the gold standard diagnosis (Table 1–5). *Sensitivity* is the proportion of study participants with the disease who have a positive test while *specificity* is the proportion of subjects without the disease who have a negative test. The higher the sensitivity and specificity, the more useful the test is.

Example 1–6 Salmon et al. (2002) compared initial neuropsychological test scores of Alzheimer's disease (AD) patients with those of normal control subjects to identify effective diagnostic measures. The diagnosis of AD was confirmed in 98 of 110 (89%) very mildly impaired patients (33/36 by autopsy, 65/74 by disease progression). The diagnosis was inaccurate in 12 patients (11%): 7 were subsequently diagnosed with other neurologic disorders, and 5 were ultimately found to be normal. The researchers concluded that neuropsychological measures of delayed recall, verbal fluency, and global cognitive status provided excellent sensitivity ($\geq$96%) and specificity ($>$93%) for differentiating between very mildly impaired AD patients and normal subjects.

Sensitivity and specificity have a trade-off that drives selection of the most useful cut point. If the cut point is set low, more of the population will screen positively and sensitivity will be high, while if the cut point is set high, more participants with the disease will be missed, lowering sensitivity but increasing specificity (decreasing false positives) (Fletcher 1988).

Occasionally, an outcome measure is used in research that has not been measured against any gold standard but has been accepted by the research community as valid, based on years of experience and use. This is true for the Kurtzke Extended Disability Status Scale (EDSS) that is routinely used in multiple sclerosis clinical research, despite known flaws (Herndon and Goodkin 1997).

Content validity refers to how well an outcome measure covers all of the characteristics of the desired outcome without including redundant or noncontributing items.

Example 1–7 Neuropsychiatric complications are common and relatively understudied manifestations of dementia. The Neuropsychiatric Inventory was developed to assess behavioral disturbances in patients with dementia. When the instrument was developed, there were no previously established methods for studying some of the behaviors being assessed. In order to evaluate content validity of this inventory, a Delphi panel of 10 internationally known experts rated the proposed questions to determine if the essential elements of the behavior were captured (Cummings et al. 1994).

Biological markers that accurately reflect disease characteristics of interest are extremely useful. Increasingly advanced techniques for neuroimaging are beginning to fulfill this role. For example, it is very difficult to assess treatment response in multiple sclerosis because of the exacerbating and remitting nature of the disease. Disease course is tremendously variable from patient to patient and it is difficult to define what constitutes an exacerbation. In a trial of the efficacy of interferon-β MRI brain scanning was used as an objective marker of new disease. It was demonstrated that the active-treatment group had fewer new lesions than the placebo group, demonstrating the utility of using a neuroimaging measure as a marker of disease activity (IFNB Multiple Sclerosis Study Group 1993; Paty and Li 1993). It is important to assess whether changes in biological markers parallel changes in clinical severity of the disease in patients. A recently reported trial of fetal cell transplants in Parkinson's disease indicated that although PET imaging indicated increased dopamine in the striatum in patients who received the transplants, there was no clinical improvement in these patients compared to those who underwent sham surgery (Freed et al. 2001).

The terms *reliability* and *precision* refer to the stability of an instrument's performance for measuring an outcome in multiple trials, including different settings, different observers, and diverse populations (see Chapter 3). Assuming no clinical change in the research participant being examined, a test instrument should yield the same score when administered by multiple observers (interrater reliability), when administered multiple times by the same observer (intrarater reliability), and when administered repeatedly over time (test–retest reliability). Reliability is enhanced when the measurement technique is standardized and anchor points on the scale are clearly defined. For example, the assessment of timed gait is well defined and would be expected to be highly reliable. Rating general *body bradykinesia*, a term used to describe slowness in the initiation and execution of body movements, as mild to severe would be expected to have less reliability due to variations in an observer's impressions of severity and drift in an observer's impression over time.

When considering the outcome to be measured, one must take into account study design. Prospective cohort studies have the advantage of accurately measuring exposures over time in a cohort that is unaffected by a disease. As the cohort is followed forward in time, data can be gathered both on continued exposures and on outcomes. Since the exposure is measured prospectively, inferences can then be made about cause and effect. But the potential for diagnostic misclassification is relatively high, especially if there is no definite diagnostic test for the disease. The effect of misclassification is to reduce the likelihood that a true relationship between the putative risk factor and the disease will be evident as a result of the study (type I error, see Chapter 3).

Example 1–8 Alzheimer's disease is an example of a neurodegenerative disorder that cannot be definitively diagnosed during life. The diagnostic accuracy from major dementia referral centers is reported to be 80% to 100% when diagnostic criteria are applied. However, in a prospective study of a community-based cohort, where new cases of AD were sought, the diagnostic accuracy was 75% using the same diagnostic criteria applied by a consensus panel. The disparity in diagnostic accuracy arose because, in the community-based cohort, most cases identified were early in the course of their illness and the diagnosis depended on a single clinical visit with the participant (Petrovitch et al. 2001).

Case–control studies enroll participants with the disease of interest and a group of control participants who are similar in characteristics to the cases. Cases and controls are then evaluated for the exposures of interest retrospectively. Because exposures are assessed in individuals with existing disease, it can be difficult to document that the exposure actually predated the onset of the disease. This is especially true of neurodegenerative diseases that have slow, gradual progression where the exact date of onset is difficult to identify. Compounding the problem of enrolling previously diagnosed cases, especially when advanced or late-stage cases are included, is the difficulty in determining whether exposures play a role in disease etiology or in disease progression and survival. This phenomenon is referred to as "prevalence-incidence bias" (see Chapter 2). One way of addressing these problems is to enroll newly diagnosed (incident) cases in case–control studies, that is, recently diagnosed cases rather than cases that have had the disease for many years. The disadvantage of enrolling only incident cases is that there is a greater chance for including some non-cases with these early cases (misclassification), as noted above with prospective studies. One approach to this dilemma is to reassess and reapply diagnostic criteria at a later time when the condition has progressed and greater diagnostic certainty can be obtained.

Natural history and prognostic studies are useful for making management decisions and for counseling patients on what to expect regarding the disease (Longstreth et al. 1987). Subjects with the disease of interest are followed over time to determine the effect of the disease on outcomes such as symptom progression or recurrence, disability, and death. The design may take the form of a simple descriptive study, where a group of patients is followed over the course of their disease and symptoms, complications, and mortality rates are assessed. Alternatively, cohort studies are an excellent design for natural history research. With this design, participants with the disease of interest as well as unaffected participants are followed over time to determine prognostic factors for the outcome of interest.

Example 1–9 Cases of myocardial infarction, coronary artery bypass surgery, and stroke were identified and followed among the participants in the prospective Honolulu Heart Program. All participants then underwent cognitive testing in late life. Men with stroke were significantly more likely than others in the cohort to have cognitive impairment, while there was no significant association between prior myocardial infarction or coronary artery bypass surgery with cognitive function test scores (Petrovitch et al. 1998).

Health services research focuses on understanding the organization, delivery, and outcomes of health-care services (see Chapter 18). This includes assessment of disease burden, measurement of the effectiveness of interventions, and measurement of the efficiency of resource utilization, including cost-effectiveness of care. Investigators often use large databases from insurance companies, health maintenance organizations, or government providers such as the Department of Veterans Affairs. The outcomes are defined from diagnostic codes such as the ICD.

Example 1–10 Patients from a commercial insurance sample and a Medicare sample with atherosclerotic vascular disease were identified through the use of ICD-9. In order to estimate the disease burden due to secondary vascular events among these patients, survival analysis was used to estimate cumulative occurrence of recurrent stroke, myocardial infarction, or peripheral arterial disease. Such information may be used to direct public health efforts toward effective prevention strategies for atherosclerotic events (Vickrey et al. 2002). This type of prevention where the target is to prevent subsequent disease events or morbidity among patients who already have a disease is *secondary prevention*. In contrast, the term *prevention* by itself is usually used to refer to *primary prevention*, where the goal is to prevent individuals from developing the disease or condition in the first place.

Outcome measures used to determine the efficacy of an intervention in clinical trials must be valid and reliable. Such measures must be responsive to and capable of quantifying clinically important changes in the patient (Hobart et al. 1996). A discussion of clinical trial design is detailed in Chapter 17. Trial patients are assessed at baseline and again after the intervention has been completed. There are several ways of studying a disease and its consequences. *Pathology* refers to the structural damage done to the body or relevant organs by the disease. Pathology may be impossible to view directly for most neurologic diseases. Instead, surrogate clinical measures or disease-specific outcome measures are used to assess disease worsening that reflects progression of the pathology (see Chapter 3).

Special Considerations for Study Conduct

Implementing a study demands as much rigor as designing a study. All research staff must be trained in the ethical principles that guide the use of human subjects in research. Before research can begin, all staff must appreciate the necessity of standardizing every procedure for data collection and management. Staff must receive detailed training on how to perform the study procedures skillfully and efficiently. Finally, awareness of the disabilities produced by the diseases, and incorporation of methods ensuring the comfort and dignity of study participants are critical.

The basic ethical principles upon which federal regulations govern the protection of human subjects are derived from the Belmont Report published in 1979 by the National Commission for the Protection of Humans Subjects. Three basic principles are set forth in this report: respect for persons, beneficence, and justice. *Respect for persons* means that individuals are autonomous and they have the right to choose what will happen to them. Those with diminished autonomy (vulnerable populations) are entitled to increased protection.

These groups include children, pregnant women, prisoners, and, of particular importance to neurologic research, those with dementia and other cognitive disorders. Respect for persons is expressed by the informed-consent process. Potential participants are invited to take part in research and are informed of study methods and risks in a manner that is fully comprehensible. Informed-consent forms must clearly state that participation in the study is strictly voluntary.

Staff who work in a medical-care environment are accustomed to dealing with patients who are seeking medical care for specific ailments and expect to get the treatment currently proven most effective. Study volunteers are not necessarily going to obtain any personal benefit from participation and are donating their time while possibly incurring risk. Research staff should be sensitive to this difference and take care that study volunteers are always fully informed about the study, are aware of all potential risks and benefits, and understand that it is their right to withdraw from the study at any time.

Beneficence means minimizing risk and maximizing potential benefits. Ongoing risk/benefit analysis is necessary, with attention to new scientific developments that have bearing on the research project. Serious consideration should be given to the balance between personal risk borne by the study participant and potential benefit to society as a whole.

Justice implies that there is fairness in selection of participants for a study. This principle includes protection of vulnerable groups such as prisoners or mentally incompetent individuals from bearing more than their share of the burden of risk in research. Also there should be no systematic exclusion of groups from potentially beneficial research on the basis of ethnicity, age, gender, or other factors.

Detailed information regarding regulations and principles governing the protection of human subjects may be found in the U.S. Department of Health and Human Services regulations for the protection of human subjects (45CFR part 46) and the Food and Drug Administration human subjects protection regulations (21CFR part 50). The ethics of research involving human participants is continuously evolving as society changes and as technology advances. More than any other field, genetics has undergone a technological explosion that, while leading to a greater understanding of disease etiology, is challenging existing concepts of informed consent and confidentiality. Investigators involved in genetics research should be familiar with published guidelines on ethical use of collected samples for DNA studies. In 1996 the American Society of Human Genetics published a report on informed consent for genetic research, providing recommendations for use of newly collected biological samples for genetics research as well as for use of existing samples. Chapter 4 contains detailed information about the ethical concerns involved in using and storing biological samples from subjects for clinical and epidemiologic research.

Future Directions and Conclusions

Replication of study results in different populations is important in assessing validity and generalizability of study findings and for building the body of evidence in a given area of research. Comparison of studies can be difficult, however, when features of the study design and methods differ. Ideally, epidemiologists will adopt similar methods whenever possible, to facilitate comparison of studies. At a minimum, the methods used to ascertain cases and controls should be clearly stated. These principles become increasingly important as the field of neuroepidemiology advances to more cross-national and cross-cultural collaborative studies. Differences in rates of disease across cultures can only yield important clues to etiology and risk factors if the design and methods are strictly standardized and diagnostic criteria verified by careful clinical–pathological studies.

One of the key difficulties in studying neurologic conditions is the lack of disease biomarkers for diagnosis and staging. Future efforts will focus on identifying genetic, imaging, chemical, and tissue biomarkers that are simple, noninvasive, and affordable. Ideally, they would enable identification of patients with the disease process prior to or in the earliest stages of the development of clinical symptoms and signs. Use of these biomarkers will reduce diagnostic misclassification and allow for valid outcome measures for interventional studies. Their identification will depend on close cooperation between scientists in the basic science fields and those in the areas of clinical research.

The long-term goal of our field is the primary prevention of neurologic disease. The most efficient approach to achieving this goal will require collaboration on many levels—among epidemiologists, to develop common methods that will facilitate comparison of studies and combined analyses, and between epidemiologists, basic scientists of many disciplines, and clinicians. Developing mechanisms to facilitate communication among researchers in diverse disciplines is challenging but critical to the speedy transition from bench to bedside. Finally, advances in understanding and preventing neurologic disease could not proceed without the generosity of thousands of volunteers—both those with the disease under study and those without the disease— for without their participation little progress would be possible.

References

American Society of Human Genetics. ASHG report. Statement on informed consent for genetic research. *Am J Hum Genet* 1996;59: 471–474.

Bower JH, Maraganore DM, McDonnell SK, Rocca WA. Influence of strict, intermediate, and broad diagnostic criteria on the age- and sex-specific incidence of Parkinson's disease. *Mov Disord* 2000;15:819–825

Bradley WG, Daroff RB, Fenichel GM, Marsden CD. Neurology in Clinical Practice, 3rd edition. Boston: Butterworth-Heineman, 1999.

Cummings JL, Mega M, Gray K, et al. The Neuropsychiatric Inventory: comprehensive assessment of psychopathology in dementia. *Neurology* 1994;44:2308–2314.

Engell T. A clinico-pathoanatomical study of multiple sclerosis diagnosis. *Acta Neurol Scand* 1988;78:39–44.

Fletcher RH. Clinical Epidemiology. Baltimore: Williams & Wilkins, 1988.

Folstein MF, Folstein SE, McHugh PR. "Mini-Mental State". A practical method for grading the cognitive state of patients for the clinician. *J Psychiatr Res* 1975;12:189–198.

Freed CR, Greene PE, Breeze RE, et al. Transplantation of embryonic dopamine neurons for severe Parkinson's disease. *N Engl J Med* 2001;344:710–719.

Goetz CG. Textbook of Clinical Neurology, 2nd edition. Philadelphia: Saunders, 2003.

Gordis L. Epidemiology. Philadelphia: W.B. Saunders, 2000.

Grandinetti A, Morens DM, Reed D, MacEachern D. Prospective study of cigarette smoking and the risk of developing idiopathic Parkinson's disease. *Am J Epidemiol* 1994; 139:1129–1138.

Graves AB, Larson EB, Edland SD, et al. Prevalence of dementia and its subtypes in the Japanese American population of King County, Washington State. The Kame Project. *Am J Epidemiol* 1996;144:760–771.

Henderson AR. Assessing test accuracy and its clinical consequences: a primer for receiver operating characteristic curve analysis. *Ann Clin Biochem* 1993;30(Pt 6):521–539.

Herndon RM. Introduction to clinical neurologic scales. In: Herndon RM, ed. Handbook of Neurologic Rating Scales. New York: Demos Vermande, 1997a, pp 1–6.

Herndon RM, Goodkin D. Multiple sclerosis and demyelinating diseases. In: Herndon RM, ed. Handbook of Neurologic Rating Scales. New York: Demos Vermande, 1997, pp 107–123.

Hobart JC, Lamping DL, Thompson AJ. Evaluating neurological outcome measures: the bare essentials. *J Neurol Neurosurg Psychiatry* 1996;60:127–130.

Hughes AJ, Ben-Shlomo Y, Daniel SE, Lees AJ. What features improve the accuracy of clinical diagnosis in Parkinson's disease: a clinicopathologic study. *Neurology* 1992;42: 1142–1146.

IFNB Multiple Sclerosis Study Group. Interferon β-1b is effective in relapsing-remitting multiple sclerosis. I. Clinical results of a multicenter, randomized, double-blind, placebo-controlled trial. *Neurology* 1993;43:655–661.

Kaatsch P, Rickert CH, Kuhl J, et al. Population-based epidemiologic data on brain tu-

mors in German children. *Cancer* 2001;92:
3155–3164.

Kagan A, Harris BR, Winkelstein W, et al. Epidemiologic studies of coronary heart disease and stroke in Japanese men living in Japan, Hawaii and California: demographic, physical, dietary and biochemical characteristic. *J Chron Dis* 1974;27:345–364.

Kandel ER, Schwartz JH, Jessell TM. Principles of Neural Science, 4th edition. New York: McGraw-Hill, 2000.

Kelsey JL, Whittemore AS, Evans AS, Thompson WD. Methods in Observational Epidemiology. New York: Oxford University Press, 1996.

Koepsell TD, Weiss NS. Epidemiologic Methods. Studying the Occurrence of Illness. New York: Oxford University Press, 2003.

Langston JW, Ballard PA, Tetrud JW, Irwin I. Chronic parkinsonism in humans due to a product of meperidine analog synthesis. *Science* 1983;219:979–980.

Longstreth WT Jr, Koepsell TD, van Belle G. Clinical neuroepidemiology. II. Outcomes. *Arch Neurol* 1987;44:1196–1202.

McDonald WI, Compston A, Edan G, et al. Recommended diagnostic criteria for multiple sclerosis: guidelines from the International Panel on the Diagnosis of Multiple Sclerosis. *Ann Neurol* 2001;50:121–127.

National Commission for the Protection of Human Subjects of Biomedical and Behavioral Research. The Belmont Report, Ethical Principles and Guidelines for the Protection of Human Subjects of Research. U.S. Department of Health, Education and Welfare, 1979.

Nelson LM, Anderson DW. Case finding for epidemiological surveys of multiple sclerosis in United States communities. *Mult Scler* 1995;1:48–55.

Paty DW, Li DK. Interferon β-1b is effective in relapsing-remitting multiple sclerosis. II. MRI analysis results of a multicenter, randomized, double-blind, placebo-controlled trial. UBC MS/MRI Study Group and the IFNB Multiple Sclerosis Study Group. *Neurology* 1993;43:662–667.

Petrovitch H, White L, Masaki K, et al. Influence of mycardial infarction, coronary artery bypass surgery, and stroke on cognitive impairment in late life. *Am J Cardiol* 1998;81:1017–1021.

Petrovitch H, White LR, Ross GW, et al. Accuracy of clinical criteria for AD in the Honolulu-Asia Aging Study, a population-based study. *Neurology* 2001;57:226–234.

Portney LG, Watkins MP. Foundations of Clinical Research, 2nd edition. Upper Saddle River, NJ: Prentice Hall, 2000.

Poser CM, Paty DW, Scheinberg L, et al. New diagnostic criteria. *Ann Neurol* 1983;227–231.

Rajput AH, Rozdilsky B, Rajput A. Accuracy of clinical diagnosis in parkinsonism—a prospective study. *Can J Neurol Sci* 1991;18:275–278.

Ross GW, Abbott RD, Petrovitch H, et al. Association of coffee and caffeine intake with the risk of Parkinson disease. *JAMA* 2000;283:2674–2679.

Rothman KJ, Greenland S. Modern Epidemiology. Philadelphia: Lippencott-Raven, 1998.

Rowland LP, ed. Merritt's Textbook of Neurology, 9th edition. Baltimore, MD: Williams and Wilkins, 1995.

Salmon DP, Thomas RG, Pay MM, et al. Alzheimer's disease can be accurately diagnosed in very mildly impaired individuals. *Neurology* 2002;59:1022–1028.

Schumacher GA, Beebe G, Kibler RF, et al. Problems of experimental trials of therapy on multiple sclerosis. *Ann NY Acad Sci* 1965;122:552–568

Squire LR, Bloom FE, McConnell SK, Roberts JL, Spitzer NC, Zigmond MJ. Fundamental Neuroscience, 4th edition. San Diego: Academic Press, 2003.

Tanner CM, Goldman SM. Epidemiology of Parkinson's disease. *Neurol Clin* 1996;14:317–335.

Tanner CM, Ottman R, Goldman SM, et al. Parkinson disease in twins: an etiologic study. *JAMA* 1999;281:341–346.

Valanis B. Epidemiology in Health Care. Stamford, CT: Appleton & Lange, 1999.

Vickrey BG, Rector TS, Wickstrom SL, et al. Occurrence of secondary ischemic events among persons with atherosclerotic vascular disease. *Stroke* 2002;33:901–906.

Victor M, Ropper AH. Adams and Victor's Principles of Neurology, 7th edition. New York: McGraw-Hill, 2001.

Wetterling T, Kanitz RD, Borgis KJ. Comparison of different diagnostic criteria for vascular dementia (ADDTC, DSM-IV, ICD-10, NINDS-AIREN). *Stroke* 1996;27:30–36.

White L, Petrovitch H, Ross GW, et al. Prevalence of dementia in older Japanese-American men in Hawaii: the Honolulu-Asia Aging Study. *JAMA* 1996;276:955–960.

Wu YW, Shek DW, Garcia PA, et al. Incidence and mortality of generalized convulsive status epilepticus in California. *Neurology* 2002;58:1070–1076.

2

Study Design, Measures of Effect, and Sources of Bias

LORENE M. NELSON AND VALERIE M. McGUIRE

Chapter 1 underscored the primary importance of defining the research question in neuroepidemiologic research and the unique challenges that neurological disorders pose for epidemiologic investigations. Two of the most important features of study design were discussed: achieving a good research definition of the neurological disorder and identifying the ideal study population with which to address the research question. In this chapter, we will provide a more in-depth description of commonly used study designs, discuss the measures of effect that reflect the associations between health predictors and neurologic outcomes, and describe the study biases that can adversely affect study validity.

Principles of Study Design

The design of a study is dictated by the research question(s) posed by the investigator(s). The goal is to design a study that will provide a valid answer to each of the research questions, and this often begins with deciding what the optimal study would be, disregarding cost, feasibility, and ethical concerns. Once the mental exercise of choosing a gold-standard study design is carried out, the investigators usually have to alter its features because of practical or ethical concerns; however, beginning with the best methods may help an investigator to judge which principles can be relaxed without compromising the ability to address the research questions.

Figure 1–3 shows the array of study design possibilities. When pursuing etiologic clues about what might cause neurologic disorders, two general types of study designs are possible: *descriptive* studies to describe the frequency of a given neurologic disorder in the population, and *analytic* studies to test specific etiologic hypotheses. In the following sections, we will discuss the study design options for each of these two research objectives, and the numeric indicators used to estimate disease frequency and the strength of associations between risk factors and neurologic outcomes (i.e., effect measures).

Descriptive Study Designs: Incidence, Prevalence, and Mortality Studies

Epidemiologic fact-finding begins with descriptive studies. The first step in understanding a neurologic disorder is to estimate how common or frequent the disorder is in the general population. Differences in disease frequency between subgroups of the population (such as those based on age, race, ethnicity, gender, and geographic location) may help identify risk factors for disease. For some disorders, such as multiple sclerosis, estimates of disease frequency in different groups have provided important clues about factors that may cause disease (see Chapter 8). In order to estimate disease frequency, an investigator must have a good "case definition" and a defined study population in which to find patients with the disease (see Chapter 1). The three primary measures of disease frequency are incidence, prevalence, and mortality.

Incidence Studies

Incidence is a measure of how quickly *new* cases of a disease are arising in a population; it is estimated by counting the number of individuals who develop or are diagnosed with a disease during a given time period in a defined population. There are two different measures of incidence, and the choice between them depends on the study design. Incidence may be estimated from either a study cohort (a fixed group of subjects) or a dynamic population (a group that is open to new subjects and allows the exit of subjects). *Cumulative incidence* can be estimated from a study design that starts with a fixed cohort of people and follows each individual over a period of time for the occurrence of the disease.

$$\text{Cumulative incidence} = \frac{\begin{array}{c}\text{number of new cases}\\\text{of disease in a}\\\text{cohort during a}\\\text{specified time period}\end{array}}{\begin{array}{c}\text{total number of people}\\\text{in the initial}\\\text{population at}\\\text{risk (cohort)}\end{array}}$$

Cumulative incidence is a proportion and is interpreted as the probability that a person in the cohort will develop the disease during a specified time period, for example, within 1 month, 1 year, or over a lifetime. Because the direct estimation of cumulative incidence requires complete follow-up of all individuals in the cohort, it is used primarily in circumstances in which the disease is very common, so that a short period of follow-up is sufficient to identify the neurologic outcome among all persons in the cohort. For example, a study that enrolled a group of newly diagnosed patients with hemorrhagic stroke and followed each patient for a 1-month period following the stroke would be able to estimate the cumulative incidence of a second hemorrhage or "rebleed" within 1 month.

A second, more commonly used measure of incidence is the *incidence rate*, which is expressed per unit of time rather than as a proportion:

$$\text{Incidence rate} = \frac{\begin{array}{c}\text{number of new cases}\\\text{of disease in a}\\\text{population during a}\\\text{given time period}\end{array}}{\begin{array}{c}\text{total amount of person-}\\\text{time contributed}\\\text{by the members of}\\\text{population}\end{array}}$$

The incidence rate can be estimated from the follow-up of a cohort but is usually estimated from a study conducted in a *dynamic* population, such as a county or a metropolitan area, where members of the population are both entering and leaving the population over the study period. When this is the case, *person-time at risk* is often estimated as the size of the population at the midpoint of the study period multiplied by the duration of the study period. The *total amount of person-time* is estimated by summing the time that each person in the population remained free of disease. The incidence rate is often expressed as cases per 10,000 people or cases per 100,000 population to avoid lengthy decimals. Incidence rate is also known as the *incidence density* or *hazard rate*.

Example 2–1 We conducted a study of the incidence of amyotrophic lateral sclerosis (ALS) in western Washington State during the years 1990–1995 (McGuire et al. 1996). We sought cases from several overlapping sources, including neurologist referrals, the coroners' offices, and patient service organizations. Over the 5-year period of study, a total of 235 cases met the case definition for ALS, and the average population size during the 5-year period was 2,559,164. The annual incidence rate was calculated as

$$[(235 \text{ cases})/((2,559,164) \times 5 \text{ study years})] \times 100,000$$
$$= 1.8 \text{ per } 100,000 \text{ per year}$$
$$(\text{or } 8/10^5 \text{ person-years})$$

Incidence rates can be calculated for a study population as a whole (crude rates) or for distinct subgroups defined by age (i.e., age-specific rates), gender (i.e., gender-specific rates), or other demographic groups. By calculating and plotting incidence rates separately for age and gender categories, researchers can draw a descriptive picture of disease incidence that yields insight into the associations of age and gender with the risk of developing the disease. Because the incidence of many neurological disorders varies according to these factors, age- and gender-specific incidence curves provide the first look at risk factors for a disorder. Figure 7–3 provides an example of age- and gender-specific incidence curves for ALS from the incidence study in western Washington State (McGuire et al. 1996). The graph clearly shows that the incidence of ALS is higher for men than for women, that ALS is rare before age 45, and that disease incidence peaks in the sixth decade of life.

Very little is known about the incidence of many rare neurologic disorders (i.e., disorders that are less frequent than 2–3 per 100,000 persons per year) because a very large study population is needed to identify enough patients to obtain a statistically precise estimate. In addition, case finding within a sufficiently large population is difficult and a low frequency of disease poses a "needle-in-a-haystack" problem. In general, descriptive studies of rare disease are not feasible unless the study population is from a country such as Finland or Sweden, where nationalized health-care systems allow the identification of individuals with a given condition. In the United States, certain health-care systems that have a uniform system of care and a large enumerated patient population, such as some health maintenance organizations (HMOs) or the Mayo Clinic unified medical records system (Kurland and Molgaard 1981), are usually the only means by which the incidence of neurologic disorders can be estimated.

Mortality Studies

Mortality indicates the rate at which individuals are dying of a condition. Mortality is estimated by counting the number of individuals who die from a disease during a given time period. As with incidence, mortality can be expressed as a cumulative proportion (e.g., cumulative mortality) or *rate* of dying (e.g., mortality rate). A *case fatality rate* is a slightly different measure, the percentage of persons that develop a disease who subsequently die of the disease.

Prevalence Studies

In contrast to disease incidence, which includes only newly diagnosed cases of disease, disease prevalence is based on all cases, both new cases and existing cases, within a population at a given point in time. *Prevalence* is an indicator of how widespread a disease is in a population, and is calculated by dividing the number of people who have the disease by the number of people in the population at a single point in time or over a defined time interval (e.g., 1 year).

$$\text{Prevalence} = \frac{\begin{array}{c}\text{number of existing cases} \\ \text{of disease at a given} \\ \text{date (or time period)}\end{array}}{\begin{array}{c}\text{total population at that} \\ \text{date (or time period)}\end{array}}$$

For example, if 10,000 people out of a population of 100,000 have dementia, then the prevalence of dementia is (10,000)/(100,000), or 10 in 100 (10%).

Prevalence may be expressed relative to different-sized populations (e.g., per 1000 persons, or per 100,000 persons). Prevalence is sometimes referred to as a *prevalence rate*, but this is incorrect because prevalence is a percentage, not a rate. The correct term is either *prevalence ratio* or simply *prevalence*. Two measures of prevalence can be estimated, depending on the definition of time that is used. If prevalence is estimated on a given day, it is referred to as *point prevalence*. When prevalence is estimated for a specified period of time, such as a year, it is *period prevalence*.

> *Example 2–2* A study of multiple sclerosis (MS) occurrence in northern Colorado provides an example of how prevalence can be estimated. Investigators doing a study of the prevalence of multiple sclerosis in two counties of northern Colorado identified 233 MS patients who met the case definition and who resided in the counties on the prevalence day, 1 January 1982 (Nelson et al. 1986). They used intensive case-finding efforts with some duplicate identification of patients; the methods included hospital discharge summaries, neurologist survey, review of 20,000 medical charts from the private neurologists in the region, and MS Society patient rolls. The population of the two counties on prevalence day (i.e., 279,163 persons) was estimated using local population census data, and point prevalence was estimated to be 84 per 100,000 population (calculated as [(233/(279,163)) × 100,000]). Sixteen people were newly diagnosed with MS during the subsequent year, for an estimated incidence of 5.7 per 100,000 during 1982.

Prevalence depends on how quickly new cases of disease arise (incidence) and how long people with disease survive (duration of disease). For two diseases with similar incidence rates, the disease with the longer survival time will have a higher prevalence. If certain assumptions are met, incidence, prevalence, and duration of disease can provide a simple estimate of one measure from the other:

Prevalence =
(incidence) × (average duration of disease)

For example, not many prevalence studies of ALS exist, however, the prevalence of ALS can be calculated if both the incidence and duration of disease are known or can be estimated. Studies of ALS incidence in North America have estimated the annual incidence of ALS as approximately 2 per 100,000 persons per year. The average duration of disease is approximately 3 years, therefore, the prevalence of ALS can be estimated as approximately 6 cases per 100,000 population.

Prevalence is useful for examining geographic patterns of low and high disease frequency and for estimating the number of patients in need of health-care services. Also, for rare disorders such as myasthenia gravis, it is often more feasible to estimate disease prevalence than incidence because there is a greater number of prevalent than incident cases and disease prevalence can be estimated with greater precision. Prevalence estimates are not optimal for determining whether a disease incidence is increasing or decreasing because apparent changes in prevalence may reflect longer or shorter survival rather than actual changes in disease incidence. It is difficult to capture the full picture of a disorder by looking solely at prevalence estimates, especially if survival or duration of disease varies according to the factors of interest such as age and gender.

Comparisons of Disease Frequency by Person, Place, and Time

Incidence rates and prevalence ratios for neurologic disorders often vary according to personal characteristics such as gender, age, and race/ethnicity. Information on how disease incidence and prevalence vary according to these factors often provides the first clues about risk factors for a neurologic disorder. For example, gender is a risk factor for MS because women have higher incidence rates than men, and age is a risk factor for dementia because incidence rates are higher in the elderly than among younger individuals. Therefore, in addition to being presented solely as crude (overall) estimates, it is very informative to present incidence and prevalence estimates for gender-specific, age-specific, and race-specific subgroups.

Information about factors that influence disease risk may also be obtained by comparing the frequency of a neurologic disorder between geographic locations (place) or calendar periods (time). Clues about putative risk factors for a disease can be obtained by identifying geographic areas where the frequency of disease is either substantially higher or lower than the average. In North America, for example, the prevalence of MS increases as the latitude increases (i.e., MS prevalence is higher in northern than in southern regions of the United States), leading some scientists to hypothesize that an infectious agent or climatic factor that varies with latitude could be a causal factor in MS (see Chapter 8).

The frequency of a neurologic disorder may increase or decrease over time, and a temporal (secular) trend may enlighten the search for parallel changes that may have occurred in the prevalence of one or more causal factors over the same time period. While decreases in disease incidence over time generally reflect real changes, increases in incidence can be more difficult to interpret because they may only reflect earlier diagnoses or improved diagnostic accuracy due to technological improvements. For example, the introduction of computed tomography (CT) and magnetic resonance imaging (MRI) has undoubtedly resulted in enhanced identification of conditions such as stroke and MS. Before concluding that the incidence of a disease is truly on the rise, investigators must therefore determine whether new diagnostic procedures that allow earlier or subclinical detection of disease have caused a spurious increase in disease incidence over time. Changes in the International Classification of Diseases (ICD) coding system sometimes produce an apparent increase or decrease in disease incidence when similar disease entities are grouped differently in the diagnostic categorization scheme.

Comparisons of Disease Frequency Between Studies

Crude (overall) incidence rates may be inappropriate for comparing different populations if age, race/ethnicity, or other factors "confound" or influence the rate differently in the comparison populations. For example, a study population that is older on average than another study population will have more incident cases of dementia despite similar incidence rates when comparing the two studies within specific age groups, but only because there are more people in the subpopulation at risk (i.e., the elderly) in one population. Because study populations from different regions may have different distributions with respect to age or gender, a statistical method called "direct standardization" is often used to allow a direct comparison of disease rates that is not confounded or influenced by these differences in population composition. A description of direct standardization and a related measure, the standardized morbidity ratio (SMR), is discussed in Chapter 3.

Factors other than differences in the demographic composition of study populations may also compromise the ability to obtain valid comparisons of disease rates across studies, including (1) differences in the research diagnostic criteria used to assess the case definition among study subjects; (2) differences in the completeness of case ascertainment or in case-finding methods and (3) differences between populations in neurological care practices, such as the number of neurologists in the region or differential availability of advanced diagnostic tests that enable early diagnosis of disease.

Analytic Study Designs: Cohort, Case–Control, and Cross–Sectional Studies

The goal of analytic studies in neurology can be reduced to one basic task: to identify associations between health predictors and neurologic outcomes. The health predictors and outcomes are selected based on the research question and the type of study design used to address the question (see Table 3–1). For example, in case–control or cohort studies, the health predictors may be an array of risk factors such as gender, age, environmental exposures, molecular or genetic markers, lifestyle behaviors, with the aim of determining whether an association exists between these factors and the likelihood of developing a given disease. When developing a new diagnostic test, the health predictor is the test itself and the outcome is the underlying presence or absence of disease. In the case of a clinical trial, the health predictor is a treatment, and the investigator's aim is to determine whether an association exists between receiving the treatment and experiencing a good clinical outcome. In this chapter, we discuss research designs and study biases in terms of this primary goal of identifying associations between health predictors and neurologic outcomes.

Prospective Study Designs

There are three types of cohort studies: randomized clinical trials (experimental studies), prospective cohort studies, and retrospective cohort studies. Prospective studies are the optimal research design because they are less prone to study biases than retrospective studies. In a prospective study, subjects are selected for study at the beginning, measurements are carried out over time, and the disease outcomes are observed in the study subjects, whether it be development of a neurologic disorder in an etiologic study or treatment outcome in a randomized clinical trial (see Fig. 1–1). In a randomized clinical trial, the investigator assigns some study subjects to receive the exposure (treatment) and others to receive no treatment (placebo control) or an alternative treatment. Subjects are then followed over time for occurrence of the neurologic outcome of interest. An important principle of randomized controlled trials is that subjects in each treatment or control

group be treated identically, except for the treatment of interest. This is typically accomplished by using a placebo or sham treatment (or an existing treatment) and keeping both subjects and investigators blinded with respect to treatment group assignment. In contrast, for observational cohort studies, investigators do not "assign" exposures but only measure the exposures (putative risk factors) of interest. Many prognostic studies use a cohort design because the optimal approach is to begin with a cohort of newly diagnosed cases (i.e., an "inception cohort"), to measure baseline characteristics that may affect prognosis, and to follow the cohort over time to observe the neurologic outcome, whether it be increased disease severity, disability, or death. Less ideally, prognostic studies may be carried out using a cross-sectional and/or retrospective study design (see Chapter 16).

Randomized Trial as the Gold Standard Study Design. The principles of randomized clinical trials (RCTs) are presented in detail in Chapter 17, and are briefly summarized here. Essentially, a randomized trial is a type of cohort study, but is often classified as an experimental design because the ability to randomize subjects to treatments involves experimental manipulation rather than just collecting data and observing outcomes in subjects. The randomization process in clinical trials is used to assign a treatment or other therapeutic intervention on a random basis to patients, making it possible to avoid many of the biases that can plague observational (nonexperimental) studies by balancing the frequency of prognostic factors that could affect the response to the treatment. Of note, however, is that even experimental studies such as randomized trials can be affected by study biases, most notably selection bias, because of differential dropout rates between patients who receive treatment versus placebo. Measurement biases may also affect randomized trials when the neurological outcome measure(s) is insensitive to the change in the clinical course of the disease (see Chapters 3 and 17).

The neurological outcome measures in a clinical trial may be dichotomous (e.g., progression to death or to disability by some criteria), ordinal (e.g., a rank-ordered disease severity or disability scale), or quantitative (e.g., timed tests of gait, grip strength). Correspondingly, the statistical analysis of clinical trial data may involve the calculation of incidence or relative risk, or may involve comparing the treatment groups with respect to average values of a quantitative measure (see Chapters 3 and 17).

A primary focus of epidemiology is to identify the determinants of disease risk, and many of the factors of interest are deleterious exposures such as cigarette smoking, excessive alcohol consumption, occupational exposures, and other factors that would not be ethical to administer in a randomized controlled clinical trial. For this reason, much of epidemiologic research uses observational (nonexperimental) designs. The randomized trial design is only used when studying interventions that are thought to prevent or reduce the incidence of a disease, such as low-fat diets, physical activity interventions, and hormone replacement therapy (i.e., the Women's Health Initiative [Writing Group for the Women's Health Initiative Investigators 2002]). In some instances, community intervention trials are carried out by assigning whole communities to receive an intervention such as a wellness campaign, and are compared on the basis of summary health measures with communities that have not received the intervention (Koepsell et al. 1992). For example, investigators from the Stanford Five-City Project randomized five communities to receive either a community-wide health education program to reduce cardiovascular risk factors (i.e., smoking, cholesterol, and blood pressure) or no community-wide health education program (Farquhar et al. 1990). After 30 to 64 months of education, the smoking rates in the treatment communities decreased by 13%, blood pressure by 4%,

and cholesterol levels by 3%, compared to the communities that did not receive the education program. Programs such as these can have a significant impact on risk factors in an entire community.

Observational Cohort Studies. Cohort studies often enroll and follow all individuals in a defined cohort because multiple risk factors (exposures) are of interest in relation to one or more neurologic outcomes. When there is only one primary exposure of interest, the investigators may enroll all exposed individuals, but only a *sample* of the unexposed individuals, because the availability of unexposed persons is often greater and not all subjects in a population need to be followed. Subjects in a cohort study may be enrolled all at the same time, or may be recruited over a time interval as they become eligible. The length of follow-up time will vary among subjects because of losses due to dropouts, losses to follow-up, or death. This process is called "censoring," and there are statistical methods (e.g., survival analysis, proportional hazards modeling) that can accommodate variable lengths of follow-up (see Chapter 3).

Cohort studies are particularly appropriate when (1) the exposure(s) of interest is rare, making it necessary to study a population that has a larger proportion of exposed individuals than in the general population; (2) the neurological disorder or outcome is fairly common, such as stroke or dementia in the elderly; and (3) when more than one neurological disorder is of interest in relation to the risk factors of interest (e.g., Alzheimer's disease and Parkinson's disease). The advantage of cohort studies is that the investigator can be certain that the risk factor preceded the development of the disease; whereas this is sometimes difficult to confirm in case–control studies. The drawbacks to cohort studies are that they are time consuming and expensive.

Example 2–3 The Framingham Study investigators examined the impact of several cardiovascular conditions on the risk of stroke in 5070 participants during a 34-year follow-up period (Wolf et al. 1991). Compared with subjects who did not have the following conditions, the incidence of stroke increased twofold in subjects who had coronary heart disease, threefold in subjects who suffered from hypertension, and more than fourfold in subjects with cardiac failure or atrial fibrillation. The effects of coronary heart disease, hypertension, and cardiac arrest on stroke risk decreased with increasing age. However, atrial fibrillation remained a powerful independent risk factor for stroke in older subjects. The risk of stroke attributable to atrial fibrillation ranged from less than 2% for subjects 50–59 years of age to 24% for those aged 80–89 years. Cohort studies with long duration of follow-up enable investigators to analyze the relative importance of each risk factor.

Ideally, the diagnosis or detection of neurologic outcomes in a cohort study will be carried out in a standardized manner using a formal case definition for the disorder(s) of interest. Neurologists or physicians who make the diagnosis should be unaware of (blinded to) the patient's exposure or risk factor status, although this is not always possible for certain exposures (e.g., smoking, body mass index). This dilemma can be addressed by having an independent neurologist review the relevant medical records and apply the case definition blinded to knowledge of the subject's exposures.

Measure of association in cohort studies. *Relative risk* (RR) is the measure of association in a cohort study between an exposure and a disease, and is calculated by dividing the cumulative incidence over the study period (risk) for the exposed group by the cumulative incidence (risk) for the unexposed group:

$$\text{Relative risk} = \frac{\text{cumulative incidence in the exposed group}}{\text{cumulative incidence in the unexposed group}}$$

In studies where the incidence rate is the measure of choice (i.e., when subjects often enter the study at different time points and may be followed for variable lengths of time), the rate ratio, rather than the relative risk, should be calculated. The *rate ratio* is the incidence rate for the exposed group divided by the incidence rate for the unexposed group. In practice, the rate ratio is often referred to as the "relative risk" even though it is computed with rates:

$$\text{Rate ratio} = \frac{\text{incidence rate in the exposed group}}{\text{incidence rate in the unexposed group}}$$

Retrospective Study Designs

Case–Control Studies. Case-control studies are used to identify risk factors for disease by comparing cases with the disease with unaffected "controls." It is useful to conceptualize every case–control study as being nested within a cohort study. For example, a case–control study can be viewed as taking two separate samples from the numbers that form an incidence rate: the *case* sample taken from the numerator and the *control* sample taken from the denominator (i.e., unaffected subjects from the whole population). In order to maximize the statistical power of a study, all cases with a neurological disorder are usually selected for study. Because controls are much more numerous in a population than cases, only a random sample is required, rather than observation of the entire population.

Case–control studies are a useful option in situations where cohort studies are difficult to perform, especially when the disease of interest is rare. Case–control studies have the advantage of selecting cases on the basis of their disease status and thereby maximizing the number of cases involved in the study so to achieve adequate statistical power. This study design is particularly helpful when there is interest in studying many different risk factors for the disorder. Case–control studies have the reputation of being quicker, easier, and less costly than cohort studies. The case–control design, however, is also more prone to study biases than is a cohort study and has the reputation of being less valued than a cohort study because of the large number of study biases that can potentially be introduced by poor choice of study methods that invoke recall bias, selection bias, or confounding. In the hands of the uninitiated, a case–control study can be plagued by a considerable number of study biases, and criticisms of weakly designed case-control studies can be merited. Many or most of the biases that affect case–control studies can be avoided by using rigorous design principles in the planning, conduct, and analysis stages of the study. Later in this chapter, we describe the various types of bias that can occur and propose methods for detecting and/or minimizing those biases.

If a *population-based* case–control study is conducted, nearly all cases are ascertained and census data are available to estimate the number of people in the underlying population, then estimating incidence rates is the first task following completion of the study. By estimating incidence rates according to age, gender, and other demographic factors such as race/ethnicity, an investigator can get a clear picture of how these factors influence the risk of developing the disease. For this and other reasons, age and gender are often used as factors to match controls to cases, because their effects are usually already understood on the basis of incidence rates (see discussion of matching later in this chapter).

One of the most challenging aspects of conducting a case–control study is the choice of appropriate control subjects. In a series of papers on the selection of controls for case–control studies, Wacholder et al. (1992a, 1992b, 1992c) emphasized that the most difficult issue is identification of the appropriate base population from which to select controls. The *base* is defined as the source population from which the cases appeared during the study period when they were eligible to become cases. In simple terms, the *controls* are individuals in the same population who had the same opportunity to be identified as cases and included in the study had they developed the disease of interest. The most commonly used control groups (and their advantages and disadvantages) are summarized in Table 2–1. The choice of control group depends on the available source population of the cases, the cost associated with recruiting the control subjects, and the resources available to the investigators carrying out the study.

Controls from defined populations. The most appropriate control group in a population-based study is a random sample of individuals from the same population as the cases. The definition of a defined population is that it is enumerated and a list or census of its members is available. Even if the underlying population is a census region such as a city, county, or metropolitan area, some method of finding controls within the region is needed because the names and addresses of individuals are not available through the census. When cases are identified from a defined population, controls should be selected from the same population, using any of the following methods: (1) those who have telephones (i.e., random digit dialing), (2) those who have driver's licenses (motor vehicle department controls), (3) those who are Medicare eligible (i.e., people 65 years and older who qualify for Medicare benefits), (4) those who vote (voter registration records), and (5) neighborhood controls. Each of these selection methods has its strengths and limitations. For example, some methods, such as random-digit dialing (RDD) or neighborhood controls result in more comprehensive coverage of the geographic region than do others such as voter registration records. Door-to-door recruitment, based on statistical sampling by blocks or census tracts, may provide the best opportunity for representative sampling, but is often prohibitively expensive.

Random-digit dialing is widely used to select controls because a large percentage

Table 2–1 Methods of Control Selection in Case-Control Studies

Method	Advantages	Disadvantages
Control Subjects from Defined Populations		
Random-digit dialing (RDD)	• Effective method if the majority of the individuals have a telephone (currently 97% of households in the U.S.) • Can contact households with unlisted numbers • Most suitable for recruiting controls under the age of 65 years	• Requires approximately 100 calls to households to recruit one eligible subject (usually matched on age ±5 years and gender) • Decrease in response rates due to screening via telephone answering machines, avoidance of telemarketers, and suspicion of calls seeking personal information such as age and gender of members • The number of households without telephones is much higher in inner cities. To allow for comparability, cases without telephones must be excluded.
Medicare-eligible controls identified from Health Care Financing Administration (HCFA) records	• More efficient than RDD for recruiting controls over age 65	• Telephone numbers are not included on HCFA lists; lists become dated. • Eligible controls on HCFA lists may have moved out of the area or died.
Individuals enrolled in a health maintenance organization	• Provides sampling frame for cases and controls • Certain health maintenance organizations have excellent computerized systems for case ascertainment.	• The health plan enrollees may not be representative of the underlying geographic population, so may limit generalizability.
Neighborhood controls: research team canvases the neighborhood of cases using a specific algorithm to select homes of control subjects.	• Provides sampling frame for cases and controls • Neighbors often seek care from the same hospital or clinic as the cases, and so may provide a valid comparison group.	• Expensive because recruitment of each control may require multiple contacts • Controls may be overmatched to cases on environmental exposures and socioeconomic factors because they are living in the same neighborhood. • Factors associated with mortality and the race/ethnicity of the neighborhood may differ between current neighbors and those who were not residents at the time of the case's diagnosis
Voter electoral rolls, motor vehicle registration departments	• Methods provides sampling frame for cases and controls	• Methods target more select populations such as voters or drivers, possibly affecting study generalizability. • Poorer coverage of geographic area (i.e., smaller percentage of residents qualify for study)
Family members such as parents, siblings, more distant relatives	• Appropriate for certain genetic study designs (see Chapter 4) • Provides some "control" for genetic background while examining environmental factors	• Can result in overmatching with respect to environmental and behavioral risk factors • Results in overmatching with respect to genetic factors, a concern in some designs

Table 2–1 *Continued*

Method	Advantages	Disadvantages
Control Subjects from Undefined Populations		
Hospitalized patients or patients from general medical care clinic	• Patients are seeking care at the same hospital or clinic as the cases. • Provides an option when other control selection methods are not feasible	• Patients without disorder of interest may not have navigated same selection forces as cases to become patients in the hospital; factors associated with referral to the hospital may be associated with risk factors of interest and could bias results.
Patients with other neurological disorders from hospital or clinic (e.g., back pain, headache)	• Patients are seeking care at the same hospital or clinic as the cases. • Convenient and low cost	• Patients with benign neurological condition are not necessarily representative of group from which neurological cases arose (i.e., may reside closer to hospital than cases, have lower socioeconomic status, other features). • Will introduce bias if control patients have conditions that are also associated with the risk factor(s) of interest. • Some neurological disorders used as control conditions may contain true cases of disease if diagnoses are not correct.
Controls recruited from media, other sources	• Controls are a "convenience sample." • Low cost	• Volunteer bias and other selection factors could have unknown effects; large biases could be introduced. • If differences between cases and controls are observed, this could be due to differences in other factors (socioeconomic factors, education) that are associated with the risk factors of interest.
Friend controls or workplace controls, unrelated family members	• Subjects are a "convenience sample." • Subjects are easy and inexpensive to identify. • Cases can identify controls.	• Can result in overmatching with respect to environmental, behavioral, and occupational risk factors; may be difficult to rectify case-control differences • Friends and coworkers chosen by cases may be a select group.

of the population in most areas have telephones (greater than 90%–97% in many regions). Random-digit dialing is conducted by choosing a random sample of telephone numbers in the study region and by calling each number to conduct a census of all household members to determine if someone is eligible to match a case in the study (usually by gender and age). Although many sampling approaches are available for RDD, a commonly used method employs a two-stage sampling scheme that minimizes the chances of calling telephone numbers such as business and government numbers that are not assigned to households (Waksberg et al. 1978). A major drawback of RDD is that a substantial proportion of potential controls may decline to participate (typically 30%–40% even in well-done studies), and the success of this method is declining over time. When this happens, participants and nonparticipants may differ in ways that could bias the study results. Despite concerns about RDD, a study from upstate New York failed to identify important biases even when the RDD refusal rate was as high as 30%–40% (Olsen et al., 1992). The potential for bias must be evaluated on a study-by-study basis.

If a neurological disorder under study affects many individuals age 65 and older, selection of controls through Medicare eligibility may be the best method because elderly individuals are less likely than younger individuals to have telephones, and the use of Medicare rolls enables the additional recruitment of controls from households with telephones as well as independent living centers and nursing homes where each individual may not have a telephone. Since approximately 90%–95% of individuals aged 65 and older are Medicare-eligible, a control sampling procedure using this criterion provides excellent coverage of this age group. A limitation of this method is that Medicare lists must be obtained through the Health Care Financing Administration (HCFA), a process that can be time consuming. Because of emerging privacy trends, it is increasingly difficult to obtain such lists, which in addition can be incomplete or out of date. Also, once a list is obtained from HCFA, subjects identified as potential controls must be contacted to determine their eligibility and willingness to participate. This process can be lengthy. If contact is by mail, participation rates may be even lower than with RDD. Moreover, if the theoretical underlying cohort is distributed over a large geographic area, the logistical aspects of identifying controls through this method are even more difficult.

Example 2–4 In a case–control study of ALS conducted in western Washington State, two controls were matched to each case according to gender and age (±5 years). Random-digit dialing proved to be an inefficient method for recruiting all the control subjects. In this study, the random-digit dialer made approximately 100 calls to recruit one control under the age of 66, but required 500 phone calls to recruit one control older than 65 years. Therefore, two methods were used to recruit population-based control subjects: RDD for 227 control subjects under 66 years of age, and Medicare rolls for 121 controls older than age 65 (McGuire et al. 1997). Had the investigators not included the Medicare rolls as part of their recruiting strategy, many older subjects would not have been matched with a suitable control and would have been excluded from the analyses.

Other methods available for selecting population-based controls, such as the use of voter registration records or motor vehicle department records, are less successful because the percentage of population coverage is less and may result in a study group that is not representative of unaffected individuals in the population region.

Controls from undefined populations. If a study selects cases from convenience sources, such as patient service organizations or through newspaper advertisements, it is not possible to define the source population from which the cases arose (i.e., no census or list of the underlying group is available). The same is true when cases are selected from hospitals, specialty clinics, or tertiary referral centers for the disease, because the underlying population of individuals who seek care from a given hospital or specialty clinic is usually not definable. When hospital or referral center cases are used, the most frequently used source of controls is patients seeking care at the same hospital as that of the cases, for conditions other than the disease of interest. If control patients are diagnosed with a condition that is associated with the exposure of interest or have had their illness for a long time, these patients should also be excluded because, like cases, the presence of the disease may have influenced their exposure to possible risk factors such as diet, physical activity, and medication use. This type of bias is called "Berkson's bias" (see Appendix 2–1).

Two other control selection methods are commonly used when cases have been assembled as a convenience sample: control selection from friends of cases and that from family members of cases. These methods seek control subjects through each of the cases enrolled in the study. Although one or more friend controls can be sought for each case, the selection of friends as controls can introduce a form of bias called "overmatching." This bias occurs because friends or family members are more likely to have exposures or risk factors similar to those of the cases, making it difficult to find differences in the antecedent factors because the two groups are artificially similar to each other. Sometimes spouses of cases are selected as controls, but this approach invites overmatching with respect to environmental exposures and lifestyle behaviors. Furthermore, the match to a spouse does not allow a match on gender and potential biological (hormonal, etc.) factors and differences between the genders can affect study results. Family members of cases such as siblings or cousins have been sought as control subjects; however, this approach also risks overmatching cases and controls in terms of both environmental and genetic factors, making it difficult to demonstrate either of these effects. The use of family controls, however, can be advantageous because it may be desirable in certain genetic association studies to select controls who come from the same genetic "population" or backgrounds from which the cases arose (see Chapter 4). Other sources for non–population-based control groups include volunteers identified through media advertisements and hospital or laboratory personnel, which were often used as control subjects in early investigations of susceptibility genes for neurological disorders. Finally, historical controls for case-control studies of genetic factors may be available through a source such as the Centre de L'Étude du Polymorphisme (CEPH), a DNA bank in France (http://locus.cmdnj.edu/nigms/ceph/ceph.html). However, even if the control group is from a defined population, biases may be invoked because the control group is not from the *same* defined population as that of the cases. While convenience samples of cases and controls may be useful to generate hypotheses or to gather preliminary data, they cannot be assumed to provide unbiased estimates of the associations between risk factors and neurologic disorders in the general population.

Measures of association in case–control studies. The *odds ratio* (OR) is the measure of association in a case–control study in which cases and controls are compared in terms of the proportion of subjects who have had the exposure of interest. The odds ratio can be calculated without information about the absolute risk (incidence) of disease—which is not available from case–control data—making it the preferred measure of association for case–control studies.

		Cases	Controls
Exposure	Exposed	a	b
Status	Not exposed	c	d

$$\text{Odds ratio} = \frac{(a \times d)}{(b \times c)}$$

Odds ratios and relative risks are not the only measures used for investigating the association of risk factors with disease occurrence. Many health outcomes, such as blood pressure and degree of carotid artery stenosis, are measured on an ordinal (ordered) or quantitative (numeric) scale. For such outcomes, the measure of association between a risk factor and the outcome may be a correlation coefficient. These concepts are summarized in Chapter 3, where statistical methods for analyzing epidemiologic data are presented.

Retrospective Cohort Studies. A study design dilemma arises when *both* the exposure and the neurologic outcome are rare. For example, both the cohort and the case–control design will be ill suited to examine the association between cadmium exposure and the risk of developing ALS, since both are relatively rare occurrences. When both the exposure and the disease are rare, conducting a cohort study with a sufficiently long period of follow-up or a case–control study with a large number of cases may be prohibitively expensive. Retrospective cohort studies can be the design of choice when both the exposure and the disease are rare. This type of association can sometimes be addressed in a retrospective cohort study conducted in a large occupational cohort that has been followed for a sufficient number of years to identify an adequate number of cases for study. For example, a retrospective cohort study in a certain industry may be possible, such as the study of polyvinyl chloride exposure and subsequent development of brain tumors in the polyvinyl chloride processing plant (Hagmar et al. 1990). In occupational cohorts, a problem in comparing disease incidence in the employed population with that in the general population is the concern that workers comprise a particularly healthy subset of the population (i.e., the "healthy worker effect"). Retrospective cohort studies are only possible in the following circumstances: (1) an existing "cohort" of exposed persons can be identified and documented, (2) data on the exposures of interest are available (e.g., in company records), and (3) the neurological disorder can be identified with assurance in the members of the cohort. Even when these three conditions exist, it may be necessary to collect information on other contributing or confounding factors (e.g., cigarette smoking, body mass index); however, members of the cohort may not be available for questioning. Following up cohort members to determine disease status is frequently a challenge in retrospective cohort studies. Furthermore, following up cohort members to determine whether they developed the disease of interest can be challenging because of the long span of time between when the cohort began and the present.

Example 2–5 Ron et al. (1988) investigated the association between radiotherapy in childhood for tinea capitis (ringworm of the scalp) and the subsequent development of tumors of the brain and nervous system among 10,834 patients treated for tinea capitis between 1948 and 1960 in Israel when records for this cohort could be obtained. Compared with 10,834 matched population-based control subjects and 5394 siblings who had not received radiation treatment, the relative risk (RR) was 8.4 (95% confidence interval [CI] 4.8–14.8) for neural tumors with increased risk for meningiomas (RR = 9.5), gliomas (RR = 2.6), nerve sheath tumors (RR = 18.8), and other neural tumors (RR = 3.4). The investigators retrospectively estimated the dose of radiation for each patient (mean dose 1.5 Gy). They reported a strong dose–response relation with a RR of 20 for doses of approximately 2.5 Gy. This cohort study was able to confirm that radiotherapy in childhood with doses of 1 to 2 Gy can significantly increase an individual's risk for neural tumors.

Cross-Sectional Studies. A cross-sectional study provides a "snapshot" of a disease and its associated characteristics at one point in time. Many clinical and epidemiologic studies are cross-sectional in design, meaning that information about both the disease and its associated factors are measured at the same time. For example, one study compared the average homocysteine levels in subjects who had had a previous stroke with levels in unaffected subjects and found that homocysteine levels were higher among subjects with a stroke (Kaye et al. 2002). The cross-sectional study design is not appropriate for making inferences about factors that cause the disease, for several reasons. First, it is not always certain that factors measured after disease diagnosis have preceded the disease (i.e., temporality), and so it may be difficult to determine whether the factor preceded or followed the disorder. Second, the presence of a neurological disorder may have caused changes in the exposure or risk factor of interest (e.g., diet, physical activity) so that the associated factor may be a result of, rather than a cause of the neurological disorder. Third, the presence of the disease may affect measurement of the exposure (e.g., blood pressure measurements after stroke). Fourth, the factor of interest may be associated with survival from the disease, and so may be underrepresented (if it hastens disease progression or death) or overrepresented (if it slows disease progression) among prevalent cases. (This type of bias, *prevalence-incidence bias* [Appendix 2–1], is particularly problematic when conducting case–control studies where the aim is to identify etiologic [causal] factors associated with the risk of developing the disease [see Chapter 1].)

Example 2–6 In the Chicago Health and Aging Project, the association of blood pressure with Alzheimer's disease (AD) was examined (Morris et al. 2000) using a cross-sectional study design. Interviews were conducted with a total of 6162 residents from a defined biracial community, and a sample of 709 of these subjects were clinically evaluated and had blood pressure measurements taken. Of these subjects, 243 (34%) had previously been diagnosed with AD. The odds ratio for AD among subjects with systolic blood pressure <130 mmHg compared to subjects with systolic blood pressure 130–139 mmHg was 2.2 (95% CI 1.2–4.1). The risk of AD among subjects with diastolic blood pressure <70 mmHg compared to subjects with diastolic blood pressure 70–79 mmHg was 1.8 (95% CI 1.1–3.1). These estimates were adjusted for age, race, gender, and education. Further adjustment for stroke, body mass index, and other factors did not affect the odds ratios. Using this design, it was not possible to conclude that blood pressure is a risk factor for AD, because the blood pressure measurements were taken after the development of AD and no prediagnosis blood pressure measures were available for either the patients with AD or their unaffected comparison group. A cohort study (longitudinal study design) would be needed to investigate whether blood pressure was a possible causal factor for AD,

because the direction of cause–effect relationship (blood pressure → AD, or AD → blood pressure) was not discernable using a cross-sectional design. Despite this concern about temporal relationship, a cross-sectional design such as the one used in this example does have merit for generating hypotheses about potential risk factors that could be investigated in future hypothesis-testing studies.

While odds ratios may be based on data from cross-sectional studies, this can be misleading because we do not know whether to interpret the association between the disease-associated risk factor as a causal (etiologic) or prognostic relationship. In prognostic studies that have a cross-sectional design, the odds ratio cannot be interpreted as an estimate of the relative risk because it is uncertain whether the exposure preceded disease, and because information differentiating etiology from prognosis is obscured. For this reason, prognostic studies with a cross-sectional design are best used for descriptive purposes, or as an effort to generate hypotheses about factors that are associated with the development and severity of disease.

Ecologic Study Designs

The objective of ecologic studies is to correlate the incidence or prevalence of disease in populations to the proportion of individuals who are exposed to a risk factor of interest in the populations. Ecologic studies make the dubious assumption that the association of exposure and disease on the population (aggregate) level reflect what is happening on an individual level among exposed and unexposed members of a population. The hallmark limitation of ecologic studies is that the proportions of the exposed and unexposed individuals who have the disorder are not known, and associations observed at the aggregate level may not represent associations when data are collected from individual subjects.

Example 2–7 For example, an ecologic study in Yorkshire, England examined the risk of brain cancer among adults with exposure to nitrate in drinking water (Barrett et al. 1998). Nitrate levels and the number of incidence cases for brain cancer were available for each of 148 water supply zones. The incidence of cancer of the brain was higher in areas with the higher average nitrate levels of 29.8 mg/L compared with the lowest quartile of nitrate of 2.4 mg/L (RR = 1.2, 95% CI 1.1–1.3). Because this is an ecologic association, unmeasured confounders could influence the association. If merited, this hypothesis-generating study would ideally be pursued in other studies, including case–control studies, where data on nitrate level exposure could be collected on an individual level for both brain cancer cases and controls.

The ecological study design can be used in populations separated temporally as well as geographically. An example is a study conducted in Rochester, Minnesota (Garraway and Whisnant 1987), where there was a striking correlation between improvement in hypertension control and a decrease in the incidence of stroke over the period from 1950 to 1979. Although a strong association was observed that was biologically plausible, it is possible that other public health and medical interventions may have occurred during this same period of time and contributed to the decrease in stroke incidence.

Collection of Information from Proxy Respondents in Case–Control Studies

When conducting case–control studies of neurologic disorders, proxy respondents are frequently sought to provide information on potential risk factors for disease when the patients themselves (*index subjects*) are unable to reliably answer survey or interview questions. Most often the proxy respondent is a spouse; however, other close relatives such as siblings, friends, or caretakers of patients can be sought as proxy respondents. Several situations may necessitate seeking information

from proxy respondents: (1) the subject is deceased, often from a rapidly progressive condition (e.g., glioblastoma–brain tumor); (2) the neurologic condition compromises the cognition of the subject, making him or her an unreliable respondent (e.g., dementia in Alzheimer's disease); or (3) the subject's communication ability is impaired due to neurologic dysfunction (e.g., slurred speech in amyotrophic lateral sclerosis) (Nelson et al. 1990).

The use of proxy respondents in case–control studies is a subject of some controversy among neuroepidemiologists because the quality of the risk factor information may be compromised when it is obtained from a proxy respondent rather than directly from the index subject. Some investigators reason that proxy respondents should be avoided at all costs because of the possible reduced quality of the information; however, this approach can result in exclusion of a potentially large proportion of study subjects and can compromise the representative nature of the case group. When the reason for needing a proxy respondent is related to disease severity or the rapidly fatal nature of the disease, the percentage of cases who remain for investigation after the deceased or impaired cases are removed can be quite substantial and may also comprise a biased subset of cases. Exclusion of cases who need proxy respondents is often a significant problem in case–control studies of prevalent cases, where patients who are longer-lived with a disease are overrepresented and patients with short duration of disease are underrepresented. Exclusion of deceased subjects or those who have substantial cognitive impairment results in the selective inclusion of patients with less severe forms of the disease. Seeking incident cases of disease for study can significantly reduce the percentage of cases for whom proxy respondents are needed.

Inclusion of proxy respondents has implications for several aspects of study design. Most importantly, when proxy respondents are required for a subset of the neurologic disease cases, what is the investigator to do when selecting age- and gender-comparable control subjects for study? Nelson et al. (1990) described several study design alternatives that are possible when proxy respondents are required for some of the index subjects. Study designs that use proxy respondents for some of the cases but none of the controls should be avoided. In particular, proxy respondents tend to underreport exposure or underestimate the level of exposure, compared to the information obtained from index subjects. If proxy respondents are used for a proportion of cases but not for control subjects, the exposure information would be underestimated on average for the cases but not for the control subjects. For exposures associated with an increased risk of disease, this can bias the results toward not finding an association when one might really exist.

The ideal study design to use in situations where proxy respondents are required for a subset of cases is to recruit proxy respondents for the comparable control subjects. If the controls are matched to cases on respondent type, then the same proportion of both study groups have data provided by proxy respondents, and the accuracy of exposure information is the same in both groups. The decision of whether to include cases who need proxy respondents is also based on other factors, including (1) the percentage of cases for whom proxy respondents will be needed, (2) whether the exclusion of impaired cases will compromise the representative nature of the case group, and (3) whether reliable information can be obtained from proxy respondents for the exposures and risk factors of interest.

Some investigators exclude all cases who require proxy respondents in a case–control study, reasoning that the quality of exposure information is not as good when obtained from proxy respondents as from index subjects themselves. Despite this concern, some studies of the reliability of proxy-provided information have indicated that the exposure information provided by proxy respondents is of surprisingly good quality when the self-reported information from the index subject is used as the standard. Nelson et al. (1994) reported that the reliability of proxy-reported data was excellent for certain characteristics such as demographic variables, information on body habitus (e.g., height, weight, body mass index), and all aspects of cigarette-smoking history (e.g., duration of smoking, number of cigarettes/day, pack-years of smoking, time since last cigarette). Example 3–9 in Chapter 3 gives results for a case–control study of Parkinson's disease in Canada where the investigators compared odds ratios that had been computed using information supplied by index subjects (e.g., cases and controls) with odds ratios obtained from proxy respondents for the same subjects. Interestingly, the odds ratio for the association of smoking with Parkinson's disease was virtually identical when the exposure information was provided by proxy respondents (OR = 0.45; 95% CI 0.27–0.75) as when the information for the same subjects was reported by the index subjects themselves (OR = 0.48; 95% CI 0.29–0.80).

Several factors affect the quality of proxy-provided information, including the method of questioning (e.g., in-person structured interviews are better than mailed questionnaires), the topic of the questions, and the amount of detail required. The reliability of proxy-provided data is good for serious health events (e.g., myocardial infarction, head injury) (Nelson et al. 1990), but is only moderate for alcohol consumption, medications and hormone preparations, and recreational physical activity (Nelson et al. 1994). In contrast, proxy-provided data tend to be of poorer quality for information collected on dietary habits from a food frequency questionnaire (Nelson et al. 1990).

Statistical approaches must be adapted when analyzing case–control data from a study that has a mix of index subjects and proxy respondents (Walker et al. 1988; Nelson et al. 1990). Odds ratios should be estimated separately for data provided by index subjects and proxy respondents. If the odds ratios are similar between the two groups, then the investigator is justified in presenting the overall odds ratio without regard to respondent type. More often than not, however, the odds ratios computed using proxy respondent data are closer to unity (i.e., no association) than are odds ratios obtained when the exposure information is reported by index subjects. This is often due to the fact that the information provided by proxy respondents is of poorer quality (i.e., has more measurement error) than that from index subjects (see Chapter 3). Therefore, it is often appropriate to "adjust" for respondent type in the data analysis to take into account the difference in odds ratio estimates; the appropriate odds ratio to report is the one that is adjusted for respondent type. In any case, it is often helpful to report the odds ratios obtained using index subject data separately from those obtained using data provided by proxy respondents so that the reader can evaluate the effect of proxy-derived information on the associations of interest. Furthermore, if the investigator collects information from a subset of control subjects and their proxy respondents, a study can be done to assess the completeness and accuracy of exposure information for proxy respondents using their index subjects as the standard. This approach can yield information about whether the proxy-provided data are of sufficient quality to include in the study. For a complete discussion of these issues, see Walker et al. (1988) and Nelson et al. (1990).

Sources of Study Bias

The conceptual simplicity and adaptability of observational study designs make them very useful for clinical and epidemiologic research. As a result, many important observational studies are performed by investigators without formal epidemiologic and biostatistical training. While the accessibility and comprehensibility of observational study designs is a nice feature, there are considerable challenges to performing such studies, and careful attention to minimizing or removing the study biases is needed to obtain valid results. Investigators who adapt a study design without knowledge of the many potential sources of bias can end up with a study that ultimately cannot provide definitive answers to the research questions they have posed. The remainder of this chapter and a section in Chapter 3 (Measurement Error) are devoted to the description of study biases and how they may be minimized or avoided altogether.

Internal and External Study Validity

The primary method of epidemiology is to take a sample or subset of subjects from a larger defined population to study factors that are linked with a health outcome such as the onset of a disease, disease severity, or death from the disease. When investigators draw a sample from a larger "source" population, they are interested in determining whether the conclusions of the research are correct for the people in the sample itself (internal validity) as well as whether the sample is a good representation of the source population (external validity).

It is natural for scientists to place great emphasis on the external validity, or representative nature, of a study population so that study findings can be generalized to the target population. In the United States, this would mean conducting the study in a group that is representative of the U.S. population with respect to characteristics such as age, gender, race/ethnicity, and socioeconomic status. Conducting epidemiologic studies of neurologic disorders in a fully representative sample of the U.S. population is very difficult and costly, and very few studies except those executed by the federal government attempt such a feat (e.g., National Health Interview Survey (NHIS; National Center for Health Statistics 2002), National Health and Nutrition Examination Survey (NHANES; National Center for Health Statistics 1996). In practice, most epidemiologic studies are conducted in smaller populations where the internal validity of the study can be achieved—that is, studies in which important biases that can affect study conclusions can be minimized or avoided altogether, but where the study population is not representative of the entire United States. An important concept in epidemiology is that a study must have internal validity before external validity or generalizability can be considered because if a study is not valid in and of itself, its representative nature is of little consequence.

Table 2–2 summarizes four common biases that can affect study validity. These are *sampling error*, or random variation in sampling subjects so that the sample does not reflect the source population's characteristics; *selection bias* that is incurred in the sampling of cases or controls from their respective underlying populations; *confounding bias,* caused by a third factor that alters the risk factor–disease association because it is correlated with both the risk factor and the disease of interest; and *infor-*

Table 2–2   Common Sources of Bias in Clinical and Epidemiologic Studies of Neurologic Disorders

Type of bias	Description	Hypothetical examples
Sampling error (sampling variation)	In the process of selecting samples of subjects from a study population, each sample will differ, purely by chance, so that no one sample is likely to be fully representative of the population.	Small randomized trial of baclofen versus placebo for the treatment of spasticity in MS: Because of small sample size, the baclofen and placebo groups differed according to the percentage who had a chronic progressive disease course: 19/40 or 48% baclofen-treated patients, versus 12/40 or 30% placebo-treated patients with chronic/progressive MS.
Selection bias	A form of sampling bias due to systematic differences between those who are selected (or agree to participate) for a study and those who are not selected (or refuse to participate)	Case–control study of stroke: Control subjects were sought through random digit dialing and who refused participation were more likely to be current cigarette smokers (25%) than were controls who participated in the study (20%), resulting in a biased (too high) OR for the smoking–stroke association.
Confounding bias	Confounding bias occurs when an effect estimate such as an OR or a RR is distorted (either accentuated or attenuated) by a third variable that is associated with both the exposure and disease.	Cohort study of stroke: Investigators examined the association of coffee consumption and stroke. Crude RR was 1.7 for drinking more than 2 cups of coffee per day, but after adjustment for cigarette smoking, the RR associated with coffee drinking was attenuated (RR = 1.1), showing no effect.
Information bias (measurement error)	Erroneous classification of an individual or an attribute (risk factor) error) into a category other than that to which it should be assigned	Case–control study of children with neural tube defects: Mothers of infants who had neural tube defects were more likely to recall having taken aspirin during pregnancy than were mothers of control infants, a type of recall bias. This reporting bias resulted in a false association between aspirin use and neural tube defects.

MS, multiple sclerosis; OR, odds ratio; RR, relative risk.

mation bias, or error in measuring either the risk factors or the disease characteristics under study. While these are the main categories of study bias, a myriad of interesting biases can affect observational and experimental studies (Appendix 2–1). Of note is that bias can be introduced at any stage of the research process, from reviewing the literature, to selecting a study sample, to collecting data, to the final steps of analyzing and presenting the data. Excellent reviews of the common sources of potential study biases can be obtained from several sources (Sackett 1979; Armstrong et al. 1992; Wacholder et al. 1992b).

Sampling Error

Some associations may occur on the basis of chance alone, that is, they may occur just because there is random variation in taking samples of study subjects so that a given sample may not reflect the source population's characteristics. This is called "sampling variability," "random error," or simply "chance." There are three primary methods for addressing sampling error: (*1*) achieve a larger sample size, (*2*) conduct collaborative reanalyses or meta-analyses to combine results from several studies, and (*3*) replicate the study results in other populations. Methods 1 and 2 are discussed in Chapter 3, and method 3 (replication) is the basic tenet of all scientific research.

Selection Bias

Selection bias occurs when subjects selected for a study are not representative of the underlying population in one or more characteristics that affect the association of interest. Selection bias can operate through improper selection of cases or controls in a case–control study. In a cohort study, selection bias can occur when the percentage of subjects lost to follow-up varies according to both the exposure of interest and the neurologic outcome. Although selection bias can affect any study design (randomized trials, cohort studies, etc.), case–control studies are more prone to selection bias than other study designs. Selection bias

can cause either overestimates or underestimates of the true associations between exposure and disease in the underlying population.

Several strategies can be implemented during the design, conduct, and analysis phases of a case-control study to minimize selection bias or to assess the impact of selection bias if it is not entirely avoidable. A clear understanding of the underlying population from which subjects are sampled is essential to understanding selection bias.

Example 2–8   Selection bias can occur at any point in the subject identification and recruitment process, and even through the point at which study data are analyzed to obtain results. Figure 2–1 provides a schematic of a hypothetical study of prognosis among patients who have sought care for MS from a specialized university (tertiary) medical center. The primary goal of a MS prognostic study is to study patients who are representative of all MS patients in the underlying geographic region. Figure 2–1 illustrates the process by which a larger sample of representative MS patients can undergo "selection forces" until the ultimate study in the study sample is whittled down to a group that is much smaller and ultimately nonrepresentative of the total MS population. Consider the scenario of patients with MS who reside in a geographic region and the likelihood that they will navigate a set of selection forces to participate in a prognostic study at a university-based MS referral and treatment center. Beginning with early symptoms of MS, most patients would seek treatment from their primary care physician, although a subset of people, perhaps those with mild symptoms, would not seek medical care. Among patients who are seen by a generalist physician, a certain number would be referred to a neurologist for a second opinion or would ask for such a referral. Other patients may not be similarly motivated, particularly lower-socioeconomic status patients with no insurance who would be less able to pay out-of-pocket expenses. Among the patients who are seen by neurologists in the region, some might be referred to a regional MS referral center because they had a questionable diagnosis with idiosyncratic features, suffered severe disability, had a complicated disease course or they were candidates for a clinical trial of a new investigational medication for MS. Once at the center, the clinical research staff may attempt to recruit all patients to participate in a long-term prognostic study; some of the referred patients would participate and others would not, their decision being based perhaps on their employment status and the ease of making repeated trips to the MS specialty center. Once enrolled and baseline data collected, certain additional patients would decline to make regular 6-month study visits for the prognostic study. In this hypothetical example, selection forces operate to "select" the final sample of patients in the study including factors such as disease severity, socioeconomic status, employment status, and other factors that likely result in a study group that is not representative of the original patient group with respect to many important factors.

In a study of referral bias in MS research conducted in northern Colorado, the authors compared the characteristics of MS patients from a population-based prevalence survey who were referred to a university-based MS referral center with MS patients from the same region who did not seek care or get referred to the university center (Nelson et al. 1988). The referral center patient group differed from the group that did not seek care at the MS university center: on average, patients in the referral center group were younger, had greater mobility impairment, and reported more recent disease worsening. It is likely that a prognostic study conducted in such a center would not result in a generalizeable sample of MS patients. Therefore, while such a referral center may be optimal as a source of patients for clinical trials or other experimental protocols, they would not be ideal for conducting studies to identify causal factors because they do not represent all patients with MS.

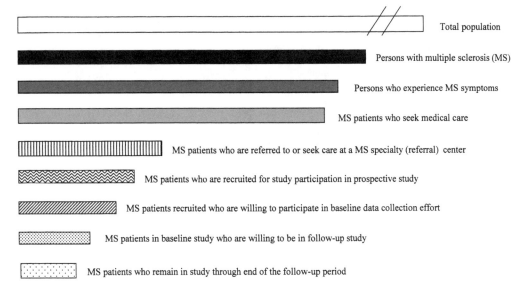

Figure 2–1 Example of selection bias (specifically, "referral bias") among patients with multiple sclerosis (MS) in the underlying population who navigate various selection forces up to enrollment in and during a study of prognostic factors in MS at a university-based MS referral center. Selection forces include willingness to seek medical care for symptoms, self or physician referral to a MS referral center, willingness to provide data for baseline prognostic study, willingness to participate in prospective portion of the study, and willingness to stay in the prospective study through the end of the study period.

In the conduct of a study, selection bias can be avoided or minimized by careful enumeration and thorough attempts at recruiting all cases within the source population. For conditions that virtually always result in a hospital admission, such as a ruptured intracranial aneurysm, one can use hospital discharge records for all hospitals serving the source population. For most neurologic conditions, however, multiple methods of case ascertainment are required (see Chapter 1). As noted above, high standards for the methods of control selection are also critical to the success of case–control studies. Random digit dialing, described above, is a reasonable alternative, particularly in areas where the proportion of households without phones is low (<5% in many areas). Other alternatives include hospital controls, friend controls, and controls from convenience samples, each of which are likely to introduce selection bias in the study.

Even with proper identification of potential subjects, selection bias can occur because of study subjects' nonresponse and refusals.

People who are difficult to reach or who refuse to participate are often different from those who enroll in a study. Minimizing nonresponse and refusal rates is therefore key to minimizing selection bias. Loss of subjects over the course of a study can also introduce selection bias; the larger the percentage of subjects lost, the greater the opportunity for selection bias to influence study results. The annual loss of subjects to follow-up can be as low as 2%–3% in rigorous cohort studies, but in practice, many cohort studies in clinical and epidemiologic research suffer annual losses of 10% or greater.

Several techniques for maximizing the participation of study subjects and not losing them to follow-up in prospective studies are available (Table 2–3). An excellent text by Bruce Armstrong and colleagues, *Principles of Exposure Measurement in Epidemiology* (1992), includes strategies for minimizing nonresponse in clinical and epidemiologic studies. Follow-up of neurologically impaired subjects presents particular challenges and usually requires a close

Table 2–3 Strategies for Reducing Participant Nonreponse and Selection Bias in Clinical and Epidemiologic Studies

Factor	Mail survey	Telephone survey	In-person interview
Advance letter or notice, or introductory letter	XX	XX	XX
Multiple mailings, requests, attempts at contact	XX	XX	XX
Follow-up using other method(s)	XX	XX	XX
Letter signed by usual physician	XX	X	X
Personalized approach	X	XX	X
A salient topic	XX	X	X
Government or university sponsorship	XX	X	X
Blanket publicity	X	X	X
Handwritten address	XX		
Colored questionnaire	XX		
Certified mailings or commemorative stamps	XX		
Incentive included with the questionnaire	XX		
Stamped return envelope	XX		
Experienced, confident interviewers		XX	XX
Careful selection/training of interviewers		X	X
Carefully constructed introduction		X	X
Verification of interviewer's credentials		X	X
Brief screening, immediate telephone interview		XX	
Use experienced interviewers for "turnarounds"		X	X
Elimination of interviewers with high refusal rates		X	X

XX, empirically supported; X, recommended.

The material in this table was adapted from Tables 11.2, 11.3, and 11.4 in Armstrong BK, White E, Saracci R. Principle of Exposure Measurement in Epidemiology. New York: Oxford University Press, 1992.

relationship with the subject's primary caretaker or family member.

Once subjects are enrolled, methods for assessing whether selection bias is present can be used. Study subjects can be compared to people in the underlying population according to characteristics for which data are available for both groups, such as age and gender and other demographic characteristics. Another technique is to compare subjects who were enrolled without difficulty to those who were very difficult to contact or who initially refused to enroll in the study, to determine if they differ in characteristics of importance for the study, the assumption being that subjects who almost did not enroll in the study will be similar to people who were eligible but were not enrolled.

Confounding Bias

Confounding occurs when the measure of the effect of exposure on disease risk (OR, RR) is distorted because of an extraneous factor (confounder) that is associated with both the exposure and the occurrence of the disease. The same variable may not be a confounder in all studies of the same exposure–disease association. As was noted earlier in the chapter, the researcher needs to eliminate the confounder as a factor that modifies the magnitude of the association before considering it a potential confounder.

The two main criteria for confounding bias are (1) among non-diseased persons, the potential confounding factor is associated with the exposure and (2) among non-exposed persons in the population, the potentially confounding factor is associated with the risk of disease. The second criterion does not require that the confounder be a true risk factor for disease (but only be correlated with disease), although that may often be the case. Other factors that are not causally associated with disease may also be confounders, such as a factor that is a correlate (or "proxy") of a cause or a factor that influences the likelihood that the disease will be detected or diagnosed (Sackett 1979) (Appendix 2–1).

Example 2–9　In a hypothetical example, alcohol consumption and cigarette smoking are primary risk factors of interest in a case–control study of hemorrhagic stroke. Figure 2–2 shows the relationship between alcohol consumption, cigarette smoking, and risk of hemorrhagic stroke. In this illustration, the risk factor of interest is heavy alcohol consumption (defined as consuming more than 2 alcoholic drinks per day), and the confounder is cigarette smoking, which is known to be a risk factor for hemorrhagic stroke. However, individuals who are heavy drinkers are more likely to be cigarette smokers than are nondrinkers or light drinkers. Therefore, any positive association between heavy alcohol consumption and hemorrhagic stroke is likely to be confounded by smoking, because cigarette smoking is a risk factor for the disease and cigarette smoking is more common among heavy drinkers (i.e., is associated with the risk factor of interest). In Figure 2–2, the crude odds ratio for the association was 4.5, but after adjustment for cigarette smoking, the odds ratio was diminished as a result of "removing" the confounding effect of smoking and was only 3.4, still a significantly increased risk but

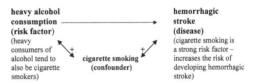

Figure 2–2　Cigarette smoking as a confounder of the alcohol–hemorrhagic stroke (HS) association. Since smoking is positively associated with alcohol consumption, and smoking itself is a very strong risk factor for HS, the "crude" odds ratio for the alcohol association is artificially inflated. It is important to adjust for the confounding effect of smoking when evaluating the alcohol–HS association. In this hypothetical example, the crude odds ratio for the association was 4.5, but after adjustment for cigarette smoking, the odds ratio was lowered to 3.4 as a result of removing the confounding effect of smoking. (See Chapter 3 for the numerical approach that was used to obtain the crude and smoking adjusted odds ratios.)

somewhat attenuated. Example 3–14 shows the numerical approach that was used to obtain the crude and the smoking adjusted odds ratios for heavy alcohol consumption.

Procedures for minimizing confounding bias can be implemented at all stages of the study, including when designing the study protocol, collecting data, and analyzing and interpreting study results. There are three primary methods for controlling confounding: restriction, matching, and stratified statistical analyses.

Use of Restriction to Control Confounding Bias. The first method for controlling confounding, restriction, is to select subjects who are homogenous with respect to the confounder. For example, by only selecting men in a study of brain tumor (glioblastoma), the associations of occupational metal exposures with brain tumor could not be confounded by gender, because the study would be comprised only of men. In practice, restriction is often not used at the study design stage because it may result in a large proportion of study subjects being excluded from study; however, even if restriction is not carried out in advance of the study, it may be applied at the statistical analysis stage even if the factor was not restricted at the design stage. For example, male gender may be a risk factor for brain tumor, resulting in a higher percentage of men than of women in a case–control study of glioblastoma. Employment in an occupation involving exposure to heavy metals may be more common among men than among women; however, gender could confound the association between occupational metal exposure and glioblastoma. If a case–control study were conducted and too few women were available to obtain an OR for this relatively rare exposure, the statistical analysis for metals exposure could be restricted to male study subjects, thus completely removing the confounding effect of gender.

Matching to Control Confounding and Increase Study Efficiency. The second method for controlling confounding is to match cases and controls on the confounding factor so that there are no differences in confounder distribution between study groups from the start of the study. When a study design requires matching cases to controls at the outset, it is important that the matching factor(s) of interest also be "adjusted" in the statistical analysis phase of the study. If the matching factor is not taken into account, confounding may still exist because the act of matching controls to cases on one factor that is itself associated with disease risk introduces a comparability that must be retained at the analysis stage so that "like" subjects in a given category of the confounder are compared with each other. Because the act of matching forces the case and control groups to be comparable with respect to the matching factor, matching variables cannot be assessed as risk factors. However, matching does not preclude examining the confounding factor as an effect modifier for other risk factor associations. Indeed, although age and gender are common matching factors, they may also be of great interest because the effects of other risk factors may vary by gender or across age groups.

In case–control studies, if the distribution of a potential confounding variable is substantially different in the case and control groups, then matching cases and controls on this variable can also increase the efficiency of adjusting for this variable in the analysis. *Efficiency* is a statistical term that indicates the relative precision of an estimate such as an incidence rate or an odds ratio. The precision of an estimate is reflected by how wide the confidence intervals are and is an indicator of the statistical uncertainty of the estimate (i.e., short, or "tight," confidence intervals signify an efficient [precise] estimate).

Age and gender are often used as matching variables in a case–control study for several reasons. First, both age and gender often meet the first criterion for confounding in that they are often associated with the risk factors of interest, such as duration of cigarette smoking or occupational exposure to heavy metals. Second, age and gender are often risk factors for disease because the incidence of most diseases varies significantly by age and often by gender as well.

Stratified Statistical Analyses and Multivariate Modeling to Control Confounding. The third method for controlling confounding is to use statistical methods such as stratified data analyses or multivariate modeling to adjust for the influence of the confounding factors. As mentioned above, statistical adjustment is needed *even if* matching has been employed in the design phase of the study. Statistical adjustment requires that the potentially confounding variable be measured in the data collection effort and also adjusted for as a covariate in the statistical analysis of study data. Confounding is detected by comparing the "crude" risk estimate (RR or OR) for the exposure–disease association with the risk estimate that is obtained after statistical adjustment for the confounding variable. Statistical methods for controlling confounding bias are presented in the last section of Chapter 3.

Information Bias (Measurement Error)

The third common type of study bias is information bias, that is, errors in the measurement of any of the factors that are under study. One of the most important study design features that an investigator has control over is the measurement quality of the two factors that are being associated with each other—the risk factor (or health predictor) and the neurological disorder or outcome under study. Information bias, also called "measurement error," can have a tremendous impact on the ability to identify an association between a risk factor and a neurological outcome, even in situations where other biases such as selection bias and confounding are under control. The ability to demonstrate a true association between a risk factor and a disease, assuming that such an association exists, is significantly hindered if either of these factors is poorly measured or "misclassified."

The classification of disease—that is, determining whether a person has a given neurologic condition or not—is largely a function of the accuracy of the clinical diagnosis. As discussed in Chapter 1, many of the neurological disorders that are commonly studied in neuroepidemiologic investigations have standardized research diagnostic criteria that are used for establishing the case definition. The degree of disease misclassification is largely determined by the "state of the art" of diagnosis of a given neurologic condition (e.g., the sensitivity and specificity of clinical signs, symptoms and laboratory tests for identifying the condition), and the investigator can do little more than select the best available case definition criteria that are feasible to apply in a given study. In contrast, the investigator has more influence over the choice of methods to assess the demographic, lifestyle, behavioral, and environmental exposures being investigated as risk factors for a given disorder. Attention to the quality of measurements for the determinants of a neurological disorder is of critical importance to the success of a study; therefore, a large section of Chapter 3 (Measurement Error and Analysis) is devoted to discussion of this concept.

Causal Reasoning and Effect Modification

Neurological diseases are complex entities, and except for diseases caused by the inheritance of a single disease-causing gene (e.g., Huntington's disease), the causes of neurologic disorders are multifactorial and likely involve the interaction of multiple genes (gene–gene interaction), environmental factors, and the combination of susceptibility genes with environmental factors (gene–environment interaction). Therefore, any given study is a simplification of a complex reality, and the relative contribution of causal factors may be very difficult to dissect.

In most experimental designs, such as randomized clinical trials, causal reasoning is based on the concept that there is a one-to-one correspondence between a given cause (treatment) and its effect. In theory, the process of randomizing research subjects to receiving either a treatment or a placebo will produce two groups that are very similar with respect to all other factors that affect the outcome except the treatment under study. If differences are observed, and no important study biases are present, the outcome of the trial is credited to either the treatment or its absence; in this way the treatment is considered to be both necessary and sufficient for causing the favorable outcome.

Causal reasoning in observational studies is more complex, and it is less reasonable to believe that there is a one-to-one correspondence between a cause (risk factor) and its effect (disease). Since most diseases are multifactorial, a given cause may be neither *necessary* (i.e., present among all individuals with a disease) or *sufficient* (i.e., itself capable of being the sole cause of disease). Consider the classic association between smoking and lung cancer. Lung cancer can arise among nonsmokers (i.e., among those exposed to asbestos), therefore, smoking is not *necessary* to cause lung cancer. Furthermore, cigarette smoking by itself is not *sufficient* to cause lung cancer, because although heavy smoking is a strong risk factor for lung cancer, only 10% of heavy smokers will develop this cancer.

An important tenet of clinical and epidemiologic research is that *association does not prove causation*. That is, the fact that a putative risk factor and the occurrence of a neurological disorder are strongly associated with each other does not provide evidence that the risk factor *causes* the disease,

only that it is *correlated* with disease occurrence. Many circumstances other than causality can underlie a given risk factor–disease association, including uncontrolled study biases or spurious correlation due to the association of noncausal factors with those that do cause disease. Before inferring that a risk factor truly causes a neurological disorder, several aspects of the risk factor–disease association must be examined.

Several scientists have developed and refined criteria for causal inference that can be used to determine whether a particular association is likely to indicate a causal relationship between a risk factor and disease (Koch 1882; U.S. Department of Health, Education and Welfare 1964; Hill 1965). A list of six cardinal criteria for causality can be assembled from these reports:

Temporal sequence—in order to be causal, events or factors that are causative must have preceded the development of disease or other neurological outcome.
Strength of association—the stronger the association, the more likely it is to be causal.
Dose–response relationship—evidence for causality is strengthened when the association is stronger at increasing levels or "doses" of the exposure.
Consistency of findings across studies using different designs strengthens the evidence for causation.
Replicability of the findings in other studies is needed before causality can be established.
Biologic plausibility—consistency with animal and laboratory research demonstrating similar cause–effect relations boosts the evidence for causality.

Making Inferences About Disease Causation

Investigators who have strong evidence for a causal relationship between a putative risk factor and the occurrence of a neurological disease are justified in calculating and reporting a figure called "attributable risk" (also know as "etiologic fraction"). From a public health perspective, the proportion of disease in a population that can be attributed to a specific risk factor is an important question that can help guide resource allocation for public health and wellness programs to prevent disease.

The *population attributable risk* (PAR) is the incidence of disease in the population that is attributable to the risk factor, and can be used to calculate the number of cases in the population that would be prevented if the risk factor were eliminated. The *population attributable risk percent* (PAR%) is an estimate of the proportion of the disease in the population that is attributable to the risk factor and by which the disease would be reduced if the exposure were eliminated. The population attributable risk is often expressed as a percent (PAR %) and can be estimated as

$$\text{Population attributable risk percent} = \frac{\begin{array}{c}\text{(rate of disease in} \\ \text{total population)} \\ \text{minus (rate of} \\ \text{disease in} \\ \text{the unexposed)}\end{array}}{\begin{array}{c}\text{rate of disease} \\ \text{in the} \\ \text{total population}\end{array}} \times 100$$

Effect Modification

Effect modification, also called statistical interaction, is present when the association between exposure and disease is stronger in certain subgroups of the study subjects than in others. If effect modification is present, additional insight into the possible causal association of the exposure and disease is possible, and it may suggest new hypotheses to explain the interaction between the characteristic that defines the subgroups and association between exposure and disease.

When differences in the magnitude of association between exposure and disease (RR or OR) are seen in different subgroups

within the study, statistical tests can be used to determine the probability that this difference occurred by chance. It is possible to test for effect modification in many different subgroups in any given study, thus increasing the possibility of a type I error (i.e., finding a significant difference when none actually exists). Therefore, deliberate testing for effect modification should generally be limited to a few subgroups, chosen a priori (prior to data analysis) on the basis of biological plausibility or on the results of previous studies. When effect modification is found in subgroups where it was not hypothesized, it should be evaluated in terms of magnitude, probability, and biological plausibility. Some researchers suggest that the criteria for reporting unexpected effect modification should be higher than the usual nominal p-value of 0.05 (e.g., a p-value of <0.10 or <0.15). Regardless, a clear distinction needs to be made in reporting between effect modification hypothesized a priori and subgroup effects discovered incidentally during data analysis.

Example 2–10 Mayeux and colleagues (1995) conducted a study of 236 community-dwelling elderly persons to determine whether the effect of head injury on the risk of Alzheimer's disease (AD) varied according to whether a person had one or more copies of the apolipoprotein epsilon 4 allele (APOE ϵ4), a genetic variant that has been shown to increase the risk of AD. Prior to the study, they hypothesized that the amount of cerebral beta amyloid precursor protein (βAPP) deposited after trauma to the brain would be greater among those subjects who had the APOE ϵ4 genotype than among those without the genotype, and that the two factors would have a synergistic effect on the risk of AD. Their findings were consistent with their hypothesis. While the overall OR for AD associated with head injury was 1.5 (95% CI 0.5–3.5), the association was different according to APOE ϵ4 allele status. Using as the referent group persons who had neither a head injury nor an APOE ϵ4 allele, the OR for those who had both a history of traumatic head injury and at least one APOE $\epsilon4$ allele was 10.5 (95% CI 1.3–87.8), and the OR among those with the presence of one or more APOE $\epsilon4$ alleles but no head injury was 2.0 (95% CI 1.1–3.5). In the absence of the APOE $\epsilon4$ allele, head injury had no association with AD (OR = 1.0, 95% CI 0.3–2.9). The OR for the combined effect of head injury and APOE $\epsilon4$ allele (OR = 10.5) was greater than an OR of 2.0, which is the OR that would be expected if each of the factors had acted independently (obtained by multiplying the OR for APOE $\epsilon4$ of 2.0 times the OR for head injury alone, 1.0). Of note is that, while the OR for the effect of head injury among those with the APOE $\epsilon4$ allele (OR = 10.5) was considerably greater than the effect of the APOE $\epsilon4$ allele alone (OR = 2.0), the test for this interaction was not statistically significant because of a relatively small sample size. A sample size nearly twice that used in this study would be needed to detect the interaction of these two factors as statistically significant. This demonstrates one of the difficulties investigators face in assessing effect modification study sample sizes must be considerably larger for detecting interactions than for detecting the *main effects* of risk factors.

The presence of effect modification is a concept that is model-dependent, that is, different conclusions can be drawn depending on whether the model for comparing subgroup effects is based on relative risks or odds ratios (i.e., the *multiplicative model*) or is based on risk differences between the subgroups (i.e., the *additive model*). In the example above, a multiplicative model based on comparison of odds ratios was used to examine the presence of effect modification between the APOE $\epsilon4$ allele and head injury in affecting the risk of AD. A full description of these two approaches is beyond the scope of this text; an excellent review is provided by Rothman et al. (1998).

In practice, if the relative risks for two or more subgroups are materially different

from one another, reporting the relative risk for study subjects as a whole would be misleading; therefore, results must be presented separately for each subgroup. As a simple theoretical example, if an exposure reduced the risk of stroke by 50% in men, but doubled the risk in women, then simply reporting the no assiciation between the exposure and the disease in the overall study (i.e., RR = 1.0) would be misleading. In this example, the relative risk estimates should be presented for men and women separately.

Future Directions and Conclusions

After recognizing the potential sources of bias in observational study designs, it may seem that no study could stand up to the various criticisms that can be leveled at such designs. Indeed, methods such as the case–control design are conceptually easy to understand but very difficult to design and execute in a manner that avoids the potential landmines of study biases that can occur. In their training, students of epidemiology and clinical research become adept at identifying potential study biases that can limit the validity of such studies. The ability to criticize study designs and identify their deficiencies is an important skill; however, finding fault is the easy part. Equally important is the ability to know which study biases are inconsequential and which biases have significant effects on the ability to draw valid conclusions from the study. This knowledge is often based on knowing where to look for study biases, determining the impact of bias on the associations that are being investigated, and deciding whether the bias is significant enough to change the conclusions of the study.

By developing a balanced approach to evaluating the design of epidemiologic studies, an investigator can ferret out the important conclusions that can be drawn and places less weight on conclusions that have a weak methodological basis. A balanced approach is particularly important in neuroepidemiology, a discipline in many senses still a frontier area for epidemiologic research. Accordingly, the science of neuroepidemiology can proceed, with each study building on the findings of previous studies and carrying forward important methodologic insights in the process.

The ability of a study to detect an association between a risk factor and the development of the disease depends on many features, including the statistical power of the study (i.e., having a sufficient number of study subjects to demonstrate a treatment effect or an association), as well as the accuracy of measurement for both the risk factor and the neurologic disorder under study. Measurement quality is the single most important aspect of design that is under the investigator's control and ideally will undergo continual improvement, to the great benefit of neuroepidemiologic research. Chapter 3 describes the various sources of measurement error that can affect research studies and posits solutions for minimizing the effects of measurement error.

References

Armstrong BK, White E, Saracci R. Principles of Exposure Measurement in Epidemiology. New York: Oxford University Press, 1992.

Barrett JH, Parslow RC, McKinney PA, et al. Nitrate in drinking water and the incidence of gastric, esophageal, and brain cancer in Yorkshire, England. *Cancer Causes Control* 1998;9:153–159.

Farquhar JW, Fortmann SP, Flora JA, et al. Effects of community-wide education on cardiovascular disease risk factors. The Stanford Five-City Project. *JAMA* 1990;264:359–365.

Garraway WM, Whisnant JP. The changing pattern of hypertension and the declining incidence of stroke. *JAMA* 1987;258:214–217.

Gregg MB. Field Epidemiology. New York: Oxford University Press, 2002.

Hagmar L, Akesson B, Nielsen J, et al. Mortality and cancer morbidity in workers exposed to low levels of vinyl chloride monomer at a polyvinyl chloride processing plant. *Am J Ind Med* 1990;17:553–565.

Hill AB. The environment and disease: association or causation? *Proc R Soc Med* 1965;56: 295–300.

Kaye JM, Stanton KG, McCann VJ, et al. Homocysteine, folate, methylene tetrahydrofo-

late reductase genotype and vascular morbidity in diabetic subjects. *Clin Sci* 2002;102: 631–637.

Koch R. The aetiology of tuberculosis. *Berlin Klin Wochenschr* 1882; 19:221. Translated and reprinted in Pinner M. The Aetiology of Tuberculosis. New York: National Tuberculosis Association, 1932.

Koepsell TD, Wagner EH, Cheadle AC, et al. Selected methodological issues in evaluating community-based health promotion and disease prevention programs. *Annu Rev Public Health* 1992;13:31–57.

Kurland LT, Molgaard CA. The patient record in epidemiology. *Sci Am* 1981;245:54–63.

Mayeux R, Ottman R, Maestre MD, et al. Synergistic effect of traumatic head injury and apolipoprotein-4 in patients with Alzheimer's disease. *Neurology* 1995;45:555–557.

McGuire V, Longstreth WT, Koepsell TD, van Belle G. Incidence of amyotrophic lateral sclerosisin the three counties in western Washington State. *Neurology* 1996;47:571–573.

McGuire V, Longstreth WT Jr, Nelson LM, et al. Occupational exposures and amyotrophic lateral sclerosis. A population-based case–control study. *Am J Epidemiol* 1997;145: 1076–1088.

Morris MC, Scherr PA, Hebert LE, et al. The cross-sectional association between blood pressure and Alzheimer's disease in a biracial community population of older persons. *J Gerontol A Biol Sci Med Sci* 2000;55: M130–M136.

National Center for Health Statistics, Division of Health Interview Statistics. 2000 National Health Interview Survey (NHIS) Public Use Data Release: HHIS Survey Description. Hyattsville, MD: Centers for Disease Control and Prevention, 2002.

National Center for Health Statistics. Third National Health and Nutrition Examination Survey (NHANES), 1988–1994: Reference Manual and Reports. Hyattsville, MD: Centers for Disease Control and Prevention, 1996.

Nelson LM, Franklin GM, Hamman RF, et al. Referral bias in multiple sclerosis research. *J Clin Epidemiol* 1988;41:187–192.

Nelson LM, Hamman RF, Thompson DS, et al. Higher than expected prevalence of multiple sclerosis in northern Colorado: dependence on methodologic issues. *Neuroepidemiology* 1986;5:17–28.

Nelson LM, Longstreth WT Jr, Koepsell TD, et al. Completeness and accuracy of interview data from proxy respondents: Demographic, medical and life-style fcators. *Epidemiology* 1994;5:204–217.

Nelson LM, Longstreth WT Jr, Koepsell TD, van Belle G. Proxy respondents in epidemiologic research. *Epidemiologic Reviews* 1990; 12:71–86.

Olson SH, Kelsey JL, Pearson TA, et al. Evaluation of random digit dialing as a method of control selection in case–control studies. *Am J Epidemiol* 1992;135:210–222.

Ron E, Modan B, Boice JD, et al. Tumors of the brain and nervous system after radiotherapy in childhood. *N Engl J Med* 1988;319:1033–1039.

Sackett DL. Bias in analytic research. *J Chron Dis* 1979;32:51–63.

Stewart R, Richards M, Brayne C, Mann A. Vascular risk and cognitive impairment in an older British, African-Caribbean population. *J Am Geriatr Soc* 2001;49:263–269.

U.S. Department of Health, Education and Welfare. Smoking and Health: A Report of the Surgeon General. Washington, DC: U.S. Government Printing Office, 1964.

Wacholder S, McLaughlin JK, Silverman DT, Mandel JS. Selection of controls in case–control studies. I. Principles. *Am J Epidemiol* 1992a;135:1019–1028.

Wacholder S, Silverman DT, McLaughlin JK, Mandel JS. Selection of controls in case–control studies. II. Types of controls. *Am J Epidemiol* 1992b;135:1029–1041.

Wacholder S, Silverman, DT McLaughlin JK, Mandel JS. Selection of controls in case–control studies. III. Design options. *Am J Epidemiol* 1992c;135:1042–1050.

Waksberg J. Sampling methods for random digit dialing. *J Am Stat Assoc* 1978;73:40–46.

Walker AM, Velema JP, Robins JM, et al. Analysis of case-control data derived in part from proxy respondents. *Am J Epidemiol* 1988;127:905–914.

Wolf PA, Abbott RD, Kannel WB. Atrial fibrillation as an independent risk factor for stroke: the Framingham Study. *Stroke* 1991; 22:983–988.

Writing Group for the Women's Health Initiative Investigators. Risks and benefits of estrogen plus progestin in healthy postmenopausal women. Principal results from the Women's Health Initiative Randomized Control Trial. *JAMA* 2002;288:321–333.

Appendix 2–1

Appendix 2–1 Catalog of Biases in Analytic Studies

Stage of research/name of bias	Description of bias
Reviewing the Literature	
One-sided reference bias	Authors restrict references to those that support their position.
Positive results bias	Authors are more likely to submit, and editors to accept, positive rather than negative results.
Hot stuff bias	When a topic is hot, authors and editors cannot resist publishing weak or preliminary results.
Specifying/Selecting Study Sample	
Referral center bias	Patients from secondary/tertiary care centers are not representative of all patients with the disease (i.e., are more severely affected, have rare clinical features, etc.).
Diagnostic suspicion bias	A physician's knowledge of a subject's prior exposure to a putative cause increases the likelihood of assigning a given diagnosis (e.g., aspirin exposure and Reye's syndrome).
Unmasking (detection) bias	An exposure may enhance a physician's ability to detect a disease early (or to falsely ascribe a diagnosis) because it causes a sign or symptom that precipitates a search for the disease.
Wrong sample size bias	Samples that are too small can prove nothing; samples that are too large can prove anything.
Admission rate (Berkson) bias	In hospital-based case–control studies, the association between exposure and disease will be distorted when hospitalization rates differ for different exposure or disease groups (e.g., positive association between smoking and hemorrhagic stroke will be underestimated when using "controls" from hospital setting who have a higher than normal smoking prevalence).
Prevalence-incidence bias	In case–control studies, the use of "prevalent" cases will result in those with short disease duration being underrepresented and those with longstanding disease being overrepresented, making it difficult to determine whether an associated risk factor has etiologic versus prognostic importance.
Diagnostic purity bias	When "pure" diagnostic groups exclude patients with comorbid conditions, the group may be nonrepresentative of all patients with the diagnosis.
Volunteer bias	Volunteer research subjects, or those that are "early comers" to a research project, may differ from non-volunteers or "late comers" (i.e., may be healthier).
Migration bias	Subjects who migrate from a region may differ systematically from non-migrators.
Membership bias	Members of certain groups (i.e., employed workers, alternative medicine clinics) may be healthier or otherwise differ systematically from all subjects with a given diagnosis.
Nonrespondent bias	"Nonrespondents" who refuse participation in a given study may have exposures or neurologic outcomes that differ from subjects who choose to participate in the study.
Administering Treatment	
Contamination or crossover bias	In a randomized trial, members of the placebo group inadvertently receive or seek active treatment; or members of the treated group(s) inadvertently receive placebo or "cross over" into the other treatment group.
Withdrawal (dropout) bias	Patients who drop out or are withdrawn from a randomized trial may differ systematically with respect to treatment outcome or adverse effects from patients who remain in the treatment (or placebo) group.

(cont.)

Appendix 2–1 Catalog of Biases in Analytic Studies *Continued*

Stage of research/name of bias	Description of bias
Administering Treatment	
Compliance bias	In a randomized trial, inadequate compliance to treatment regimen influences the efficacy or effectiveness of the treatment.
Unblinded observer bias	When an investigator is not blinded to treatment assignment, investigator convictions about a given treatment may systematically influence measurement of treatment outcomes.
Measuring Exposures, Outcomes	
Insensitive measure bias	Outcome measures are incapable of detecting clinically significant changes or differences.
Missing clinical data bias	Data on risk factors, clinical features, or diagnostic tests that are missing from medical records may be missing because they have never been assessed, are normal (or absent), or were assessed/performed but never recorded in the medical record.
Recall bias	In a case–control study, cases may ruminate about possible causes for their illness and thus exhibit better or different recall of prior exposures.
Apprehension bias	Certain physiological measures, such as blood pressure or pulse rate, may differ from the usual value because the subject is apprehensive.
Unacceptability bias	Measurements or questions that hurt, embarrass, or invade a subject's privacy may be systematically refused or evaded.
Obsequiousness bias	Subjects may alter questionnaire responses in a direction they perceive as desired responses.
Exposure suspicion bias	Knowledge of a subject's disease status on the part of the investigator or interviewer may influence the intensity or outcome of a search for exposure to a putative cause or risk factor.
Hawthorne effect revisited	Study subjects may systematically alter their behavior or their responses when they know they are being observed.
Interviewer bias	Study interviewers may be biased or persist in eliciting certain answers from subjects when they believe they know the underlying cause(s) of a disease.
Instrument bias	Defects in measuring instruments or improper calibration may lead to measurements that systematically deviate from the true values.
Data Analysis and Interpretation	
Data dredging biases	When data are reviewed and analyzed for all possible associations or subgroup effects without a priori hypotheses, results are suitable for "hypothesis-generating" purposes only.
Tidying-up biases	Exclusion of data "outliers" or other inexplicable results that are not justified on statistical grounds may lead to biased study conclusions.
"Repeated looks" bias	In a randomized trial, repeated analyses of data as they accumulate are not independent tests and may lead to inappropriate conclusions about treatment efficacy or termination of trial.
Cognitive dissonance bias	An investigator's belief in a given treatment, disease mechanism, or risk factor association may increase rather than decrease in the face of contradictory evidence.
Correlation bias	The investigator may equate correlation with causation (see Causal Reasoning).
Significance bias	The confusion of statistical significance with biological or clinical significance may cause an inappropriate conclusion of an important effect (for very large studies with minimal biological or clinical effects), or may discourage future studies (when a statistically underpowered study with inadequate sample size fails to demonstrate an association that does exist).

Adapted with permission from Sackett DL. Bias in analytic research. *J Chron Dis* 1979;32:51–63.

3

Measurement and Analysis

STEPHEN K. VAN DEN EEDEN, BEATE RITZ, AND KRISTIN COBB

The success of a neuroepidemiologic study is defined by how close the estimate of association between a risk, preventive, or prognostic factor and an outcome gets to the true association. While the discovery of complete "truth" is never possible, careful attention to validity of the study design, accuracy in the measurement of the factors under study, and validity of the outcome definition will greatly enhance the ability of the researcher (and his or her readers) to interpret the results of a research study. This chapter focuses on measurement (and mismeasurement) of exposures, risk factors, prognostic factors, and intermediate and confounding variables, as well as statistical analysis. The reader is referred to Chapters 16, 17, and 18, which cover prognosis, clinical trials, and health services research, for more detailed discussions of prognostic, treatment and health delivery predictors, and outcome measures for these fields.

Outcome Measures in Neuroepidemiology Studies

In all neuroepidemiologic research the outcome to be studied must be carefully defined and precisely measured. Laboratory or other definitive testing is not available to confirm diagnoses for many neurological disorders, making accurate disease classification difficult in neurologic studies. Disease status as an outcome measure is discussed in detail elsewhere (Chapters 2 and 4–15). Outcomes in prognostic and other studies include disease severity, functional status, and general health measures. These will be discussed in more detail in this chapter.

Appropriate Outcome Measures

The direct measurement of health is impossible since health is an abstract concept that often means different things to different people. Patients may assess health differently than their providers, for example, and perceptions of health may vary from patient to patient and from provider to provider. Thus health or disease must be measured with a variety of scales. Such measures include pathological ratings of the state of disease, such as the stage and grade of a glioma; quantitative measures, such as nerve conduction velocities in diabetic neuropathy or limb strength in multiple sclerosis; and measures of the impact of disease on functional status and quality of life, such as the quality of life scales used to assess headache-related disability. Table 3–1 shows a variety of study types and outcome measures.

> *Example 3–1* Duncan et al. (2000) reviewed all published randomized trials of drug intervention in stroke ($n = 51$) and found a range of end points: impairment in 42 studies, activity level in 39 studies, death in 34 studies, and pathophysiological measures in 9. Outcome measures included 14 different measures of impairment (including 8 different stroke scales), 11 measures of activity, 1 quality of life instrument, and 8 other miscellaneous instruments. Patients were followed from 1 week to 1 year before outcomes were measured. These authors recommended that considerable effort be given to standardizing the use of various instruments, outcomes, and follow-up times to improve study comparability.

The choice of an appropriate outcome measure is driven by the research question under study. Questions about prognosis demand the use of outcomes such as changes in disease severity, changes in quality of life (such as changes in mobility aid dependence or in activities of daily living), or death. Studies of the course of chronic progressive diseases may have outcomes such as the rate of clinical decline over time, whereas studies of exacerbating-remitting disease courses may have outcomes such as "attack frequency" or "exacerbation rate."

Disease Severity Measures

A sound measure of disease severity is critical to many studies. Obvious examples

would be clinical trials of therapeutic agents that may seek to identify how the agent arrests disease progression or even halts the disease process. For example, evaluating how well neuroprotective agents improve the course of Alzheimer's disease or Parkinson's disease requires accurate measures of the severity of these diseases. Disease severity can also be an important confounding factor in treatment studies where mortality is the outcome if the randomized groups are not comparable with respect to disease severity at the onset of the study.

For most diseases or conditions there are one or more instruments used to measure disease severity. In choosing an instrument to use for disease severity, the researcher needs to know the original purpose for which the instrument was designed. In many cases, an instrument's use has been historical and while used currently, it may be viewed as inadequate or in need of updating.

> *Example 3–2* The two most common disease severity measures for Parkinson's disease (PD) are the United Parkinson's Disease Rating Scale and the Hoehn and Yahr scale. While there is now clear recognition of sleep disturbance problems in many patients with PD, neither of these scales included a sleep assessment item. There are suggestions to modify one or both of these instruments to include a component of sleep to better capture the range of impact of PD (Askenasy 2001).

It needs to be kept in mind that not all aspects of a 'validated' scale perform the same way. Measurement of objective parameters tend to be better replicated than parameters that are based on subjective observational data. Similarly, measures that have a clinical anchor are better replicated by a single observer than across observers.

> *Example 3–3* The Unified Parkinson's Disease Rating Scale motor examination is used to rate motor signs in persons with Parkinson's disease. Interrater reliability studies have found that those items with clear anchor points for each possible score

Table 3-1 Overview of Outcome Measures by Study Goal

Study Goal	Outcomes among persons with disease	OUTCOME MEASURE						
		Disease onset as outcome	Disease cure as outcome	Severity of disease, disease features	Mortality outcomes	Quality of life measures	General health status measures	Functional status measures	Utilization and/or cost measures
Disease distribution	X	X			X				
Disease etiology		X			X				
Disease prevention	X	X	X	X	X				X
Disease prognosis			X	X	X	X	X	X	
Health services			X	X	X	X	X	X	X
Disease treatment			X	X	X	X	X	X	X

such as gait and arising from a chair have the highest agreement. Items with no clear clinical anchor point for scoring such as speech disorder and facial immobility have poor agreement.

Disease severity can be defined in a number of aspects or domains—for example, pathologic markers of disease stage, clinical signs or symptoms, and behavioral measures. Caution is indicated when interpreting the results of clinical trials with outcomes that measure only progression of symptoms or signs. A statistically significant improvement on a scale does not necessarily reflect meaningful clinical improvement. Measures of impairment or functional disability, and quality of life, while more conceptually abstract, may provide better information regarding how a disease affects a patient.

Since no outcome measure is perfect, multiple outcome measures are commonly used in clinical trials. Multiple measures are especially useful for assessing progression of disorders that affect more than a single domain of neurological function.

Example 3–4 Huntington's disease is characterized by the slow onset and gradual progression of dementia and chorea. There is presently no treatment available that can alter progression of this disease. In a trial designed to test the ability of two agents to slow progression of Huntington's disease, coenzyme Q10 and remacemide, the primary outcome measure was the total functional capacity scale (Huntington Study Group 2001). This measure assesses work ability, financial management, household chore performance, and self-care capacity, as well as independent living potential. Additional secondary outcomes included the Unified Huntington's Disease Rating Scale (Huntington Study Group, 1996), which measures functional capacity, motor function, and behavior/cognition, and other measures of cognition including the Stroop test (Jensen and Rohwer 1966) and the Hopkins Verbal Learning Test (Huntington Study Group 2001).

It is beyond the scope of this chapter to go into great detail on each disease severity measure for each condition. For the pathologic and clinical instruments of disease severity, a review of the literature on clinical trials and clinical epidemiological studies usually will provide a quick introduction to the range of instruments available for a specific disease.

General Health and Quality of Life Measures

Although general health measures are not the focus of most neuroepidemiologic studies, they may serve several secondary purposes. These measures are often inappropriate for the assessment of subtle improvements or decrements in disease status in impaired individuals since they will quickly reach the top or bottom of these scales. In addition, some scales meant for some other purpose may inappropriately record nonexistent symptoms. For example, a general depression scale may misinterpret the masked facies often found in Parkinson's disease as depression. Widely used general instruments, such as the Medical Outcome Study's (MOS) short form SF-12 or SF-36, for which population norms are available, can serve as a yardstick for how the study population compares to a general population. In fact, many studies include both a disease-specific quality of life instrument as well as a general health measure. These can be used to see if health status changes are both disease-specific and encompass broader concepts of health. One measure of well-being is how the patient is impacted by a disease.

Quality of life measurements have improved greatly during the last two decades. Several good sources of information for quality of life instruments exist, including *Compendium of Quality of Life Instruments, Vol. 1–5* (Salek 1998), *Quality of Life Assessment in Clinical Trials. Methods and Practice* (Staquet et al. 1998), *Measuring Disease: A Review of Disease-Specific Quality of Life Measurement Scales* (Bowling 2001), and online at http://www.qolid. org. Two other texts, *Measuring Health. A*

Guide to Rating Scales and Questionnaires (McDowell and Newell 1996) and *Health Measurement Scales. A Practical Guide to Their Development and Use* (Streiner and Norman 1995), include detailed information on a range of disease-specific and general health measures. They also provide guidance on how to develop one's own instruments and how to use existing instruments.

Functional Status Measures

In some prognostic studies or clinical trials, functional status may be more important than a pathological or clinical measure of disease severity. These types of measures are likely to be particularly important for conditions that affect mobility and cognition. Some of the better-known functional status measures are presented in Table 3–2. Many other measures are described in the texts cited in the preceding paragraph.

Measuring Risk Factors and Predictors of Disease Outcome

General Issues in Choice of Exposures and Risk Factors

Exposures and risk factors are chosen for study on the basis of scientific factors (prior research and biologic plausibility), practical matters (resources available, and degree of difficulty in obtaining the information or biological sample), and the specificity of the information being sought. It is usually not enough to assess exposure as an ever-versus-never variable—for example, whether a participant ever smoked or was ever exposed to a drug or pesticide. Details related to amount or dose of exposure and to the timing of exposure are critical to properly investigating these types of associations. Thus, to the extent feasible, details such as age at first exposure, termination of exposure, and dose should be measured. For intermittent exposures such as occupational or home exposure to pesticides, or anti-inflammatory medications used for symptom relief, a complete history should be ascertained that includes information on frequency of use and dose for each episode of exposure. For some exposures, such as occupational exposures, the precise dose is rarely known. In such cases, proxy measures such as proximity to an exposure, use of protective equipment, or other such factors are often used to create categories that can be ordered from high to low exposure. A detailed discussion of these issues can be found in a number of resource books, such as *Principles of Exposure Measurement* (Armstrong et al. 1994), *Research Methods in Occupational Epidemiology* (Checkoway et al. 1989), and *Nutritional Epidemiology* (Willett 1998).

Assessment and Uncertainties of Disease Onset

For some conditions, such as traumatic brain injury, the timing of onset is evident.

Table 3–2 Commonly Used Functional Status Instruments

Name of instrument	Areas covered
Index of Independence in Activities of Daily Living (ADL) (Katz and Akpom 1976)	6 questions rated by staff
Barthel Index (Collin et al. 1988)	10 or 15 questions on activities in the house and personal hygiene tasks rated by self or staff
The Physical Self-Maintenance Scale (Lawton and Brody 1969)	31 questions in 8 activities of daily living rated by self or staff
Stanford Health Assessment Questionnaire (Wolfe et al. 1988)	24 questions on daily functioning rated by self or staff
A Rapid Disability Rating Scale (Linn 1967)	8- or 18-item questionnaire on daily activities or functions rated by staff
Functional Independence Measure (Stineman et al. 1996)	18-item questionnaire on physical and functional status rated by staff

In other neurologic conditions, however, the disease process may have preceded the event. As an example, a patient may have been having transient ischemic attacks for years before a stroke manifests itself. For some studies it would be important to consider such issues. For many neurologic conditions, there is no clear onset date.

> *Example 3–5* Amyotrophic lateral sclerosis (ALS, or Lou Gehrig's disease) results from the loss of motor neurons over time, but patients don't show clinical signs of disease until about 50% or more neurons are lost (McGeer and McGeer 2002). In diseases with insidious onset such as ALS, the disease was clearly present, albeit in an occult form, prior to diagnosis. Thus, in studying such conditions, defining exposure periods of greatest relevance becomes extremely important, and the investigator may need to exclude periods close in time to the diagnosis from etiologic consideration.

Data Collection Approaches

Data for research may come from many sources and may include existing or newly collected data. Medical records are a potentially rich source of data that may have advantages over data obtained from participants themselves; for example, the patient may have difficulty in recalling events or the data may be technical in nature and may never have been routinely available to the participant. In many cases, however, individuals themselves are likely to be the best source of data—for example, for lifestyle or quality of life factors.

For virtually all studies, the more standardized or structured the data collection process or instrument is, the more uniform data collection will be. Even for studies that rely on medical records, a source frought with the vagaries of what data are recorded, a structured instrument is highly desirable. It is similarly important that structured instruments and administration procedures be used when directly collecting data from the subject through the use of questionnaires. In all cases, it is important to pilot test the instruments to ensure that they are understandable. Whenever possible, it is of great value to validate a questionnaire, or to at least assess its reliability in the context of the study that is underway.

Questionnaires

Questionnaires are frequently used in all types of studies and may be self-administered or administered by an interviewer or research nurse involved in the study. Questionnaires generally are used when the data sought can only reliably, or more completely be obtained from the respondents themselves. Examples of this kind of data include residential history, long-term use of nonsteroidal anti-inflammatory (NSAID) medications, occupational history, lifestyle factors (e.g., smoking, diet, physical activity), compliance to various treatments, and quality of life or disease impact responses. In some cases, the resources to directly obtain data from other sources (i.e., employment records) are not available and a questionnaire format may be used. Decisions regarding the selection or design of questions are often related to practical concerns such as resources, time, and complexity. In general, the more complex the questionnaire, the more critical it is to have a professional interviewer administer the questionnaire. An interview may be administered in person or over the telephone. Table 3–3 provides some advantages and disadvantages to each approach.

Since most areas of inquiry are not new, it behooves the researcher to find and use standardized questionnaires or portions of questionnaires. Increasingly, there is a move to develop and use modules of questionnaires. For example, the National Cancer Institute (see http://dceg.cancer.gov/QMOD/) has sought to develop standardized questionnaires that can be used in epidemiologic studies. Table 3–4 shows some national surveys for which questionnaires are available on the Web at the National Center for Health Statistics (NCHS) of the Centers for Disease Control and Prevention (CDC).

Table 3–3 Strengths and Limitations of Various Methods of Administering Questionnaires

Type	Cost	Potential biases	Response rate	Complexity/time to complete	Control and ability for prompting
Mailed (self-administered) questionnaire	Less expensive	Response bias Respondent may be helped by others Respondent needs to read and write	Lowest response	Low to high, moderate is best	Low
Telephone interview	Moderately expensive	Interviewer	Moderate to high response	Low to moderate (getting more difficult)	High
In-person interview	Most expensive	Interviewer	Moderate to high response	Low to high	High

Table 3–4 National Surveys with Available Questionnaires

Survey	Source	Types of questions
Behaviorial Risk Factor Surveillance Survey (BRFSS)	CDC	Health behaviors
National Health and Nutrition Examination Survey (NHANES)	CDC	Health behaviors and nutrition
National Health Interview Survey (NHIS)	CDC	Health assessment and functional status
National Survey of Family Growth (NSFG)	CDC	Family composition and size, family planning services and choices, prenatal care
Longitudinal Study of Aging	CDC/NIA	Aging, health, activity, functional status, living arrangements
National Health Care Survey (NHCS)	CDC	Survey of health-care providers

CDC, Centers for Disease Control and Prevention; NIA, National Institute of Aging

The use of such questionnaires facilitates the direct comparison of results across studies and the pooling of data across studies.

Direct Observation and Biological Measures

Researchers may directly observe their subjects to obtain data, such as in behavioral studies. Other forms of direct observation include various assessments of functional status or disease severity (for example, the quality or level of movement in Parkinson's disease that would be used in the Unified Parkinson's Disease Rating Scale). Physiological measures such as blood pressure, blood flow, bone lead levels, and nerve conduction velocities may be used as predictors of disease onset or progression. Tissue for biological measures may be derived from blood samples (e.g., serum proteins, DNA, antibodies to infectious agents), affected tissue (e.g., tumor, brains of Alzheimer's disease patients), or even toenails (e.g., repository for trace metals). Biologically derived data are often critical in all types (e.g., etiologic, progression, mortality, etc) of studies and the importance of these data is increasing. The temporal pattern of exposure and outcome is an important consideration in interpreting biological data. For example, it is not informative to have postdiagnostic blood pressure to use as a predictor of stroke. However, since somatic DNA essentially does not change, obtaining and analyzing susceptibility genes from DNA ob-

tained after diagnosis would not affect the results.

Quality Control Issues in the Conduct of Clinical and Epidemiologic Studies

Effective research technicians appreciate the critical importance of standardizing procedures. Technicians should perform the study procedures identically and consistently to minimize variation in participant measurements. This is especially important for multicenter studies, as staff may be under different supervision.

Strict attention to standardization can be difficult for research staff members who are from a patient-care setting, as they may be accustomed to tailoring patient management to the specific medical problems of each patient. The use of a script for all data collection can help to ensure standardization.

Instructional videotapes and standard operating procedure manuals can help train research staff to perform specific procedures for the study. Newly trained staff should practice the procedures on non-study volunteers to develop their skills. The training should include observation and immediate feedback by more experienced staff. Staff members may also be required to acquire formal certification by passing a written or performance examination. Retraining and recertification at regular intervals are critical to prevent drift in procedure techniques over time.

Types of Measures

Data may be collected as categorical (qualitative) or continuous (quantitative) variables. Categorical variables have a countable number of possible values, e.g., ethnicity or sex. When a categorical variable has only two possible values, e.g., male or female, it is referred to as a binary, or dichotomous, variable. Errors in the measurement of binary variables are called *classification errors,* or *misclassification.* When the values of a categorical variable have a meaningful order, such as mild, moderate, and severe head trauma or number of cigarettes smoked per day, they are called *ordinal variables.* Ordinal variables confer more information than simple (nominal or nonordered) categories, but assessing the effects of potential measurement errors for ordered categories is more difficult than for binary variables. The most information is conveyed by a quantitative or continuous measure, such as blood lipid content or blood pressure, for which the number of possible values is only limited by the sensitivity of our measurement instruments. Such measures have a rational interval to them that has meaning, for example, a systolic blood pressure of 150 mmHg is 50% higher than one of 100 mmHg. Continuous measures allow the use of the most powerful statistics (such as regression analysis), but for practical or clinical purposes these variables are often reduced to categories for the analysis; for example, high blood pressure may be defined as a diastolic pressure above 90 mmHg, or a cut point of <24 in Mini-Mental State Examination scores may be used to screen for a clinical diagnosis of Alzheimer's disease (Salmon et al. 2002).

Measurement Error

Every observational epidemiologic study (case–control or cohort) must identify study subjects (diseased cases and nondiseased controls) and obtain and compare relevant information pertaining to all subjects. Etiological cohort studies usually start with a large group of (nondiseased) people. For a prognostic study, the cohort is usually a group of patients with the disease of interest, ideally identified and followed from diagnosis. During the follow-up period, some of them will be diagnosed with the disease of interest or the prognostic end point of interest (e.g., advanced disease, mortality). All risk or prognostic factor information is assembled prior to disease diagnosis or end point. For case–control studies, one seeks to identify from a defined population all cases and a sample of nondiseased (matched or randomly selected) controls at the time of case identification. Then information about prior exposures and risk factors is extracted from interviews or records for both cases and controls. Measurement error can occur when exposure or predictive factors are incorrectly measured or disease status is misclassified. Measurement error can have a dramatic effect on study results.

As highlighted in Chapter 2, it is extremely important that the investigator strive for the highest measurement quality for the risk (exposure) factor or health predictor and the neurologic condition under study. The ability to demonstrate a true association between a risk factor and a disease (assuming one exists) can be substantially impaired if either of these factors is poorly measured. In the following section, we will concentrate on the influence that measurement quality of the health predictors or risk factors has on the success of a study.

Types of Measurement Error

In neuroepidemiologic observational studies, two types of measurement error can lead to a reduction of statistical power and/or to distorted estimates of effect: random error and systematic error. Random error reduces study precision, whereas systematic error reduces study validity.

Random Error

Random error is influenced by study size and determines statistical power. In principle, random error could be reduced to zero if one could take an infinite number of measurements. For example, when weighing a postmortem brain on a scale, one may get different readings (either too high or too low) depending on who is performing the task and when and how the scale is read. Averaging these randomly different estimates of weight for the same brain tends to give a weight that is not too high or too low; when repeated indefinitely, the average weight will approach the true weight.

Systematic Error (Bias)

Accuracy is the degree to which a measurement actually represents what it intends to represent. Accuracy is affected by systematic errors of measurement, such as those stemming from a miscalibrated instrument that systematically over- or underrecords. For example, if a scale used to weigh postmortem brains is tipped so that it systematically adds weight, all brains will appear heavier. Systematic error is also called *bias,* and increasing the sample size or the number of measurements cannot offset bias; that is, the scale will overreport the weight of all brains systematically until we calibrate it. Note that if the goal of a study is to compare the difference of brain weights from patients and normal subjects, such a biased scale will still give a valid measure of the difference between the groups, as long as the same biased scale is used to weigh all brains. Systematic error is also known as *information bias* in epidemiologic studies, because it most often arises when information collected about or from a subject is inaccurate or erroneous. Certain patients may systematically over- or underreport certain exposures, depending on other factors such as disease severity, age, sex, and time since last use or exposure.

Misclassification of Exposure

Misclassification is a type of measurement error that occurs when a subject is placed into the wrong category of a categorical exposure; for example, a heavy drinker might be misclassified as a non- or moderate drinker. The concept of misclassification, however, also extends to measurements taken on a continuous scale. In epidemiologic research, it is important to evaluate whether exposure misclassification occurs differentially or nondifferentially with respect to an outcome of interest. Exposure misclassification is called *differential* when it is influenced by disease status and *nondifferential* when it is independent of disease status.

Differential Misclassification. Differential information bias is especially a concern in studies collecting exposure information retrospectively (case–control studies); it is also known as *recall bias* (for further discussion of recall bias, see below). Consider a case–control study of head trauma and epilepsy. Cases may have more actively searched their past to identify potential causes for their disease and thus may be more likely to remember or identify all events they suspect to be causally related to their disease. Nondiseased subjects may not have had any reason to search their past and thus will be less likely to recollect such events and are more likely to underreport them. This type of misclassification can affect prognostic studies as well.

Nondifferential Misclassification. Misclassification is nondifferential when there is little reason to believe that the measurement error differs systematically for patients and control subjects. For example, if we could access medical records of a health maintenance organization (HMO) for periods prior to the diagnosis of epilepsy and determine whether and when head traumata occurred in patients and non-patient controls, we would not expect to encounter differential exposure misclassification bias. This is because there is no a priori reason to believe that these traumata would be recorded differentially for HMO enrollees according to whether they are diagnosed with the disease of interest (Parkinson's or epilepsy) at a later time. Even if we suspect that these files only record severe head traumata leading to hospitalization or medical treatment at the HMO and tend to underreport less severe head traumata or those treated elsewhere, the underreporting error would be expected to be the same for epilepsy patients and non-patients and thus be considered nondifferential.

The more pervasive type of measurement error in observational studies is nondifferential misclassification, which mostly leads to a dilution of the effect estimates—i.e., an odds (OR) or risk ratio (RR) is closer to its null value of 1.0 or a correlation coefficient approaches its null value of zero even when a true association exists. Specifically, in the case of a dichotomous exposure, nondifferential misclassification is likely to bias measures of association towards the null or no difference value (e.g., OR = 1 or RR = 1), obscuring real differences (Kleinbaum et al., 1982). More generally, nondifferential exposure misclassification biases effect estimates towards the null when measurement errors for exposure and for disease are conditionally independent of each other, or "uncorrelated." Assuming that misclassification is nondifferential and no error occurred in disease measurement, misclassifying only 10% of the exposed subjects as unexposed and vice versa can reduce a true odds ratio from 3.00 to an observed odds ratio of 2.20 (Salmon et al. 2002).

Measurement errors for exposure and disease are more likely to be correlated if both the information concerning disease and the information concerning exposure status have been derived from the same sources, e.g., if both were obtained in interviews or abstracted from medical records. If disease and exposure information has been obtained from the same source, measurement accuracy of exposure and disease might be influenced by the same psychological, cultural, or social attributes of the participant or the data collector, or the specific circumstances surrounding data collection and can result in a seriously biased result. Thus, it is critical that the investigator invest time and effort in avoiding this situation.

Example 3–6 Benedetti et al. (2001) used the medical records–linkage system of the Rochester Epidemiology Project to identify incident cases of Parkinson's disease (PD) in Olmsted County, Minnesota. Between 1976 and 1995, they identified 72 women who developed PD and matched each incident case by age to a general population control subject without PD at the time of diagnosis of the case. The researchers collected exposure data concerning hysterectomy, early menopause, and estrogen replacement therapy through a review of the complete medical records of cases and control subjects in the system. The cases were identified and the risk factor information was collected from the same medical records system over a 20-year period. Thus, some information may have been subject to correlated recording errors—for example, errors may have been correlated for variables such as age at menopause, smoking behavior, length of hormone replacement therapy, and time of first diagnosis of PD, all of which may be similarly influenced by social status attributes of the woman or attitudes of the recording medical personnel.

If separate sources of information are not available to determine exposure and outcome status, it has been recommended that investigators (1) conduct quantitative sensitivity analyses in which observed results are corrected for a range of plausible misclassification scenarios, taking potential correlation of classification errors into account, or (2) identify shared determinants of measurement accuracy for both exposure and outcome and control for these in the analysis (Brenner et al. 1993).

Impact of nondifferential exposure misclassification. The impact of misclassification is quantified by the specificity (the probability of a false negative) and sensitivity (the probability of a false positive) of exposure assessment; if both sensitivity and specificity are 100%, there is no misclassification. In case–control studies, exposure misclassification will bias the odds ratio a smaller amount, in general, when the specificity of exposure classification is high (i.e., above 90%–95%) even if the exposure sensitivity is quite low (as low as 60%). When specificity drops to about 50%, even perfect sensitivity does not prevent the odds ratio from dropping from 3.00 to 1.59, while perfect specificity but low sensitivity (about 50%) results in much less strong bias of the odds ratio (the odds ratio drops from 3.00 to 2.53).

Furthermore, the size of the bias of an effect estimate such as an odds or risk ratio depends strongly on the prevalence of exposure. If the exposure prevalence is low in the general population (less than 10%), sensitivity operates only on a small exposed proportion of the population, while specificity operates on a much larger unexposed part of the population. In case–controls studies, bias increases dramatically with decreasing specificity of exposure classification because cases are by definition rare events in the population from which they arise.

Example 3–7 We are currently conducting a study of PD and residential exposures to pesticides in Central California (Rull and Ritz, 2003). We recently investigated the potential for exposure misclassification when comparing California pesticide use report data alone with a more detailed exposures assessment based on a combination of pesticide and agricultural land use data (gold standard). We classified a home as exposed, for example, when the common pesticide para-quat was applied within a 500 m buffer. We observed almost 100% specificity but only about 35% sensitivity using paraquat pesticide data alone; the exposure prevalence (application within 500 m of homes) in a random sample of residential parcels was found to be 11%. Under these conditions a hypothetical true odds ratio of 2 for paraquat exposure and PD would be reduced by 25% to 1.75 using the less detailed exposure assessment method. However, for a pesticide used much more rarely such as maneb (exposure prevalence in a random sample of residential parcels was only 0.9%), a hypothetical

true odds ratio would be reduced by 55% from 2 to 1.45 when using the less detailed pesticide application information.

Impact of differential misclassification. While under the assumptions described above we can expect nondifferential misclassification to bias results towards the null, the direction of the bias resulting from differential misclassification is not easily predictable. Thus, researchers are generally more concerned about this kind of measurement error. Differential misclassification can bias results either towards or away from the null, either underestimating or exaggerating an effect. As stated previously, one goal of exposure assessment in epidemiology is to provide a valid estimate of effect such as an odds ratio or relative risk. In many diseases, timing of exposure may be essential and the most relevant window of exposure in chronic diseases with long latency may lie in the past. Thus, in many cases the only measurements possible are those retrospectively obtained via questionnaires or interviews; exceptions are when historical exposure samples or records exist (such as the serum obtained and stored for the women in Example 3–8 before they developed multiple sclerosis).

Example 3–8 A recent nested case–control study linked increased Epstein-Barr virus antigen in the serum to risk of developing late-onset multiple sclerosis in women. Interestingly, the effect estimate was much stronger when blood was obtained prior to rather than after diagnosis: fourfold differences in titers were found to be associated with a relative risk of multiple sclerosis of 3.9 (95% CI 1.1–13.7) when blood was obtained 2 months to 6 years prior to diagnosis, compared to a relative risk of only 1.6 (95% CI 1.2–2.1) when blood was collected and tested after onset of disease (Ascherio et al., 2001). The authors also suggested that age at primary infection with the virus might contribute to increased risk.

Differential misclassification bias has been of particular concern in interview-based case–control studies, since cases with the disease may ruminate about prior exposure and report it more completely than nondiseased controls—i.e., cases might exaggerate exposure while nondiseased comparison subjects may be less likely to recall even a true exposure. These differences in the accuracy of subject recall are known as *recall-bias*, which is one of the major concerns to the validity of case–control studies that use interviews to retrospectively obtain exposure data; the net effect, if present, is to exaggerate the magnitude of the difference between cases and controls in reported rates of exposure to risk factors under investigation. While in most cases investigators might be concerned that recall bias leads to an inflation of the ratio estimate, differential recall bias can also cause an attenuation of the effect estimate. An example of the latter case is presented in Example 3–9 for proxy respondents (relatives) in situations when cases cannot be interviewed, such as when they are dead or demented (see also Chapter 2 and Walker et al., 1988).

> *Example 3–9* Semchuk and Love (1995) examined how using proxy respondents (spouses, children, or other relatives answer interview questions instead of the study subject) to derive risk factor data from interviews can influence PD risk estimates in a case–control study. They found substantial attenuations of risks for some relatively rare risk factors such as family history of essential tremor (7% exposure prevalence in the control group, which represented the population distribution of exposure) or herbicide use (5% exposure prevalence in the control group), factors for which sensitivity of proxy responses compared to subject responses was as low as 25%–50% but specificity was still quite reasonable at 90%–97%. The odds ratio derived from the gold standard (the study subject's own response) compared to that obtained from a proxy respondent for family history of essential tremor was 2.37 (95% CI 1.20–4.69) vs.

1.37 (95% CI 0.67–2.80) and for herbicide use was 3.06 (95% CI 1.34–7.00) vs. 2.36 (95% CI 1.10–5.04), thus showing a strong reduction of the risk estimates when using proxy respondents. The authors also showed that the odds ratios for a common exposure such as smoking (74% exposure prevalence in the control group), which had a sensitivity of 91%–98% and a specificity of 85%–94%, had only a minor influence on the effect estimates (OR of 0.48, 95% CI 0.29–0.80) when the subjects reported smoking, compared to when a proxy reported smoking (OR of 0.45, 95% CI 0.27–0.75). Thus, with low-exposure prevalence it is a priority to achieve high specificity of exposure assessment, i.e., to reduce the possibility that unexposed subjects are erroneously included in the exposed group.

Differential misclassification of disease. Differential recall does not only impact case–control studies or exposure classification (Neugebauer and Ng, 1990). Rather, differential recall can influence measurement of outcomes as a function of exposure status in cohort studies (leading to detection bias) if disease detection depends on the subject's reports. For example, Hertzman et al. (1987) reported that hazardous waste site workers said they had more health problems after receiving information about the hazards of a landfill. A similar symptom exaggeration might be expected after highly publicized and visible exposure scenarios; for example, one might suspect that exposure to oil fires may trigger Gulf War veterans who witnessed the fires and followed discussions about potential adverse health effects due to toxics from the combustion to report higher rates of neurological symptoms when enrolled in a study. In studies relying on subjective disease and symptom reports, whether recorded in interviews or abstracted from medical charts, exposure status might potentially influence recall and/or recognition and reporting of the outcome of interest and thus produce differential bias leading to a form of detection bias (Neugebauer and Ng, 1990).

Methods to Assess and Improve Measurement Quality

The discussions and examples above show how much effect estimates derived in an epidemiologic study could suffer from lack of precision or accuracy. Thus, methods have been proposed to assess and improve measurement quality or even to correct for measurement error. Table 3–5 displays the interplay between precision and validity with an example of each.

Assessing Reliability

A precise or reliable measurement results in nearly the same value if repeated; thus, precision is also referred to as *reproducibility*. Statistically, precision is evaluated by the standard deviation of repeated measurements or the coefficient of variation—the standard deviation divided by its mean—when several variables are being compared. Precision can also be assessed by examining the consistency of results from paired measurements using a simple correlation coefficient for continuous variables or a kappa coefficient for categorical variables. The kappa coefficient is best known for use in the assessment of agreement (reliability) for two or more independent observers. Kappa calculates agreement between ob-

servers over and above what might be expected by chance alone and thus is also referred to as the *degree of concordance* beyond that due to chance or the *chance-corrected agreement*. For two observers kappa lies in the range −1 to 1. (For more than two observers, the minimum value will tend towards 0.) A kappa coefficient of < 0 indicates agreement worse than chance (i.e., the observers disagree), a coefficient of 0 indicates agreement no better (worse) than chance, and a coefficient of > 0 indicates agreement better than chance (i.e., the observers agree). Armstrong et al. (1994) provide an excellent review of methods for computing reliability measures such as the kappa statistic or the intraclass correlation coefficient.

Improving Reliability

Methods recommended for improvement of reliability or precision are standardizing the measurement methods (through instruction or calibration), training and certifying observers or interviewers, and automating and refining instruments and repetition, i.e., repeating measurements. Determining which of these strategies is most appropriate hinges most likely as much on feasibility and costs as on the re-

Table 3–5 Differences Between Precision and Validity

	Precision (lack of random error)	Validity (accuracy)
Definition	Consistency of measurement; is the value similar when repeatedly measured?	The extent to which the measure represents what is intended.
Assessment	Repeat measurements and compare the values; indefinite repetitions will in principle reduce the error to zero.	Compare the measure to a gold standard (a true reference); if no gold standard is available, use the best possible measure as a reference (alloyed gold standard).
Example	Weigh postmortem brain several times.	Weigh postmortem brains on different scales in different laboratories; once a month, compare measurement obtained from a calibrated scale with those from the scales used in the different labs.
Value	Increased power to detect an effect; lack of precision requires more measurements before an effect becomes evident.	Study conclusions can be questioned when a measure seems to lack validity or no attempt has been made to validate it, i.e., to ensure that it measures what is intended.
Error type	Random error (increased variance)	Systematic error (bias)

Adapted with permission from Hulley SB, Cummings SR. Designing Clinical Research. Baltimore, MD: Williams and Wilkins, 1988.

quired precision or the magnitude of a problem anticipated if precision were limited.

Example 3–10 Sevillano et al. (2002) evaluated an instrument for screening for prevalence of parkinsonism in a door-to-door community survey. A nine-item questionnaire aimed at identifying parkinsonism-related symptoms was administered and collected door-to-door by laypeople, and the process was repeated by specialists at a medical facility before patients underwent neurological examination. Diagnoses were then established and confirmed after a 3-year follow-up. Concordance was found to be ≥64% with kappa ≥0.316 for six questions. The authors also reported that the instrument's sensitivity, determined by different cut-off scores, had a high impact on PD detection, the observed male/female ratio, severity, and the mean age at onset in the community survey.

Assessing Validity

Good precision, or reliability, is necessary but not sufficient to achieve good measurement quality. Even if a variable is measured very reliably, it might not be valid, i.e., measuring what is intended. Returning to postmortem brain weights as an example, an unbalanced scale can be very reliable while never reporting the true weight until calibrated (calibration is one strategy to avoid instrument bias). While precision and accuracy often go hand in hand, validity more often determines the degree to which findings will lead to correct inferences.

Validity can only be assessed against an external gold standard that is known to be more accurate than the measurement being assessed (also called *criterion-related validity,* i.e., different measures of the same variable are compared with each other, such as self-report and spousal report of smoking behavior). *Face validity* is a subjective judgment based on intuitive reasoning that a measure is making sense.

Example 3–11 A study assessed the validity of three parent-rated measures of health-related quality of life (HRQOL) scales for pediatric epilepsy by means of evaluating differences across epilepsy severity groups and correlations between HRQOL scales and neurologic variables (seizure severity, epilepsy duration, current/prior antiepileptic medications) and psychosocial measures (emotional functioning, IQ, social skills, adaptive behavior) (Sherman et al. 2002). The researchers found that the HRQOL measures were moderately to highly intercorrelated and that the scales differed in terms of their associations with criterion measures: for example, the Hague Restrictions in Epilepsy Scale was related to the highest number of neurologic variables and the Impact of Child Neurologic Handicap Scale to the fewest. All three scales were related to psychosocial functioning and to global quality of life. The authors concluded that the three scales are adequate measures of HRQOL for use in intractable childhood epilepsy.

Example 3–12 Barquet et al. (1997) developed a prognostic model to predict significant morbidity or mortality from meningococcal disease, based on clinical findings. In a total of 907 patients with microbiologically proven and diagnosed meningococcal disease, they developed the prognostic model based on those patients diagnosed in 1987–1990, and then used those diagnosed in 1991–1992 to validate the model. In multivariate analyses, independent predictors of death were hemorrhagic diathesis (OR = 101, 95% CI 30–333), focal neurologic signs (OR = 25, 95% CI 7–83), and age 60 years or older (OR = 10, 95% CI 3–34), whereas receipt of adequate antibiotic therapy prior to admission was associated with reduced likelihood of death (OR = 0.09, 95% CI 0.02–0.4). Hemorrhagic diathesis was scored with 2 points, presence of focal neurologic signs with 1 point, age of 60 years or older with 1 point, and preadmission antibiotic therapy was scored as −1. The scores of −1, 0, 1, 2, and 3 or more points were associated with a probability of death of 0%, 2.3%, 27.3%, 73.3%, and 100%, respectively.

Improving Validity

When validity is threatened because study subjects or the observer may change behavior and influence data collection, all measurements should be made as unobtrusive as possible and both observer and subject should be blinded to the true hypothesis of the study (a recommendation that may be impractical or impossible in observational field research).

Assessing and Correcting for Recall Bias

As mentioned above, recall bias is regarded as one of the major threats to the validity of case–control studies that employ interviews to retrospectively obtain exposure data. If previous research is not available to determine sensitivity and specificity of recall and to estimate selection probabilities for the factors under investigation, it is often recommended that validation substudies be used. In a validation substudy, the exposure status (or disease status) of each subject is measured by two methods: first, by the *primary* but error-prone method used for all study subjects; and, second by a *criterion* method that is error-free (gold standard) or at least one much more reliable (alloyed gold standard) than the primary method (Wacholder et al. 1993; Brenner 1996). The validation substudy, thus, provides information on the performance of the best (better) method that then can be used to evaluate and correct the results obtained with the less valid (cruder or less expensive) measure used in a larger study population.

Factors that are important for assessing accuracy of subject recall are (*1*) the time interval that passed since exposure occurred and the degree of detail required to be recalled (less time having passed and less detail required tend to produce more reliable answers); (*2*) personal attributes of the study subjects such as age, educational attainment, and socioeconomic status; (*3*) the significance, duration, frequency, and meaningfulness of the events asked to be recalled; (*4*) social desirability or non-desirability of the reported behavior (illegal drug use); and (*5*) interviewing techniques, design of questionnaires, and the motivation of the respondent (Coughlin 1990).

Some methods have been proposed to determine whether recall bias exists in a given study and, if it does, to correct for it. One method often recommended to reduce recall bias is to select controls not just randomly from the base population, but with certain restrictions, so that the selected control informants have the same motivation to report events and exposures as case informants, e.g., selecting as control subjects patients suffering from types of disease other than the ones under study. However, Pearce and Checkoway (1988) warned that the use of restricted controls might produce selection bias if the exposure under study is related to inclusion in the restricted control group. Furthermore, selecting controls with other conditions does not guarantee elimination of case–control differences in recall.

Drews et al. (1993) showed that even when recall bias exists, the observed association can be closer to the true association when using a population-control series instead of a restricted control group: in a number of situations even relatively large differences in recall accuracy failed to bias the association away from the null value of association. Furthermore, the use of restricted control-series did not eliminate nondifferential misclassification resulting in bias towards the null. The effects of recall bias and nondifferential misclassification may cancel each other out under many circumstances, resulting in relatively little bias in studies relying on population-based controls (Drews and Greenland 1990). In fact, these authors concluded that it is possible that the use of restricted controls creates more bias than it prevents. Since the impact of differential recall depends on a fair number of ancillary parameters (such as sensitivity, specificity, and prevalence of exposure), they recommend that investigators concerned about recall bias evaluate the influence of misclassification and selection bias in their study through sensitivity analysis. Changing classification rates and estimating the impact of such changes on the effect estimates of interest such as the odds or rate ratio is a form of sensitivity analysis. These analyses should be based on parameter values reasonable for a study and can be based on the knowledge or suspicion of the investigator concerning misclassification rates, e.g., under most circumstances it will not be reasonable to assume that 80% or more of all smokers will be misclassified as nonsmokers.

Greenland (1988) argued that it may be more cost-efficient to conduct a smaller study that applies the criterion (best) exposure measure to all subjects than to conduct a validation substudy. He supplied a formula to aid detecting such a situation or to estimate the extent of validation (criterion measurement) that needs to be performed. He also noted that a fully validated design has the added advantage of not needing any of the analytic assumptions required for adjusting all subject exposure estimates according to the validation substudy results.

Raphael (1987) furthermore recommended the construction of a validity scale to estimate the general propensity of a study subject to over- or underreport exposures. This method requires adding to an interview exposures that have been previously evaluated and ruled out as risk factors for the disease under study ("fake" risk factors) but are as plausible to the study subject as putative risk factors of interest. When case respondents positively endorse an excessively large number of items (fake risk factors) in comparison to control respondents, it is likely that the endorsement is due to overreporting-recall bias rather than actual higher rates of exposure. If other plausible factors previously ruled out as disease risk factors do not exist, one could try to construct a validity scale using any type of exposure for which independent records exist, such as medical records of medication use. Discrepancies between respondent reports and validated medical records can be used to estimate the extent to which respondent reports are biased by recall.

Methods for Correcting Study Results for Mismeasured Variables

Many published methods for correcting bias created by misclassification require the use of a gold standard that allows one to classify the true exposure of interest with complete accuracy for all subjects or a representative subgroup, and often they also require that the misclassification be nondifferential (Greenland and Kleinbaum 1983, Walter and Irwig 1988). If a gold standard is available, one can estimate the sensitivity and specificity of the imperfect measure and use these to calculate corrected effect estimates. If misclassification is shown or suspected to be differential, one can apply different correction factors for those diagnosed with the disease and nondiseased control subjects.

Furthermore, if no gold standard is available but a second, potentially imperfect, source of information can be obtained for exposure assessment, it has been shown that one can use both classification schemes in combination to correct effect estimates for bias as long as exposure misclassification is nondifferential (Hui and Walter 1980, Drews et al. 1993). For example, medical charts might be regarded as an "alloyed gold standard" since they do not provide an error-free gold standard for exposure assessment because of random (nondifferential) recording errors. Flanders et al. (1995) extended bias correction methods to situations when exposure misclassification may be differential—e.g., when medical records are suspected to contain recording errors that depend on a physician's perception of a subject's risks for a disease (Neugebauer and Ng 1990). Flanders' approach, however, has large limitations—most importantly it requires a substantial amount of data for the resulting estimates to be stable (more than 500 cases and controls).

Statistical Analysis of Epidemiologic Data

Analyses for Descriptive Aims

Comparing Disease Rates Between Studies.
Disease frequency is described by incidence, prevalence, or mortality; these measures were defined in Chapter 2, therefore, this chapter will focus on how measures can be compared between studies. Incidence and mortality rates may vary across age, gender, race, and time. For example, women have higher rates of multiple sclerosis than men, and dementia occurs more frequently in the elderly. Therefore, incidence and mortality rates may be given as age-specific, gender-specific, race-specific, or calendar period–specific rates, rather than as crude rates. The *age-specific rate* is the rate of disease or death for a particular age group in the population, whereas the *crude rate* is the overall rate in the population.

Standardization. Crude incidence rates may be inappropriate for comparing different populations if there is confounding by age. For example, a population that is older on average than another population will have more incident cases of dementia despite similar rates within age groups.

Incidence and mortality rates are typically reported as age-standardized rates. An *age-standardized rate* is the overall rate that would be expected if a study population had the age structure of a reference population. Rates that are standardized to the same reference (for example, the U.S. population in 2000) can be directly compared. Age-standardized weights are calculated as the weighted average of the age-specific rates from the study population, using as weights the age distribution of the standard population—usually from published data (see Appendix 3–1).

Standardized Mortality Ratios. A ratio is a measure of comparison. *Standardized mortality ratios* (SMRs) compare mortality in a study population to mortality in a reference population. The SMR is calculated by dividing the observed number of deaths in a defined period in the study population by the expected number of deaths (as calculated by standardization to the reference population), multiplied by 100.

$$\text{SMR} = (\text{observed deaths}/\text{expected deaths}) \times 100$$

For example, a researcher might be interested in whether a particular U.S. city has higher or lower age-adjusted death rate from traumatic brain injury than that of the general U.S. population. An SMR close to 100 would indicate that the mortality rate from traumatic brain injury in the city was similar to that in the rest of the country, whereas an SMR >100 would indicate a higher rate in the city, and an SMR <100 would indicate a lower rate in the city.

Statistical Analyses for Analytic Aims in Epidemiology

Hypothesis Testing. Statistical tests evaluate whether observed associations in a study population are likely to be real or are simply due to chance. For example, if a drug-treatment group improves its performance on a test of cognitive function more than a placebo group does, does this reflect a true benefit for the drug or natural fluctuation? A formal statistical test requires the specification of a *null hypothesis*, or a hypothesis of "no effect," such as, the treatment-drug has no effect on cognitive function. If the observed outcome is highly unlikely under the assumption that the null hypothesis is true, the null hypothesis may be rejected.

P-value. A p-*value* is the probability that one would have seen an observation as extreme or more extreme than one did if the null hypothesis was true. Small *p*-values are deemed *statistically significant* and provide evidence for rejecting the null hypothesis. By convention, *p*-values <0.05 are often considered statistically significant. This preset significance level is called the α-*level* or the Type I error.

Epidemiologists and clinicians should be reminded of the limitations of hypothesis testing. Hypothesis testing only gives information about whether an association is likely to exist under the statistical testing paradigm employed. Hypothesis testing should be complemented by estimates of the effect size whenever possible (see parameter estimation discussion below).

Type I and Type II Errors. The *Type I error* is the probability of a false positive, or the probability that an investigator will erroneously reject the null hypothesis when in fact no effect exists. Investigators generally try to keep this error rate low, because concluding that an effect exists when it doesn't may lead to harmful health recommendations and/or policy decisions. On the flip side, if investigators fail to reject a null hypothesis when they should, this is called a *Type II* (or β) *error*. Generally, researchers are willing to accept a higher false-negative rate. Failing to reject the null hypothesis is not the same as concluding that no effect exists; studies may miss effects if they are insufficiently powered.

Multiple Comparisons. In epidemiologic studies, multiple-comparison concerns are evoked when a large number of exposures (e.g., risk factors, candidate genes, prognostic factors) are examined with respect to risk of a given disease or progression. If 100 associations are examined, based on random error one would expect to find 5 of them significant using the standard α level of 0.05. In general, there are two camps regarding this issue. One side takes a strictly statistical approach, stating that adjustments in, say, the *p*-value are needed to ensure protection against a Type I error; an example of this approach is the Bonferroni method. However, some advocate a different approach that does not assign a statistical penalty. Proponents of this approach suggest that the proper course is to conduct careful analyses and place the results in the context of prior research and biological plausibility; namely, if an association is the first one reported in the literature, it is appropriate to note it as such, be cautious and

self-critical, and provide any biological background that would support the finding. If, in fact, the association is to be added to a body of literature of many similar associations, the researcher can interpret it within that context, regardless of whether it was a primary hypothesis or not.

Statistical Power and Sample Size. *Statistical power* is the probability of correctly detecting a real effect; it is the complement of the type II error:

$$Power = 1 - \beta$$

Ensuring sufficient statistical power is an integral part of designing an ethical study, as underpowered studies may waste resources and expose subjects to unnecessary risks. Studies have more power to detect an effect when the effect is large, when the sample size is large, and when the measurement is precise—such that associations are more easily distinguished from chance fluctuations.

Statistical Decision	True State of Null (H_0) Hypothesis	
	H_0 True	H_0 False
Reject H_0	Type I error (α)	Correct
Do not reject H_0	Correct	Type II error (β)

Sample Size Considerations. Sample size is a function of the difference being sought, the variability of measurement, and the levels set for α (the Type I error) and β or power. For a given α and β, the sample size will increase with smaller differences that are expected or decrease with bigger differences with similar variability. With the same differences but high variability, a large sample size would be needed.

Sample size calculations aim to give a study sufficient statistical power to detect a clinically relevant effect. Larger sample sizes are needed to detect smaller effects and when the background variability of the outcome measurement is high. Lowering the α or the preset Type I error level (thereby decreasing the chance of a false positive) will also increase the required sample size.

Statistical versus Clinical Significance. Statistical significance does not necessarily imply clinical significance. A study with a huge sample size may have adequate power to detect very small differences between groups, but these differences may not be clinically meaningful. The magnitude of the effect size should be considered along with the size of the p-value when drawing conclusions. For example, if a 10-subject study shows that a new drug lowers patients' blood pressure by an average of 20 mmHg compared with placebo, the p-value may not be statistically significant, but the drug certainly merits further study. However, if a 10,000-subject study shows that a drug lower blood pressure by 1 mmHg compared with placebo, the p-value will be highly statistically significant, but the drug has no meaningful effect. P-values provide no information about the size of an effect, only about whether or not an effect exists; therefore, when estimating effect, confidence intervals (see below), which give information about both the effect size and whether or not an effect exists, should be reported.

Example 3–13 Kasner et al. (2002) conducted a randomized clinical trial of the effectiveness of acetaminophen on reducing core body temperature in acute stroke. During acute stroke, elevated core body temperature (hyperthermia) may aggravate neuronal injury, whereas hypothermia may protect neurons. Thirty-nine acute stroke patients were randomized to acetaminophen ($n = 20$) or placebo ($n = 19$). Patients treated with acetaminophen were more often hypothermic (14% of the study period) than patients given placebo (5% of the study period), but the difference was not statistically significant, $p = 0.09$. The lack of statistical significance should not be taken as evidence of a lack of benefit for acetaminophen. The odds ratio estimate and associated confidence interval provide more information than the p-value. The odds ratio for hypothermia in acetaminophen versus placebo was 3.4 (95% CI 0.83–14.2). The large confidence intervals indicate the lack of precision in the estimates due to the small sample size. The authors concluded that acetaminophen was unlikely to have a clinical benefit for lowering body temperature, however, the trend seems large enough to warrant further study despite the lack of statistical significance. Indeed, if the same findings had been obtained with a 50% increased sample size (e.g., $n = 30$ acetaminophen patients and $n = 30$ placebo-treated patients), the p-value for the comparison of acetopinophen and placebo (e.g., 14% vs. 5% hypothermic) would have been <0.05.

Epidemiology and neurology, as well as the scientific journals in these two fields, have different perspectives regarding the importance of the p-value in drawing conclusions from statistical analyses. Neurology journals, as well as journals for other clinical specialties, often place an undue amount of emphasis on the importance of the cutoff of "$p < 0.05$" when determining whether a research finding is "significant" or not. This approach can limit the proper interpretation of study findings because many published clinical studies have too few subjects to obtain precise estimates and, as a result, do not have enough statistical power to detect a result as significant at the $p < 0.05$ level. As in Example 3–13 above, it is common practice in neurology journal articles for authors to discount borderline p-values (e.g., p-values between 0.06 and 0.10) as "not statistically significant." Indeed, many researchers believe that it is fruitless to submit a journal article or report a result that is not statistically significant at the $p < 0.05$ level; many valuable findings may be missed when such an approach is used. This perspective is limiting because it does not consider whether the study was statistically underpowered in the first place, or that adding just a few more subjects may have produced a more precise estimate.

Epidemiologists often use an approach that does not place primary importance on the p-value but instead emphasizes the *magnitude* of the association together with an assessment of the *precision* (or conversely, the variability) of the estimate as indicated by the confidence limits. The width of the confidence interval reflects the range of values for the association and is a measure that conveys more information than does the p-value about the variability of the estimation process. While a p-value $p < 0.05$ does indicate that the confidence limits for an odds ratio or relative risk exclude unity, it does not give much information about how broad or narrow the confidence bounds are to assess the effect on sampling variability on the estimate. The reader may observe the greater reliance of epidemiology on reporting confidence limits when reading epidemiology journals, where fewer p-values are reported in favor of reporting confidence bounds. As noted earlier in this chapter, it is important to place one's research in the context of the existing literature. For example, an association with an odds ratio of 3.0 with wide confidence intervals in which that effect estimate is consistent with the existing literature should be judged differently from the same odds ratio and confidence interval when it conflicts with existing studies or is new. For more detail discussion of this and related matters see Gardner and Altman (1986), Feinstein (1998), and Rothman and Greenland (1998).

Parameter Estimation. Often researchers are more interested in estimating a *parameter* rather than calculating a p-value. Parameters of interest include summary statistics such as a population mean or the difference between two means, and measures of association, such as an odds ratio. The researcher calculates a *point estimate* for the parameter, and then must specify a *confidence interval* (CI) around the point estimate. Over many experiments, the 95% confidence interval will fall around the true parameter 95% of the time, giving researchers 95% certainty that they have captured

the true parameter somewhere in their interval. Smaller sample sizes and greater measurement variability decrease the certainty of an observed point estimate, thereby widening the confidence interval. Confidence intervals have duality with hypothesis tests. If a 95% confidence interval contains the null value (0 for a difference of means or 1.0 for an odds ratio or relative risk), then a hypothesis test at the 0.05 significance level would fail to reject the null hypothesis.

Statistical Tests

Table 3–6 displays the appropriate statistical tests for analyzing different types of data. Typically, it is convenient to divide variables into *predictor variables* and *outcome variables* (also known, respectively, as *independent* and *dependent* variables). For clinical trials, this nomenclature makes sense—the treatment determines the outcome. However, it is important to recognize that these terms do not always imply order or causality. For example, statistical tests of association such as the chi-square test and the correlation coefficient treat "predictor" and "outcome" variables equally.

Comparison of Groups

Epidemiologists and clinical researchers often compare groups, such as exposed and unexposed, treatment and control, male and female, or cases and controls. The outcome or characteristic to be compared may be categorical (e.g., recovered/did not recover or has 0, 1, or 2 copies of the ApoE-ϵ4 polymorphism) or continuous (e.g., weight or systolic blood pressure). Categorical variables require a comparison of proportions and continuous variables require a comparison of means.

Comparing Proportions. When both the predictor and outcome variables are categorical, they may be cross-classified in a *contingency table* and compared using a *chi-square test* of independence. A contingency table with R rows and C columns is an R × C contingency table. An example of

Table 3–6 Choice of Appropriate Statistical Test or Measure of Association for Various Types of Data by Study Design

TYPES OF VARIABLES TO BE ANALYZED		
Predictor (independent) variable(s)	Outcome (dependent) variable(s)	Statistical procedure or measure of association
Cross-sectional or Case–Control Studies		
Categorical	Continuous	ANOVA*
Dichotomous	Continuous	t-test*
Continuous	Continuous	Simple linear regression
Multivariate (categorical and continuous)	Continuous	Multiple linear regression
Categorical	Categorical	Chi-square test†
Dichotomous	Dichotomous	Odds ratio, Mantel-Haenszel odds ratio
Multivariate (categorical and continuous)	Dichotomous	Logistic regression
Cohort Studies		
Dichotomous	Dichotomous	Relative risk
Categorical	Time to event	Kaplan-Meier curve or log-rank test
Multivariate (categorical and continuous)	Time to event	Cox-proportional hazards model

*Nonparametric tests are used when the outcome variable is clearly non-Gaussian.

†Fischer's exact test is used when the sample size is very small, such that any observed or expected cells contain less than five subjects.

a hypothetical 2×2 contingency table, with the marginal totals (column and row totals) presented, is as follows:

	male	female	
exposed	20	30	50
unexposed	30	20	50
	50	50	100

If gender and exposure are unrelated—or, in statistical lingo, if they are *independent*—the proportion of males who are exposed should be similar to the proportion of females who are exposed. In the example, 60% (30/50) of females are exposed, compared with 40% (20/50) of males. The chi-square test evaluates whether this difference is real or simply an artifact of chance (see Appendix 3–1).

When comparing more than two groups, a significant chi-square test indicates that at least two groups differ, but does not pin down which groups are different. When the sample size is very small, *Fischer's exact test*

is used as an alternative to the chi-square test.

Comparing Group Means. If the outcome variable to be compared between groups is continuous and reasonably normally distributed (i.e., bell-shaped), the data can be analyzed using a *t-test* (for two groups) or an *analysis of variance (ANOVA) test* (for two or more groups). If the outcome data are clearly non-normal, *nonparametric tests* of comparison should be used.

t-test. A *two-sample t-test* compares means from two samples that are independent. For example, a two-sample *t*-test might be used to compare the average ages or average isometric muscle strengths between a treatment and control group. The *t*-test evaluates whether the means of two groups are statistically different. The *paired t-test* is used when a single group of individuals is compared at two different time points. For example, in a crossover randomized controlled trial, each person serves as his or her own control, i.e., treatment and control are compared within individuals.

Analysis of variance test. The ANOVA is used for testing differences in means across two or more groups. The ANOVA is a generalization of the *t*-test. Statistically, ANOVA compares the variability of the outcome between study groups to the variability within groups. The idea is that, within groups, any fluctuation in outcome reflects random variation, and between-group differences in outcome must surpass this background variability to be considered real. If the variability between groups is much greater than the variability within groups, this suggests that at least two of the groups have different means.

Statistical Methods for Continuous Data

Epidemiologists are often interested in the relationship between two continuous variables, such as weight and blood pressure, or antioxidant intake and free radical concentrations in cerebrospinal fluid. Methods to evaluate *linear* relationships between two variables are discussed here. Recall that a line follows the equation $y = mx + b$, with m denoting the slope and b denoting the y-intercept. If two variables x and y are linearly related, their relationship can be described by this equation; conceptually, this means that as x changes, y changes proportionally.

Correlation Coefficient. The *Pearson's product-moment correlation coefficient (r)* is a measure of the strength of the linear association between two variables. The correlation coefficient takes on a unit-less value between -1 and $+1$, with -1 indicating perfect negative correlation, 0 indicating no correlation, and $+1$ indicating perfect positive correlation.

Squaring the correlation coefficient gives the *coefficient of determination* (R^2), which is useful because it has a straightforward interpretation. The coefficient of determination takes on values from 0 to 1 and is a measure of the proportion of the total variability in the outcome that is explained by a linear relationship with the predictor. For example, if the R^2 value for the relationship between height and weight was 0.50 (or 50%), this would mean that height explained half of the variation in weight, leaving other factors, including chance and diet, to account for the rest of the variation.

Simple Linear Regression. If two variables are correlated and their relationship is known, then having information about one variable yields valuable information about the second. For example, if serum cholesterol level and carotid artery thickness (a risk factor for stroke) are related, then knowing that a person has high cholesterol may help one to better guess one's level of carotid stenosis. Whether used for filling in unknown information or for forecasting future events, this practice is called *prediction*.

The aim of *simple linear regression* is to find the linear equation that best describes the relationship between a predictor variable and an outcome variable (the *best-fit line*). This equation can be used to make quantitative predictions about the outcome. The best-fit line is the line that minimizes the squared differences between the observed and predicted values of an outcome variable. This line may be written as

$$Y = \alpha + \beta x$$

The term α represents the y-intercept, or the expected value of y when x is zero. The coefficient β, which represents slope, is called the *regression coefficient*. A one-unit increase in the independent variable (x) yields a β-unit increase in the dependent variable (Y). Note that β is unit-dependent; for example, a regression coefficient for the relationship between weight and height that is calculated in pounds/foot will be 12 times greater than the same β estimated in pounds/inch.

Evaluating the equation at each level of x gives the expected value of Y at that level.

For example, in the Tromso Study, a prospective follow-up study of cardiovascular disease risk factors in Tromso, Norway, the regression equation predicting millimeters of intima-media carotid thickness (IMT) from serum cholesterol (measured as standard deviations) in men was IMT (mm) = 0.87 + 0.019 (cholesterol) (Stensland-Bugge et al. 2000); this indicates that for every 1 standard deviation increase in cholesterol, the expected increase in IMT for men is 0.019 mm. Note that, unlike the correlation coefficient, which makes no distinction between the variables to be compared, linear regression requires that a dependent variable and independent variable (also called the *predictor variable*) be unambiguously specified.

Multiple Linear Regression. Multiple linear regression is an extension of simple linear regression which allows for multiple predictors in the model.

$$Y = \alpha + \beta_1 x_1 + \beta_2 x_2 + \beta_3 x_3 + \beta_4 x_4 \ldots$$

For example, the multiple linear regression equation for predicting mm IMT in men from the Tromso study included

mm IMT = 0.87 + 0.04 (age) + 0.013 (total cholesterol) + 0.02 (blood pressure) + −0.012 (physical activity low/medium/high) + 0.02 (body mass index) + 0.049 (smoking yes/no)

Each regression coefficient from multiple linear regression can be interpreted as the amount of change in the outcome variable that would be expected per one-unit change of the predictor, if all other variables in the model were held constant. In this way, potential confounders may be accounted for simply by their inclusion in the model. Note that the effect of cholesterol is reduced— the regression coefficient decreases from 0.019 to 0.013—after controlling for factors that may confound the relationship between cholesterol and IMT, such as physical activity and body mass index (BMI).

Two variables that measure the same thing or similar things should not both be included in a multiple regression model, because they in effect cancel each other out; this problem is called *multicollinearity*. For example, once BMI has been included in a model, it would be inappropriate to also include weight.

Linear regression methods require a continuous, reasonably normally distributed independent (outcome) variable, but predictors may be categorical or continuous. Sometimes, mathematical transformations of the data, such as the logarithmic transformation, are needed to meet the assumptions of the linear regression model.

Statistical Analysis of Cohort Studies

Cohort studies follow subjects over time to compare disease occurrence between different exposure groups. Because subjects are selected on exposure status rather than disease status, absolute disease risks can be estimated. Also, because time is taken into account, cohort studies can be used to estimate disease rates and rate ratios and to predict how long a disease or death event will take to occur.

The Relative Risk. If a cohort study is evaluating the association between a single dichotomous exposure and a single dichotomous outcome, the risk (cumulative incidence over the study period) for each exposure group and the ratio of the two risks (relative risk [RR]) can be directly calculated from the 2 × 2 table:

	case	control	
exposed	a	b	$a + b$
unexposed	c	d	$c + d$

$$RR = \frac{a/(a + b)}{c/(c + d)}$$

The 95% confidence interval for the relative risk is

$$95\% \text{ confidence interval} = \left(RR^* \exp\left[-1.96\sqrt{\frac{1 - a/(a + b)}{a} + \frac{1 - c/(c + d)}{c}}\right], \right.$$
$$\left. RR^* \exp\left[-1.96\sqrt{\frac{1 - a/(a + b)}{a} + \frac{1 - c/(c + d)}{c}}\right]\right)$$

For example, suppose a cohort study to examine the relationship between diabetes and subsequent stroke generated the following hypothetical 2 × 2 table:

	stroke	no stroke	
diabetes	8	92	100
no diabetes	4	96	100

The relative risk would be estimated as

$$RR = \frac{8/100}{4/100} = 2.0$$

The 95% confidence interval would be (0.62–6.42). A confidence interval that crosses unity indicates that chance may be an explanation for this observation.

When any of the cells of the 2 × 2 table are small, the estimate of association between exposure and disease is imprecise. For example, if twice as many subjects had developed stroke in the same proportions (perhaps if the subject were followed-up for a longer time period or older subjects were studied), the 2 × 2 table would be

	stroke	no stroke	
diabetes	16	84	100
no diabetes	8	92	100

The relative risk is the same (2.0), but the 95% confidence interval is now narrower: 0.90–4.45.

The relative risk is valid when the amount of follow-up time between the exposed and unexposed groups is comparable. In reality, however, subjects often enter the study at different time points and may be followed for variable amounts of times. If follow-up times vary widely, the *rate ratio*, rather than the relative risk, should be calculated. The rate ratio is the incidence rate for the exposed group divided by the incidence rate for the unexposed group; recall that incidence rates are calculated using total person-years of follow-up rather than total persons followed.

Time-to-event Analysis (Survival Analysis)

Analytic methods that consider time to event as the dependent variable are called *survival analyses* or *time-to-event analyses.*

Kaplan-Meier Curves. The *Kaplan-Meier curve* graphically displays the time period between each death (or disease) event. The horizontal axis represents time and the vertical axis represents a probability between 0% and 100%. The curve is a step-function that starts at a vertical height of 100% and steps down each time a subject *fails*— that is, gets the disease or dies. The height of the curve at a given time point is the probability of surviving beyond that time point. For example, suppose an investigator was tracking stroke incidence in 100 patients with carotid stenosis who were being treated with a new drug. At the start of the study (time = 0), 100% of the subjects would be stroke-free. If the first subject had a stroke at 1 month, the graph would step down to 99/100, or 99%, at 1 month, and the probability of remaining stroke-free beyond 1 month would be estimated at 99%.

Variable follow-up times are easily incorporated into Kaplan-Meier analysis. Subjects that drop out of the study prematurely are said to be *censored*, and they are ignored in the calculation of survival probabilities beyond their censorship. For example, if three subjects from the hypothetical example were lost to follow-up between the beginning of the study and the first death at 1 month, then the survival probability at 1 month would be given as 96/97 rather than 99/100.

Kaplan-Meier curves are excellent for visually comparing the survival of several different exposure groups. For example, a curve for patients with carotid stenosis being treated with a new drug could be compared with a second curve that represented patients with carotid stenosis being treated surgically. The *log-rank test* is a formal statistical test that compares survival curves of different groups. Kaplan-Meier techniques are limited to categorical predictors.

Cox Proportional-Hazards Model. The *Cox proportional hazards model* is a multivariate technique that has time to event as the dependent variable. Similar to multiple linear regression, multiple potential confounders and multiple risk factors, both continuous and categorical, can be included in the model. The coefficients from this model can be used to calculate the adjusted risk ratio.

Statistical Analysis of Case–Control Studies

The statistical analysis of case–control data differs depending on whether subjects were sampled in an unmatched or a matched approach. The following discussion considers techniques for analyzing data from unmatched studies.

Case–control studies test for associations between disease occurrence and risk factors or "exposures." In a case–control study, the numbers of cases and controls are fixed by design, making disease status (yes/no) the predictor variable and exposure status the outcome. Of course, epidemiologists are interested in predicting disease-risk from exposure status, not exposure-risk from disease status. Fortunately, the odds ratio allows an easy swap between these two perspectives.

The Odds Ratio. The odds differs from probability (risk) in that *odds* is the probability of an event happening divided by the probability of it not happening. For example, if the probability of an event occurring is 1 in 3, the odds of it happening are 1 to 2. The odds ratio can be calculated without information about the absolute risk of disease—which is not available from case–control data—making it the preferred measure of association for case–control studies. The *odds ratio* is the ratio of the odds of exposure among cases to the odds of exposure among controls, *which is mathematically equivalent to the ratio of the odds of disease among the exposed to the odds of disease among the unexposed.* The general 2×2 table from a case–control study with a dichotomous exposure is as follows:

	case	control
exposed	a	b
unexposed	c	d

The odds ratio is calculated as

$$OR = \frac{ad}{bc}$$

The 95% confidence interval for the odds ratio is based on the natural log of the odds ratio and is given by

95% confidence interval
$$= \left(OR * \exp\left[-1.96\sqrt{\tfrac{1}{a} + \tfrac{1}{b} + \tfrac{1}{c} + \tfrac{1}{d}}\right]\right),$$
$$\left(OR * \exp\left[+1.96\sqrt{\tfrac{1}{a} + \tfrac{1}{b} + \tfrac{1}{c} + \tfrac{1}{d}}\right]\right)$$

A confidence interval for the odds ratio that crosses unity indicates insufficient evidence for an association between exposure and disease.

The *rare disease assumption* says that, if the disease in question is rare, then the odds ratio is a good approximation of the *relative risk,* or the ratio of the probability of disease among the exposed to the probability of disease among the unexposed. This derives from the mathematical fact that if the probability of an event *not* happening is almost 1 (e.g., the chance of *not* having a rare disease is almost 100%), then probability and odds are nearly identical.

Controlling for Confounding in Statistical Analysis

Confounders are a major concern in case–control studies and in some clinical research studies where two disease subgroups are compared (e.g., in prognostic studies and cross-sectional clinical studies). Many case–control studies will try to control for confounding in the design phase through techniques such as matching. Confounders can also be accounted for during the data-analysis phase.

Stratification. In general, any time that data are partitioned by age group, race, gender, smoking status, or any other categorical variable, this is called *stratification*. By stratifying case–control data into subgroups corresponding to levels of a putative confounder, separate odds ratios can be calculated at each level of the confounder, thereby removing the confounder's effect. The *Mantel-Haenszel procedure* combines the stratum-specific odds ratios into a summary odds ratio. The Mantel-Haenszel odds ratio is the weighted average of the stratum-specific odds ratios, each weighted by the size of the stratum (see Appendix 3–1).

Example 3–14 For example, in a case–control study of smoking, alcohol consumption, and hemorrhagic stroke (HS), there might be concern about the confounding effect of smoking on the alcohol association. Consider the following hypothetical data:

	HS	controls
heavy alcohol use	217	73
no alcohol use	283	427

The crude odds ratio is (217*427)/(73*283) = 4.5, suggesting a strong positive association of heavy alcohol use and hemorrhagic stroke. However, many drinkers of excessive alcohol are also smokers, and smoking is a strong risk factor for hemorrhagic stroke. When stratified by smoking status (ever/never), the data might appear as follows:

	smokers	
	HS	controls
alcohol	175	28
no alcohol	175	112

	nonsmokers	
	HS	controls
alcohol	42	45
no alcohol	108	315

The odds ratio from the smokers' stratum is (175*112)/(28*175) = 4.0 and the odds ratio from the nonsmokers' stratum is (42*315)/(45*108) = 2.7. The Mantel-Haenszel summary odds ratio is 3.4, showing a strong effect for heavy alcohol consumption. If the Mantel-Haenszel odds ratio differs substantially from the crude odds ratio, confounding is present and the adjusted odds ratio should be reported.

Although the Mantel-Haenszel procedure is easy to interpret and calculate, it can only be used to control for categorical confounders and continuous confounders that have been divided into intervals. The procedure also becomes cumbersome if more than a single confounder needs to be taken into account. In these circumstances, a multivariate technique called *logistic regression* is used.

Logistic Regression. Logistic regression is a multivariate technique that can be used to calculate an adjusted odds ratio when there are multiple confounders, and/or continuous confounders. Logistic regression is similar to multiple linear regression, but is used when the outcome variable is binary (dichotomous) rather than continuous. The odds ratio is modeled as the natural log of the odds ratio:

$$\ln (OR) = \alpha + \beta_1 x_1 + \beta_2 x_2 + \beta_3 x_3 \ldots$$

When exponentiated, each regression coefficient β_i represents the increase in the odds of disease for a one-unit increase in the exposure x_i, controlling for all other predictors in the model. Logistic regression must be done by computer, and is a standard component of most statistical software packages.

References

Armstrong BK, White E, Saracci R. Principles of Exposure Measurement. New York: Oxford University Press, 1994.

Ascherio A, Munger KL, Lennette ET, et al. Epstein-Barr virus antibodies and risk of multiple sclerosis: a prospective study. *JAMA* 2001;286:3083–3088.

Askenasy JJ. Approaching disturbed sleep in late Parkinson's disease: first step toward a proposal for a revised UPDRS. *Parkinsonism Relat Disord* 2001;8:123–131.

Barquet N, Domingo P, Cayla JA, et al. Prognostic factors in meningococcal disease. Development of a bedside predictive model and scoring system. Barcelona Meningococcal Disease Surveillance Group. *JAMA* 1997; 278:491–496.

Benedetti MD, Maraganore DM, Bower JH, et al. Hysterectomy, menopause, and estrogen use preceding Parkinson's disease: an exploratory case–control study. *Mov Disord* 2001;16:830–837.

Bowling A. Measuring Disease: A Review of Disease-specific Quality of Life Measurement Scales, 2nd edition. Buckingham, England: Open University Press, 2001.

Brenner H. Correcting for exposure misclassification using an alloyed gold standard. *Epidemiology* 1996;7:406–410.

Brenner H, Savitz D, Gefeller O. The effect of joint misclassification of exposure and disease on epidemiologic measures of association. *J Clin Epidemiol* 1993;46:1195–1202.

Checkoway, H, Pearce NE, Crawford-Brown DJ. Research Methods in Occupational Epidemiology (Monographs in Epidemiology and Biostatistics (Vol. 13). New York: Oxford University Press, 1989.

Collin C, Wade DT, Davies S, Horne V. The Barthel ADL Index: a reliability study. *Int Disability Study* 1988;10:61–63.

Coughlin SS. Recall bias in epidemiologic studies. *J Clin Epidemiol* 1990;43:87–91.

Drews CD, Greeland S. The impact of differential recall on the results of case–control studies. *Int J Epidemiol* 1990;19:1107–1112.

Drews C, Greenland S, Flanders D. The use of restricted controls to prevent recall bias in case–control studies of reproductive outcomes. *Ann Epidemiol* 1993;3:86–93.

Duncan PW, Jorgensen HS Wade DT. Outcome measures in acute stroke trials. A systematic review and some recommendations to improve practice. *Stroke* 2000;31:1429–1439.

Feinstein AR. P-values and confidence intervals: two sides of the same unsatisfactory coin. *J Clin Epidemiol* 1998;51:355–360.

Flanders D, Drews C, Kosinski A. Methodology to correct differential misclassification. *Epidemiology* 1995;6:152–156.

Gardner MJ, Altman DG. Confidence intervals rather than P values: estimation rather than hypothesis testing. *Br Med J* 1986 15;292: 746–750.

Greenland S. Statistical uncertainty due to misclassification: implications for validation substudies. *J Clin Epidemiol* 1988;42:167–174.

Greenland S, Kleinbaum DG. Correcting for

misclassification in two-way tables and matched-pair studies. *Int J Epidemiol* 1983; 12:93–97.

Hertzman C, Hayes M, Singer J, Highland J. Upper Ottawa street landfill site health study. *Environ Health Perspect* 1987;75:173–195.

http://dceg.cancer.gov/QMOD/. Questionnaire Modules. Division of Cancer Epidemiology and Genetics, National Cancer Institute, 2003.

http://www.qolid.org. Quality of Life Instrument Database. MAPI Research Institute, 2003.

Hui SL, Walter SD. Estimating the error rates of diagnostic tests. *Biometrics* 1980;36:167–171.

Hulley SB, Cummings SR. Designing Clinical Research. Baltimore, MD: Williams and Wilkins, 1988.

Huntington Study Group. Unified Huntington's Disease Rating Scale: reliability and consistency. Huntington Study Group. *Mov Disord* 1996;11:136–142.

Huntington Study Group. A randomized, placebo-controlled trial of coenzyme Q10 and remacemide in Huntington's disease. *Neurology* 2001;57:397–404.

Jensen AR, Rohwer WD. The Stroop color-word test: a review. *Acta Psychol* 1966;25:36–93.

Kasner SE, Wein T, Piriyawat P, et al. Acetaminophen for altering body temperature in acute stroke: a randomized clinical trial. *Stroke* 2002;33:130–134.

Katz S, Akpom CA. A measure of primary sociobiological functions. *Int J Health Serv* 1976;6:493–508.

Kleinbaum DJ, Kupper LL, Morgenstern H. Epidemiologic Research: Principles and Quantitative Methods. New York: Van Nostrand/Reinhold, 1982.

Lawton MP, Brody EM. Assessment of older people: self-maintaining and instrumental activities of daily living. *Gerontologist* 1969; 9:179–186.

Linn MW. A rapid disability rating scale. *J Am Geriatr Soc* 1967;15:211–214.

McDowell I, Newell C. Measuring Health. A Guide to Rating Scales and Questionnaires, 2nd edition. New York: Oxford University Press, 1996.

McGeer PL, McGeer EG. Inflammatory processes in amyotrophic lateral sclerosis. *Muscle Nerve* 2002;26:459–470.

Neugebauer R, Ng S. Differential recall as a source of bias in epidemiologic research. *J Clin Epidemiol* 1990;43:1337–1341.

Pearce N, Checkoway H. Case–control studies using other diseases as controls: problems of excluding exposure-related diseases. *Am J Epidemiol* 1988;127:851–856.

Raphael K. Recall bias: a proposal for assessment and control. *Int J Epidemiol* 1987;16: 167–170.

Rothman KJ, Greenland S. Approaches to statistical analysis. In: Rothman KJ, Greenland S, eds. *Modern Epidemiology,* Philadelphia, PA: Lippincott, Williams and Wilkins, 1998, pp. 183–100.

Rull R, Ritz B. Historical pesticide exposure in California using pesticide use reports and land-use surveys: an assessment of misclassification error and bias. Unpublished manuscript, 2003.

Salek S, ed. Compendium of Quality of Life Instruments, Vol. 1–5. Chichester, UK: John Wiley and Sons, 1998.

Salmon DP, Thomas RG, Pay MM, et al. Alzheimer's disease can be accurately diagnosed in very mildly impaired individuals. *Neurology* 2002;59:1022–1028.

Semchuk KM, Love EJ. Effects of agricultural work and other proxy-derived case–control data on Parkinson's disease risk estimates. *Am J Epidemiol* 1995;141:747–754.

Sevillano MD, de Pedro-Cuesta J, Duarte J, Claveria LE. Field validation of a method for population screening of parkinsonism. *Mov Disord* 2002;17:258–264.

Sherman EM, Slick DJ, Connolly MB, et al. Validity of three measures of health-related quality of life in children with intractable epilepsy. *Epilepsia* 2002;43:1230–1238.

Staquet M, Hays RD, Fayers PM, eds. Quality of Life Assessment in Clinical Trials. Methods and Practice. Oxford: Oxford University Press, 1998.

Stensland-Bugge E, Bonaa KH, Joakimsen O, Njolstad I. Sex differences in the relationship of risk factors to subclinical carotid atherosclerosis measured 15 years later: the Tromso Study. *Stroke* 2000;31:574–581.

Stineman MG, Shea JA, Jette A, et al. The Functional Independence Measure: tests of scaling assumptions, structure, and reliability across 20 diverse impairment categories. *Arch Phys Med Rehabil* 1996;77:1101–1108.

Streiner DL, Norman GR. Health Measurement Scales. A Practical Guide to Their Development and Use, 2nd edition. Oxford: Oxford Medical Publications, 1995.

Wacholder S, Armstrong B, Hartge P. Validation studies using an alloyed gold standard. *Am J Epidemiol* 1993;137:1251–1258.

Walker AM, Velma JP, Robins JM. Analysis of case–control data derived in part from proxy respondents. *Am J Epidemiol* 1988;127:905–914.

Walter SD, Irwig LM. Estimation of test error rates, disease prevalence and relative risk from misclassified data: a review. *J Clin Epidemiol* 1988;41:923–937.

Willett W. Nutritional Epidemiology (Monographs in Epidemiology and Biostatistics Series, Vol. 30), 2nd edition. New York: Oxford University Press, 1998.

Wolfe F, Kleinheksel SM, Cathey MA, et al. The clinical value of the Stanford Health Assessment Questionnaire Functional Disability Index in patients with rheumatoid arthritis. *J Rheumatol* 1988;15:1480–1488.

Appendix 3–1

Formulas for the odds ratio and relative risk, from a 2×2 table.

Odds Ratio

$$OR = \frac{ad}{bc}$$

95% confidence limits:

$$OR^* \exp\left[-1.96\sqrt{\tfrac{1}{a} + \tfrac{1}{b} + \tfrac{1}{c} + \tfrac{1}{d}}\right], \; OR^* \exp\left[+1.96\sqrt{\tfrac{1}{a} + \tfrac{1}{b} + \tfrac{1}{c} + \tfrac{1}{d}}\right]$$

Mantel-Haenszel Summary Odds Ratio

For k strata with T subjects in each stratum:

$$OR_{MH} = \frac{\sum_{i=1}^{k} \dfrac{a_i d_i}{T_i}}{\sum_{i=1}^{k} \dfrac{b_i c_i}{T_i}}$$

Relative Risk

$$RR = \frac{a/(a+b)}{c/(c+d)}$$

95% confidence limits:

$$RR^* \exp\left[-1.96\sqrt{\tfrac{1 - a/(a+b)}{a} + \tfrac{1 - c/(c+d)}{c}}\right], \; RR^* \exp\left[-1.96\sqrt{\tfrac{1 - a/(a+b)}{a} + \tfrac{1 - c/(c+d)}{c}}\right]$$

4

Genetic Epidemiology of Neurologic Disease

MARIEKE C.J. DEKKER, LORENE M. NELSON,
AND CORNELIA M. VAN DUIJN

Genetic epidemiology is a discipline that covers a broad spectrum of research, ranging from studies of disease aggregation in families to studies of the specific molecular origin of a disorder. Many developments have contributed to the rapid growth of genetic epidemiology in the past decade, including the sequencing of the human genome, the identification of common genetic variants, and advances in the vast armamentarium of high throughput methods for studying the human genome. In recent years, research interest has shifted from genetic disorders that are caused by a single gene (e.g., Huntington's disease) to common multifactorial disorders or complex diseases such as Alzheimer's disease that are likely to result from the interaction of genes and the environment.

This chapter will begin with a discussion of Mendelian versus complex (non-Mendelian) neurological disorders, followed by an overview of the structure of DNA and the molecular basis of disease. We will discuss the methods of genetic epidemiology,

differentiating family-based studies from population-based studies of unaffected individuals. The options for genetic epidemiology study designs will be presented, with a discussion of strengths and limitations of each approach. Finally, we will summarize recent technological developments and outline the important ethical and social implications of genetic epidemiologic research in the study of neurological disorders.

Genetic Transmission of Disease

Mendelian versus Non-Mendelian (Complex) Diseases

As a first step in examining the genetic transmission of a disease, classical genetic approaches are used to estimate disease heritability, that is, the proportion of the total variance in a trait (or percentage of disease) that can be explained by the additive effects of genes. Twin studies are the classic method for estimating heritability, and studies of the degree of clustering or, *familial aggregation,* of disease are also valuable. A distinction is often made between Mendelian and non-Mendelian traits. Mendelian disorders are usually single gene disorders caused by either a single dominant or two recessive autosomal mutations. Autosomal disease genes are located on one of the 22 autosomes, whereas "sex-linked" genes are on either the X or Y sex chromosomes.

For a Mendelian disorder, examining the transmission patterns of the disease through a family may yield clues to the nature of the mutation involved in the disease. If a disorder is *autosomal dominant,* the disease is expected to be present in multiple generations, because having one copy of the mutation is sufficient to lead to disease pathology. Since subjects carrying two dominant mutations (homozygotes) are rare and often incompatible with life, most patients carry only one copy of the mutation (so-called heterozygotes). For a dominant mutation, disease risk is thus conferred when an individual receives one mutant form of a gene from either parent (Speer 1998). Affected parents will pass on disease to approximately 50% of the offspring since the probability that the mutant or normal gene is transmitted to offspring is equal (Figure 4–1). Huntington's disease is an example of an autosomal dominant disorder.

If two defective copies of an autosomal gene are needed to develop disease, a mutation is referred to as *autosomal recessive.* Parents of patients with a recessive disorder are most often heterozygous and therefore are not affected. Recessive disorders typically emerge in consanguineous matings, since these matings increase the probability that both parents are carriers of the same mutation. A classical example of an autosomal recessive neurological disorder is Kennedy's disease, a motor neuron disease characterized by muscle weakness and atrophy.

Genetic disorders that are linked to the sex chromosomes may also occur. In particular, since males only possess one X-chromosome, a recessive mutation may lead to disease when only one copy is present whereas in women two defective copies are needed. Duchenne's muscular dystrophy (DMD) is a sex-linked recessive disease that shows a typical clustering of disease in males, with no male-to-male transmission.

A problem in examining Mendelian transmission of disease is that mutations may not always lead to disease. The cumulative incidence of disease among a mutation carrier (*penetrance,* or the probability that the person develops the disease during life) may depend on age, sex, and other factors. For many Mendelian diseases, the reason for reduced penetrance is unknown, but may be related to other genetic or environmental factors. The presence of a number of dominant or recessive mutations with reduced age- or sex-related penetrance may result in a disorder that appears to be non-Mendelian.

In contrast to the Mendelian inheritance patterns discussed thus far, the inheritance of a non-Mendelian or multifactorial (complex) disorder is more difficult to investigate. Complex diseases, which comprise the majority of neurological conditions, are likely to result from several low penetrance "susceptibility genes," each of which constitutes a minor contribution to pathogenesis. The relationship between a given genotype and phenotype (the observable trait) is not straightforward. In complex disorders, disease etiology is likely explained by the interaction between multiple susceptibility genes (gene–gene interaction) or the combination of one more susceptibility genes with environmental factors (gene–environment interaction). Most common neurologic disorders such as Alzheimer's disease, epilepsy, Parkinson's disease, and multiple sclerosis exhibit complex inheritance patterns that may be the result of expression of different genes in combination with exogenous (environmental) exposures.

Assessment of familial aggregation is the first step in dissecting the genetic components of a neurological disorder. Knowledge of the transmission of disease (Mendelian versus non-Mendelian) is crucial for determining the most powerful strategy for studying the

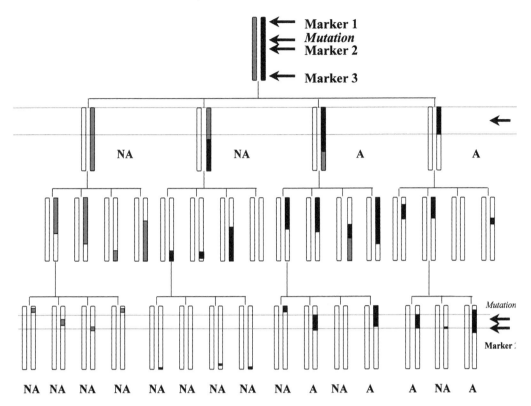

Figure 4–1 Linkage analysis to localize a mutation transmitted through generations. This figure depicts two homologous chromosomes of a founding parent (black and grey). In one of them (indicated in black), a mutation occurred, which will be passed down to 50% of the progeny. Each carrier receiving the mutation may pass it down to offspring with a 50% probability. Along with the mutation, an amount of flanking DNA is transmitted. Because of recombination, the piece of DNA shared by patients consecutively becomes smaller over generations. In the figure, three markers (1, 2, 3) flanking the mutation are shown. In a genomic search, patients in the third generation may no longer share markers 1 and 2 of the mutated chromosome, but marker 2 still flags the mutation.

molecular basis of disease. However, familial aggregation rarely comprises more than 10%–15% of a neurological disorder, and the remaining individuals affected are *sporadic* in nature, with no apparent genetic or environmental causes. The disease etiology of sporadic cases is likely to be a complex combination of genetic and environmental factors.

Molecular Basis of Neurological Disease

Genetic information is stored by deoxyribonucleic acid (DNA). At the molecular level, DNA is made up of a sugar, a phosphate, and a base. The DNA sequence is described by the order of the bases (adenine, guanine, cytosine, thymine), represented by their initials A, G, C, and T. Three-base nucleotides form a *codon*, which codes for 1 of the 20 amino acids that can be synthesized in the human body. In a process called *transcription*, a string of codons is joined together and copied into single-stranded ribonucleic acid (RNA), which is then processed into protein. Proteins are the building blocks of the body's structures such as bone, muscle, vasculature, neurons, enzymes, hormones, and neurotransmitters.

In the nineteenth century, without knowledge of underlying molecular biology, Mendel introduced the term *gene* as the fundamental unit that transmits traits from parents to offspring (Speer 1998). The most straightforward definition of a gene is the part of DNA that encodes for a protein. Genes actually comprise no more than 5% of human chromosomes (Nowak 1994); therefore, the large majority of DNA (>90%) does not code for proteins. *Exons* are the parts of a gene that are translated into proteins. DNA in the area next to the exons is involved in the regulation and transmission of gene expression. Between exons, noncoding regions called *introns* occur and are later removed (spliced out) when messenger RNA (mRNA) translates the coding regions (codons) to protein. The function of the DNA in intronic regions is not well understood. The largest quantity of genomic material lies between genes (intergenic) and the DNA in this region has no known function.

At present, the human genome is estimated to contain 30,000 genes. Mutations in exons leading to a change in amino acid in a protein may be pathogenic due to loss or gain in the function of the protein. Although introns do not encode for protein, mutations in the intronic regions may affect gene splicing and may subsequently change the structure or synthesis of the protein. Nucleic acid changes in the *promoter* region that regulate gene expression can change the level, location, or timing of gene expression.

The genetic code is *degenerate*, meaning that several triplets can code for the same amino acid (e.g., the codons A-C-T and A-G-T both code for same amino acid). Hence, point mutations do not always result in changes at the level of the amino acid; these silent mutations may be dispersed throughout the population. At one particular locus in the human genome, several forms of the same gene (alleles) may therefore exist. These genetic variants are called *alleles,* and when a variant occurs in more than 1% of the population, it is called a *polymorphism.*

A distinction commonly encountered in the genetics literature is that between mutations and polymorphisms. At a molecular level, however, this distinction is not clear-cut. Mutations have low frequency (generally less than 1%, as high as 5%) but are thought to be highly penetrant, resulting in disease pathogenesis in a majority of carriers. For example, in virtually all carriers, mutations of the presenilin 1 (PSEN1) gene lead to Alzheimer's disease with an onset before 55 years of age (Van Broeckhoven et al. 1992). In contrast to disease-causing mutations, polymorphisms may not be related to the risk of disease or may be associated with only a modest increase in disease risk; these polymorphisms are said to be disease-associated rather than disease-causing variants.

The number of affected nucleotides in a genetic variant can range from a single base pair to thousands of base pairs such as in the Huntington disease gene. There are several types of polymorphisms including nucleotide insertions and deletions and nucleotide repeat polymorphisms, but most polymorphisms in the genome are single-nucleotide polymorphisms (SNPs). Table 4–1 provides a summary of the predicted relative risks for single-nucleotide polymorphisms in candidate gene association studies according to type and location of genetic variant. This table illustrates how polymorphisms can be prioritized for study based on the nature of a variant and its predicted functional effect on its protein product.

Example 4–1 An example of a disease-associated polymorphism is the apolipoprotein ε4-allele (APOE*4), which has an allele frequency of approximately 17% in Caucasians. The risk of developing Alzheimer's disease for carriers of the APOE*4 allele is 1.5- to 2.5-fold increased (Slooter and Van Duijn 1997). Nevertheless, APOE*4 is neither necessary nor sufficient to develop Alzheimer's disease (Farrer et al. 1997).

Table 4–1 Predicted Relative Risks for Single-nucleotide Polymorphisms in Candidate Gene Association Studies According to Type, Location, and Functional Effect of Genetic Variant

Type of genetic variant	Location	Functional effect	Frequency in genome	Predictive relative risk of phenotype
Nonsense	Coding sequence (exon)	Premature termination of amino acid sequence	Very low	Very strong
Missense/nonsynonymous	Coding sequence (exon)	Changes in amino acid in protein to one with similar properties	Low	Weak to very strong, depending on location
Insertion/deletions (frameshift)	Coding sequence (exon)	Changes the frame of the protein-coding region, usually with very negative consequences for the protein	Low	Very strong, depending on location
Insertion/deletions (in frame)	Coding or noncoding	Changes amino acid sequence	Low	Weak to very strong
Sense/synonymous	Coding sequence (exon)	Does not change the amino acid sequence in the protein, but can alter splicing	Medium	Weak to strong
Promoter/regulatory region	Promoter, untranslated regions	Does not change the amino acid but can affect the level, location, or timing of gene expression	Low to medium	Weak to strong
Splice site/intron–exon boundary	Within 10 base pairs of exon	Might change the splicing pattern or efficiency of introns	Low	Weak to strong
Intronic	Deep within introns	No known function, but might might affect expression or mRNA stability	Medium	Weak
Intergenic	Noncoding regions between genes	No known function, but might might affect expression through enhancer or other mechanisms	High	Very weak

Adapted with permission from Tabor HK, Risch NJ, Myers RM. Opinion: candidate-gene approaches for studying complex genetic traits: practical considerations. *Nat Rev Genet* 2002;3:391–397.

Methods in Genetic Epidemiology in Neurological Disorders

The primary goals of genetic epidemiology are to identify specific genes that contribute to the pathogenesis of neurologic disorders and to quantify the impact of a given gene or genetic variant on the occurrence of a disease in the general population. Table 4–2 summarizes the research objectives of genetic epidemiology and the study designs that address those objectives. The strength of the association between a genetic variant and disease may be obtained either from a cohort study that compares disease incidence in carriers to that in noncarriers or from a case–control study that contrasts the frequency of the genetic variant among cases and controls (Rothman and Greenland 1998). In this section, we describe two different strategies for discovering susceptibility genes: genome screening and candidate gene studies.

Genome Screening

A genome screen may be conducted to achieve a partial or complete search of the genome for genes involved in a disorder. This approach often begins with no a priori knowledge of the genes that are involved; however, in some cases, linkage studies can provide some information that certain regions on certain chromosomes are more suspect than others. Genome screening is carried out by genotyping a set of polymorphic markers that are distributed across the genome. Usually, these markers cover all chromosomes and are approximately equally distributed across the genome. In some studies, however, markers are distributed more densely in "gene-rich" regions of certain chromosomes or in regions where previous studies have indicated the likely presence of a disease-associated gene. These markers are not necessarily located in a gene, but often are located in noncoding areas not involved in any biological process.

The rationale behind genome screening is that a causally related mutation or poly-morphism should be found more often in patients with a neurogenetic disorder than in controls. However, given that the genome contains over 3 billion base pairs (van Ommen 1999), the probability that a random marker is located at a disease mutation by chance is virtually zero. The basic principle underlying genome screening is that our genetic information is linearly arranged in chromosomes. Loci that are physically close together on a chromosome are likely to be transmitted together from parent to offspring. Therefore, patients who inherit a disease gene from a common ancestor often not only receive the disease mutation but also adjacent parts of the chromosome. Any marker that is physically located near a causal mutation should be present more often in cases than in unaffected relatives or unrelated controls and can serve to flag the mutation. Using this principle, disease genes can be identified by screening the genome of patients by means of a limited number of markers covering the genome.

Example 4–2 A recent study used pooled DNA samples to screen the whole genome for disease-associated markers in a study of multiple sclerosis (MS) patients and controls (Sawcer et al. 2002). The genome scan was conducted with microsatellite markers spaced 0.5 centimorgans apart using DNA pools (i.e., combined DNA samples) from 216 MS cases, 219 controls, and trio families (745 affected individuals and their 1490 parents). Ten markers were associated with MS, including three markers previously identified within the HLA region on chromosome 6p (D6S1615, D6S2444, and TNFα), four markers from regions previously identified in linkage studies, and three markers from novel sites not yet found with linkage analysis (D1S1590 at 1q, D2S2739 at 2p, and D4S416 at 4q). This study provided evidence to support MS-linked regions on chromosomes 6p, 17q, 19q, and 1p.

Candidate Gene Studies

Candidate gene studies offer an alternative to genome screening. Investigators who use

Table 4–2 Research Goals and Objectives in Genetic Epidemiology, Descriptions of Study Designs

Research objective	Study design(s) used to address objective
Goal: To determine the extent to which the disease aggregates in families, percentage of variation due to genetic factors	
Determine extent to which the disease aggregates in families	Collect family history data for family members of cases (probands) and for family members of unaffected individuals (controls) to estimate the prevalence of the disease in each group
Estimate percentage of disease etiology caused by heritability	Studies to compare disease concordance rates in monozygotic (identical) twins and dizygotic (fraternal) twins
Goal: To quantify the prevalence of disease-associated variants and their associations with disease risk	
Estimate prevalence of a gene variant in general population	Cross-sectional survey with DNA collection, demographic and racial/ethnic information on study subjects
Assess magnitude of association between a genetic variant and occurrence of a neurological disorder	Prospective cohort studies Population-based case–control studies Twin studies
Assess gene–gene and gene–environment interactions in determination of disease risk	Prospective cohort studies or case-control studies with DNA collection and additional information on environmental risk factors
Goal: To identify new disease-causing mutations or disease-associated gene polymorphisms	
Conduct studies in families with multiple affected members to segregate disease trait and link genetic loci with disease occurrence	Segregation studies Linkage studies Positional cloning Affected sib-pair studies
Identify gene variants, single-nucleotide polymorphisms (SNPs) for candidate gene investigations	Cross-sectional survey of general population or selection of a series of cases with disease, use DNA sequencing to identify SNPs
Study genetic isolates to identify disease-associated gene variants, or "founder effects"	Studies of genetically isolated populations
Goal: To identify the biochemical mechanism(s) by which disease-associated gene variants cause neurologic dysfunction	

Conduct animal studies to examine the effect of a gene variant on disease pathogenesis	Genetic studies in animals:
	  Transgenic models
	  Knock-out models

Examine functional effect of gene-associated variants on protein structure and function; relate to disease pathogenesis	Laboratory studies:
	  Functional genomic studies
	  Gene expression arrays
	  Proteomics

Develop treatment interventions to reverse or ameliorate biochemical effect of genetic variant on disease onset or outcome	Animal studies of potential treatments Clinical trials
Goal: To examine the utility of genetic tests in clinical populations and for disease screening in the general population	
Assess validity and utility of a genetic test in clinical setting	Diagnostic accuracy study
Evaluate efficacy of genetic screening test in different populations	Screening effectiveness study

this strategy begin with a knowledge of disease pathogenesis and identify promising "candidate" genes that may be expected to play a role in disease pathogenesis based on the gene product, the protein, or homology to a gene that is known to be involved in the disease. Candidate genes chosen by this method are then "sequenced" from chromosomes (DNA) obtained from a number of individuals, with the purpose of identifying specific mutations or polymorphisms of a nucleic acid that differ from the normal ("wild-type") sequence. If a gene has two or more variants (alleles), then a group of cases with a neurologic disease can be compared with a control group to determine whether the allele occurs more frequently in one group than in the other (i.e., an allelic association). Gene–disease associations can also be examined according to the *genotype* of an individual, that is, whether the person carries one normal allele and one variant allele (heterozygote), or two variant alleles (homozygote), using the group with two normal alleles (wild type) as the comparison group. A *dose-response relationship* is said to occur if the relative risk for homozygotes (2 variant alleles) is higher than the relative risk for heterozygotes (1 variant allele); this finding strengthens the evidence of a causal relationship between the marker and disease risk.

A major challenge of the candidate gene approach is that a priori knowledge of the pathogenesis of the disease is required, and good evidence must be present that a given protein plays a role in the pathogenic process before justifying the large expense of genotyping assays. For a large number of neurologic disorders, knowledge of proteins involved in the etiology is limited or absent. For example, before cloning of the PSEN genes involved in early-onset Alzheimer's disease, the presenilin protein and its function were unknown (Van Broeckhoven et al. 1992).

Another problem in studies of candidate genes is that having a large number of candidate genes may create a multiple testing problem because a certain number of associations, even those that are not true, will arise on the basis of chance alone. For genome screening in families with multiple affected generations, established criteria are available to adjust for multiple testing based on the number of tests that can be made given the size of the genome and the linkage between regions. In contrast, adjustment methods for the multiple-comparison problem is not as straightforward in the context of candidate gene studies because a large number of candidate genes, each of which may have several polymorphisms of interest, may quickly accumulate a large number of associations that require statistical tests of significance.

Example 4–3 A great number of proteins may be hypothetically involved in diseases such as Parkinson's disease, on the basis of proteins detected postmortem in brain tissue, or the large number of dopamine-regulating proteins in the substantia nigra and striatum such as the dopamine transporter, dopamine receptors, and the enzymes monoamine oxidase-B and tyrosine hydroxylase. Given the large number of genes that can be tested in this context, adjustment of statistical significance levels for multiple testing is necessary. If hundreds of tests are performed, testing using a significance level of 0.05 will yield a large number of false-positive findings (approximately 5 false-positive findings for every 100 genetic markers tested). For candidate gene studies, the debate on how to adjust for multiple testing is ongoing (Lander and Schork 1994; Lee 2002) because standard corrections for multiple comparisons such as the Bonferoni method are too conservative.

Although adjustment for multiple testing is necessary in candidate gene studies, the need for replication of findings in different populations is even more important. False-negatives may also pose problems for candidate gene association studies, especially when the frequency of the variant alleles is less than 5%–10%. In this case, only large association studies will have enough statistical power to detect associations. It may be argued, however, that it is most important to identify polymorphic genes of relatively high frequency (e.g., ApoE*4, 17%) because a greater percentage of the population risk will be attributable to such genes.

Study Designs in Genetic Epidemiology

Family-based Study Designs

Family-based study designs are of great importance to the identification of new genes and have been the traditional backbone of genetic epidemiologic research. Several excellent reviews of study design options in genetic epidemiology, including family-based designs, are available (Zhao et al. 1997; Whittemore and Nelson 1999). Using linkage studies of extended pedigrees from affected families, remarkable progress has been made in unraveling the etiology of several monogenetic neurological disorders in which there is a clear-cut relation between a genetic factor and occurrence of disease (e.g., Huntington's disease, Duchenne muscular dystrophy).

The objective of a linkage study is to find markers of alleles that are preferentially transmitted to affected individuals within a family. Linkage is based on the concept that relatives who develop a disease due to the same mutation are expected to share alleles on DNA markers that flank the disease mutation. Linkage analysis uses the principle of *recombination* to localize the disease mutation transmitted in a family that confers the disease risk.

During the process of meiosis, homologous pieces of chromosomes may cross over, which results in an exchange or recombination of the genetic information encoded on the two chromosomes. Two loci close together on a chromosome will more frequently be transmitted together, whereas for two loci located far apart, recombination is likely to occur. The closer two loci are, the less likely it is that recombination will occur between them, and as a result,

the two loci are "linked" to each other. By using genetic markers spaced throughout the genome, linkage analysis capitalizes on this closeness or linking to identify disease-associated regions by identifying markers that are shared by family members affected with the disease.

Detailed statistical aspects of linkage studies are beyond the scope of this chapter. Basically, in a linkage analysis the number of recombinations between disease status and a marker allele (observed in a family) is compared to the expected number of recombinations under the null hypothesis. The test statistic for linkage is the log odds (LOD) score. The *LOD score* is the log of the likelihood ratio of linkage of the disease to the studied marker, versus the likelihood of no linkage. By convention, significant evidence for linkage is found when LOD scores exceed 3, whereas LOD scores below -2 imply exclusion of the region.

As it is often impossible to clinically distinguish between patients who developed the disease because of a specific mutation and those who have a different etiology, recombination between the disease and marker may be falsely inferred; therefore the power of linkage analysis in complex disorders is low. Family members share environment in addition to genes, and the polymorphism-associated risk may depend heavily on the presence of other genetic or environmental risk factors, a situation that makes linkage studies unfeasible. In this situation, linkage studies are not informative regarding the cause of disease.

An alternative approach to linkage studies for studying complex disorders is a family-based study using affected sib-pairs. Siblings share a high proportion (50%) of their genetic material, including large segments of DNA. The a priori probability of a patient sharing 0 alleles with any other sib is 25%; 1 allele is 50%; 2 alleles is again 25%. For markers located close to the disease mutation, affected sibs are expected to share more alleles than the average of 1 allele. The test statistic for the analysis is based on counting alleles shared by a pair of affected siblings. Counts exceeding the expected value under the null hypothesis (1 allele shared) are compatible with a disease locus nearby the marker examined.

An advantage of the sib-pair design is that two siblings with the same common disease are more likely to have developed the disease due to the same mutation than two distantly related subjects. Furthermore, siblings share not only a high proportion of DNA but also large chromosomal regions. In principle, the disease gene may thus be detected with a limited number of markers. The statistical power of sib-pair studies is limited, particularly if multiple genes are involved (Lander and Schork 1994), and detecting linkage in such disorders will require thousands of (affected) sibling-pairs.

Choice of the most powerful study design (linkage versus sib-pair approach) requires studies on clustering of disease in families to determine whether the disorder is segregated as a Mendelian or non-Mendelian trait. The most powerful design for a Mendelian disorder is linkage analysis, whereas for a non-Mendelian trait, sibpair analysis is more suitable. Among patients with a common non-Mendelian disorder, however, subgroups with distinctly Mendelian segregation may be identified. For example, linkage analysis has been successful at identifying single gene mutations for early-onset forms of Alzheimer's disease, Parkinson's disease, and migraine with aura (May et al. 1995). Although these traits are rare and may only explain a minor fraction of disease in the population, knowledge of the molecular genetic origin of the disease in these early-onset cases may yield clues toward key proteins involved in pathogenesis. These proteins may serve as targets in development of therapy for early-onset as well as late-onset forms.

When examining familial aggregation, clustering of a disease may be due not only to genetic factors but also environmental factors. For instance, nutritional habits cluster in families and may explain familial aggregation of disease, as might other characteristics such as cigarette smoking and occupational exposures. Hypertension, a major risk factor for stroke, is a complex condition showing strong familial aggregation and high heritability. Salt sensitivity is known to be a genetically determined risk factor for hypertension. For example, in a population with a uniformly low salt consumption, genetic contribution to the incidence of hypertension will appear to be low because the trait will be less likely to be expressed, whereas in populations with larger variation in salt intake the contribution of genetically conferred salt sensitivity may be considerable. For complex disorders, familial aggregation is therefore not a fixed property of a trait but can vary with the environmental determinants of disease risk.

Estimating the risk of a disease mutation in families requires ascertainment of a random group of unrelated families. Such studies are expensive and time consuming, and this study design is rarely used to estimate gene-associated risk. For mutations that are extremely rare in the population, such as mutations involved in early-onset Alzheimer's or early-onset Parkinson's disease, an astronomical sample size would be needed to observe enough cases of disease. Studies of genetic and environmental factors that modify the penetrance of disease may only be feasible in those few families segregating the rare diseases.

Population-based Studies

Family-based studies are the classic approach to determine the genetic etiology of a trait; however, only in monogenic (single gene) Mendelian disorders is this approach feasible. With the exception of rare and conspicuous phenotypes, a family-based approach rarely yields sufficient power to detect a genetic cause for common disorders. The affected sib-pair design might seem to provide an alternative for genetic linkage analysis, however, large numbers of affected sib-pairs are required to gain sufficient statistical power to detect genes involved. For disorders with a high mortality and/or late onset, affected sib-pairs are difficult to trace, which further limits feasibility. For these reasons, much of the current focus of neurogenetic research is on individuals without affected relatives (i.e., sporadic cases). Migraine, epilepsy, Alzheimer's disease, and Parkinson's disease are among the diseases in this category.

Recent years have seen the growth of population-based gene association studies because some of the limitations of family based-designs can be avoided through the use of population-based study designs. The rationale behind population-based studies is similar to that of family-based studies, in that the DNA of the disease-associated gene is flanked by DNA that is passed to the next generation and is thus dispersed throughout the population. As a result, a mutation related to disease risk can be ascertained in a genomic screen by identifying chromosomal regions shared by patients (Fig. 4–1). This unique alignment of genes along the chromosome is called a *haplotype*.

In the general population, it is difficult to perform a genomic screen for markers in linkage disequilibrium with a disease because there is only a small probability that any two patients with a common complex disorder have inherited a gene from a common ancestor. People with a common trait, randomly derived from the general population, are expected to be only very distantly related, and as a result, any two people share only a small amount of DNA. As shown in Figure 4–2, the amount of DNA shared progressively diminishes over generations. Thus, in order for a disease-associated marker to identify a region that may contain a disease-associated gene, the marker and disease locus must be very close together. A large number of markers with dense spacing and an extensive number of patients are therefore needed for whole genome screens to be successful (Risch and Merikangas 1996).

Although samples derived from the general population are very suitable for candi-

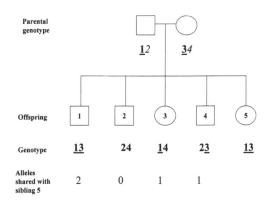

Figure 4–2 Expected allele sharing in affected and unaffected siblings. This figure show a pedigree of two parents and five children. Squares indicate males and circles indicate females. Since parents pass one of two alleles to offspring with equal probability, siblings share 50% of DNA on average. On average, two siblings share one allele.

date gene studies, such studies have been widely criticized because of the repeated failure to replicate results.

Example 4–4 Extensive candidate gene studies have been conducted on Parkinson's disease. Impairment of enzyme detoxification capacity has long been thought to account for an increased susceptibility to Parkinson's disease (McCann et al. 1997), possibly because of impaired ability to handle environmental neurotoxins. Two genes encoding detoxification enzymes, the *CYP2D6* gene (encoding for debrisoquine 4-hydroxylase cytochrome P450) and the *NAT2* gene (encoding for N-acetyltransferase 2) have been studied as candidate genes for Parkinson's disease. Because of their function in detoxification, these genes were studied as obvious candidates. Initial findings were positive but could neither be replicated in individual studies nor in a pooled reanalysis of study data (Nicholl et al. 1999).

Candidate gene studies have sometimes proved more successful when used as follow-up studies after linkage or sib-pair studies identify a chromosomal region that may contain a disease-associated variant.

Example 4–5 APOE*4, the most common genetic factor implicated in Alzheimer's disease, was discovered primarily by means of the candidate gene approach after linkage analysis suggested an Alzheimer's disease gene on chromosome 19 (Pericak-Vance et al. 1991). APOE was considered a "positional candidate," because its gene product, apolipo-protein E, was found to be associated with senile plaques in brains of patients with Alzheimer's disease.

The Importance of Population-based Genetic Epidemiology Studies. Population-based studies play a pivotal role in the assessment of risks associated with genetic factors. Population studies are needed to assess the frequencies of disease-causing mutations and disease-associated polymorphisms so that the proportion of disease attributable to genetic factors can be estimated. Furthermore, population-based association studies are of critical importance for estimating the strength of the association between a given genetic variant and the occurrence of a neurologic disorder (i.e., the odds ratio or relative risk associated with a given disease-associated polymorphism) and for determining whether environmental or lifestyle factors interact with the disease-associated genotype to increase the risk of the disease.

Risk estimation for genetic factors follows the classical approach of epidemiologic studies described in Chapters 1 and 2. Relative risks of disease may be derived from studies comparing risk of disease in carriers to that in noncarriers. Alternatively, relative risks may be estimated by obtaining odds ratios for the disease-associated genotypes in case–control studies using incident patients derived from a single study base, as described in Chapters 1 and 2. To obtain absolute measures of risk, cohort studies are needed to estimate the difference in disease incidence between carriers and noncarriers of a disease-associated variant (Rothman and Greenland 1998).

Example 4–6 Studies aiming to quantify the incidence of disease associated with common polymorphisms are lagging behind developments in molecular genetics. After initially finding the association of the APOE*4 allele with Alzheimer's disease (AD) in 1991, many case–control studies examining this association used prevalent AD patients from clinic-based series (Farrer et al. 1997). Recently, several population-based cohort studies have been done to estimate the incidence of AD in carriers and noncarriers of the APOE*4 allele. In a prospective cohort study begun in 1994 and conducted in a large health maintenance organization, 2356 subjects were followed for at least 1 year. Of these, 151 cases were diagnosed with AD. The investigators reported a twofold increase in risk for AD and carrying a single copy of APOE*4 and a sixfold increase in risk carrying two copies of APOE*4, after adjusting for age (Kukull et al. 2002). Several other cohort studies showed similar results (Myers et al. 1996; Slooter et al. 1998; Havlik et al. 2000). For clinical as well as public health purposes, unbiased risk estimates are essential.

The Importance of Assessing Gene–Environment Interactions

For complex genetic disorders in which multiple genetic and environmental factors contribute to the development of the disease, it is unlikely that a gene effect is independent of that of other risk factors. A key aim of neuroepidemiologic studies is to examine how environmental factors act against certain genetic backgrounds to increase the risk of developing a neurologic disorder. It is believed that many complex neurologic disorders result from one or more environmental factors acting on a background of (or in the presence of) common disease-associated genetic variants. Large-scale epidemiologic studies are therefore needed that collect data on genes and environmental factors to dissect the complex etiology of complex neurological diseases.

Challenges in the Conduct of Genetic Associations Studies

Genetic association studies often face the same challenges as other epidemiologic studies and may fail to identify true associations because of factors such as small (underpowered) studies, poor choice of control group in case–control studies, over-interpretation of study results, and unwarranted conclusions that a disease-associated genetic variant is a causal factor in disease prior to study replication (Cardon and Bell 2001). In addition to the usual study challenges, population-based genetic associations studies may be influenced by *population admixture* or *population stratification,* a problem that may occur when two or more distinct genetic subgroups are included in a study. For example, the odds ratio from a case–control study can be biased if the frequency of the disease-associated genetic variant is more common in certain ethnic subgroups than in others and the case and control groups have different ethnic compositions. Bias due to population admixture may occur in any genetic association study, whether it be a cohort (follow-up) study or a case-control study. In a case-control study, cases and controls may be drawn from different subpopulations. Population stratification bias may occur in any study where cases and controls are not matched for their race/ethnicity, because many genetic variants differ in frequency between individuals from different ancestral backgrounds. Several methods have been proposed for minimizing or controlling for population stratification bias, including (1) statistical methods to induce comparability, (2) the use of family controls from the same genetic background as cases, (3) the use of unlinked genetic markers to determine whether cases and controls have a similar genetic background ("genomic controls"), and (4) conducting studies in a genetically isolated population in which the genetic background of the residents is homogenous.

Addressing the Admixture Problem by Using Statistical Control for Race/Ethnicity. Critics of population-based genetic association studies conducted in heterogenous ethnic populations have suggested that population stratification (the mixture of indi-viduals from heterogeneous genetic ancestries) undermines the validity of these studies. Many epidemiologists believe that the problem of admixture is more of a theoretical concern and does not introduce material biases into a study in most real-life circumstances. They propose that population stratification can be adequately addressed by collecting information on the genetic (ancestral) background of cases and controls in the study and controlling for this potential confounder in the same way that other confounding variables are treated in epidemiologic studies (see Chapter 2).

Example 4–7 Using empirical data on the frequency of *N*-acetyltransferase (NAT2) slow acetylation genotypes and incidence rates of bladder cancer among U.S. Caucasians from eight different European ancestries, Wacholder et al. (2000) showed that the relative risk for the NAT2–bladder cancer association was minimally biased if the subjects' ethnicities were not adjusted in the statistical analysis. The investigators concluded that U.S. studies restricted to non-Hispanic U.S. Caucasians of European origin are unlikely to be significantly biased, even when statistical methods that adjust for different European ancestral backgrounds are not applied.

Despite this empirical evidence, many believe the statistical control method is inadequate for controlling for the diverse genetic backgrounds of subjects who participate in a study, and other approaches are proposed, such as the use of family controls.

Addressing the Admixture Problem by Using Family Controls. To overcome the problem of population admixture, the transmission disequilibrium test (TDT) can be used. Originally, the TDT was used in family-based studies, but it has been adapted for use in population-based studies (Pritchard and Rosenberg 1999). Rather than ascertaining a control group, alleles of parents not transmitted to the patients can be used to construct a "virtual" control genotype (Ewens and Spielman 1995). A disease-associated allele will more frequently than not be transmitted to the affected individual. The TDT approach requires ascertainment of DNA from the parental generation. For late-onset disorders, this approach is of limited value because parents are often deceased. Although variations of the TDT for sibling controls have been developed to overcome this problem, the power of the sib-TDT is significantly lower than that of a case–control approach (Slager et al. 2000).

Addressing the Admixture Problem by Using Genomic Controls. Another method for dealing with the problem of population admixture is to use genetic markers that differ in frequency according to a person's genetic ancestry but are "unlinked" (not associated) with the disease of interest (Ardlie et al. 2002). While the genomic control method can identify situations in which the diseased and nondiseased groups are similar or dissimilar with respect to population admixture, statistical adjustment for differences in population admixture between groups is not straightforward.

Addressing the Admixture Problem by Studying Genetic Isolates. Another way of circumventing distortions due to admixture is to select genetically isolated populations for study. The population of a genetically isolated community originates from a limited number of ancestors (founders). Such a founder population limits the degree of genetic diversity introduced, leading to a more homogeneous population. Genetic drift, a random process occurring in small populations, further reduces the number of putative susceptibility genes in these populations. Studies of genetic isolates also merit discussion because of their potential value in finding disease susceptibility genes.

Studies of Genetic Isolates

In genetically isolated populations, there is a higher probability that patients have developed the disease because of a mutation inherited from a common ancestor. Finland is a prototypic population that is widely studied as a "genetic isolate" because it has experienced isolation for over 100 generations and expanded from a small group of founders into the 5 million inhabitants of today, resulting in a genetically homogeneous population (Lander and Schork 1994). Another example of a genetic isolate is Iceland (McInnis 1999). In contrast to studies in the general population, genome screens have proven to be useful in genetic isolates (Lander and Schork 1994).

In addition to studies of populations of prolonged isolation, some studies in more recently isolated populations have been successful. In these populations, the founder effect is the major determinant of the limited genetic variation (Houwen et al. 1994). Using populations isolated for as little as 300–400 years (i.e., up to 20 generations), genetic loci associated with genetically complex disease have been identified, including genetic loci associated with manic depression in Costa Rica (Freimer et al. 1996) and susceptibility loci for mycobacterial infection in Malta (Newport et al. 1996). The method *haplotype sharing*, as depicted in Figure 4–3, has been applied with success in studies of recent genetic isolates (Houwen et al. 1994).

One drawback of studying genetically isolated populations is the limited value of extrapolation of study results from genetic isolates to other populations. Isolation that spans over 100 generations may have caused a population like Finland to have obtained a more or less "private" makeup of the genome (De La Chapelle and Wright 1998). An advantage of studies in populations of more recent isolation is that genetic makeup of the isolated population may more closely resemble that of the general population. However, it remains to be determined whether disease-related mutations or polymorphisms detected in an isolated population will also be present in the general population.

Mendelian inheritance can explain only a minor fraction of neurologic disease in the general population. The challenge for the future of genetic epidemiologic research will be the identification of genes involved

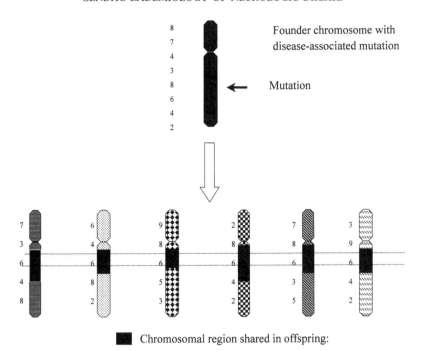

Figure 4–3 Allele sharing in a genetically isolated population. *Above:* Founder chromosome with disease-associated mutation. *Below:* Region surrounding the disease locus, shared by patients with the same phenotype. These affected individuals are all descendants from a common ancestor.

in the etiology of common sporadic neurologic disorders. With the shift in genetic epidemiologic research from monogenetic to complex disorders, design of genetic epidemiologic studies will change dramatically. As discussed earlier, the study of complex disorders will see a shift from family-based designs to sib-pair and population-based studies. This in turn implies a shift in data collection towards ascertainment of large series of patients and affected siblings to reach sufficient statistical power in a study (Risch and Merikangas 1996). Such studies require large-scale genotyping, thus developments in genetic epidemiology will depend heavily on advances in high-throughput molecular genotyping techniques.

Impact of the Human Genome Project on Neuroepidemiology

One of the most important developments in molecular genetics to boost genetic epidemiologic research is the recent completion of the draft of the Human Genome Project. This accomplishment has resulted in an enormous amount of information on genes and genetic variation that will greatly benefit genetic research on complex diseases. Along with growing insight into biology of neurological disease, the Human Genome Project will create opportunities for candidate genes studies. If major improvements in study design can be achieved, then candidate gene studies may capture a prominent position in genetic epidemiologic research. Another possibility created by the Human Genome Project is that of including markers for all human genes in a genome screen. This approach differs from a classical genome screen because it emphasizes the use of markers more likely to have a functional effect on the protein (approximately 5% of DNA) (Risch and Merikangas 1996).

A technical development important for the feasibility of such large-scale genetic epidemiologic research is the introduction of microarrays that include (binary) information on the presence or absence of polymorphism in a gene, enabling thousands of SNPs to be tested for association with a neurologic condition (see Table 4–1). These technical devices will create the opportunity to rapidly screen for DNA mutations or variations in large series of affected individuals (Cheung et al. 1998; Wang et al. 1998). Identification of SNP maps throughout the human genome is crucial to this effort (Risch and Merikangas 1996). Needless to say, major progress is anticipated in this field within the next decade.

Ethical, Legal, and Social Issues in Genetic Epidemiology Studies

The ethics of research involving human participants are continuously evolving as society changes and technology advances. More than any other field, genetics has undergone a technological explosion leading to greater understanding of disease etiology but also has challenged existing concepts of informed consent and confidentiality. Investigators involved in genetics research should be familiar with published guidelines on the ethical use of collected samples for DNA studies. The American Society of Human Genetics published a report in 1996 on informed consent for genetic research. This statement provides recommendations for use of newly collected biological samples for genetics research as well as for use of existing samples.

Future Directions and Conclusions

Genetic epidemiology is a young but rapidly developing science. Although its early years have been largely dedicated to family-based research in monogenetic disorders, modern genetic epidemiologic research will focus on complex multifactorial disorders, and large-scale population-based studies will be of increasing importance. Perhaps the most dramatic aspects of genetic epidemiologic research arising from the switch of emphasis from Mendelian dis-

orders to complex disorders are the implications for clinical medicine and public health. In contrast to the limited number of subjects at risk for monogenetic disorders such as Huntington's disease, the clinical and public health implications in studies of complex genetic disorders are relevant for a large number of subjects. Future studies on genetics of multifactorial diseases will therefore require close integration of genetic and epidemiologic research. The identification of previously unknown proteins involved in disease pathogenesis will enable the development of diagnostic tests for neurologic disorders and the investigation of protein targets for drug development to benefit individuals who suffer from neurologic diseases.

References

Ardlie KG, Lunetta KL, Seielstad M. Testing for population subdivision and association in four case–control studies. *Am J Hum Genet* 2002;71:304–311.

ASHG report. Statement on informed consent for genetic research. The American Society of Human Genetics. *Am J Hum Genet* 1996; 59:471–474.

Cardon LR, Bell JI. Association study designs for complex diseases. *Nat Rev Genet* 2001;2: 91–99.

Cheung VG, Gregg JP, Gogolin-Ewens KJ, et al. Linkage disequilibrium mapping without genotyping. *Nat Genet* 1998;18:225–230.

De La Chapelle A, Wright F. Linkage disequilibrium mapping in isolated populations: the example of Finland revisited. *Proc Natl Acad Sci USA* 1998;95:12416–12423.

Ewens WJ, Spielman RS. The transmission/disequilibrium test: history, subdivision, admixture. *Am J Hum Genet* 1995;57:455–464.

Farrer LA, Cupples LA, Haines JL, et al. Effects of age, sex, and ethnicity on the association between apolipoprotein E genotype and Alzheimer disease: a meta-analysis. *JAMA* 1997;349:1349–1356.

Freimer NB, Reus VI, Escamilla M, et al. An approach to investigating linkage for bipolar disorder using large Costa Rican pedigrees. *Am J Med Genet* 1996;67:254–263.

Havlik RJ, Izmirlian G, Petrovitch H, et al. APOE-ε4 predicts incident AD in Japanese-American men: the Honolulu-Asia Aging Study. *Neurology* 2000;54:1526–1529.

Houwen RH, Baharloo S, Blankenship K, et al.

Genome screening by searching for shared segments: mapping a gene for benign recurrent intrahepatic cholestasis. *Nat Genet* 1994;8:380–386.

Kukull WA, Higdon R, Bowen JD, et al. Dementia and Alzheimer's disease incidence: a prospective cohort study. *Arch Neurol* 2002; 59:1737–1746.

Lander ES, Schork NJ. Genetic dissection of complex traits. *Science* 1994;265:2037–2048.

Lee WC. Testing for candidate gene linkage disequilibrium using a dense array of single nucleotide polymorphisms in case–parents studies. *Epidemiology* 2002;13:545–551.

May A, Ophoff R, Terwindt G, et al. Familial hemiplegic migraine locus on 19p13 is involved in the common forms of migraine. *Hum Genet* 1995;96:604–608.

McCann SJ, Pond SM, James KM, Le Couteur DG. The association between polymorphisms in the cytochrome P-450 2D6 gene and Parkinson's disease: a case–control study and meta-analysis. *J Neurol Sci* 1997;153: 50–53.

McInnis MG. The assent of a nation: genethics and Iceland. *Clin Genet* 1999;55:234–239.

Myers RH, Schaefer EJ, Wilson PW, et al. Apolipoprotein E ε4 association with dementia in a population-based study: the Framingham study. *Neurology* 1996;46:673–677.

Newport MJ, Huxley CM, Huston S, et al. A mutation in the interferon-gamma-receptor gene and susceptibility to mycobacterial infection. *N Engl J Med* 1996;335:1941–1949.

Nicholl DJ, Bennett P, Hiller L, et al. A study of five candidate genes in Parkinson's disease and related neurodegenerative disorders. *Neurology* 1999;53:1415–1421.

Nowak R. Mining treasures from "junk" DNA. *Science* 1994;263:608–610.

Pericak-Vance MA, Bebout JL, Gaskell PC Jr, et al. Linkage studies in familial Alzheimer's disease: evidence for chromosome 19 linkage. *Am J Hum Genet* 1991;48:1034–1050.

Pritchard JK, Rosenberg NA. Use of unlinked genetic markers to detect population stratification in association studies. *Am J Hum Genet* 1999;65:220–228.

Risch N, Merikangas K. The future of genetic studies of complex human diseases. *Science* 1996;273:1516–1517.

Rothman KJ, Greenland S. Modern Epidemiology. Philadelphia: Lippincott-Raven, 1998.

Sawcer S, Maranian M, Setakis E, et al. A whole genome screen for linkage disequilibrium in multiple sclerosis confirms disease associations with regions previously linked to susceptibility. *Brain* 2002;125:1337–1347.

Slager SL, Huang J, Vieland J. Effect of allelic heterogeneity on the power of the transmission disequilibrium test. *Genet Epidemiol* 2000;18:143–156.

Slooter AJ, Cruts M, Kalmijn S, et al. Risk estimates of dementia by apolipoprotein E genotypes from a population-based incidence study: the Rotterdam Study. *Arch Neurol* 1998;55:964–968.

Slooter AJ, van Duijn CM. Genetic epidemiology of Alzheimer's disease. *Epidemiol Rev* 1997;1:107–119.

Speer MC. Basic concepts in genetics. In: Haines J, Pericak-Vance MA, et al., eds. Approaches to Gene Mapping in Complex Human Diseases. Wiley-Liss, 1998, pp 17–49.

Tabor HK, Risch NJ, Myers RM. Opinion: candidate-gene approaches for studying complex genetic traits: practical considerations. *Nat Rev Genet* 2002;3:391–397.

Van Broeckhoven C, Backhovens H, Cruts M, et al. Mapping of a gene predisposing to early-onset Alzheimer's disease to chromosome 14q24.3. *Nat Genet* 1992;2:335–339.

van Ommen GJ. Commentary on the current role of human genetics in health care. *Cytogenet Cell Genet* 1999;86:140–141.

van Ommen GJ, Bakker E, Den Dunnen JT. The human genome and the future of diagnostics, treatment, and prevention. *Lancet* 1999; 354(Suppl I):5–10.

Wacholder S, Rothman N, Caporaso N. Population stratification in epidemiologic studies of common genetic variants and cancer: quantification of bias. *J Natl Cancer Inst* 2000;92:1151–1158.

Wang DG, Fau JB, Siao CJ, et al. Large-scale identification, mapping, and genotyping of single-nucleotide polymorphisms in the human genome. *Science* 1998;280:1077–1082.

Whittemore AS, Nelson LM. Study design in genetic epidemiology: theoretical and practical considerations. *J Natl Cancer Inst Monogr* 1999;26:61–69.

Zhao LP, Hsu L, Davidov O, et al. Population-based family study designs: an interdisciplinary research framework for genetic epidemiology. *Genet Epidemiol* 1997;14:365–388.

5

Alzheimer's Disease and Vascular Dementia

AMY BORENSTEIN GRAVES

Dementia is an acquired, persistent loss of intellectual abilities that includes significant impairments in memory and in at least one other sphere of mental activity. This chapter explores the frequency with which dementing illnesses, particularly the most common forms of dementia (Alzheimer's disease and vascular dementia), occur in populations, their distributions by personal characteristics, and what is known about their causes and potential protective factors.

At least half of the dementias, and some estimate close to 70% (Breteler et al. 1992; Graves and Kukull 1994), are caused by Alzheimer's disease (AD). Dementia occurs only rarely as a result of vascular lesions alone (Snowdon and Markesbery 1999), around 2%–3%, but occurs more frequently in combination with AD (10%–20%) (Meyer et al. 1988; Galasko et al. 1994). The two disorders overlap considerably: between 18% and 46% of dementia cases share both Alzheimer and vascular lesions (Tomlinson et al. 1968; Launer 2002). This overlap increases with age (Snowdon et al. 1997).

More than 70 disease states can result in the clinical characteristics of dementia (for a more detailed discussion of the types and causes of dementia, the reader is referred to Cummings and Benson 1992; Morris 1994). Table 5–1 shows the many etiologies of dementia. Dementia can be one symptom of diseases that have other clinical and pathologic features (e.g., Parkinson's disease [PD], Huntington's disease [HD], multiple sclerosis), or it can be a distinct syndrome for which a specific cause is known (e.g., slow viruses, medications, toxicants, trauma, anoxia, neoplasms). In a small percentage of cases, dementia may be treatable and reversible (as in hypothyroidism, vitamin B_{12} deficiency, or medication-induced dementia).

Clinical and Pathologic Features of Alzheimer's Disease and Accuracy of Clinical Diagnosis

The initial symptoms of AD involve difficulties in remembering recent events and in learning new material. Language and math-

Table 5–1 Taxonomy of the Major Causes of Dementia

Cortical Dementias

Alzheimer's disease (AD)
Pick's disease and other frontal lobe dementias

Subcortical Dementias

Extrapyramidal syndromes

Parkinson's disease
Huntington's disease
Progressive supranuclear palsy
Wilson's disease
Spinocerebellar degenerations
Idiopathic basal ganglia calcification
Amyotrophic lateral sclerosis/parkinsonism-dementia complex on Guam (ALS/PDC)
Normal-pressure hydrocephalus
Dementia syndrome of depression

White matter diseases

Multiple sclerosis
HIV/AIDS encephalopathy

Vascular dementias

Lacunar state
Binswanger's disease

Combined Cortical and Subcortical Dementias

Multi-infarct dementias

Slow virus dementias

Creutzfeldt-Jakob disease
Neurosyphilis/paresis
Generalized Lewy body disease

Toxic and metabolic encephalopathies

Systemic illnesses
Endocrinopathies
Deficiency states
Medication intoxication
Heavy metal exposures
Alcoholic dementia
Industrial dementias (solvents, insecticides, carbon monoxide, etc)

Other dementia syndromes

Post-traumatic
Postanoxic
Neoplastic

Adapted with permission from Cummings JL and Benson DF. A Clinical Approach, 2nd edition. Boston: Butterworth-Heineman, 1992.

ematical ability (such as balancing a checkbook) as well as judgment may also be diminished. As AD progresses, individuals experience impairment in remote memory and may lose purposeful movement (apraxia), language (aphasia), and the ability to carry out everyday activities. Finally, individuals may become mute and incontinent, have seizures, and lose their abilities to walk, feed themselves, and recognize close relatives.

The clinical diagnosis of AD is based on criteria such as the *Diagnostic and Statistical Manual of Mental Disorders,* 4th ed. (DSM-IV) (American Psychiatric Association 1994; previous versions exist) and the National Institute of Neurological and Communication Diseases and Stroke/Alzheimer's Disease and Related Disorders Association (NINCDS-ADRDA) (McKhann et al. 1984). The clinical evaluation consists of a history (most commonly from an informant), mental status testing, and physical and neurological examinations. A blood test can exclude dementias due to causes such as deficiency states, medication abuse, or syphilis. Neuroimaging, with computed tomography (CT) or magnetic resonance imaging (MRI), can exclude obvious brain tumors and vascular disorders. A consensus committee of neurologists, geriatricians, internists, and/or neuropsychologists weighs the evidence and decides whether AD is the most likely diagnosis. A clinical diagnosis of AD is not definitive and must be supplemented with evidence of neuropathologic signs at autopsy. The hallmark of the neuropathology of AD is the presence of neuritic plaques and neurofibrillary tangles in the brain (Mirra and Gearing 1994). Neuritic plaques are extracellular and consist of abnormal accumulation of β/A4-amyloid in the neuropil. Neurofibrillary tangles are fibrillar structures inside the neuron that occupy the cell body and apical dendrites. Importantly, tangles are not specific for AD. They are found in cognitively normal and in mildly impaired persons in the entorhinal cortex, and are present in other neurodegenerative conditions such as dementia pugilistica and amytrophic lateral sclerosis–parkinsonism dementia complex (ALS-PDC) of Guam. Neuropil threads (individual thickened neurites distinct from plaques) are also seen in AD pathology; the density of these threads appears to be better correlated with cognitive function than either plaques or tangles (Mirra and Gearing 1994). The degree of synaptic loss has also been reported to correlate well with severity of cognitive decline (DeKosky and Scheff 1990; Terry et al. 1991). Nerve cell loss has been shown to occur in AD with up to a 60% reduction (Mann 1985) in large neurons; in the hippocampus, Ball (1977) reported a 47% decrease in hippocampal neurons.

The accuracy of the clinical diagnosis is evaluated by comparison to the neuropathologic diagnosis. The positive predictive value (PPV) of the clinical diagnosis for the neuropathologic diagnosis is quite high (80%–90%) (Corey-Bloom et al. 1995), but varies depending on where the diagnosis is made (e.g., at a specialized memory disorder/Alzheimer clinic, the PPV will be higher than in general medical practice) and which clinical and neuropathologic criteria are used. In one study from the San Diego Alzheimer's Disease Research Center, the PPV for the diagnosis of AD (using NINCDS-ADRDA clinical and Khachaturian neuropathological criteria [Khachaturian 1985]) was 89.3% (Galasko et al. 1994).

Neuropathologic studies are complicated by the bias inherent in autopsied samples. A case of clinical AD seen at an Alzheimer center may be more likely to receive an autopsy than one seen in general practice. Additionally, the proportion of persons who have clinical AD who never receive a diagnosis may be substantial (Ross et al. 1997), and the proportion who are clinically but never pathologically diagnosed is also high.

Example 5–1 One study that is not biased with regard to autopsy donation is the Nun Study (Snowdon et al. 1997). At study inception, each nun agreed to be evaluated every year and to donate her brain upon death. This study evaluated the false-negative rate, or the proportion of persons who do not present with dementia during life who are found to meet neuropathologic criteria. Table 5–2 shows results from the study (Snowdon et al. 1997). Remarkably, 19/61 or 31% of the nuns who met neuropathologic criteria for AD were not demented prior to death (Mortimer 1997). In four other studies, the false-negative rate ranged between 10% and 67% (Blessed et al. 1968; Crystal et al. 1988; Katzman et al. 1988; Morris et al. 1996). Factors that may preserve mental function and prevent clinical expression in the face of disease pathology will be discussed later.

Clinical and Pathologic Features of Vascular Dementia

Vascular dementia (VaD) may result either from multiple discrete infarcts (so-called multi-infarct dementia) or from dementing syndromes that have cerebrovascular origins, such as diffuse subcortical white matter disease (Geldmacher and Whitehouse 1997). Because of these different vascular pathologies, no single set of clinical criteria developed for VaD has become widely accepted (Chui et al. 1992; Roman et al. 1993; American Psychiatric Association 1994), making epidemiologic studies of VaD challenging.

To satisfy the clinical criteria for VaD, patients must fulfill criteria for dementia and demonstrate evidence of cerebrovascular disease. Usually, such evidence is

Table 5–2 Results from the Nun Study*

	AD Neuropathology	No AD Neuropathology	Total
Demented	42	3	45
Not demented	19	38	57
Total	61	41	102

*Sensitivity = 69%; specificity = 93%; positive predictive value = 93%; negative predictive value = 67%; false-negative = 31%; false-positive rate = 6.7%.
Source: Snowdon et al. (1997).

gleaned from clinical information and/or neuroimaging. Some sets of criteria also require that a temporal relationship exist between the infarct(s) and the onset of dementia (Roman et al. 1993); others do not specify this criterion (Chui et al. 1992). However, it has become widely recognized that dementia may result from subclinical cerebrovascular disease that is evident only upon neuropathologic examination of the brain and/or quantitation of white matter hyperintensities on MRI (Snowdon et al. 1997). It has been estimated that 50% of cases attributed to VaD are actually mixed with AD (Galasko et al. 1994).

In the case of overt vascular events, the timing of the stroke relative to the onset of cognitive deficits must be carefully assessed. Proxy informants may have difficulty recalling the timing of vascular events relative to the onset of cognitive deficits, making it hard to assess causality. Using the most common criteria for VaD, the sensitivity of the clinical diagnosis vis-à-vis the neuropathologic diagnosis has been shown to range between 0.20 for the National Institute of Neurological Disorders and Stroke and Association Internationale pour la Recherche et l'Enseignment en Neurosciences (NINDS-AIREN) criteria (Roman et al. 1993) and 0.70 using the Alzheimer's Disease Diagnostic and Treatment Centers (ADDTC) criteria (Chui et al. 1992); specificity ranges from 0.78 to 0.93, respectively (Gold et al. 2002). However, these figures do not take into account the more prevalent and subclinical type of cerebrovascular events, namely those characterized by multiple or strategic lacunar infarcts and diffuse white matter lesions linked with small vessel disease (Pantoni and Inzitari 2002).

Alzheimer's Disease and Vascular Dementia: Are They Really Two Distinct Disorders?

Because of the difficulties involved in the clinical diagnoses of AD and VaD, the fact that these two disorders often coexist, and that overlap is further accentuated with in-

creasing age, diagnostic misclassification is an important issue in the epidemiology of dementia. The combination of vascular components and Alzheimer-like symptoms may result in a final clinical diagnosis of AD only, VaD only, or mixed (AD + VaD) dementia. Thus, depending on the study's methods—screening criteria, country in which it was conducted (medical culture and stigma of the dementia diagnosis), age distribution, inclusion of institutionalized patients, as well as the specific clinical criteria being used—results from different studies may not be comparable. Furthermore, in recent years, research on risk factors for AD and VaD has consistently implicated cardiovascular risk factors, such as atherosclerosis, diabetes, hypertension, and homocysteinemia as factors associated with both conditions. Because of the difficulties in distinguishing between AD and VaD, and because they share many risk factors and clinical features, this chapter does not separate the discussions of AD and VaD, but presents information about both conditions.

Descriptive Epidemiology

It is widely accepted that the prevalence of dementia and AD rises exponentially with age, with rates doubling every 5.1 years (Jorm et al. 1987). In the twentieth century, mortality rates in developed countries declined sharply, leading to a large increase in the population over age 65, and an even larger increase in those 85 or older. This trend will continue in the twenty-first century. Because the frequency of dementia increases exponentially with age, many have predicted an epidemic of dementia. However, along with increasing longevity, factors related to being able to tolerate neuropathological brain lesions without showing clinical symptomatology (brain reserve, see Risk and Protective Factors for Disease Expression, below) have become more common, namely increases in head/brain size, IQ, height, fetal and childhood nutrition, and socioeconomic status (including higher education). At the same time, stroke rates in industrialized nations have declined. Thus, while dementia and AD will play an important role in the first half of this century, the dementia "epidemic" may not be as extensive as has been forecasted (Evans 1990; Mortimer 1997).

Methodologic Challenges

Methodologic issues in the descriptive epidemiology of AD and VaD render comparisons between studies and inferences to populations difficult. Among the challenges are the identification of representative populations, variable participation rates, the need to include institutionalized as well as community-dwelling populations, the nonstandardized use of cognitive tests to screen for dementia, and the complexities of the diagnostic process itself as well as case definitions. Also hampering the quantification of prevalence and incidence rates are small numbers of elderly, particularly in the very old (90+) age stratum. The insidious nature of the clinical presentation of AD has made accurate dating of the age at onset as well as the distinction between prevalent and incident cases challenging. In addition, the common co-occurrence of strokes in old age can contribute to difficulties in making an accurate differential diagnosis.

Although many epidemiologic studies strive to obtain pathologic confirmation of clinical dementia diagnoses, the acquisition of brains for postmortem examination depends on the type of population studied (referral/memory disorder clinic–based vs. population-based) as well the participants' religious and cultural beliefs. The lack of autopsy confirmation necessitates confidence in clinical diagnostic criteria, which are frequently unreliable for dementia subtypes. A final problem in comparing prevalence and incidence rates across studies is the lack of adjustment for differences in age distributions. Because age is such a strong risk factor for dementia and AD, age-specific rates must use narrow age categories (maximum 5-year groups) to ensure comparability; the use of wider categories (e.g., 10 years) almost guarantees confounding by age. Differences in survival rates within age groups further render prevalence ratios incomparable; for example, comparing men with women is problematic since women live longer and also live longer with disease. The comparison of overall crude rates within and between studies should therefore be interpreted with caution.

Multiphase designs are critical for complete ascertainment of dementia cases in communities; however, these designs are difficult to implement and may underestimate disease rates. In the first phase of such a study, defined populations undergo a cognitive screening test to identify individuals who may have dementia. Two methods may be used after initial screening: (1) those who fail the screen receive a battery of clinical and neuropsychological evaluations and are subsequently diagnosed. This method will underestimate prevalence/incidence rates because false negatives will be missed; or (2) a complex sample of those who do and do not fail the screen are selected for a full clinical evaluation, but this sampling of screen negatives is expensive and a large sample must be taken to provide reliable estimates (Edland et al. 1999).

Prevalence and Incidence

Example 5–2 In 1989, a study in the *Journal of the American Medical Association* reported higher rates of AD in a community population than had previously been published (Evans et al. 1989). From this study, an extrapolation was made to the U.S. population that 4 million Americans are affected with AD. Subsequently, this number has been used to represent the burden of AD in this country. However, in 1998, the General Accounting Office (U.S. General Accounting Office [GAO] 1998) made a report to the Secretary of Health and Human Services, in which 18 prevalence studies were reviewed. This report estimated that 1.9 million Americans aged 65 and over were afflicted with AD. This lower number was supported in another analysis (Brookmeyer et al. 1998), which estimated that

2.32 million Americans had AD (range 1.09–4.58). The study by Evans et al. (1989) included all levels of clinical severity in their case definition and did not adhere strictly to the NINCDS/ADRDA research criteria; thus their prevalence ratios may have been overestimated.

Although age-specific prevalence ratios of dementia vary substantially among studies, overall prevalence is about 2% between ages 65 and 74, 8% from 75 to 84, and 30% for ages 85 and over. Approximately 5%–8% of persons aged 65 and over have dementia (Graves and Kukull 1994), although studies in Asia tend to report lower rates, and some studies (Evans et al. 1989) report rates closer to 10% (Graves et al. 1996a). Approximately 60%–80% of all dementia patients reside in the community and the remainder are institutionalized. Of all institutionalized persons in the United States, roughly 50% are demented (Graves and Kukull 1994). The clinical course typically lasts between 3 and 20 years, with a mean of about 7 years; but this estimate is imprecise because age at onset is difficult to pinpoint accurately. Persons with AD have a 1.4- to 3-fold excess risk of mortality (Aronson et al. 1991; Evans et al. 1991). An estimated 7.1% of all deaths in the United States in 1995 were due to AD, tying AD with cerebrovascular diseases as the third leading cause of death that year (Ewbank 1999). Alzheimer's disease is estimated to cost the United States $112 billion annually (in year 2000 dollars; Katzman and Fox, 1999).

Incidence and Age. The age-specific incidence curves for dementia and AD have been shown to be equivalent (Gao et al. 1998). Figure 5–1 shows age-specific inci-

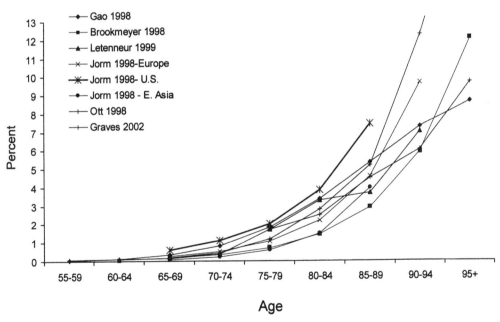

Figure 5–1 Annual incidence rates, in percent, for dementia and AD. In Gao et al. (1998), rates are estimated from a meta-analysis of 12 studies of dementia. In Brookmeyer et al. (1998), rates are for AD and are smoothed for four U.S. studies. In Letenneur et al. (1999), rates are for AD among women (no overall statistics are given). In Jorm and Jolley (1998), rates from a meta-analysis of 23 studies are summarized for AD (mild +) from three parts of the world: Europe, the United States, and East Asia, and in Ott et al. (1998) rates (in percent) were calculated for both sexes for dementia. In Graves (2002) rates are shown for Japanese Americans.

dence rates for dementia and AD. Despite the use of disparate methodologies for case identification and definition, the trends for incidence mirror those for prevalence, with rates increasing steeply with age.

There has been much discussion as to whether incidence rates plateau in the oldest age group (90 and over) (Mortimer et al. 1981; Brookmeyer et al. 1998). Although most studies report a continuing increase in incidence through the tenth decade of life, few data are available in the very old age strata and rates may be unreliable. One study (Gao et al. 1998) showed that, while the incidence rate continues to climb with age, the increase in rate slows with age: for every 5-year increase in age, both dementia and AD incidence rates tripled before age 65, doubled between age 65 and 75, and increased by only 1.5 times after age 85. Data from the Nun Study demonstrate that, while the prevalence of AD pathology declines in the tenth decade, the rate with which sisters develop the clinical syndrome of dementia continues to rise (Mortimer et al. 2001).

The development of dementia may be determined by an individual trajectory or rate of decline, and this rate may be steeper among persons who have a single gene or a susceptibility gene and more gradual for persons without genetic or other pathologic predisposition (such as head injury) (see Fig. 5–2). The alternative possibility is that only those persons who are genetically or otherwise susceptible to the pathology are destined to get AD, and other individuals will not be susceptible to getting either the pathologic or clinical disease, no matter how long they live.

Age at Onset. Alzheimer's disease was historically distinguished by age into "early-onset" cases (usually ≤65) and "late-onset" cases (>65). As in many other disorders, genetic factors appeared to be more important in early-onset cases. Today, single gene mutations are known to produce early-onset AD (Price et al. 1998). The ε4 variant of apolipoprotein E (ApoE), a

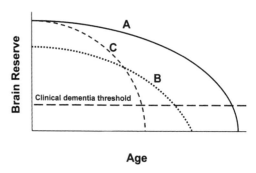

Figure 5–2 Solid line (*A*) represents the trajectory for most individuals in the population who do not develop dementia or AD in their lifetime. In this example, neurons are lost at a slow rate over the life course and the clinical dementia threshold is reached only after death from another cause. Dotted line (*B*) represents the trajectory for individuals who have the same rate of neuron loss and accumulation of Alzheimer lesions and contributing causes for dementia as (*A*) but have less brain reserve to start (poorer development of neurons in early life and interconnectivity). Dashed line (*C*) represents the trajectory of a person with the same relative brain reserve capacity as (*A*) but who has a genetic or other predisposition to dementia/AD.

cholesterol-carrying protein, leads to an earlier clinical onset of AD (see section on Risk Factors for Pathology, below). The age at onset of clinical dementia/AD is likely dependent upon the trajectory of brain reserve (Fig. 5–2), which in turn is related to several risk factors discussed below.

Gender. Many incidence studies have found that women are at increased risk for AD (Li et al. 1991; Bachman et al. 1993; Kokmen et al. 1993; Letenneur et al. 1994; Paykel et al. 1994; Yoshitake et al. 1995; Aevarsson and Skoog 1996). However, some of these studies failed to find a statistically significant association or stated that their results were 'suggestive' without providing statistical power or significance levels. Other studies (Hebert et al. 1992; Johansson and Zarit 1995; McDowell et al. 1998; Rocca et al. 1998) have found no effect of gender on the risk of dementia or AD. Recent studies (Fratiglioni et al. 1997;

Gao et al. 1998; Jorm and Jolley 1998; Ott et al. 1998; Letenneur et al. 1999; Ruitenberg et al. 2001) demonstrate that women are at higher risk than men for AD in the oldest age groups. Lower education, lower occupational status, smaller head circumference, and lower circulating levels of estrogens may place women at higher risk for manifesting clinical symptoms of dementia and AD, even though the two sexes may be at equal risk for developing AD pathology.

Geography and Ethnicity. Despite the use of different methodologies, most studies have reported similar overall rates of dementia. However, the relative proportions attributed to AD and vascular causes have differed markedly (Graves et al. 1996a). Studies performed in East Asia have typically attributed 30%–60% of the dementias to vascular etiologies, and approximately half as many to AD (Jorm 1990; Graves et al. 1996a). In the West, approximately 50%–75% of the dementias are attributed to AD. Some of the reduced risk for AD in the East has been proposed to be due to a lower population frequency of the apolipoprotein E-ε4 (ApoE-ε4) allele (about 9%–10%; Davignon et al. 1988).

Example 5–3 Since the clinical diagnoses of AD and VaD are in part subjective, differences in diagnostic styles across cultures could lead to a difference in diagnoses, with VaD being a more acceptable diagnosis than AD in the East. These opposing trends have led to a cross-national study of dementia and its subtypes among Japanese living in Hi-

roshima, Japan; Honolulu, Hawaii; and Seattle-King County, WA (the Ni-Hon-Sea Project). Age- and gender-specific prevalence ratios from these studies (Table 5–3) (White et al. 1996; Graves et al. 1996a; Yamada et al. 1999) show that, using standardized methodology, the proportions attributable to AD did not differ to the extent seen in studies in which the methodologies were nonstandardized. However, since prevalence is confounded by duration of disease, incidence rates from these studies will be more informative for comparing risks of AD and VaD.

Another methodologically standardized cross-cultural study that compared African Americans in Indianapolis, Indiana, with black Africans in Ibadan, Nigeria, reported that the overall prevalence of dementia was 3.6 times higher in the U.S. black sample than in the Nigerian sample: 8.29% (95% confidence interval [CI] 7.1–9.4) vs. 2.29% (95% CI 1.2–3.4) (Hendrie et al. 1995a). The low prevalence in Nigerian blacks occurred despite a twofold higher population frequency of the ApoE-ε4 allele (30%) (Hendrie et al. 1995b) compared with other populations (15%) (Davignon et al. 1988). Although previous studies reported a strong association between ApoE-ε4 and dementia/AD in the Indianapolis African-American sample (Hendrie et al. 1995b), there was no relationship between the presence of ApoE-ε4 and AD in the Nigerian sample (Osuntokun et al. 1995).

Tang et al. (1998) followed 1079 Medicare recipients for 5 years and found that the cumulative risk for AD to age 90, adjusting for education and gender, was 4.4

Table 5–3 Prevalence Ratios of Alzheimer's Disease in the Ni-Hon-Sea Project, by Age and Gender

Age (years)	Hiroshima men	Honolulu men	Seattle men	Hiroshima women	Seattle women
65–69	0.5	—	0.5	0.2	0.9
70–74	0	0.5	0.9	1.4	1.7
75–79	2.5	1.7	2.4	2.6	4.1
80–84	4.8	5.9	3.8	1.9	8.6
85–89	10.5	15.2	15.7	26.6	18.5
90–94	27.3	—	19.6	22.7	42.1

times higher for African Americans (95% CI 2.3–8.6) and 2.3 times higher for Hispanics (95% CI 1.2–4.3) compared with whites. The presence of the ApoE-ε4 allele did not predict AD in African Americans or in Hispanics (RR = 1.0 and 1.1, respectively), while in whites it did (relative risk [RR] = 2.5; 95% CI 1.1–6.4). A meta-analytic case–control study of the association between the ε4 allele and AD (Farrer et al. 1997) showed inconsistent relationships in African American and Hispanic populations. These studies have incited interest in the potential role played by cholesterol in the association between ApoE-ε4 and AD (Jarvik et al. 1995; Chandra and Pandav 1998).

Analytic Epidemiology of Alzheimer's Disease/Dementia

Methodologic Issues

With the evolution of the epidemiology of dementia/AD from case–control studies to prospective cohort studies has come a new set of methodologic dilemmas. Early case–control studies of AD included only cases of "pure" AD; thus atherosclerotic risk factors such as hypertension were excluded from discovery by study design. Many of these studies had small sample sizes and limited statistical power to detect more subtle risk factors. They also relied on proxy respondent reports of exposures and on estimates of the year of onset of AD. Since dementia and AD occur late in life, the relationship of the proxy respondent to the patient (e.g., spouse or child) greatly affects the accuracy of exposure reports. Although spouses are usually considered the "best" reporter of adult exposures, they do not always provide the most valid and reliable data, especially if the marriage was recent and/or the exposures occurred in the distant past. The shift to prospective cohort studies has helped to clarify the role of factors such as cardiovascular risk factors and education; however, these studies are hampered by adequately defining population cohorts, eliminating prevalent cases to follow nondemented cohorts through time,

and differential attrition over the follow-up period. Several characteristics of incidence studies of dementia and AD may bias observed relative risks toward the null value in comparison with prevalence studies, as we shall see in the next example.

Example 5–4 Studies that aim to characterize incidence must first adequately detect and eliminate prevalent cases from the cohort. Since AD is an insidious disease, there will always be individuals who qualify as "nondemented" in a cohort because they do not meet clinical criteria for the disease at the prevalence phase (baseline) but nevertheless harbor the disease (Kawas et al. 1994; Plassman et al. 1995a). It is likely then, that individuals who during follow-up will become incident cases, already have minor memory loss at baseline, and therefore may report exposures with some degree of misclassification. In fact, some studies that have found risk factors for prevalent disease that are otherwise well established in the AD literature have been unable to replicate these findings using incident series. This seems counterintuitive, since all epidemiology textbooks state that incidence is more desirable than prevalence when studying etiologic factors. This problem may underlie disparate findings in the Canadian Study of Health and Aging (CSHA). From their prevalence data, the odds ratio (OR) for AD associated with a family history of dementia was strong (OR = 2.6, 95% CI 1.5–4.5) (Canadian Study 1994). In their incidence data, the relative risk (RR) was 1.02 (95% CI 0.6–1.8) (Lindsay et al. 2002). In a meta-analysis of four incidence studies in Europe European Studies of Dementia (EURODEM), 528 cases of dementia were identified in 28,768 person-years of follow-up time (Launer et al. 1999). The RR for dementia associated with a family history of dementia was, for one first-degree family member, 0.9 (95% CI 0.6–1.3) and for two family members, 1.4 (95% CI 0.8–2.7). Both CHSA and EURODEM acknowledge that family history is a well-known and well-characterized risk factor for dementia and AD. Both discuss their null findings for family history in light of deficiencies of case–control studies, i.e., that proxy respondents for cases must have overreported family history of dementia, and/or proxy respondents for controls underreported such a family history. The possibility that self-reports of family history are biased in incidence studies was not considered but is equally likely as an explanation for the disappearance of this risk factor in prospectively collected data.

Risk Factors for Alzheimer's Disease/Dementia

Risk Factors for Pathology

Genetic Causes. One of the earliest and most robust risk factors identified for AD is a family history of dementia (Heston et al. 1981; Graves and Kukull 1994). The etiology of AD clearly has important genetic origins, and the lifetime risk of developing AD likely involves a large genetic component (Breitner and Welsh 1995). While some genetic mechanisms have been uncovered (Table 5–4), others are suggestive (Reynolds et al. 1999a) and still others remain to be found (Breitner et al. 1995).

A family history increases the risk for AD two- to fourfold, with risk decreasing with increasing age and increasing with the number of affected relatives (van Duijn et al. 1991a). The definition of what constitutes a family history has been problematic in studies of familial aggregation. Large, long-lived families contribute more information than families with few members; studies have also used differing definitions of how many relatives must be affected and how many generations must be considered as having a positive family history of dementia (Graves and Kukull 1994). Familial aggregation connotes more than just genetic aggregation; it also involves early-life exposures. Thus, studies of family history may overestimate the genetic contribution to disease. A type of design that is able to tease out the environmental from the genetic variation is a study of twins reared apart versus those reared together (Lichtenstein et al. 1993). It is clear that in some very rare forms of AD (approximately 1%–5% of all AD cases) (Cummings et al. 1998; Roses 1998), single gene mutations

Table 5–4 Risk Factors, by Type: Pathologic and Disease Expression

Risk factors for pathology	RISK FACTORS FOR DISEASE EXPRESSION				Protective factors
	Early-life brain development	Reserve remaining at any given age	Anti-cognitive reserve		
• Chromosome 21 βAPP mutations	• Head circumference/ brain size	• Atherosclerotic risk factors	• Achieved education/ income/IQ		• Nonsteroidal anti-inflammatory drugs
• Chromosome 14 Presenilin 1 mutations	• Height	• Exposures to neurotoxins			• Hormone replacement therapy
	• IQ	• Smoking			
• Chromosome 1 Presenilin 2 mutations	• Linguistic ability	• Alcohol			• Antioxidants
• Chromosome 19 ApoE-ε4 polymorphism		• Mental stimulation (e.g., occupation)			
• Other genes as yet undiscovered (making family history a major risk factor)					
• Down's syndrome					
• Head injury*					

*Perhaps only in combination with one or more ApoE-ε4 alleles.

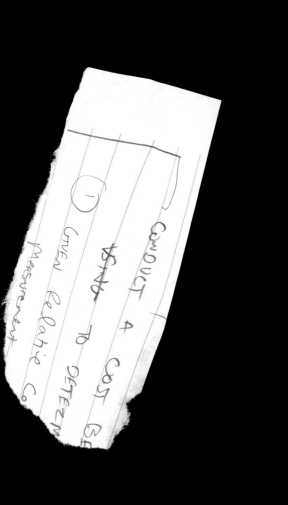

occur (chromosomes 1, 14, and 21, with 1 being the most common (Reynolds et al. 1999a). These forms of disease usually affect individuals in their 40s and 50s (for reviews, see Lendon et al. 1997; Price et al. 1998; Reynolds et al. 1999a). Pedigree studies suggest that transmission of these mutations in very early–onset AD is consistent with a 100% penetrant autosomal dominant model, implying that everyone with such mutations will express the disease if they live long enough. Mutations on chromosomes 1, 14, and 21 lead to rapid deposition of Aβ in the brain. Other than the ApoE-ε4 allele, gene association studies of late-onset sporadic cases have not been consistent (Combarros et al. 2002).

Down's syndrome. Patients with Down's syndrome (DS) are known to express clinical AD beyond the age of 40 and to have Alzheimer pathology on autopsy (Geller and Potter 1999). The three copies of chromosome 21 possessed by DS patients are thought to account for an abnormally high deposition of Aβ (Reynolds et al. 1999a).

The heritability of AD is estimated at between 0.28 and 0.74 (Reynolds et al. 1999a). Disparities in age at onset within monozygotic twin pairs (Breitner et al. 1995) suggest that some of the inherited risk can be modulated by environmental risk factors or factors that inhibit the clinical appearance of dementia/AD (see Risk and Protective Factors for Disease Expression, below).

Since the first report of the predisposing genetic locus on chromosome 19 (Strittmatter et al. 1993) and the subsequent demonstration of a dose–response relationship between the number of ApoE-ε4 alleles and age at onset of AD (Corder et al. 1993), many studies have reproduced the association between the ApoE-ε4 allele and AD (Breitner et al. 1995; Reynolds et al. 1999a; Tol et al. 1999). This association is specific to late-onset AD. The proportion of AD cases with one or two ApoE-ε4 alleles is between 30% and 40%, while it is about 11%–15% among controls (Farrer et al. 1997). However, estimates of risk derived

from clinic-based samples, which are enriched with family history–positive patients, may be overestimates (Mullan et al. 1996). It also has been proposed that ApoE-ε4 does not influence whether one gets AD, but only when it begins (Breitner et al. 1998). Additionally, women may be at a higher risk than men if they possess an ApoE-ε4 allele (Farrer et al. 1995). However, this has not been firmly established (Ghebremedhin et al. 2001). ApoE-ε4 status also may interact with age (the effect declines with age; Jarvik 1997) and with other environmental risk factors, such as head injury and smoking (see below). Tol et al. (1999) have proposed that between 12% and 17% of AD is explained by the ApoE-ε4 allele, although other estimates are as high as 40%–50% (Combarros et al. 2002). Farrer et al. (1995) reported that more than half of individuals possessing one or more ε4 alleles failed to develop AD in their lifetime. Thus, ApoE testing for genetic counseling is not recommended, although ε4 status could be used as a diagnostic adjunct (Lendon et al. 1997). Mohs et al. (1987) have shown that by age 90, the risk to relatives of AD probands is around 50%. This suggests an autosomal dominant mechanism with full penetrance only in the nineties. The etiology of AD is certain to involve a complex interaction of genetic and environmental factors.

Head Injury. Head injury was found to be a risk factor for AD in the early case–control studies conducted in the 1980s (Mortimer et al. 1991) with an OR of around 1.8 (95% CI 1.3–2.7). Studies using a prospective design generally have supported this finding (Schofield et al. 1997a; Nemetz et al. 1999), although some studies failed to demonstrate an association (Launer et al. 1999). Nemetz (1999) found that traumatic head injury does not increase the risk for acquiring AD but is a risk factor for earlier onset of the disease. Two studies have suggested that ApoE genotype may interact with head injury in a multiplicative manner (Mayeux et al. 1995; Jordan et al. 1997). Another study reported a trend, which was not statistically significant (O'Meara et al. 1997). Lastly, a large meta-analysis of case–control studies with 2233 probands with probable or definite AD compared with 14,668 first-degree family member controls showed an OR of 9.9 (95% CI 6.5–15.1) for head injury with loss of consciousness. However, when stratified by the ApoE-ϵ4 allele, this study found an elevated OR for AD and head injury in the ApoE-ϵ4 negatives (OR = 3.3) that was not present in the ApoE-ϵ4 positives (Guo et al. 2000). Therefore, the interaction between head injury and ApoE-ϵ4 necessitates further work. Mechanisms by which head injury can contribute to AD risk include increased β-amyloid deposition following a head injury (McKenzie et al. 1994); increased synthesis of ApoE after injury; and close binding of ApoE-ϵ4 to the β-amyloid peptide (Strittmatter et al. 1993). Wisniewski and Frangione (1992) have proposed that ApoE-ϵ4 chaperones β-amyloid into brain cells. Graham et al. (1999) have found that Aβ aggregates in the brain among approximately 30% of patients who die after a single episode of severe head injury, and that ϵ4 is overrepresented in head-injured patients showing Aβ pathology. This evidence is the first to link genetic susceptibility to AD with an environmental risk factor.

Risk and Protective Factors for Disease Expression

As early as 1966, Roth et al. noted that dementia does not usually occur until a critical number of Alzheimer lesions or critical volume of brain softening (secondary to strokes) is evident. This theory has been further developed by Mortimer (Mortimer 1980, 1995, 1997; Mortimer and Graves 1993). He has proposed that the clinical expression of AD requires two elements: (1) a propensity, which may be largely genetic, to accumulate AD lesions over the life span at a rate sufficient to meet neuropathologic criteria at death, and (2) the attainment of a critical threshold of "brain reserve" be-

low which normal cognitive function can not be sustained (Mortimer 1995). Three scenarios, which differ in the initial level and the rate of loss of brain reserve, are shown in Figure 5–2. Dementia/AD may be prevented either through slowing of the rate of accumulation of Alzheimer lesions or through preservation of brain reserve. Factors that enhance brain reserve (good childhood environment and nutrition, adult mental stimulation) and interventions that interrupt the cascade of events leading to clinical presentation of disease (estrogen replacement therapy, nonsteroidal anti-inflammatory drugs, anti-oxidant therapy) are promising candidates for prevention. Conversely, environmental and experiential risk factors may accelerate the accumulation of lesions and the rate of loss of brain reserve, thereby hastening the clinical onset of disease (atherosclerotic risk factors, exposures to neurotoxins).

Mortimer (1997) has proposed three types of brain reserve: (1) the number of neurons and/or the density of their interconnections in youth when the brain is fully developed (early-life brain development)—this corresponds to the difference between trajectories A and B in Figure 5–2; (2) the amount of functional brain tissue remaining at any age, which determines whether or not one is cognitively intact—this corresponds to the point at which each line (A, B, or C in Fig. 5–2) crosses the clinical dementia threshold; and (3) the collection of cognitive strategies for solving problems and taking neuropsychological tests (cognitive reserve)—this corresponds to the ability to compensate cognitively for the pathologic load of plaques and tangles. The discussion of risk and protective factors for disease expression will be divided into three sections: early-life development, reserve remaining at any age, and cognitive reserve (Table 5–4).

Early-Life Development. Many studies have found that low education predicts prevalent and incident dementia and AD (Mortimer and Graves 1993; Evans et al. 1997;

Letenneur et al. 1999). Years of education are easy to measure but education is opportunistic; i.e., some individuals may be able to seek an education by virtue of their situation in childhood while others may not. Therefore, the effect of education in predicting dementia/AD may be underestimated. However, education is closely related to intelligence and other early-life factors such as childhood socioeconomic status and achieved head circumference/brain size, height, and linguistic ability.

Recent studies support the idea that early-life conditions that maximize growth in childhood and adolescence diminish or delay the clinical expression of dementia and AD. Brain growth occurs predominantly during the latter part of gestation and the first 2–3 years of life (Graves et al. 1996b) and is the major determinant of cranial growth, which is complete by age 6. Brain size is positively associated with final attained IQ (Andreasen et al. 1993).

Small head size has been associated with earlier age at onset of AD (Schofield et al. 1995) and impaired global function using the Cognitive Abilities Screening Instrument (CASI) among prevalent AD cases (Graves et al. 1996b). A threefold increased risk of AD (OR adjusted for age, education, and ethnicity: 2.9 [95% CI 1.4–6.1]) was observed with the lowest 20th percentile of head circumference (HC) in women in a population-based prevalence study; the OR for men was 2.3 (95% CI 0.6–9.8) (Schofield et al. 1997b). Smaller HC was also associated with poor cognitive performance among nondemented individuals in a community-based study (Reynolds et al. 1999b). More recently, a population-based study showed an increased risk for AD among individuals carrying ApoE-ϵ4 allele who also had a HC in the lowest tertile in the population (hazard ratio [HR] = 14.1, 95% CI 3.0–65.2); the HR in the other three categories were as follows: ApoE-ϵ4 positive, higher two tertiles HC: OR 3.9, 95% CI 1.1–14.1; ApoE-ϵ4 negative, lowest tertile HC: HR = 1.9, 95% CI 0.4–8.1; and ApoE-ϵ4 negative, higher two

tertiles HC: HR = 1.0, implying multiplicative interaction between the lowest tertile of HC and the presence of the ApoE-ϵ4 allele (Borenstein Graves et al. 2001). Subsequently, Edland et al. (2002) were unable to replicate these findings in a case–control study from the Mayo clinic in Rochester, Minnesota. The mean education level was not given in this study, but the educational levels are typically high in the population served by the Mayo Clinic. Mortimer et al (2003) have recently shown that HC is not important when other brain reserve factors are present, such as high education levels. In their study, only those individuals with both low education and small head size were at increased risk for dementia.

Similar associations have been reported between height and AD. Abbott et al. (1998) reported a higher prevalence of AD among men who were 154 cm or shorter (4.7%) compared with taller men (2.9%).

Example 5–5 Additional support for risk of AD being set early in life comes from the Nun Study (Snowdon and Markesbery 1999). Among members of the School Sisters of Notre Dame born before 1917, 1027 nuns were invited to participate in a prospective study in which they would have annual physical evaluations and donate their brain for autopsy upon death. Of these, 66% agreed to participate. Hand-written autobiographies written at an average age of 22, as well as cognitive and neuropathologic data were available for 93 sisters. Idea density was defined as the average number of ideas expressed per 10 words in the last 10 sentences of the essay. Ideas included elementary propositions, such as a verb, adjective or adverb, or a prepositional phrase. Associations between idea density and outcomes occurring an average of 60 years later, including the Mini-Mental State Examination score and mean numbers of neurofibrillary tangles per 0.586 mm^2 in different brain regions, were reported among 93 sisters for the clinical outcome and 25 sisters with neuropathologic information. Table 5–5 shows the re-

Table 5-5 Association Between Low Idea Density (Lowest Tertile) and Neuropathologic Alzheimer's Disease Among 25 Nuns in Milwaukee and Other Convents

	MILWAUKEE CONVENT ODDS RATIO		OTHER CONVENTS ODDS RATIO		COMBINED CRUDE ODDS RATIO	
	NAD	No NAD	NAD	No NAD	NAD	No NAD
Lowest tertile idea density	5	0	4	2	9	2
Upper two tertiles idea density	0	9	1	4	1	13
Total	5	9	5	6	10	15
Odds ratio and p-value	$45/0 = \infty$ ($p < 0.001$)		$16/2 = 8$ ($p = 0.14$)		$117/2 = 58.5$ ($p < 0.001$)	

NAD, met criteria for neuropathologic Alzheimer's disease.
Source: Snowdon et al. 1996.

sults when idea density was categorized into tertiles and the outcome of whether the neuropathologic criteria for Alzheimer's disease (NAD) were satisfied on post-mortem examination of the brain. While the numbers in the combined crude table are small, it can be seen that the association between low idea density and NAD is extremely strong (OR = 58.5, $p < 0.001$). Because low idea density was so highly predictive of AD neuropathologic lesions, the authors proposed that low linguistic ability in early life may be an early expression of AD neuropathology itself and not just a factor related to decreased brain reserve.

The findings we have discussed on achieved brain/head size, height, and linguistic ability suggest that early life deprivation, in the form of poverty, poor nutrition, parental education, and occupation predispose to an earlier manifestation of dementia/AD. Mortimer et al. (1998) have shown that AD cases with a family history of AD who had a low socioeconomic status during childhood had 32 times the risk of AD compared to a group with no family history and higher socioeconomic status (95% CI 6.9–147). No association was present in those without a family history of AD, indicating that only persons who are at genetic risk for the disease may be protected.

Individuals with higher IQ in early life perform better on cognitive tests in late life (Plassman et al. 1995a). IQ has been shown to better predict incident dementia (Schmand et al. 1997) and cognitive decline

(Graves et al. 1996c) than education. Persons with higher IQ likely have more mental stimulation as adults. Mental exercise in adulthood may play a neuroprotective role (Swaab 1991). Therefore, protection conferred in childhood is likely to carry through adulthood by virtue of continued mental activity (see Cognitive Reserve, below).

Reserve Remaining at Any Age. Specific insults to the brain determine the relative amount of functional brain tissue at any age (Mortimer 1997). The risk factors that have been examined in dementia and AD include cardiovascular factors, exposure to neurotoxins such as aluminum and solvents, as well as electromagnetic fields, cigarette smoking, and alcohol consumption. Head injury also fits under this rubric, although it is followed by amyloid deposition, and has been treated here as a risk factor for pathology. Other factors may provide neuroprotection. Some examples are exposure to nonsteroidal anti-inflammatory drugs, estrogens, and antioxidants.

Cardiovascular Risk Factors. Early case–control studies of AD restricted case definitions to patients with "pure AD"; those with a vascular contribution were excluded. With community-based prospective studies, new data have emerged, demonstrating that the presence and severity of cognitive impairment in AD is affected by the presence of vascular lesions (Snowdon et al. 1997; Heyman et al. 1998).

Some convincing evidence suggests that a reduction in cardiovascular risk factors reduces the likelihood of clinically expressing dementia. In the Nun Study, nuns with no subcortical brain infarcts at autopsy who did not meet neuropathologic criteria for AD had a mean Mini-Mental Examination Score (MMSE, scored out of a maximum of 30 points) of 26 adjusted for age, time of death, and education, similar to the adjusted mean MMSE of 25 for those who had such infarcts but did not meet neuropathologic criteria. In contrast, the adjusted mean for women who met AD criteria but had no infarcts was 15, and those nuns having both AD at autopsy and subcortical infarcts had a mean MMSE of 3 (Snowdon et al. 1997). This study suggests that if AD lesions are accompanied by vascular lesions, it is much more likely that the dementia threshold will be reached.

The ApoE-ϵ4 allele is a risk factor for cardiovascular disease (Jarvik 1997). Studies have since investigated the role of cardiovascular risk factors in dementia and AD, and whether these are modified by the ϵ4 allele. Haan and colleagues (Haan et al. 1999) showed that the rate of cognitive decline was higher among persons with high systolic blood pressure, atherosclerosis of the internal carotid artery, and diabetes mellitus, and that these associations were amplified in persons with an ϵ4 allele. In another population-based study, Hofman et al. (1997) compared 284 dementia patients (207 with AD) with 1698 nondemented individuals. The odds ratios for AD were 3.0 (95% CI 1.5–6.0) in persons with severe atherosclerosis and 3.9 (95% CI 1.6–9.6) in persons who also possessed an ϵ4 allele. For vascular dementia, persons who had atherosclerosis and an ϵ4 allele incurred an estimated risk of 19.8 (95% CI 4.1–95). Midlife hyperglycemia and hypertension have also been shown to be related to cognitive decline in male twins, but these risk factors did not interact with the ϵ4 allele (Carmelli et al. 1998).

In a large, population-based study in Rotterdam, diabetes mellitus was found to predict prevalent dementia status. This association was strong among insulin-dependent diabetics (OR = 3.2, 95% CI 1.4–7.5) and strongest when vascular dementia was considered as the outcome (OR = 5.4, 95% CI 1.2–23.8) (Ott et al. 1996). In the Honolulu-Asia Aging Study (HAAS), diabetes was positively associated with incident AD (RR = 1.8, 95% CI 1.1–2.9), and individuals who also possessed an ϵ4 allele were at particularly high risk (RR = 5.5, 95% CI 2.2–13.7) (Peila et al. 2002). Individuals who were both diabetic and were ϵ4 carriers also showed a higher number of hippocampal neuritic plaques (RR = 3.0, 95% CI 1.2–7.3) and neurofibrillary tangles in the cortex (RR = 3.5, 95% CI 1.6–7.5) and hippocampus (RR = 2.5, 95% CI 1.5–3.7). In New York, a multiethnic study demonstrated that diabetes was associated with a higher incidence of AD (RR = 1.6, 95% CI 1.2–2.1). However, in the Canadian Study on Health and Aging, diabetes was associated with vascular dementia (RR = 2.0, 95% CI 1.2–3.6) but not with AD (RR = 0.9, 95% CI 0.3–2.2) and not with all dementia types (RR = 1.3, 95% CI 0.9–1.8). Therefore, we see that even among similarly designed studies of a prospective nature, conflicting results continue to pervade the literature on dementia and AD. The HAAS is an especially appealing study, since many exposures, such as diabetes, were measured in midlife, and dementia outcomes are available 30 years or more later.

Systolic blood pressure also has been found to increase the risk for poor cognitive function in late life (Launer et al. 1995) and to predict brain atrophy, low brain weight, and neuropathologic AD (Swan et al. 1998, Petrovitch et al. 2000). Launer (2002) has proposed that the conflicting evidence for the relation between hypertension and AD arises from the use of different study designs. In general, studies that have a long follow-up, such as the HAAS, show that hypertension is associated with an increased risk for AD and its neuropathology (Petrovitch et al. 2000).

In the Rotterdam study, total fat intake was associated with a 2.4-fold increase in the risk of dementia (95% CI 1.1–5.2), which was more pronounced for vascular dementia (Kalmijn et al. 1997). Fish consumption was inversely related to incident dementia and AD (RR = 0.3, 95% CI 0.1–0.9). There is evidence that a high-fat diet up-regulates ApoE activity in animals (Knight et al. 2001). In the North Manhattan Study, 980 individuals were followed for a mean of 4 years, and 242 cases of dementia developed. Caloric intake was measured by semiquantitative food frequency questionnaires at baseline. The hazard ratio (HR) in the highest quartiles of calorie intake was 1.5 (95% CI 1.0–2.2) for AD; in those with an ε4 allele, it was 2.3 (95% CI 1.1–4.7) (Luchsinger et al. 2002). Since these confidence intervals overlap, there was no effect-modification by ε4 status: also, the analyses compared the highest to the lowest quartiles—data from the middle quartiles should have been included.

Plasma homocysteine, a major vascular risk factor, also has been shown to increase risk for AD. In a prospective study of 1092 men and women from the Framingham Study followed for a median of 8 years, 111 subjects developed dementia, including 83 AD cases. The RR for AD was doubled for individuals who had levels >14 μmol per liter (Seshadri et al. 2002). Increasing evidence also links hypercholesterolaemia to the etiology of AD (Kivipelto et al. 2002).

An emerging area of research is the examination of statins in AD. Several lines of research indicate that individuals who are prescribed statins (lipid-lowering agents) are at reduced risk for AD (RR = 0.29, 95% CI 0.13–0.63) (Jick et al. 2000); in the Canadian Study of Health and Aging, a similar RR was reported (RR = 0.26, 95% CI 0.08–0.88) (Rockwood et al. 2002). This is a promising area for pharmacological intervention, although it remains unclear whether individuals who have normal levels of cholesterol should take statins as a preventive agent for AD. Also, the independent roles of high cholesterol and ApoE need to be clarified.

Exposures to Neurotoxins.

Aluminum. The question of whether aluminum (Al) is a risk factor for AD has been heavily debated. Even one of the first findings on which the hypothesis is based (elevated concentrations of Al in plaques and tangles) is controversial, and recent work shows that brain Al is not elevated in AD (Bjertness et al. 1996). Since exposure to aluminum is pervasive, it is difficult to study. Epidemiologic studies have included case–control studies of occupation and studies correlating Al in drinking water with prevalence of AD. The case–control studies generally show no effect (Salib and Hillier 1996), despite the use of differing methodologies (Martyn et al. 1997). In two studies, an industrial hygienist blindly rated exposures based on job descriptions (Graves et al. 1998); in the second study, a job-exposure matrix (JEM) also was used (Gun et al. 1997). A JEM is a two-entry data matrix depicting information about an individual's job on one axis, such as occupation, job title, and tasks; on the other axis risk factors (such as aluminum) to evaluate are shown. Sir Richard Doll has eloquently reviewed the evidence for and against the aluminum hypothesis (Doll 1993). He concluded that Al is indeed neurotoxic, but is probably not a cause of AD. Others agree (Munoz 1998), but some feel that the evidence is sufficient that Al should not be dismissed as a possible risk factor for AD (Forbes and Hill 1998).

Solvents. Early occupational studies found a relation between the use of solvents and neurobehavioral deficits. In 1991, a meta-analysis of pooled data from case–control studies (Graves et al. 1991a) found no association between occupational solvent exposure and AD (OR = 0.76, 95% CI 0.47–1.23). However, a case–control study comparing 193 probable AD cases with 243 controls enrolled in a large health maintenance organization (HMO) in Seattle, Washington, later reported an elevated OR of 2.3 (95% CI 1.1–4.7), which was strongest among men (OR = 6, 95% CI

2.1–17.2). This latter study asked proxy informants to provide specific solvent exposure histories as well as job descriptions likely to involve solvent use (Kukull et al. 1995). Gun et al. (1997) compared 170 AD patients with 170 medical practice–based controls. They obtained occupational histories from informants, and exposures were rated by a panel of occupational hygienists using a JEM and blinded to case-control status. This study found no statistically significant associations. Also, Graves et al. (1998) reported a slightly elevated risk for AD among those exposed to solvents in their jobs (OR = 1.8; 95% CI 0.8–3.9), but the OR and dose–response effect were not statistically significant.

Electromagnetic fields. Sobel and colleagues have proposed that electromagnetic fields (EMF) exposure may initiate an inflammatory process that may be involved in the cascade of pathologic events that results in selective neuronal death in AD (Sobel et al. 1995). In 1995, Sobel et al. published findings from three separate case–control studies showing statistically significant odds ratios of about 3.0 for probable AD associated with EMF. Occupational history was not collected in a comparable manner for AD cases and controls, and data were obtained from a proxy respondent for cases and by direct interview for controls. The authors replicated their result (OR = 3.9, 95% CI 1.5 to 10.6) in a subsequent case–control study using controls with dementia other than vascular dementia (Sobel et al. 1996). Savitz at al. (1998) found no association between EMF and mortality from AD in a cohort study of electric utility workers, but mortality from AD is poorly reported on death certificates. In a third study, Feychting et al. (1998) compared 77 dementia cases ascertained from the Swedish twin registry with two groups of controls. Elevated odds ratios were found for the last occupation with exposure levels at or exceeding 2 microT but for the job with the highest magnetic field exposures, odds ratios were close to

1.0. Lastly, Graves et al. (1999b) evaluated EMF by means of occupational ratings by two industrial hygienists (IHs) who were blinded to case-control status. No associations were found (OR ever/never exposed for first IH = 0.74, 95% CI 0.29–1.92; OR for second IH = 0.95, 95% CI 0.27–2.43; kappa for two IHs was good at 0.57), nor were any dose–response effects noted. Further study will be necessary, using prospective data, to substantiate observed associations.

Smoking. Findings for the smoking–AD association are complex. Case–control studies have generally found an inverse association between smoking and AD (Graves et al. 1991b; Lee 1994; Tyas 1996), although these results are not always consistent (Tyas et al. 2000). Prospective studies either showed no effect (Wang et al. 1999) or showed that smoking is a factor that increases the risk of AD (Ott et al. 1998). In one meta-analysis of pure AD cases (Graves et al. 1991b), the pooled odds ratio using raw data from eight case–control studies was 0.78 (95% CI 0.62–0.98). A second meta-analysis yielded an OR of 0.64 (95% CI 0.58–0.79) (Lee 1994), and a more recent meta-analysis reported a pooled OR of 0.74 (95% CI 0.66–0.84) (Almeida et al. 2002). In case–control studies, the inverse association was modified by a family history of dementia or ApoE-ε4 (van Duijn et al. 1995; OR = 0.1, 95% CI 0.01–0.87). Among families with a strong genetic background, the onset of AD was later among smokers than among nonsmokers (van Duijn and Hofman 1991b).

It has been postulated that the inverse association from case–control studies is due to selective mortality (Riggs 1993; Graves and Mortimer 1994). Patients with AD who smoke may die faster than AD cases who do not smoke or controls who do or do not smoke, resulting in an underestimation of the association from case–control studies. The observed protective effect in case–control studies may also be a result of confounding by genetic constitution. As argued by Riggs (1993), given that smokers who live long enough to get AD may be genetically different from those who do not, the genetic pools of older prevalent cases and older controls may be mismatched. Supporting this idea, Plassman et al. (1995b) showed that among dizygotic twins (who share half their genes), the OR for AD associated with smoking was 0.55 (95% CI 0.18–1.59) and among monozygotic twins (who share all their genes), the OR was 2.0 (95% CI 0.45–10.06).

Prospective studies generally show that smoking is associated with poor cognitive performance (Launer et al. 1996; Galanis et al. 1997) and a higher risk of AD (Ott et al. 1998, Merchant et al. 1999), although some do not find the association (Hebert et al. 1992; Wang et al. 1999). Wang et al. (1999) reported that demented smokers were 3.4 times more likely to die over a 3-year follow-up period than demented nonsmokers, lending support to the differential survival theory, but not all studies have found this effect.

In incident series, it is possible that a prevalence–incidence bias renders the initially nondemented sample enriched in smokers who have not yet displayed symptoms and who will display such symptoms only when they become older and have more vascular lesions. This may be one reason why smoking is a risk factor for cognitive impairment and AD in many incident series.

Two prospective studies have found that smokers without an ApoE-ϵ4 allele incurred a higher risk for AD (RR = 2.1, 95% CI 1.2–3.7 [Merchant et al. 1999]; RR = 4.6, 95% CI 1.5–14.2 [Ott et al. 1998]) than those with the allele (RR = 1.4, 95% CI 0.6–3.3 [Merchant et al. 1999]; RR = 0.6, 95% CI 0.1–4.8 [Ott et al. 1998]). Thus, in prospective studies, as in case-control studies, smoking diminishes the effect of ϵ4 on AD. The smoking debate may involve two sides of the same coin: in persons who have the ϵ4 allele or are otherwise genetically at risk for AD, smoking may be protective, while smoking

may be a risk factor in persons without the allele who accumulate vascular lesions. Therefore, while retrospective case–control and prospective studies may on the surface disagree, they both may be consistent with different biologic mechanisms that depend on cofactors (such as genes and vascular disease).

Alcohol. Alcohol consumption in low to moderate amounts may reduce the accumulation of cardiovascular pathology, either through an inhibitory effect of ethanol on platelet aggregation or by altering the serum lipid profile (Ruitenberg et al. 2002). Given that excessive alcohol abuse may result in a loss of cognition and can be a primary component of dementia (Renner and Morris 1994), studies have also found that low to moderate consumption may be protective for cognitive function (Launer et al. 1996; Carmelli et al. 1999) and dementia (Orgozozo et al. 1997). A case–control study of 98 late-onset AD cases compared high alcohol consumption with no alcohol and found an increased risk (OR = 4.4, 95% CI 1.4–13.8) (Fratiglioni et al. 1993) controlling for smoking. Many studies have found no association (Graves et al. 1991b; for an excellent review, see Tyas 2001). In particular, early case–control studies using case definitions that excluded alcohol abusers ensured a null result (Graves et al. 1991b). Recent studies have examined the role of alcohol in cognitive function. A study of 14,000 middle-aged adults participating in The Atherosclerosis Risk in Communities Study (ARIC) examined delayed memory, digit symbol, and word fluency in 1990–1992. In a cross-sectional analysis, alcohol drinkers performed better than nondrinkers on the digit symbol subtest and in word fluency (Cerhan et al. 1998). The Rotterdam study has examined the association between alcohol consumption and risk for dementia, AD, and VaD (Ruitenberg et al. 2002). They identified 197 cases of dementia (146 AD, 29 VaD) over 6 years of follow-up of 7983 participants. Adjusting for age, gender, systolic blood pressure, education, smoking, and body mass index, they found that light to moderate drinking of any type of alcohol was associated with a HR of 0.58 (95% CI 0.38–0.90) for any type of dementia, which was more pronounced for vascular dementia (HR = 0.29, 95% CI 0.09–0.93) and the association was not present for AD. Further longitudinal examination of this hypothesis is warranted.

Possible Protective Factors

Nonsteroidal anti-inflammatory drugs. Post-mortem findings in AD indicate that immune-mediated autodestructive processes occur in AD, and that reactive microglia and cytokines are contained within neuritic plaques (McGeer and McGeer 1999). These and other findings have given rise to the hypothesis that anti-inflammatory agents may protect against AD and retard disease progression. Nonsteroidal anti-inflammatory drugs (NSAIDs) suppress the cyclooxygenases (COX). One isoform of COX induces inflammation after being induced by interleukin 1β (IL-1β) and related cytokines; IL-1β is elevated in AD brain (Breitner 1996). Studies of twins discordant for AD have shown that the use of NSAIDs can delay the onset of AD by 5–7 years, essentially reducing the incidence by half (Breitner et al. 1994, 1995; McGeer and McGeer 1999). A double-blind, placebo-controlled trial of 28 AD patients randomized for 6 months to indomethacin found that treated patients improved 1.3% on the Mini-Mental State Examination, whereas those on placebo declined by 8.4% ($p < 0.003$) (Rogers et al. 1993). Many observational studies have found a protective effect of NSAIDs against cognitive decline (Rozzini et al. 1996) or AD (Rich et al. 1995; Stewart et al. 1997), although not all results have been statistically significant (Beard et al. 1998; in't Veld et al. 1998; Peacock et al. 1999). In the Baltimore Longitudinal Study on Aging, Stewart et al. (1997) reported on 1686 participants, seen biennially beginning in 1979. At each visit, participants were asked to list all medicines used since their last visit. Use of aspirin, NSAIDs, and acetaminophen were defined as time-dependent cumulative exposure variables in Cox proportional hazards models. Of the three, only NSAIDs were significant in these models (RR = 0.46, 95% CI 0.24–0.86). The Rotterdam Study followed 6989 subjects age 55 and over for an average of 7 years: 394 subjects developed dementia, including 293 with AD. There was a dose–response effect for the association between use of NSAIDs and development of AD (RR = 0.95, 95% CI 0.7–1.3 for 1 month or less of cumulative use; RR = 0.83, 95% CI 0.6–1.1 for use between 1 and 24 months; RR = 0.20, 95% CI 0.05–0.8 for more than 24 months of use). An analysis of the type of NSAID that may be specific to this association was not evident from this study, but subsequent work by the same group showed that some NSAIDs, such as ibuprofen, indomethacin, and sulindac, may lower the production of amyloid-β-42. (Breteler et al. 2002). A large prevention trial is ongoing (ADAPT), which is testing celecoxib and naproxen (Martin et al. 2002).

Hormone replacement therapy among women. The role of estrogens in memory, cognition, and the central nervous system has been studied extensively. Several reviews are available (Birge et al. 1997; Rice et al. 1997; Yaffe et al. 1998; McEwen and Alves 1999). Early case–control studies generally found no association for estrogen use and AD (Yaffe et al. 1998). It is of concern that these studies included the use of proxy respondents and the occasional use of direct control interviews. Results from two case–control studies that used pharmacy records to ascertain exposures are conflicting, one showing no association (Brenner et al. 1994), the other showing an OR of 0.42 (95% CI 0.18–0.96) (Waring et al. 1999). Yaffe et al. (1998) state that few of these studies adjusted for education, a known confounder of the association. A recent nested case–control study among 2816 women in Italy found an OR of 0.28

(95% CI 0.08–0.98), adjusted for age, education, ages at menarche and menopause, smoking, alcohol consumption, body weight at 50 years old, and number of children (Baldereschi et al. 1998). This study also questioned proxy informants for suspected dementia cases and unaffected women themselves about their hormone replacement therapy (HRT) use, possibly enhancing the association in this way. Yaffe et al. (1998) conducted meta-analyses from eight case–control studies. This yielded a summary OR for any dementia and AD of 0.8 (95% CI for AD 0.56–1.12). Two prospective studies elicited information about HRT from nondemented women at entry (Tang et al. 1996; Kawas et al. 1997). Cox proportional hazards models were used to estimate the RR for AD. In the first study (Tang et al. 1996), the RR was 0.40 (95% CI 0.22–0.95), and in the second (Kawas et al. 1997), it was 0.46 (95% CI 0.21–0.98). However, while the first study found that women who used HRT longer were at an advantage (RR = 0.13, 95% CI 0.02–0.92), the second did not find an effect for duration. Tang et al. (1996) found that women who had an ApoE-ε4 allele and were on HRT were most protected from AD (RR = 0.13, 95% CI 0.02–0.95). Most of the HRT in these studies also included progesterone. Preliminary data from a prospective study (Rice et al. 1998) show that progesterone may reduce the beneficial effect of estrogen and that estrogen may be most beneficial to women having multiple other disclosing risk factors such as low income, family history of memory problems, and mild cognitive impairment (Rice et al. 1999). A large prospective cohort study in Cache County, Utah showed that HRT reduced the risk of AD over an average of 3 years by 41% with an adjusted HR of 0.59 (95% CI 0.36–0.96), but this effect was only evident in women who had used HRT in the past and for more than 10 years (Zandi et al. 2002). Recent evidence including this study suggests that a reduction in incidence of AD may be limited to women who initiate HRT at menopause.

Thus, remaining questions about HRT use and dementia include whether unopposed estrogen alone will have more favorable outcomes than estrogen combined with progesterone; what the critical time window is for onset of use, and what duration of use is necessary to achieve a reduction in risk.

Antioxidants, folate, and gingko biloba. There is substantial evidence to implicate oxidative stress as being involved in the cascade of events that lead to AD (see Rosler et al. 1998 for a review). A small trial of selegiline, α-tocopherol (vitamin E), or both, showed significant delays in outcomes for AD for all treatment groups compared with placebo (Sano et al. 1997). Data using the third wave of the National Health and Nutrition Examination Survey (NHANES) showed a cross-sectional association between decreasing serum levels of vitamin E per unit of cholesterol and increasingly poor memory across three ethnic groups after adjusting for relevant variables (Perkins et al. 1999). However, other antioxidants were not associated with poor performance (vitamins A and C and β-carotene). Another study has found, despite a relatively small sample size, that both vitamin E and vitamin C supplement users had a reduced incidence of AD over a mean follow-up period of 4 years (Morris et al. 1998). These are difficult exposures to measure and are subject to reporting biases, compliance issues, and time-dependent use. While not all studies have shown a protective effect, antioxidants show promise in reducing the incidence of dementia and AD. Ongoing large trials will clarify these issues in the near future.

Oken et al. (1998) have conducted a meta-analysis of the efficacy of ginkgo biloba on cognition in AD. They report a small but significant effect of 3- to 6-month treatments with 120 to 240 mg of ginkgo biloba extract. This is a burgeoning area of research and more investigation is necessary to explore these associations.

Other agents of interest include folate, homocysteine, and melatonin (Clarke et al.

1998, Liu et al. 1999). The next 5 years will bring enhanced scientific activity to find agents that can retard the pathologic progression of AD, thereby delaying the clinical onset of AD-type dementia.

Cognitive Reserve

As mentioned previously, low education is a risk factor for dementia/AD and dementia due to vascular events (Skoog 1998). Several studies have also found that other factors related to adult education and income (Evans et al. 1997; Graves et al. 1999a) and occupational status (Stern et al. 1994; Mortel et al. 1995) are similarly related to the risk of dementia and AD. Animal studies show that environmental and mental enrichment inhibits spontaneous apoptosis and protects against excitotoxic injury (Young et al. 1999). Epidemiologic studies have shown that frequent participation in cognitively stimulating activities reduces the risk of incident AD (Wilson et al. 2002).

Several studies have found that, while individuals with higher socioeconomic indices do not present with clinical dementia as soon as those with lower SES, when they do, their pathology is more advanced (Stern et al. 1992, 1995; Alexander et al. 1997). This phenomenon may be due to cognitive reserve; when persons have developed multiple cognitive strategies for solving problems and taking neuropsychological tests, they may perform within normal limits despite the presence of underlying pathology (Mortimer 1997). Cognitive reserve has major implications for screening for dementia in the community. A low probability of finding cases within the upper strata of cognitive performance necessitates that a disproportionate amount of resources be invested to find them.

Future Directions and Conclusions

Understanding of the epidemiology of dementia and AD has increased rapidly over the last two decades. Many risk factors have been identified, both genetic and en-

vironmental, and with this has come an increased understanding of their interactions. The appearance of clinical symptoms of dementia in life depends on many risk and protective factors, some of which are under genetic control, such as genes for cardiovascular and cerebrovascular disease, and apolipoprotein E, and many of which are not, such as socioeconomic status in early life, attained education and adult socioeconomic conditions, a healthy lifestyle, head trauma, and chemical exposures. Some factors are dependent on both genetic and environmental factors, such as IQ and final brain size. The pursuit of prevention of dementia and AD will likely involve exposures throughout the life course.

The prevention of dementia and AD will require input from many disciplines. In epidemiology, prospective cohort studies begun in the 1990s (and some older studies that have added dementia outcomes, such as the Framingham and Honolulu Heart Program [now Honolulu Asia Aging Study]) will continue to clarify associations found in earlier case–control studies and offer data on new risk factors, such as the role of cardiovascular and cerebrovascular diseases in AD. It is important that these prospective studies have sufficient follow-up time to allow cause-and-effect inferences to be made. It should also be recognized that if AD is a lifelong process beginning in childhood and if early-life exposures are as important as they appear to be in recent studies, epidemiologists may need to link these two periods of life. Prospective studies using overlapping cohorts may be one viable strategy.

Many risk factors for the dementia of AD and VaD overlap. Studies of VaD have often not separated risk factors for the underlying stroke(s) from risk factors for the dementia among persons with stroke. Those who have studied risk factors for dementia in stroke find that many factors related to brain reserve (including the location and volume of brain infarcted with respect to VaD) are also related to dementia with stroke, such as age, ethnicity, and education (Nyenhuis and Gorelick 1998). Since our goal as epidemiologists is to prevent disease, perhaps a more global view toward reducing risk factors for dementia as a whole should be taken.

Future research should explore which factors—clinical, environmental, genetic and experiential—render individuals vulnerable to expressing dementia symptoms and which factors increase brain reserve and delay the appearance of clinical symptoms. If symptoms of dementia can be delayed by 5 years, the incidence rate of AD would be reduced by half. Reducing exposures to known and modifiable risk factors, improving adult health status, and enhancing growth potential in infancy and childhood are steps that can be taken to improve brain reserve and reduce the incidence of dementia.

ACKNOWLEDGMENT

I would like to thank Dr. James A. Mortimer for his thoughtful contributions over the years, and for his comments in the revision of this chapter.

References

Abbott RD, White LR, Ross GW, et al. Height as a marker of childhood development and late-life cognitive function: the Honolulu-Asia Aging Study. *Pediatrics* 1998;102:602–609.

Aevarsson O, Skoog I. A population-based study on the incidence of dementia disorders between 85 and 88 years of age. *J Am Geriatr Soc* 1996;44:1455–1460.

Alexander GE, Furey ML, Grady CL, et al. Association of premorbid intellectual function with cerebral metabolism in Alzheimer's disease: implications for the cognitive reserve hypothesis. *Am J Psychiatry* 1997;154:165–172.

Almeida OP, Hulse GK, Lawrence D, Flicker L. Smoking as a risk factor for Alzheimer's disease: contrasting evidence from a systematic review of case–control and cohort studies. *Addiction* 2002;97:15–28.

American Psychiatric Association. Diagnostic and Statistical Manual of Mental Disorders, Fourth Edition. Washington DC: American Psychiatric Association, 1994, pp. 143–147.

Andreasen NC, Flaum M, Swayze V, et al. Intelligence and brain structure in normal individuals. *Am J Psychiatry* 1993;150:130–134.

Aronson MK, Ooi WL, Geva DL, et al. Dementia: age-dependent incidence, prevalence and mortality in old old. *Arch Intern Med* 1991;151:989–992.

Bachman DL, Wolf PA, Linn RT, et al. Incidence of dementia and probable Alzheimer's disease in a general population: the Framingham Study. *Neurology* 1993;43:515–519.

Baldereschi M, Di Carlo A, Lepore V, et al. Estrogen-replacement therapy and Alzheimer's disease in the Italian Longitudinal Study on Aging. *Neurology* 1998;50:996–1002.

Ball MJ. Neuronal loss, neurofibrillary tangles and granulovacuolar degeneration in the hippocampus with ageing and dementia. A quantitative study. *Acta Neuropathol* 1977;37:111–118.

Beard CM, Waring SC, O'Brien PC, et al. Nonsteroidal anti-inflammatory drug use and Alzheimer's disease: a case–control study in Rochester, Minnesota, 1980 through 1984. *Mayo Clin Proc* 1998;73:951–955.

Birge SJ, Mortel KF. Estrogen and the treatment of Alzheimer's disease. *Am J Med* 1997;103(3A):36S–45S.

Bjertness E, Candy JM, Torvik A, et al. Content of brain aluminum is not elevated in Alzheimer's disease. *Alzheimer Dis Assoc Disord* 1996;10:171–1744.

Blessed G, Tomlinson B, Roth M. The association between quantitative measures of dementia and of senile change in the cerebral gray matter of elderly subjects. *Br J Psychiatry* 1968;114:797–811.

Borenstein Graves A, Mortimer JA, Bowen JD, et al. Head circumference and incident Alzheimer's disease: modification by apolipoprotein E. *Neurology* 2001;57:1453–1460.

Borenstein Graves A, Wu Y, McCormick W, Bowen JD, McCurry S, Larson EB. Incidence rates of dementia, Alzheimer's disease and vascular dementia in the Kame Project: roles of age, gender, education and apolipo-protein E. *Neurobiol Aging* 2002;23(1S):S419.

Breitner JC. The role of anti-inflammatory drugs in the prevention and treatment of Alzheimer's disease. *Annu Rev Med* 1996;47:401–411.

Breitner JCS, Gau BA, Welsh KA, et al. Inverse association of anti-inflammatory treatments and Alzheimer's disease. *Neurology* 1994;44:227–232.

Breitner JC, Jarvik GP, Plassman PL, et al. Risk of Alzheimer disease with the ϵ4 allele for apolipoprotein E in a population-based study of men aged 62–73 years. *Alzheimer Dis Assoc Disord* 1998;12:40–44.

Breitner JCS, Welsh KA. Genes and recent development in the epidemiology of Alzheimer's disease and related dementia. *Epidemiol Rev* 1995;17:39–47.

Breitner JCS, Welsh KA, Helms MJ, et al. Delayed onset of Alzheimer's disease with nonsteroidal anti-inflammatory and histamine H2 blocking drugs. *Neurobiol Aging* 1995;16: 523–530.

Brenner DE, Kukull WA, Stergachis A, et al. Postmenopausal estrogen replacement therapy and the risk of Alzheimer's disease: a population-based case–control study. *Am J Epidemiol* 1994;140:262–267.

Breteler MMB, Claus JJ, van Duijn CM, et al. Epidemiology of Alzheimer's disease. *Epidemiol Rev* 1992;14:59–82.

Breteler MMB, in't Veld B, Hofman A, Stricker B. A β-42 peptide lowering NSAIDs and Alzheimer's disease. *Neurobiol Aging* 2002; 23:S286.

Brookmeyer R, Gray S, Kawas C. Projections of Alzheimer's disease in the United States and the public health impact of delaying disease onset. *Am J Public Health* 1998;88:1337–1342.

Canadian Study of Health and Aging: risk factors for Alzheimer's disease in Canada. *Neurology* 1994;33:2074–2080.

Carmelli D, Swan GE, Reed T, et al. Midlife cardiovascular risk factors, ApoE, and cognitive decline in elderly male twins. *Neurology* 1998;50:1580–1585.

Carmelli D, Swan GE, Reed T, et al. The effect of apolipoprotein E4 in the relationships of smoking and drinking to cognitive function. *Neuroepidemiology* 1999;18:125–133.

Cerhan JR, Folsom AR, Mortimer JA, et al. Correlates of cognitive function in middle-aged adults. Atherosclerosis Risk in Communities (ARIC) Study Investigators. *Gerontology* 1998;44:95–105.

Chandra V, Pandav R. Gene–environment interaction in Alzheimer's disease: a potential role for cholesterol. *Neuroepidemiology* 1998;17:225–232.

Chui HC, Victoroff JI, Margolin D, et al. Criteria for ischemic vascular dementia proposed by the State of California Alzheimer's Disease Diagnostic and Treatment Centers. *Neurology* 1992;42:473–480.

Clarke R, Smith AD, Jobst KA, et al. Folate, vitamin B_{12}, and serum total homocysteine levels in confirmed Alzheimer disease. *Arch Neurol* 1998;55:1449–1455.

Combarros O, Alvarex-Arcaya A, Sanchez-Guerra M, et al. Candidate gene association studies in sporadic Alzheimer's disease. *Dement Geriatr Cogn Disord* 2002;14:41–54.

Corder EH, Saunders Am, Strittmatter WJ, et al. Gene dosage of apolipoprotein E type 4 allele and the risk of Alzheimer's disease in late onset families. *Science* 1993;261:921–923.

Corey-Bloom J, Thal LJ, Galasko D, et al. Diagnosis and evaluation of dementia. *Neurology* 1995;45:211–218.

Crystal H, Dickson D, Fuld P, et al. Clinico-pathologic studies in dementia: nondemented subjects with pathologically confirmed Alzheimer's disease. *Neurology* 1988; 38:1682–1687.

Cummings JL, Benson DF. Dementia: A Clinical Approach, 2nd edition. Boston: Butterworth-Heinemann, 1992.

Cummings JL, Vinters HV, Cole GM, et al. Alzheimer's disease: etiologies, pathophysiology, cognitive reserve, and treatment opportunities. *Neurology* 1998;51(Suppl 1): S2–S17; discussion S65–S67.

Davignon J, Gregg RE, Sing CF. Apolipoprotein E polymorphism and atherosclerosis. *Arteriosclerosis* 1988;8:1–21.

DeKosky ST, Scheff SW. Synapse loss in frontal cortex biopsies in Alzheimer's disease: correlation with cognitive severity. *Ann Neurol* 1990;27:457–464.

Doll R. Review: Alzheimer's disease and environmental aluminium. *Age Ageing* 1993;22: 138–153.

Edland SD, Graves AB, McCormick WC, Larson EB. Estimation and sample design in prevalence surveys of dementia. *J Clin Epidemiol* 1999;52:399–403.

Edland SD, Xu Y, Plevak M, et al. Total intracranial volume: normative values and lack of association with Alzheimer's disease. *Neurology* 2002;59:272–274.

Evans DA. Estimated prevalence of Alzheimer's disease in the United States. *Milbank Q* 1990;68:267–289.

Evans DA, Funkenstein HH, Albert MS, et al. Prevalence of Alzheimer's disease in a community population of older persons: higher than previously reported. *JAMA* 1989;262: 2551–2556.

Evans DA, Hebert LE, Beckett LA, et al. Education and other measures of socioeconomic status and risk of incident Alzheimer disease in a defined population of older persons. *Arch Neurol* 1997;54:1399–1405.

Evans DA, Smith LA, Scherr PA, et al. Risk of death from Alzheimer's disease in a community population of older persons. *Am J Epidemiol* 1991;134:403–412.

Ewbank DC. Death attributable to Alzheimer's disease in the United States. *Am J Public Health* 1999;89:90–92.

Farrer LA, Cupples A, Haines JL, et al. Effects of age, sex and ethnicity on the association between apolipoprotein E genotype and Alzheimer disease: a meta-analysis. *JAMA* 1997;278:1349–1356.

Farrer LA, Cupples LA, van Duijn CM, et al. Apolipoprotein E genotype in patients with Alzheimer's disease: implications for the risk of dementia among relatives. *Ann Neurol* 1995;38:797–808.

Feychting M, Pedersen NL, Svedberg P, et al. Dementia and occupational exposure to magnetic fields. *Scand J Work Environ Health* 1998;24:46–53.

Forbes WF, Hill GB. Is exposure to aluminum a risk factor for the development of Alzheimer's disease? *Arch Neurol* 1998;55:737–739.

Fratiglioni L, Ahlbom A, Viitanen M, Winblad B. Risk factors for late-onset Alzheimer's disease: a population-based, case–control study. *Ann Neurol* 1993;33:258–266.

Fratiglioni L, Viitanen M, von Strauss E, et al. Very old women at highest risk of dementia and Alzheimer's disease: incidence data from the Kungholmen Project, Stockholm. *Neurology* 1997;48:132–138.

Galanis DJ, Petrovitch H, Launer LJ, et al. Smoking history in middle age and subsequent cognitive performance in elderly Japanese-American men: the Honolulu-Asia Aging Study. *Am J Epidemiol* 1997;145:507–515.

Galasko D, Hansen LA, Katzman R, et al. Clinical–neuropathological correlations in Alzheimer's disease and related dementias. *Arch Neurol* 1994;51:888–895.

Gao S, Hendrie HC, Hall KS, Hui S. The relationships between age, sex and the incidence of dementia and Alzheimer disease: a meta-analysis. *Arch Gen Psychiatry* 1998;55:809–815.

Geldmacher DS, Whitehouse PJ Jr. Differential diagnosis of Alzheimer's disease. *Neurology* 1997;48(Suppl 6):S2–S9.

Geller LN, Potter H. Chromosome missegregation and trisomy 21 mosaicism in Alzheimer's disease. *Neurobiol Dis* 1999;6:167–179.

Ghebremedhin E, Schultz C, Thal DR, et al. Gender and age modify the association between ApoE and AD-related neuropathology. *Neurology* 2001;56:1696–1701.

Gold G, Bouras C, Canuto A, et al. Clinico-pathological validations study of four sets of clinical criteria for vascular dementia. *Am J Psychiatry* 2002;159:82–87.

Graham DI, Gentleman SM, Nicoll JA, et al. Is there a genetic basis for the deposition of beta-amyloid after fatal head injury? *Cell Mol Neurobiol* 1999;19:19–30.

Graves AB, Kukull WA. The epidemiology of dementia. In: Morris JC, ed. Handbook of Dementing Illnesses. New York: Marcel Dekker, 1994, pp 23–69.

Graves AB, Larson EB, Edland SD, et al. Prevalence of dementia and its subtypes in the Japanese American population of King County, Washington State. *Am J Epidemiol* 1996a;144:760–771.

Graves AB, Larson EB, Wenzlow A. Protective factors for cognitive decline in a Japanese American community. *Neurobiol Aging* 1996c;17(Suppl):S40.

Graves AB, Mortimer JA. Does smoking reduce the risks of Parkinson's and Alzheimer's diseases? *J Smoking-Related Disord* 1994; 5(Suppl 1):79–90.

Graves AB, Mortimer JA, Larson EB, et al. Head circumference as a measure of cognitive reserve: association with severity of impairment in Alzheimer's disease. *Br J Psychiatry* 1996b;169:86–92.

Graves AB, Rajaram L, Bowen JD, et al. Cognitive decline and Japanese cultures in a cohort of older Japanese Americans in King County: the Kame Project. *J Gerontol B Psychol Sci Soc Sci* 1999a;54(3):S154–S161.

Graves AB, Rosner D, Echeverria D, et al. Occupational exposures to solvents and aluminium and estimated risk of Alzheimer's disease. *Occup Environ Med* 1998;55:627–633.

Graves AB, Rosner D, Echeverria D, et al. Occupational exposures to electromagnetic fields in Alzheimer's disease. *Alzheimer Dis Assoc Disord* 1999b;13:165–170.

Graves AB, van Duijn CM, Chandra V, et al. Occupational exposures to solvents and lead as risk factors for Alzheimer's disease: a collaborative re-analysis of case–control studies. *Int J Epidemiol* 1991a;20(Suppl 2):S58–S61.

Graves AB, van Duijn CM Chandra V, et al. Alcohol and tobacco consumption as risk factors for Alzheimer's disease: a collaborative re-analysis of case–control studies. *Int J Epidemiol* 1991b;20(Suppl 2):S48–S57.

Graves AB, Wu Y, McCormick W, et al. Incidence rates of dementia. Alzheimer's disease and vascular dementia in the Kame Project: roles of age, gender, education and Apolipoprotein E. *Neurobiol Aging* 2002;23(1S):S419.

Gun RT, Korten AE, Jorm AF, et al. Occupational risk factors for Alzheimer disease: a case–control study. *Alzheimer Dis Assoc Disord* 1997;11:21–27.

Guo Z, Cupples LA, Kurz A, et al. Head injury and the risk of AD in the MIRAGE study. *Neurology* 2000;54:1316–1323.

Haan MN, Shemanski L, Jagust WJ, et al. The role of APOE4 in modulating effects of other risk factors for cognitive decline in elderly persons. *JAMA* 1999;282:40–46.

Hebert LE, Scherr P, Beckett LA, et al. Relation of smoking and alcohol consumption to incident Alzheimer's disease. *Am J Epidemiol* 1992;135:347–355.

Hendrie HC, Hall KS, Hui S, et al. Apolipoprotein E genotypes and Alzheimer's disease in a community study of elderly African Americans. *Ann Neurol* 1995b;37:118–120.

Hendrie HC, Osuntokun B, Hall KS, et al. Prevalence of Alzheimer's disease and dementia in two communities: Nigerian Africans and African Americans. *Am J Psychiatry* 1995a;152:1485–1492.

Heston LL, Mastri AR, Anderson VE, White J. Dementia of the Alzheimer type: clinical genetics, natural history and associated conditions. *Arch Gen Psychiatry* 1981;38:1085–1090.

Heyman A, Fillenbaum GG, Welsh-Bohmer KA, et al. Cerebral infarcts in patients with autopsy-proven Alzheimer's disease: CERAD, part XVIII. *Neurology* 1998;51:159–162.

Hofman A, Ott A, Breteler MMB, et al. Atherosclerosis, apolipoprotein E, and prevalence of dementia and Alzheimer's disease in the Rotterdam Study. *Lancet* 1997;349:151–154.

in't Veld BA, Launer LA, Hoes AW, et al. NSAIDs and incident Alzheimer's disease: the Rotterdam Study. *Neurobiol Aging* 1998;19:607–611.

Jarvik GP. Genetic predictors of common disease: apolipoprotein E genotype as a paradigm. *Ann Epidemiol* 1997;7:357–362.

Jarvik GP, Wijsman EM, Kukull WA, et al. Interactions of apolipoprotein E genotype, total cholesterol level, age and sex in prediction of Alzheimer's disease: a case–control study. *Neurology* 1995;45:1092–1096.

Jick H, Zornberg GL, Jick SS, et al. Statins and risk of dementia. *Lancet* 2000;356:1627–1631.

Johansson B, Zarit SH. Prevalence and incidence of dementia in the oldest old: a longitudinal study of a population-based sample of 84–90 year-olds in Sweden. *Int J Geriatr Psychiatr* 1995;10:359–366.

Jordan BD, Relkin NR, Ravdin LD, et al. Apolipoprotein E-e4 associated with chronic traumatic brain injury in boxing. *JAMA* 1997;278:136–140.

Jorm AF. The Epidemiology of Alzheimer's Disease and Related Disorders. New York: Chapman and Hall, 1990.

Jorm AF, Jolley D. The incidence of dementia: a meta-analysis. *Neurology* 1998;51:728–733.

Jorm AF, Korten AE, Henderson AS. The prevalence of dementia: a quantitative integration of the literature. *Acta Psychiatr Scand* 1987;76:465–479.

Kalmijn S, Launer LJ, Ott A, et al. Dietary fat intake and the risk of incident dementia in the Rotterdam Study. *Ann Neurol* 1997;42:776–782.

Katzman R, Fox PJ. The world-wide impact of dementia, projections of prevalence and costs. In: Mayeux R, Christen Y, eds. Epidemiology of Alzheimer's Disease: From Gene to Prevention. New York: Springer-Verlag, 1999, pp 1–17.

Katzman R, Terry R, DeTeresa R, et al. Clinical, pathological, and neurochemical changes in dementia: a subgroup with preserved mental status and numerous neocortical plaques. *Ann Neurol* 1988;23:138–144.

Kawas C, Resnick S, Morrison A, et al. A prospective study of estrogen replacement therapy and the risk of developing Alzheimer's disease: the Baltimore Longitudinal Study of Aging. *Neurology* 1997;48:1517–1521.

Kawas C, Segal J, Stewart WF, et al. A validation study of the Dementia Questionnaire. *Arch Neurol* 1994;51:901–906.

Khachaturian ZS. Diagnosis of Alzheimer's disease. *Arch Neurol* 1985;42:1097–1105.

Kivipelto M, Laasko M, Tuomilehto J, et al. Hypertension and hypercholesterolaemia as risk factors for Alzheimer's disease: potential for pharmacological intervention. *CNS Drugs* 2002;16:435–444.

Knight DS. Mahajan DK. Qiao X. Dietary fat up-regulates the apolipoprotein E mRNA level in the Zucker lean rat brain. *Neuroreport* 2001;12:3111–3115.

Kokmen E, Beard CM, O'Brien PC, et al. Is the incidence of dementing illness changing? A 25-year time trend study in Rochester, Minnesota (1960–1984). *Neurology* 1993;43:1887–1892.

Kukull WA, Larson EB, Bowen JD, et al. Solvent exposure as a risk factor for Alzheimer's disease: a case–control study. *Am J Epidemiol* 1995;141:1059–1071.

Launer LJ. Demonstrating the case that AD is a vascular disease: epidemiologic evidence. *Ageing Res Rev* 2002;1:61–77.

Launer LJ, Andersen K, Dewey ME, et al. Rates and risk factors for dementia and Alzheimer's disease: results from EURODEM pooled analyses. *Neurology* 1999;52:78–84.

Launer LJ, Feskens EJM, Kalmijn S, Kromhout D. Smoking, drinking and thinking: the Zutphen Elderly Study. *Am J Epidemiol* 1996;143:219–227.

Launer LJ, Masaki K, Petrovitch H, et al. The association between midlife blood pressure levels and late-life cognitive function. *JAMA* 1995;274:1846–1851.

Lee PN. Smoking and Alzheimer's disease: a review of the epidemiological evidence. *Neuroepidemiology* 1994;13:131–144.

Lendon CL, Ashall F, Goate AM. Exploring the etiology of Alzheimer disease using molecular genetics. *JAMA* 1997;277:825–831.

Letenneur L, Commenges D, Dartigues JF, Barberger-Gateau P. Incidence of dementia and Alzheimer's disease in elderly community residents of southwestern France. *Int J Epidemiol* 1994;23:1256–1261.

Letenneur L, Gilleron V, Commenges D, et al. Are sex and educational level independent predictors of dementia and Alzheimer's disease? Incidence data from the PAQUID project. *J Neurol Neurosurg Psychiatry* 1999; 66:177–183.

Li G, Shen YC, Chen CH. A three-year follow-up study of age-related dementia in an urban area of Beijing. *Acta Psychiatr Scand* 1991;83:99–104.

Lichtenstein P, Harris JR, Pedersen NL, Mc-Clearn GE. Socioeconomic status and physical health, how are they related? An empirical study based on twins reared apart and twins reared together. *Soc Sci Med* 1993; 36:441–450.

Lindsay J, Laurin D, Verreault R, et al. Risk factors for Alzheimer's disease: a prospective analysis from the Canadian Study of Health and Aging. *Am J Epidemiol* 2002;156:445–53.

Liu RY, Zhou JN, van Heerikhuize J, et al. Decreased melatonin levels in postmortem cerebrospinal fluid in relation to aging, Alzheimer's disease, and apolipoprotein E-ε 4/4 genotype. *J Clin Endocrinol Metab* 1999; 84:323–327.

Luchsinger JA, Tang MX, Shea S, Mayeux R. Caloric intake and the risk of Alzheimer disease. *Arch Neurol* 2002;59:1258–1263.

Mann DMA. The neuropathology of Alzheimer's disease: a review with pathogenetic, aetiological and therapeutic considerations. *Mech Ageing Dev* 1985;31:213–255.

Martin BK, Meinert CL, Breitner JC. ADAPT Research Group. Double placebo design in a prevention trial for Alzheimer's disease. *Control Clin Trials* 2002;23:93–99.

Martyn CN, Coggon DN, Inskip H, Lacey RF, Young WF. Aluminum concentrations in drinking water and risk of Alzheimer's disease. *Epidemiology* 1997;8:281–286.

Mayeux R, Ottman R, Maestre G, et al. Synergistic effects of traumatic brain injury and apolipoprotein-ε 4 in patients with Alzheimer's disease. *Neurology* 1995;45:555–557.

McDowell I, Hill GB, Lindsay JP, Helliwell B. The Canadian Study of Health and Aging: incidence of dementia. *Neurobiol Aging* 1998;19:S170.

McEwen BS, Alves SE. Estrogen actions in the central nervous system. *Endocr Rev* 1999; 20:279–307.

McGeer PL, McGeer EG. Inflammation of the brain in Alzheimer's disease: implications for therapy. *J Leukoc Biol* 1999;65:409–415.

McKenzie JE, Gentleman SM, Roberts GW, et al. Increased numbers of β-APP-immunoreactive neurones in the entorhinal cortex after head injury. *Neuroreport* 1994;6:161–164.

McKhann G, Drachman D, Folstein M, et al. Clinical diagnosis of Alzheimer's disease: report of the NINCDS-ADRDA Work Group under the auspices of the Department of Health and Human Services Task Force on Alzheimer's disease. *Neurology* 1984;34: 939–944.

Merchant C, Tang M-X, Albert S, et al. The influence of smoking on the risk of Alzheimer's disease. *Neurology* 1999;52:1408–1412.

Meyer JS, McClintic KL, Rogers R, et al. Aetiological considerations and risk factors for multi-infarct dementia. *J Neurol Neurosurg Psychiatry* 1988;51:1489–1497.

Mirra SS, Gearing M. The neuropathology of dementia. In: Morris JC, ed. Handbook of Dementing Illnesses. New York: Marcel Dekker, 1994, pp 189–226.

Mohs RC, Breitner JCS, Silverman JM, et al. Alzheimer's disease: morbid risk among first-degree relatives approximates 50% by 90 years of age. *Arch Gen Psychiatry* 1987;44: 405–408.

Morris JC, Ed. Handbook of Dementing Illnesses. New York: Marcel Dekker, 1994.

Morris MC, Beckett LA, Scherr PA, et al. Vitamin E and vitamin C supplement use and risk of incident Alzheimer disease. *Alzheimer Dis Assoc Disord* 1998;12:121–126.

Morris JC, Storandt M, McKeel DW, et al. Cerebral amyloid deposition and diffuse plaques in "normal" aging: evidence for presymptomatic and very mild Alzheimer's disease. *Neurology* 1996;46:707–719.

Mortel KF, Meyer JS, Herod B, Thornby J. Education and occupation as risk factors for dementias of the Alzheimer and ischemic vascular types. *Dementia* 1995;6:55–62.

Mortimer JA. Epidemiological aspects of Alzheimer's disease. In: Maletta GJ, Pirozzolo FJ, eds. The Aging Nervous System. New York: Praeger Publishers, 1980, pp. 307–332.

Mortimer JA. The continuum hypothesis of Alzheimer's disease and normal aging: the role of brain reserve. *Alzheimer's Res* 1995; 1:67–70.

Mortimer JA. Brain reserve and the clinical expression of Alzheimer's disease. *Geriatrics* 1997;52:S50–S53.

Mortimer JA, Fortier I, Rajaram L, Gauvreau D. Higher education and socioeconomic status in childhood protect individuals at genetic risk of AD from expressing symptoms in late life: the Saguenay-Lac-St-Jean Health and Aging Study. *Neurobiol Aging* 1998;19:S215.

Mortimer JA, Graves AB. Education and other socioeconomic determinants of dementia and Alzheimer's disease. *Neurology* 1993; 43:(Suppl 4):S39–S44.

Mortimer JA, Schuman LM, French LR. Epidemiology of dementing illness. In: Mortimer JA, Schuman LM. eds. The Epidemiology of Dementia. New York: Oxford University Press, 1981, pp 3–23.

Mortimer JA, Snowdon DA, Markesbery WR. Pathological correlates of dementia at advanced ages: findings from the Nun Study. *Neurology* 2001;56(Suppl 3):A181.

Mortimer JA, Snowdon DA, Markesbery WR. Head circumference, education and risk of dementia: findings from the Nun Study. *J Clin Exp Neuropsychol* 2003;25:671–679.

Mortimer JA, van Duijn CM, Chandra V, et al. Head trauma as a risk factor for Alzheimer's disease: a collaborative re-analysis of case–control studies. *Int J Epidemiol* 1991; 20 (Suppl 2):S28–S35.

Mullan M. Scibelli P. Duara R, et al. Familial and population-based studies of apolipoprotein E and Alzheimer's disease. *Ann NY Acad Sci* 1996;802:16–26.

Munoz DG. Is exposure to aluminum a risk factor for the development of Alzheimer's disease? *Arch Neurol* 1998;55:737–739.

Nemetz PN, Leibson C Naessens JM, et al. Traumatic brain injury and time to onset of Alzheimer's disease: a population-based study. *Am J Epidemiol* 1999;149:32-40.

Nyenhuis DL, Gorelick PB. Vascular dementia: a contemporary review of epidemiology, diagnosis, prevention and treatment. *J Am Geriatr Soc* 1998;46:1437–1448.

Oken BS, Storzbach DM, Kaye JA. The efficacy of Ginkgo biloba on cognitive function in Alzheimer's disease. *Arch Neurol* 1998;55: 1409–1415.

O'Meara ES, Kukull WA, Sheppard L, et al. Head injury and risk of Alzheimer's disease by apolipoprotein E genotype. *Am J Epidemiol* 1997;146:373–384.

Orgozozo JM, Dartigues JF, Lafont S, et al. Wine consumption and dementia in the elderly: a prospective community study in the Bordeaux area. *Rev Neurol (Paris)* 1997; 153:185–192.

Osuntokun BO, Sahota A, Ogunniyi AO, et al. Lack of an association between apolipoprotein E4 and Alzheimer's disease in elderly Nigerians. *Ann Neurol* 1995;38:463–465.

Ott A, Stolk RP, Hofman A, et al. Association of diabetes mellitus and dementia: the Rotterdam Study. *Diabetologia* 1996;39:1392–1397.

Ott A, Slooter JC, Hofman A, et al. Smoking and risk of dementia and Alzheimer's disease in population-based cohort study: the Rotterdam Study. *Lancet* 1998;351:1840–1843.

Pantoni L, Inzitari D. Pathological examination in vascular dementia. *Am J Psychiatry* 2002; 159:1439–1440.

Paykel ES, Brayne C, Huppert FA, et al. Incidence of dementia in a population older than 75 years in the United Kingdom. *Arch Gen Psychiatry* 1994;51:325–332.

Peacock JM, Folsom AR, Knopman DS, et al. Association of nonsteroidal anti-inflammatory drugs and aspirin with cognitive performance in middle-aged adults. *Neuroepidemiology* 1999;18:134–143.

Peila R, Rodriguez BL, Launer LJ. Type 2 diabetes, APOE gene, and the risk for dementia and related pathologies: the Honolulu Asia Aging Study. *Diabetes* 2002;51:1256–1262.

Perkins AJ, Hendrie HC, Callahan CM, et al. Association of antioxidants with memory in a multiethnic elderly sample using the Third National Health and Nutrition Examination Survey. *Am J Epidemiol* 1999;150:37–44.

Petrovitch H, White LR, Izmirilian G, et al. Midlife blood pressure and neuritic plaques, neurofibrillary tangles, and brain weight at death: the Honolulu-Asia Aging Study. *Neurobiol Aging* 2000;21:57–62.

Plassman BL, Helms MJ, Welsh KA, et al. Smoking, Alzheimer's disease and confounding with genes. *Lancet* 1995b;345:387.

Plassman BL, Welsh KA, Helms M, et al. Intelligence and education as predictors of cognitive state in late life: a 50-year follow-up. *Neurology* 1995a;45:1446–1450.

Price DL, Tanzi RE, Borchelt DR. Sisodia SS. Alzheimer's disease: genetic studies and transgenic models. *Annu Rev Genet* 1998; 32:461–493.

Renner JA, Morris JC. Alcohol-associated dementia. In: Morris JC, ed. Handbook of Dementing Illnesses. New York: Marcel Dekker, 1994, pp 393–412.

Reynolds CA, Wetherell JL, Gatz M. Heritability of Alzheimer's disease. In: Vellas B, Fitten LJ, eds. Research and Practice in Alzheimer's Disease. Paris: Serdi Publisher, 1999a, pp 175–191.

Reynolds MD, Johnston JM, Dodge HH, et al. Small head size is related to low Mini-Mental State Examination scores in a community sample of nondemented older adults. *Neurology* 1999b;53:228–229.

Rice MM, Graves AB, McCurry SM, Larson EB. Estrogen replacement therapy and cognitive function in postmenopausal women without dementia. *Am J Med* 1997;103(3A):26S–35S.

Rice MM, Graves AB, McCurry SM, et al. Progesterone, but not ApoE, modifies the beneficial effect of estrogen on cognitive decline. *J Am Geriatr Soc* 1998;46:S8.

Rice MM, Graves AB, McCurry SM, et al. The influence of risk factors for cognitive decline on the association between estrogen replacement therapy and cognitive change. *Gerontologist* 1999;39:515–516.

Rich JB, Rasmusson DX, Folstein MF, et al. Nonsteroidal anti-inflammatory drugs in Alzheimer's disease. *Neurology* 1995;45:51–55.

Riggs JE. Smoking and Alzheimer's disease: protective effect or differential survival bias? *Lancet* 1993;342:793–704.

Rocca WA, Cha RH, Waring SC, Kokmen E. Incidence of dementia and Alzheimer's disease: a reanalysis of data from Rochester, Minnesota, 1975–1984. *Am J Epidemiol* 1998;148:51–62.

Rockwood K, Kirkland S, Hogan DB, et al. Use of lipid-lowering agents, indication bias, and the risk of dementia in community-dwelling elderly people. *Arch Neurol* 2002;59:223–227.

Rogers J, Kirby LC, Hempelman SR, et al. Clinical trial of indomethacin in Alzheimer's disease. *Neurology* 1993;43:1609–1611.

Roman GC, Tatemichi TK, Erkunjuntti T, et al. Vascular dementia: diagnostic criteria for research studies: report of the NINDS-AIREN International Workshop. *Neurology* 1993;43:250–260.

Roses AD. Alzheimer diseases: a model of gene mutations and susceptibility polymorphisms for complex psychiatric diseases. *Am J Med Genet* 1998;81:49–57.

Rosler M, Retz W, Thome J, Riederer P. Free radicals in Alzheimer's dementia: currently available therapeutic strategies. *J Neural Transm Suppl* 1998;54:211–219.

Ross GW, Abbott RD, Petrovitch H, et al. Frequency and characteristics of silent dementia among elderly Japanese-American men: the Honolulu-Asia Aging Study. *JAMA* 1997;277:800–805.

Roth M, Tomlinson BE, Blessed G. Correlation between scores for dementia and counts of 'senile plaques' in cerebral gray matter of elderly subjects. *Nature* 1966;209:109–110.

Rozzini R, Ferrucci L, Losonczy K, et al. Protective effect of chronic NSAID use on cognitive decline in older persons. *J Am Geriatr Soc* 1996;44:1025–1029.

Ruitenberg A, Ott A, van Swieten JC, et al. Incidence of dementia: does gender make a difference? *Neurobiol Aging* 2001;22:575–580.

Ruitenberg A, van Swieten JC, Witteman JCM, et al. Alcohol consumption and risk of dementia: the Rotterdam Study. *Lancet* 2002; 359:281–286.

Salib E, Hillier V. A case–control study of Alzheimer's disease and aluminium occupation. *Br J Psychiatry* 1996;168:244–249.

Sano M, Ernesto C, Thomas RG, et al. A controlled trial of selegiline, alpha-tocopherol, or both as treatment for Alzheimer's disease. *N Engl J Med* 1997;336:1216–1222.

Savitz DA, Checkoway H, Loomis DP. Magnetic field exposure and neurodegenerative disease mortality among electric utility workers. *Epidemiology* 1998;9:398–404.

Schmand B, Smit JH, Geerlings MI, Lindeboom J. The effects of intelligence and education on the development of dementia. A test of the brain reserve hypothesis. *Psychol Med* 1997;27:1337–1344.

Schofield PW, Logroscino G, Andrews HF, et al. An association between head circumference and Alzheimer's disease in a population-based study of aging and dementia. *Neurology* 1997b;49:30–37.

Schofield PW, Mosesson RE, Stern Y, et al. The age at onset of Alzheimer's disease and an intracranial area measurement. *Arch Neurol* 1995;52:95–98.

Schofield PW, Tang M, Marder K, et al. Alzheimer's disease after remote head injury: an incidence study. *J Neurol Neurosurg Psychiatry* 1997a;62:119–124.

Seshadri S, Beiser A, Selhub J, et al. Plasma homocysteine as a risk factor for dementia and Alzheimer's disease. *N Engl J Med* 2002; 346:476–483.

Skoog I. Status of risk factors for vascular dementia. *Neuroepidemiology* 1998;17:2–9.

Snowdon DA, Greiner LH, Mortimer JA, et al. Brain infarction and the clinical expression of Alzheimer disease. The Nun Study. *JAMA* 1997;277:813–817.

Snowdon DA, Kemper SJ, Mortimer JA, et al. Linguistic ability in early life and cognitive function and Alzheimer's disease in late life. *JAMA* 1996;275:528–532.

Snowdon D, Markesbery W. The prevalence of neuropathologically confirmed vascular dementia: findings from the Nun Study. In: Korczyn A, ed. Proceedings of the First International Conference on Vascular Dementia. Bologna, Italy: Monduzzi Editore, 1999, pp 19–24.

Sobel E, Davanipour Z, Sulkava R, et al. Occupations with exposure to electromagnetic fields: a possible risk factor for Alzheimer's disease. *Am J Epidemiol* 1995;142:515–524.

Sobel E, Dunn M, Davanipour Z, et al. Elevated risk of Alzheimer's disease among workers with likely electromagnetic field exposure. *Neurology* 1996;47:1477–1481.

Stern Y, Alexander GE, Prohovnik I, Mayeux R. Inverse relationship between education and parietotemporal perfusion deficit in Alzheimer's disease. *Ann Neurol* 1992;32:371–375.

Stern Y, Alexander GE, Prohovnik I, et al. Relationship between lifetime occupation and parietal flow: implications for a reserve against Alzheimer's disease pathology. *Neurology* 1995;45:55–60.

Stern Y, Gurland B, Tatemichi TK, et al. Influence of education and occupation on the incidence of Alzheimer's disease. *JAMA* 1994; 271:1004–1010.

Stewart WF, Kawas C, Corrada M, Metter EJ. Risk of Alzheimer's disease and duration of NSAID use. *Neurology* 1997;48:626–632.

Strittmatter WJ, Saunders AM, Schmechel D, et al. Apolipoprotein E: high-avidity binding to β-amyloid and increased frequency of type 4 allele in late-onset familial Alzheimer disease. *Proc Natl Acad Sci USA* 1993:90: 1977–1981.

Swaab DF. Brain aging and Alzheimer's disease, "wear and tear" versus "use it or lose it". *Neurobiol Aging* 1991;12:317–324.

Swan GE, DeCarli C, Miller BL, et al. Association of midlife blood pressure to late-life cognitive decline and brain morphology. *Neurology* 1998;51:986–993.

Tang MX, Jacobs D, Stern Y, et al. Effect of oestrogen during menopause on risk and age at onset of Alzheimer's disease. *Lancet* 1996; 348:429–432.

Tang MX, Stern Y, Marder K, et al. The APOE-ε4 allele and the risk of Alzheimer disease among African Americans, Whites and Hispanics. *JAMA* 1998;279:751–755.

Terry RD, Masliah E, Salmon DP, et al. Physical basis of cognitive alterations in Alzheimer's disease: synapse loss is the major correlate of cognitive impairment. *Ann Neurol* 1991;30:572–580.

Tol J, Slooter JC, van Duijn CM. Genetic factors in early- and late-onset Alzheimer's disease. In: Mayeux R, Christen Y, eds. Epidemiology of Alzheimer's Disease: From Gene to Prevention. New York: Springer-Verlag, 1999, pp 33–39.

Tomlinson BE, Blessed G, Roth M. Observations on the brains of non-demented old people. *J Neurol Sci* 1968;7:331–356.

Tyas SL. Are tobacco and alcohol use related to Alzheimer's disease? A critical assessment of the evidence and its implications. *Addiction Biol* 1996;1:237–254.

Tyas SL. Alcohol use and the risk of developing Alzheimer's disease. *Alcohol Res Health* 2001;25:299–306.

Tyas SL, Pederson LL, Koval JJ. Is smoking associated with the risk of developing Alzheimer's disease? Results from three Canadian data sets. *Ann Epidemiol* 2000;10: 409–416.

U.S. General Accounting Office. Alzheimer's Disease: Estimates of Prevalence in the United States. Report to the Secretary of Health and Human Services. 1998, GAO/HEHS-98-16.

van Duijn CM, Clayton D, Chandra V, et al. Familial aggregation of Alzheimer's disease and related disorders: a collaborative re-analysis of case–control studies. *Int J Epidemiol* 1991a;20:S13–S20.

van Duijn CM, Havekes LM, van Broeckhoven C, et al. Apolipoprotein E genotype and association between smoking and early onset Alzheimer's disease. *BMJ* 1995;310:627–631.

van Duijn CM, Hofman A. Relation between nicotine intake and Alzheimer's disease. *BMJ* 1991b;302:1491–1494.

Wang HX, Fratiglioni L, Frisoni G, et al. Smoking and the occurrence of Alzheimer's disease: cross-sectional and longitudinal data in a population-based study. *Am J Epidemiol* 1999;149:640–644.

Waring SC, Rocca WA, Petersen RC, et al. Postmenopausal estrogen replacement therapy and the risk of AD: a population-based study. *Neurology* 1999;52:965–970.

White L, Petrovitch H, Ross GW, et al. Prevalence of dementia in older Japanese-American men in Hawaii: the Honolulu-Asia Aging Study. *JAMA* 1996;276:995–960.

Wilson RS, de Leon CFM, Barnes LL, et al. Participation in cognitively stimulating activities and risk of incident Alzheimer's disease. *JAMA* 2002;287:742–748.

Wisniewski T, Frangione B. Apolipoprotein E: a pathological chaperone protein in patients with cerebral and systemic amyloid. *Neurosci Lett* 1992;135:235–238.

Yaffe K, Sawaya G, Lieberburg I, Grady D. Estrogen therapy in postmenopausal women: effects on cognitive function and dementia. *JAMA* 1998;279:688–695.

Yamada M, Sasaki H, Mimori Y, et al. Prevalence and risks of dementia in the Japanese population: RERF's adult health study Hiroshima subjects. Radiation Effects Research Foundation. *J Am Geriatr Soc* 1999;47:189–195.

Yoshitake T, Kiyohara Y, Kato I, et al. Incidence and risk factors of vascular dementia and Alzheimer's disease in a defined elderly Japanese population: the Hisayama study. *Neurology* 1995;45:1161–1168.

Young D, Lawlor PA, Leone P, et al. Environmental enrichment inhibits spontaneous apoptosis, prevents seizures and is neuroprotective. *Nat Med* 1999;5:448–453.

Zandi PP, Carlson MC, Plassman BL, et al. Hormone replacement therapy and incidence of Alzheimer's disease: the Cache County Study. *JAMA* 2002;288:2123–2129.

6

Movement Disorders

CAROLINE M. TANNER AND KAREN MARDER

Movement disorders are a distinct group of neurologic disorders characterized by abnormal involuntary movements. Although the term *movement disorders* suggests any disorder causing a problem of movement, in fact the majority of disorders causing difficulty moving (such as weakness or frank paralysis) do not involve abnormal involuntary movements and thus are not included in the category of movement disorders. The movement disorders are characterized phenomenologically (Table 6–1). While the observable phenomena are distinct, many of these disorders are thought to result from dysfunction of the same brain region, generally termed the *extrapyramidal system.* This system includes the brain areas outside the pyramidal system, which comprises the primary motor pathways. Although abnormal involuntary movements are primary features, many movement disorders also include changes in cognition and/or mood.

In this chapter we have chosen to focus on five movement disorders: Parkinson's disease, dystonia, tic disorders, Hunting-ton's disease, and essential tremor. We believe that these five demonstrate many of the most common challenges encountered in the epidemiologic investigation of movement disorders.

Parkinson's Disease

Parkinson's disease (PD) is one of the most common late-life neurodegenerative disorders. Because it is increasingly common with increasing age, its prevalence in the United States is expected to triple over the next 50 years with the aging of the population. Despite intensive research during the past several decades, the cause or causes of Parkinson's disease remain unknown. Nonetheless, significant progress is being made in elucidating genetic and environmental risk factors and neurodegenerative processes contributing to Parkinson's disease.

Disease Description

James Parkinson described a clinical syndrome that remains today the cornerstone

Table 6–1 Definitions of Common Abnormal Involuntary Movement

Tremor	A rhythmic oscillation of one or more body parts
Postural tremor	A tremor maximal when sustaining a fixed posture of the affected part (such as holding arms outstretched)
Resting tremor	A tremor maximal when the affected part is at rest (such as hands in lap)
Action or kinetic tremor	A tremor maximal during movement of the affected part (such as writing)
Bradykinesia	An abnormal slowness of voluntary movement
Akinesia	The absence of voluntary movement
Dystonia	A syndrome of sustained abnormal muscle contractions, frequently causing twisting and repetitive movements or abnormal postures of affected body parts
Cervical dystonia	Torticollis, retrocollis, spasmodic torticollis; sustained or intermittent neck and shoulder turning
Laryngeal dystonia	Spasmodic dysphonia; forced or whispering speech
Blepharospasm	Sustained or intermittent dystonic eye closure
Oromandibular dystonia	Sustained or intermittent jaw opening or closing, facial grimacing
Chorea	Unpredictable, nonstereotypic, continuous, brief, rapid, involuntary movements of a body part
Tic	A stereotypic, sudden, purposeless, involuntary movement that may be transiently suppressed and that resembles purposeful behavior
Myoclonus	Rapid, lightning-like jerk sufficient to move the joint

of clinical diagnostic criteria: bradykinesia, resting tremor, cogwheel rigidity, and postural reflex impairment (Parkinson 1817; Gelb et al. 1999). Pathologically, the hallmarks of Parkinson's disease are loss of pigmented neurons, most prominently in the substantia nigra, with associated characteristic α-synuclein-positive inclusion bodies (Lewy bodies). *Secondary parkinsonism* refers to the syndrome of parkinsonism but with an identifiable exogenous cause, such as neuroleptic drugs or carbon monoxide exposure. Typically, these conditions involve additional signs of more extensive brain injury. Neurodegenerative disorders may include the syndrome of parkinsonism along with abnormalities (often termed *atypical parkinsonism* or *parkinsonism plus*). These syndromes may not be easily distinguished from Parkinson's disease without an autopsy. Most recently, specific genetic causes of parkinsonism have been identified. While these disorders are commonly also referred to as Parkinson's disease, in fact, the gene-associated familial syndromes described to date often have clinical and/or pathologic features that are different from classical Parkinson's disease.

The uncertainty of clinical diagnosis is an important factor in the design and critical analysis of epidemiologic studies of Parkinson's disease. There is no diagnostic test for Parkinson's disease. Diagnosis is dependent entirely on the neurologic history and examination. Thus, the experience of diagnosticians can affect diagnostic accuracy.

Example 6–1 Computerized prescription records of 74 general medical practices were used to identify presumed Parkinson's disease in a Welsh community (Meara et al. 1999). Parkinsonism was confirmed in 74% of 402 cases examined, but only 53% met diagnostic criteria for Parkinson's disease. The remainder had other causes of parkinsonism or questionable features (21%) or no parkinsonism (26%). In the 26% without parkinsonism, 48% had essential tremor, 36% had gait disorders without parkinsonism, and 16% had primary dementia. Because this study used drug prescription to find disease, milder or more questionable cases were likely not identified, as these would be less likely to receive treatment. These findings and others suggest that significant disease misclassification may occur if expert review is not used to diagnose Parkinson's disease (Marttila and Rinne, 1976; Mutch et al. 1986).

Additionally, individuals who are clinically diagnosed with Parkinson's disease do not always show typical pathologic changes at postmortem. Surveys of postmortem findings in cases clinically diagnosed as Parkinson's disease found typical postmortem neuropathology in only 80% of cases (Rajput et al. 1991a; Hughes et al. 1993). In future studies, some of these diagnostic dilemmas may be improved by new imaging techniques, careful exclusion of cases with known genetic forms of parkinsonism, and, ultimately, development of sensitive and specific biomarkers of disease.

Descriptive Studies

In all populations studied, Parkinson's disease is rare before age 50 and increases with increasing age thereafter (Zhang and Roman 1993; Tanner and Goldman 1996; Melcon et al. 1997; Van den Eeden et al. 2003). This pattern could reflect either the cumulative effects of an environmental exposure or an age-associated genetic factor. Parkinson's disease is also more common

in men than in women. Male-associated environmental exposures or X chromosome–linked genetic susceptibility factors could explain such a pattern. Parkinson's disease may differ in frequency internationally, with North America and Europe showing higher rates of disease, but too few comparable studies have been published to allow a definitive conclusion.

Age. Increasing age is unequivocally associated with increasing risk for Parkinson's disease. This is true in all community-based studies, with annual incidence increasing dramatically from fewer than 10 per 100,000 at age 50 to at least 200 per 100,000 at age 80 (Tanner and Aston 2000). Although Parkinson's disease is intimately related to aging, it has been well documented that its underlying process is distinct from natural aging (McGeer et al. 1988; Fearnley and Lees 1991; Gibb and Lees 1991).

Gender. Men are diagnosed with Parkinson's disease about twice as often as women, irrespective of geographic location or race (Tanner and Goldman 1996; Baldereschi et al. 2000). This pattern is seen in both prevalence and incidence studies (Fig. 6–1). This increased risk in men may

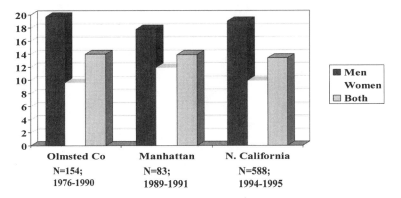

Figure 6–1 Age- and gender-specific incidence for Parkinson's disease was estimated for three U.S. populations: Olmsted County, Minnesota (Rocca et al. 2001), the Upper West Side of Manhattan (Mayeux et al. 1995), and northern California (Van Den Eeden et al. 2003). The pattern of male preponderance of disease and the magnitude of disease are similar in all three populations. The overall rates are age and gender adjusted; gender-specific rates are age adjusted.

reflect biological differences between men and women, such as the effects of sex hormones or X chromosome–linked susceptibility genes. Alternatively, culturally determined differences in male and female behavior, with associated differences in exposure to risk factors, could explain the pattern. The latter hypothesis is supported by a large Finnish study showing a dramatic increase in the male-to-female relative risk from 0.9 in 1971 to 1.9 in 1992 (Kuopio et al. 1999). Further epidemiologic studies, along with experimental laboratory studies, are needed to explain this pattern.

Race. Parkinson's disease may be more common in nations with primarily white populations, although the evidence is far from clear. Lower prevalence has been reported in non-whites (Tanner and Goldman 1996), but whether these differences were real or related to shorter survival or diagnostic differences is not clear. Recent incidence studies in multiethnic populations did not find differences among racial or ethnic groups (Fig. 6–2) (Mayeux et al. 1995; Morens et al. 1996; Van den Eeden et al.

2003). However, the actual numbers of non-whites in these studies were small, and precision of the estimates was consequently poor.

Temporal Variation. Changing incidence over time has been estimated in only two locations. In Olmsted County, Minnesota, there was no apparent change in age-specific Parkinson's disease incidence in recent decades (Rocca et al. 2001). In contrast, a large Finnish study found a dramatic demographic shift when comparing 1971 incidence to that of 1992, with a strong male and rural predominance not previously observed (Kuopio et al. 1999). It is difficult to be certain whether these variations in disease frequency represent actual changes, or instead represent other determinants, such as improved diagnosis or record keeping, or relative changes in mortality from competing diseases (Riggs 1993). Identification of changes in disease frequency over time could provide clues to the cause of disease. For example, increasing incidence over time could be due to increased exposure to causative agents.

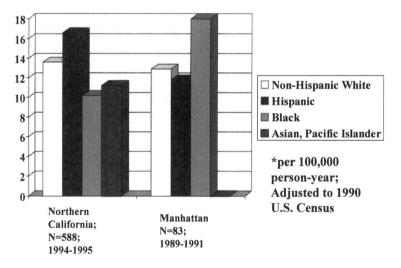

Figure 6–2 Parkinson's disease incidence by ethnicity was estimated for 2 U.S. populations: the Upper West Side of Manhattan (Mayeux et al. 1995) and northern California (Van Den Eeden et al. 2003). For comparison, rates were ad-

justed to the 1990 U.S. census. Incidence in non-Hispanic whites is similar. Incidence in the other ethnic groups is not statistically different from that for non-Hispanic whites, but numbers are small and precision is poor.

Geography. Geographic variation can be traced primarily from prevalence estimates, as few incidence studies have been performed. Estimated prevalence varies widely across countries, from 31 per 100,000 persons in Libya to 657 per 100,000 in Buenos Aires, Argentina (Tanner and Ben-Shlomo 1999). Many of these inconsistencies may be explained by demographic differences in the underlying populations, by methodologic differences in the individual studies, or by differences in access to health care or disease survival rates. However, international variation in Parkinson's disease frequency is seen even after adjusting for many of these inconsistencies (Zhang and Roman 1993). If there are international differences in Parkinson's disease frequency, underlying factors could be either differences in the genetic characteristics of the underlying populations or differences in exposure to causative and protective environmental factors.

Analytic Studies

Many potential environmental and genetic risk factors for Parkinson's disease have been identified. Exposure to environmental toxins may interrupt energy production in the mitochondria or cause increased levels of oxidative stress that in turn might lead directly to nerve cell injury or death. An individual's ability to respond to these insults may be determined by genetic polymorphisms that code for metabolic enzymes with reduced or increased ability to metabolize environmental toxins. Other environmental factors such as dietary antioxidants, caffeine, or nicotine-like substances may protect neurons from these injuries.

Environmental Risk Factors. Environmental causes of Parkinson's disease have been suspected for many years. In 1983, investigation of a cluster of parkinsonism in northern California narcotic addicts identified the neurotoxicant 1-methyl-4-phenyl tetrahydropyridine (MPTP) (Langston et al. 1983). MPTP-induced parkinsonism is clinically and pathologically very similar to Parkinson's disease. These findings prompted the search for an environmental cause for Parkinson's disease, guided by numerous laboratory studies investigating MPTP toxicology (Langston 1996). MPTP exposure is uncommon, but agents similar to MPTP in structure or function are possible environmental exposures. For example, the pesticide paraquat is structurally similar to MPTP and causes parkinsonism in animals (Thiruchelvam et al. 2000; McCormack et al. 2002). Other compounds causing parkinsonism in animals share the mechanism of mitochondrial complex I inhibition, such as the pesticide rotenone (Betarbet et al. 2000). These observations have directed epidemiologic investigations of risk factors for Parkinson's disease.

Pesticides. Pesticides are of particular interest because of the similarities of some pesticides to MPTP. Also, an association between Parkinson's disease and farming or rural living indirectly supports pesticides as risk factors (see below). Case–control studies also implicate specific pesticides. A meta-analysis of 19 published studies found a combined odds ratio (OR) of 1.94 (95% confidence interval [CI] 1.49–2.53) for pesticide exposure (Priyadarshi et al. 2000). Specific compounds or compound classes have only rarely been identified, however. Two autopsy studies detected increased levels of the insecticide dieldrin in Parkinson's disease brain (Fleming et al. 1994; Corrigan et al. 2000). Liou et al. (1997) reported increased risk of Parkinson's disease in association with paraquat (OR = 3.22) in Taiwan. In other studies, exposure to herbicides, insecticides, alkylated phosphates, organochlorines, and wood preservatives have all been reported to be associated with increased risk of Parkinson's disease, but the categories or specific agents differed among these reports (Semchuk et al. 1992; Butterfield et al. 1993; Seidler et al. 1996; Gorell et al. 1998).

Rural living and farming. Case–control studies conducted throughout the world have identified rural living, farming, gardening, and well water drinking as risk factors for Parkinson's disease (Ho et al. 1989; Stern et al. 1991; Morano et al. 1994; Gorell et al. 1998; Marder et al. 1998; McCann et al. 1998). Although the precise nature of the association with putative rural risk factors varies across studies, the consistency of these findings is remarkable considering the different methods and locations. It is unclear how rural factors other than pesticide exposure may be related to Parkinson's disease.

Other occupations. A higher frequency of Parkinson's disease has been reported among teachers (Schulte et al. 1996; Tsui et al. 1999), health workers (Schulte et al. 1996; Tsui et al. 1999), carpenters and cleaners (Fall et al. 1999), and in workers chronically exposed to metals (Gorell et al. 1999). However, associations were not consistently observed among the studies. Most studies did not employ uniform methods of determining occupation. Only one study systematically investigated occupation-associated exposure to any toxicant (Gorell et al. 1999). Future studies will need to employ more rigorous methods to determine occupational risks for Parkinson's disease.

Infection. A unique form of parkinsonism was caused by an epidemic of encephalitis in the early 1900s, but many subsequent studies have failed to identify an infectious cause of Parkinson's disease. Although a handful of sporadic associations have been published, these have rarely been confirmed (Tanner and Goldman 1996). Parkinsonism in an animal model has been caused by the common soil pathogen *Nocardia asteroides* (Kohbata and Beaman 1991). To date, this has not been associated with Parkinson's disease in humans (Hubble et al. 1995). Theoretically, an infectious process could explain the familial nature of Parkinson's disease. Because *Nocardia* is commonly found in soil, it could also provide an alternate explanation for

the rural preponderance of Parkinson's disease. However, other supportive data are lacking.

Smoking. Not smoking cigarettes is the most consistently observed risk factor for Parkinson's disease. An inverse association between cigarette smoking and Parkinson's disease has been observed in studies spanning more than 30 years, involving diverse populations, and including several large prospective investigations (Doll et al. 1994; Grandinetti et al. 1994; Benedetti et al. 2000; Willems-Giesbergen et al. 2000). Overall, disease risk in cigarette smokers appears to be about half that of nonsmokers, and is reduced with greater doses of cigarette smoke (Sugita et al. 2001). Animal studies suggest that nicotine may protect against experimental parkinsonism (Janson et al. 1993; Prasad et al. 1994). Alternatively, decreased smoking in Parkinson's disease could be a manifestation of the conservative personality that has been observed in Parkinson's disease patients prior to their diagnosis (Menza 2000).

Alcohol. Alcohol use has been found by some to be inversely associated with Parkinson's disease even after controlling for possible confounding by smoking (Hellenbrand et al. 1996; Fall et al. 1999; Paganini-Hill 2001). One study found that fewer cases with Parkinson's disease had a diagnosis of alcoholism than controls (Benedetti et al. 2000). A biologic explanation for this observation has not been articulated. Alternatively, the low consumption of alcohol in Parkinson's disease has commonly been attributed to the reserved personality that has been observed before Parkinson's disease manifests itself (Menza 2000).

Diet. Differences in diet could explain the geographic variability in Parkinson's disease prevalence or the clustering of the disease within families. Several case–control studies have investigated dietary factors, providing associations for further evaluation. Because antioxidant-containing foods and vitamin supplements may be neuroprotective, several studies have examined the association of these with Parkinson's disease. However, dietary or supplementary intake of antioxidants does not appear to lower risk of Parkinson's disease (Tanner and Goldman 1996). Eating foods high in animal fat has been associated with increased risk of Parkinson's disease in several case–control studies (Logroscino et al. 1996; Gorell et al. 1997; Anderson et al. 1999), as has higher total caloric intake (Hellenbrand et al. 1996; Logroscino et al. 1996). Oxidative stress, a proposed pathogenetic mechanism for Parkinson's disease, is thought to be increased by lipid consumption and higher caloric intake. Moreover, dietary restriction has been found to prevent loss of dopaminergic neurons in rats given the neurotoxin MPTP (Duan and Mattson 1999). Further investigation of this association seems merited.

Coffee and caffeine. An inverse association of both coffee and caffeine consumption and Parkinson's disease has been reported in case–control and cohort studies (Fall et al. 1999; Benedetti et al. 2000; Ross et al. 2000; Ascherio et al. 2001; Paganini-Hill 2001). The effect appears to differ between men and women, with a direct dose–response association in men (higher consumption associated with lower risk) but a U-shaped pattern in women, although fewer women have been studied. Caffeine may be neuroprotective through its antagonist action on the adenosine A2A receptor (Chen et al 2001), providing biologic plausibility for this observation.

Head trauma. Prior head trauma has been associated with Parkinson's disease in numerous case–control studies (Tanner and Goldman 1996). The head injury typically occurs decades before the diagnosis of Parkinson's disease, minimizing the chance that disease-related disability caused the injury (Factor et al. 1991; Seidler et al. 1996; Taylor et al. 1999). While recall bias could

explain observed associations, Bower et al. (2002) report a similar association when comparing injury documented in the medical record before the diagnosis of disease. Further investigation in prospective cohorts will be important.

Genetic Risk Factors

Hereditary risk factors for Parkinson's disease have been an active research focus for more than a century. This research has taken three primary directions: (1) familial studies and genetic linkage analysis, (2) twin studies, and (3) single gene associations.

Modern molecular methods have led to exciting discoveries of genetic mutations that cause parkinsonism, although these are rare (Table 6–2). Investigations of genetic forms of parkinsonism must overcome a number of methodologic difficulties. First, diagnosis of many, if not most, "affected" individuals is by family-derived historical information rather than by examination. Because onset is in late life, uniform methods of ascertainment cannot usually be used across generations. Information available historically may be incomplete or inaccurate. Second, autopsy confirmation is uncommon. As a result, it is not possible to be certain that the familial disorder fulfills the diagnostic gold standard provided by postmortem examinations. In most families, the clinical or pathological features of at least some of the cases are not fully consistent with those of typical Parkinson's disease. Therefore, extrapolation of findings in these cases to nonfamilial cases may not be appropriate. Despite these limitations, several genes have been identified. Investigation of these genes in the laboratory has already provided important clues to the cause of Parkinson's disease.

Other Studies of Familial Aggregation. Case–control studies have implicated a genetic contribution to the cause of Parkinson's disease. A positive family history for Parkinson's disease is more frequently reported by Parkinson's disease cases than

Table 6–2 Studies of the Genetics of Parkinsonism

Study	Mode of inheritance	Genetic defect	Approximate no. of cases affected	Onset age (years)
Polymeropoulous et al. 1997; Papadimitriou et al. 1999	Autosomal dominant	Ala 53 Thr mutation of α-synuclein gene, chromosome 4q PARK1	60 in 5 families	20–85
Kruger et al. 1998	Autosomal dominant	Ala 30 Pro mutation of α-synuclein gene, chromosome 4q PARK1	3 definite, 2 possible in 1 family	30–56
Hattori et al. 1998a; Kitada et al. 1998; Lücking et al. 1998	Autosomal recessive	Linkage: chromosome 6q25.2–27 parkin gene PARK2	Unknown; 100s to 1000s worldwide	Most common before age 30
Wsolek et al. 1995; Gasser et al. 1998	Autosomal dominant	Linkage: chromosome 2p13 PARK3 Reduced penetrance (est. 40%)	57 in 6 families	36–82
Farrer et al. 1999	Autosomal dominant	Linkage: chromosome 4p14–16.3 PARK4 Reduced penetrance	2 large U.S. families with common ancestor	<20–50s
Leroy et al. 1998; Farrer et al. 2000	Autosomal dominant	Chromosome 4p14–15 Ubiquitin carboxyhydrolase L1 (UCH-L1) gene PARK5 Reduced penetrance	3 cases in 2 families	49, 51
Valente et al. 2001, 2002	Autosomal recessive	Linkage: chromosome 1p35–36 PARK6	1 Sicilian family	32–48
Van Duijn et al. 2001	Autosomal recessive	Linkage: chromosome 1p36 PARK7	1 Dutch family	≤40
Funayama et al. 2002	Autosomal dominant	Linkage: chromosome 12p11.23–q13.11 PARK8 Low penetrance	1 Japanese family	
Hicks et al. 2001	Autosomal recessive	Linkage: chromosome 1p32 PARK10	117 patients in 51 Icelandic families	Similar to sporadic Parkinson's disease

control subjects, with odds ratios ranging from 2.7 to 14.6 (Payami et al. 1994; Rybicki et al. 1999; Taylor et al. 1999; Autere et al. 2000; Kuopio et al. 2001). This risk factor appears to be stronger in those with younger onset of disease. Methodologic challenges encountered in performing case–control studies such as these include the possibility of family bias. Because cases are more likely to be aware of disease in family members than are unaffected controls, disease may be underestimated in controls if family members are not examined. A recent validation study of family history in the context of a population-based case–control study has shown significant family bias. Elbaz and colleagues (2002) found underreporting of disease in relatives of controls and overreporting in relatives of cases, causing a fourfold overestimation of the odds ratio. In many studies, cases were identified from referral centers. Familial parkinsonism may be more common in these centers than in the community. Also, it is important to consider family composition when comparing disease frequency in cases and controls. Differences in family size, age, or gender could result in an over- or underestimation of disease risk.

Example 6–2 A large study by Marder et al. (1996), which used community-based case identification methods, also found a significantly increased risk of Parkinson's disease in first-degree relatives of Parkinson's disease cases, but the magnitude of risk was considerably less than in studies using clinic-based populations. Controlling for gender, ethnicity, and relationship to proband, they found that first-degree relatives of cases were 2.3 times as likely to develop Parkinson's disease than relatives of controls, and that male relatives were at twice the risk of female relatives. The lifetime incidence (to age 75) in first-degree relatives of cases was only 2% vs. 1% in control families, suggesting that, although there is a significant familial component, idiopathic Parkinson's disease may not be due to simple Mendelian inheritance.

The population of Iceland provides a unique means for investigating the role of genetics in Parkinson's disease, because genealogic information is known for over 11 centuries (Sveinbjornsdottir et al. 2000). Relatedness was determined for 772 living and dead Icelanders with parkinsonism (diagnosed over a 50-year period). Parkinson's disease risk was increased 6.7 times in siblings, 3.2 in offspring, and 2.7 in nieces and nephews of later onset (after age 50) disease. Parkinson's disease cases were more closely related than the controls. This pattern supports a complex heredity, with multiple genes and/or gene–environment interaction contributing to both early- and late-onset disease. The increased risk in siblings compared with children of cases supports a common early environmental factor or, alternatively, recessively inherited modifying genes. In fact, a recessively inherited gene causing parkinsonism has recently been described in this population (Hicks et al. 2002). Because Icelanders in general may be considered to constitute a partial genetic isolate, the degree to which these findings can be extended to other populations is uncertain. In contrast to population-based studies in other regions, the number of young-onset cases was very high (more than 25%) in this report. The estimated prevalence of younger-onset disease (≤ 50 years) was much greater than older-onset disease, while typically prevalence and incidence increase with increasing age. These observations could reflect incomplete ascertainment of older-onset cases, or a different pattern of disease in Iceland than in other countries. Aggregation of disease in families does not always imply a genetic cause, however. Since families share behaviors and environments, familial occurrence cannot necessarily be attributed to an underlying genetic mechanism.

Genome-wide Scans. Genome-wide scans provide a method for comprehensively examining chromosomal regions that may influence risk for Parkinson's disease. In two studies, the most compelling association was with chromosome 6 within the parkin gene (*PARK2*), seen in families with at least one individual with onset younger than 40 years. Linkage was also identified to chromosomes 17q, 8p, 5q, and 9q in families with later-onset disease (Scott et al. 2001) and on chromosomes 1, 9, 10, and 16 (DeStefano et al. 2001). Taken together, these results highlight the difficulties encountered in such studies. Because the results are not overlapping, significant heterogeneity is suggested. Alternatively, some results, while meeting the prespecified statistical criteria for linkage, may prove to be biologically invalid. Another possibility is that distinct populations of familial atypical parkinsonism may be included in each study. Further replications using this potentially powerful tool will help to clarify this conundrum.

Twin Studies. Twin studies have also been used to test the hypothesis of a genetic contribution to the etiology of Parkinson's disease (Table 6–3). Similar to other genetic approaches, studies in twins have not supported a major genetic determinant in later-onset disease. However, in earlier-onset parkinsonism, genetic factors are prominent. Because observations in twins have been primarily cross-sectional, important information may have been missed. Follow-up studies will be critical to understanding the genetic and environmental contribution to disease.

Future Directions and Conclusions

Recent advances in epidemiological, genetic, and basic science research are generating plausible hypotheses regarding the cause of Parkinson's disease. These advances, rather than narrowing the focus to a single genetic or environmental cause, suggest that Parkinson's disease is a complex disorder with multiple causes, likely due to the interaction of genes and environment. While determining the many potential causes of Parkinson's disease will be challenging, the development of successful future therapies and preventive measures will depend on a sound understanding of the interaction of environmental, molecular, and genetic factors involved in Parkinson's disease.

Dystonia

Dystonia, a syndrome of sustained muscle contractions, frequently causing twisting and repetitive movements or abnormal postures, is a disabling, clinically heterogeneous disorder affecting individuals throughout the lifespan (Fahn 1988). Dystonia has adverse health effects, and also poses a significant socioeconomic burden (Butler et al. 1998). Although dystonia is the third most common movement disorder, little is understood about many aspects of dystonia, including the descriptive epidemiology of the disease and the causes of most forms of dystonia. This lack of knowledge has limited progress in identifying treatments or cures for this disabling disorder.

Disease Description

Dystonia may be grouped into two broad etiologic categories: primary and secondary (Table 6–4) (Fahn et al. 1998). This section will focus on primary dystonia (also called *primary torsion dystonia*). Primary dystonia is distinguished from most secondary dystonias by the absence of signs other than dystonia and dystonic tremor. Primary dystonia has no consistent neuropathologic lesion or neurochemical abnormality. In a minority of cases, once dystonia is identified, a genetic test may confirm presence of a dystonia-associated mutation (see below). In the remainder, there is no diagnostic test. The initial diagnosis of dystonia relies solely on the recognition of the signs during a clinical examination. The clinical spectrum of primary dystonia is remarkably variable. Dystonia may begin at any age from early childhood to the eighth decade and may vary anatomically from involvement of a single muscle (focal, or spasmodic dysphonia) to contractions of numerous limb, axial, and cranial muscles (general-

Table 6-3 Twin Studies of Parkinson's Disease Concordance

Study	Ascertainment diagnosis	CONCORDANT PAIRS		Risk ratio (95% CI)	Methodologic concerns
		MZ	DZ		
Duvoisin et al. 1981 Ward et al. 1983	Clinical practice; advertisement Expert exam	4/48	1/19	1.58 (0.19–13.27)	Small sample size; selection bias possible; examiners knew zygosity; young ages; only MZ twins followed
Marsden 1987	Advertisement Family doctor	1/11	1/11	1.00 (0.07–14.05)	Small sample size; selection bias possible; diagnosis uncertain; cross-sectional
Marttila et al. 1988	Records linkage National Health database	0/18	1/14	0 (0–14.06)	Small sample size; diagnosis uncertain
Vierregge et al. 1992	Advertisement Expert exam	3/9	3/12	1.33 (0.35–5.13)	Small sample size; selection bias possible; examiner knew zygosity; cross-sectional
Tanner et al. 1999	Direct screen; unselected twin cohort Expert consensus based on exam	11/61	10/90	1.39 (0.63–3.10)	Cross-sectional

DZ, dizygotic; MZ, monozygotic; CI, confidence interval.

Table 6–4   Causes of Dystonia

Primary (or idiopathic) Dystonia

Clinical signs of dystonia only
No exogenous cause
No other neurologic disease
Includes inherited dystonias with generalized or
focal phenotypes

Secondary Dystonia

Associated with other neurologic disorders
Due to acquired/exogenous causes

ized dystonia). It is common for persons with dystonia of any type to seek medical attention without receiving the correct diagnosis for years before encountering an expert familiar with the disorder, complicating epidemiologic studies of disease frequency.

Descriptive Studies

Few studies have estimated the prevalence of dystonia, only one estimated incidence (Tanner and Goldman 1994; Duffy et al. 1998; Epidemiologic Study of Dystonia in Europe Collaborative Group 2000), and no study has estimated incidence or prevalence in age-, gender-, and race/ethnicity-specific strata including all clinical subtypes. The prevalence of generalized primary dystonia has been estimated to range from 0.96 per 100,000 in Israel to 11 per 100,000 in New York (Korczyn et al. 1980; Risch et al. 1995). Estimated prevalence of focal dystonia ranges from 6.1/100,000 in Yonago, Japan (Nakashima et al. 1995) to 225 per 100,000 in Bruneck, Italy (Muller et al. 2002). In the few studies in which the frequency of both primary focal and generalized primary dystonia have been estimated, focal dystonia is 9–14 times more frequent than generalized primary dystonia. (Li et al. 1985; Nakashima et al. 1995). Precision in these studies is poor; the community surveys cited all had identified fewer than 40 primary dystonia cases. More cases are found in surveys derived from botulinum toxin clinics (Duffy et al. 1998; Epidemiologic Study of Dystonia in Europe Collaborative Group 2000; Konkiewitz et al.

2002), although the fact that botulinum toxin is most effective for only a few forms of dystonia (torticollis and blepharospasm) makes these estimates more uncertain.

All of these studies are likely underestimating the true frequency of primary dystonia, because a significant proportion of disease is likely not diagnosed. For example, Risch et al. (1995) observed that 50% of the family members of persons with genetic dystonia who had dystonic findings on neurologic examination had not been previously diagnosed. Efforts to increase awareness of dystonia symptoms in healthcare workers and patients will be important components of future studies.

Age. The age at onset distribution is bimodal, with modes at age 9 (early-onset) and 45 (late-onset), divided by a nadir at age 27 (Bressman et al. 1989). The focal dystonias present most often in adult life (e.g., writer's cramp, occupational hand dystonias) and generalized primary dystonia begins most commonly in children.

Gender. No consistent gender effect on primary dystonia has been observed. In 957 adults with primary dystonia attending botulinum toxin clinics, cervical ocular and laryngeal dystonia occurred earlier in men, while writer's cramp onset was earlier in women (Epidemiological Study of Dystonia in Europe [ESDE] Collaborative Group 1999).

Race. While primary dystonia has been reported in all races (Tanner 1991), the relative distribution of dystonia across racial groups is not known. An excess of early-onset primary dystonia is observed in Ashkenazi Jews, due to a presumed single founder mutation (Risch et al. 1995). Only one report, derived from a large tertiary referral center, has investigated the distribution of primary dystonia by race or ethnicity (Almasy et al. 1997). In this New York–based practice, the clinical features of dystonia appeared to vary with race/ethnicity. Ashkenazi Jews had an earlier age at onset and a greater frequency of limb onset than did non-Jewish Caucasians. African Americans appeared to have intermediate age at onset and a tendency to cranial and laryngeal involvement at onset, but only 29 cases were observed. The numbers of Asians and Hispanics were too few to allow analysis. No other report has investigated the racial or ethnic distribution of primary dystonia.

Genetic Risk Factors

While at least 13 genetic dystonia syndromes have been described, only 4 mutations have been identified (Table 6–5; Klein and Ozelius 2002). Of these, only one mutation causes primary generalized dystonia. This mutation, DYT1, alters the protein product, torsinA (Ozelius et al. 1997). DYT1 is dominantly inherited. Penetrance is low (30%–40%), but the environmental or genetic factors influencing the manifestation of clinical signs remain unknown. The DYT1 GAG deletion is most important in the Ashkenazi population, where it accounts for about 90% of early limb-onset cases. In non-Jewish people, only 40%–65% of early limb-onset primary dystonia cases carry the mutation.

Environmental Risk Factors

Investigation of environmental risk factors for primary dystonia has been limited, but the low penetrance of the one causative gene identified argues that this work is critically important to an understanding of the disorder. Nongenetic risk factors theoretically include both those factors causing dystonia to manifest in gene carriers (to date, only DYT1 mutations are associated with primary dystonia) and those risk factors causing dystonia in the absence of a genetic predisposition.

Trauma and Primary Dystonia. The risk factor for dystonia most frequently proposed is trauma. Typically, the trauma is described as an injury to the dystonic body part, preceding dystonia onset by months or longer (Gowers 1888; Jankovic 2001). Commonly reported injuries in clinical series include "whiplash" from a motor vehicle accident, reported in up to 20% of spasmodic torticollis patients, hand trauma in up to 10% with focal hand dystonias, and ocular lesions such as keratitis in 10%–20% with blepharospasm (Fletcher et al. 1991; Jankovic 1994; Defazio et al. 1998). The injury is proposed to alter sensory input and induce central nervous system reorganization, resulting in a movement disorder (Jankovic 2001).

Antecedent Illness. Because the DYT1 gene encoded a protein in the heat shock family, it was suggested that the expression of torsinA may be modulated by infection or fever. Saunders-Pullman et al. (2000) com-

Table 6–5 Genes Causing Dystonia

Gene, chromosome	Mode of inheritance	Clinical features
DYT1, 9q34	Autosomal dominant	Generalized dystonia
DYT2, unknown	Autosomal recessive	Generalized dystonia
DYT3, Xq13.1	X-linked	Dystonia plus
DYT4, unknown	Autosomal dominant	Generalized dystonia; laryngeal dystonia
DYT5, 14q22.1–q22.2	Autosomal dominant	Dystonia plus
DYT6, 8p21–8p22	Autosomal dominant	Focal or segmental dystonia
DYT7, 18p	Autosomal dominant	Focal dystonia
DYT8, 2q33–q25	Autosomal dominant	Dystonia plus
DYT9, 1p21–p13.3	Autosomal dominant	Dystonia plus
DYT10, 16p11.2–q12.1	Autosomal dominant	Dystonia plus
DYT11, 7q21–31	Autosomal dominant	Dystonia plus
DYT12, 19q	Autosomal dominant	Dystonia plus
DYT13, 1p36.13	Autosomal dominant	Cervical and cranial dystonia

pared antecedent severe febrile illness and trauma in manifesting and nonmanifesting *DYT1* carriers. Early-onset childhood illness was associated with manifesting dystonia, but peripheral trauma was not. More studies are needed.

Cigarette Smoking. One case–control study of 202 adults with primary dystonia and 202 controls found an inverse association of cigarette smoking and primary dystonia (Defazio et al. 1998). The magnitude of the association (OR = 0.66, 95% CI 0.4, 1.07) was similar to that repeatedly observed in Parkinson's disease (Marras and Tanner 2002). Dystonia is presumed to be mediated by the same general brain circuitry as in Parkinson's disease (Tanner 1991). Dystonia may occur in Parkinson's disease and alterations of central dopaminergic systems can cause both Parkinson's disease and dystonia (Bressman 2000). Therefore, shared risk factors for the disorders are not implausible. Identifying an inverse association of smoking and primary dystonia may provide important clues to involvement of cholinergic mechanisms in primary dystonia and clues to prevention.

Occupation and Repetitive Movement. Focal hand dystonia is commonly associated with occupations involving repetitive movements, such as typing or playing a musical instrument (Chen and Hallett 1998). These dystonias can be devastating and may cause career change. Similarly, childhood-onset *DYT1* generalized dystonia frequently presents with focal signs, often manifesting only with prolonged task-specific activity (e.g., writing, running). If specific occupations, hobbies, or characteristic physical activities are shown to be associated with dystonia, avoidance of these could be important in those at risk (for example, nonmanifesting *DYT1* carriers).

Future Directions and Conclusions

Further epidemiologic studies in differing populations are important to define the international distribution of dystonic disorders. Epidemiologic studies are also needed to elucidate the etiology of the disorder to guide the development of treatments or cures. The study of many large kindreds using linkage analysis may help to clarify questions about the hereditary pattern of dystonia and the homo- or heterogeneity of dystonic disorders as well as provide for understanding the pathophysiology of the disorder.

Tic Disorders

Disease Description

A *tic* is a stereotypic, sudden, purposeless, involuntary movement that may be transiently suppressed and that resembles purposeful behavior. Tic disorders may be classified as *simple tic,* which is a single stereotypic involuntary movement (such as an eyeblink or throat clearing), or *chronic multifocal tic disorder,* which comprises multiple different simple and complex motor and vocal stereotypic movements (such as head tossing, kicking, snorting, and involuntary expletive speech [coprolalia]). Both simple tic and chronic multifocal tic disorder may resolve over time or may be lifelong. If chronic multifocal tic disorder is lifelong, it is referred to as *Tourette syndrome.*

A major difficulty in the epidemiological study of tic disorders is the lack of a diagnostic test. At present, there is no diagnostic test for any tic disorder, so diagnosis is dependent on clinical examination and history. The epidemiologic investigation of tic disorders is challenging for several reasons. First, while Tourette syndrome is by definition a lifelong disorder, tic severity waxes and wanes over time. Tics often are most obvious in childhood. Cross-sectional observational studies will likely underestimate the "true" disease frequency. An individual correctly classified as having Tourette syndrome in a survey during childhood might not be thus identified as an adult, when tic severity is typically less.

Second, tics may not be recognized as abnormal movements by cases, family members, teachers, or health professionals. In studies in which expert examinations are not performed and cases are identified by history only, many cases may be missed. Third, tics are intermittent, and the specific phenomenology of tics may change. In addition, tics are suppressible, and cases commonly will suppress the abnormal movements in social situations, such as during an epidemiologic study. Thus, tics may be missed if diagnostic criteria require their observation by the examiner. Also, because diagnosis of Tourette syndrome requires multifocal tics, cross-sectional investigations may misclassify those manifesting single tics when evaluated. On the other hand, in studies in which examinations are not performed and cases are identified by interview only, many cases may be missed because affected persons or their relatives may be unaware of the tics. Differences in interviewing technique could produce inflated or deflated estimates of disease.

Behavioral disorders such as attention deficit disorder and obsessive-compulsive disorder appear to be associated with motor and vocal tics, although the relationship is not understood (Erenberg et al. 1986; Comings and Comings 1987; Spencer et al. 1995; Nolan et al. 1996; Walkup et al. 1996). As a result, when determining Tourette syndrome frequency, some investigators might include individuals with attention deficit disorder, obsessive-compulsive disorder, or simple tics, while others might include only those with motor or vocal tics.

The identification of a Tourette syndrome gene or genes using molecular genetic techniques may allow accurate diagnosis in the future, but until then diagnostic uncertainty may lead to erroneous conclusions about such important observations as the frequency, natural history, and clinical syndrome of Tourette syndrome.

Descriptive Studies

Since tics vary both in frequency and severity, any attempt to determine the true incidence or prevalence of tics in a single session is destined to be inaccurate. Similarly,

the distinction of simple tic from chronic multifocal tic must be made through clinical examination and history and often may not be determined at one visit. Several studies have assessed the prevalence of tics or Tourette syndrome in groups of school-age children and adolescents in defined communities (Lapouse and Monk 1964; Rutter et al. 1970; Burd et al. 1986; Caine et al. 1988; Comings et al. 1990b; Apter et al. 1993; Costello et al. 1996; Landgren et al. 1996; Verhulst et al. 1997; Mason et al. 1998). These studies have reported a tremendous range of prevalence estimates for Tourette syndrome, likely the result of differences in study design. While features such as the source of the sample, the age range of the sample, the sample size, and the diagnostic criteria employed likely all contribute, differences in ascertainment appear to be important determinants of the magnitude of prevalence estimates.

Studies determining the numbers of cases in a population by self-identified volunteers or by individuals seeking medical treatment for tics most likely underestimate prevalence, particularly for mild or infrequent tics. For example, investigators identifying cases by advertisement and voluntary registries in Monroe County, New York, estimated prevalence at 3/10,000, based on 41 cases (Caine et al. 1988). In Nebraska, prevalence of Tourette syndrome was estimated at 5/10,000, based on voluntary registry and mailed survey to physicians (Burd et al 1986). Use of more intensive ascertainment methods is associated with higher estimated prevalence.

Example 6–3 Costello et al. (1996) used a two-stage design to ascertain cases of tic disorders and Tourette syndrome living in an 11-county area of North Carolina. DSM-III diagnostic criteria were used. First, a random group of about 4000 children was assembled from among 11,758 children in three age cohorts (9-, 11-, and 13-year-olds). A 57-item questionnaire about behavioral problems was completed by each child's parents. The 1009 children with highest severity scores were classified as "screen positive," the others, "screen negative." From these groups, nearly 800 screen positives and 260 screen negatives were selected for more intensive evaluation. Both parents (the primary informant) and children were interviewed about psychiatric symptoms and level of functioning. Data collected estimated 3-month prevalence. Prevalence was estimated as 420 per 10,000 for all tic disorders collectively and 10 per 10,000 for Tourette syndrome. Because this study identified Tourette syndrome and tics only from those with the most severity of externalizing symptoms, children without disruptive behavior problems would have been missed. Consequently, this is likely an underestimate of the frequency of Tourette syndrome and tics.

A similar study design investigated tics in adolescents (Verhulst et al. 1997) and also estimated 10 cases per 10,000 for Tourette syndrome and 400/100,000 for all tic disorders. Even more intensive ascertainment methods resulted in the highest reported estimate of Tourette syndrome prevalence.

Example 6–4 Using school rosters masked for confidentiality, Kurlan et al. (2001) recruited a random sample of children from special education classrooms and a comparison sample of children from regular education classrooms (frequency matched by age and gender). Research technicians trained to identify tics performed the standardized evaluations of each child. Teachers and parents were interviewed. Despite the random sampling frame, only 11% of those recruited actually participated. Participants were more likely to be in special education (21% participants vs. 17% nonparticipants) and less likely to be from an urban school district (22% participants vs. 42% nonparticipants). For any tic disorder, weighted prevalence was 23.4% in special education and 18.5% in regular classrooms. Using full DSM-IV diagnostic criteria, Tourette syndrome frequency was 1.5% for special education and 0.8% for regular education classrooms. Excluding a

controversial criterion requiring significant impairment, Tourette syndrome frequency for special education classrooms was 7% (7.8% weighted) and 3.8% for regular education classrooms (3.1% weighted). This study illustrates several points regarding the challenges involved in studying tic disorders. First, in-person evaluation was associated with the highest reported tic frequency. Use of expert observers likely increased recognition of tics, especially mild tics without associated behavior problems, providing a more accurate picture of the distribution of disease in the community than is seen in estimates derived from medical care settings. Second, a change in diagnostic criteria from DSM-III to DSM-IV caused a significant difference in estimated prevalence. One new (and controversial) criterion introduced into the DSM-IV, requiring marked distress or significant functional impairment to diagnose Tourette syndrome, resulted in a fourfold reduced prevalence estimate. Third, despite a random sampling design, the very low participation rates suggest that participation may have been nonrandom. If more children participated because they were known or suspected to have tics, prevalence could be overestimated.

While it is possible that selection bias artificially inflated prevalence in this study, two other studies involving direct observation of school populations had similar results, despite different sampling strategies. Mason et al. (1998) used systematic observation of ninth-grade classrooms as well as interviews. Tourette syndrome prevalence was estimated at 2.9%. In a 4-year follow-up of Swedish schoolchildren and those in a tic disorder clinic, 1.1% met criteria for Tourette syndrome (Kadesjo and Gillberg 2000). This 100-fold difference in published estimates of Tourette syndrome prevalence highlights the challenge posed in the epidemiologic investigation of tic disorders. Ascertainment through medical-care systems rather than through community surveys may be particularly critical in determining the number of cases identified. More studies using direct observation to ascertain tics will be important to determine whether Tourette syndrome is a rare disorder, as has been believed, or a common disorder that only comes to medical attention when symptoms are severe.

Gender. Boys are more likely to have Tourette syndrome than girls. This is most apparent in clinical series. For example, in their clinical series of 200 subjects, Erenberg et al. (1986) reported a 4.7 to 1 ratio of males to females. Similar findings been reported in other clinical series (Park et al. 1993; Spencer et al. 1995; Nolan et al. 1996). An international database found a 4.3:1 male/female ratio, but with wide variation across sites (Freeman et al. 2000). Community-based samples show similar patterns, but the magnitude of the gender difference varies across studies (Table 6–6). Thus, as is true for the prevalence of Tourette syndrome in the population, the source of sample and case definition strongly influence the resulting male-to-female ratio. Nonetheless, it is evident that boys are at greater risk for Tourette syndrome and chronic tic disorder than girls.

Geography. Tourette syndrome appears to be worldwide in distribution. Clinical series and case reports have been published from numerous countries, including the United States (Shapiro et al. 1978), Europe (Abuzzahab et al. 1976; Lees et al. 1984), Japan (Nomura et al. 1982), China (Bai et al. 1983), Hong Kong (Leih et al. 1982), the Middle East (Robertson and Trimble 1991; Apter et al. 1992), and India (Abuzzahab et al. 1976). Differences in disease frequency across populations are likely if Tourette syndrome is determined primarily by genetic factors, but the methodological difficulties discussed above and small numbers of population-based studies performed to date do not permit conclusions.

Analytic Studies

The chief risk factors for Tourette syndrome and chronic multifocal tic disorder are familial predispostion (Kurlan et al. 1986; Pauls and Leckman 1986; Caine et al. 1988; Comings et al. 1990a; Robertson et al. 1991) and male gender (see above). However, identification of a specific gene remains elusive. Recently, a severe form of exacerbating and remitting disease has been proposed to be a sequelae to infection with group A β-hemolytic streptococci (Swedo and Leonard 1998). Whether this association is actually causal has been disputed, however (Kurlan et al. 2001). Careful epidemiologic studies are needed to clarify this association.

The identification of other risk factors, if they exist, will be facilitated by the identification of the underlying genetic factors. An attempt to identify specific risk factors for persistent severe tics in adulthood found no specific clinical sign to be associated with persistent severe tics in adulthood (Goetz et al. 1992). Gender may be a risk factor for comorbid conditions, such as an association between female gender and obsessive-compulsive disorder (Noshirvani et

Table 6–6 Gender Differences in Tics and Tic Disorders—Selected Studies

Study	Population sampled; age	Tourette syndrome prevalence (%)	Male/female ratio
Burd et al. 1986	State TS Registry, Nebraska; 7–18	0.05	9:1
Comings et al. 1990b	Pupils in 3 schools; 5–14	0.6	10:1
Apter et al. 1993	Israeli army inductees; 16–17	0.05	2:1
Costello et al. 1996	Community survey of school children; 9–13	0.1	1.9:1
Mason et al. 1998	Single school grade 9; 167; 13–14	2.9	4:1
Kadesjo and Gillberg 2000	Community school children, registry; 7–11	1.1	4:1

al. 1991) and male gender and attention deficit disorder (Biederman et al. 1991).

Future Directions and Conclusions

The identification of a Tourette syndrome gene or genes could lead to greatly increased understanding of tic disorders. Other necessary studies include prospective studies documenting the natural history of tic disorders and the search for clinical or biologic markers relating to clinical course.

Huntington's Disease

Huntington's disease is an autosomal dominant disease caused by an expanded CAG repeat at the 5′ end of the IT-15 gene, located at chromosome 4p16.3 (Huntington's Disease Collaborative Research Group 1993). There is a triad of symptoms, consisting of (1) a movement disorder, (2) cognitive impairment, and (3) psychiatric symptoms. The movement disorder is characterized by chorea, dystonia, myoclonus, tremor and sometimes rigidity, and a disorder of voluntary movements such as impairment in saccadic and smooth eye movements, gait, swallowing or speech. Although classically defined by the extrapyramidal movement disorder, due to selective vulnerability of the caudate and putamen, the two other arms of the triad are often more disabling. The cognitive impairment progresses to dementia. In addition, a host of psychiatric features such as depression, mania, anxiety, obsessive-compulsive disorder, and psychosis may occur.

Age of onset may occur anytime between the ages of 2 and 80. Approximately 10% of cases occur below the age of 20 years and have been termed *juvenile Huntington's disease*. These patients have features that resemble idiopathic Parkinson's disease including tremor, rigidity, dystonia, and bradykinesia. They may also have learning disability and seizures. Huntington's disease has been reported throughout the world. Longer CAG repeat lengths are associated with earlier age of onset. This relationship is most apparent for the juvenile-onset cases

who generally have more than 60 CAG repeats. CAG repeat length is believed to account for 50%–60% of the variance in age of onset (Andrew et al. 1993; Duyao et al. 1993; Stine et al. 1993; Ranen et al. 1995; Brinkman et al. 1997) for the majority of adult-onset Huntington's disease cases (90%) with fewer than 60 repeats. There may be other genetic modifiers of age of onset. A polymorphism in linkage with the kainate receptor (GluR6) was associated with younger age of onset of Huntington's disease (MacDonald et al. 1999). In another study, the apoE4 allele was associated with a later age of onset (Panas et al. 1999). It is unclear whether CAG repeat length affects progression of the disease after onset (Illarioshkin et al. 1994; Kieburtz et al. 1994; Brandt et al. 1996).

Pathology is initially most evident in the basal ganglia (putamen and caudate), which may show up to 60% loss of mass. As the disease progresses, other areas including the white matter, thalamus, subthalamic nucleus, and cortex may atrophy to a lesser extent (20%). The cell type that has been shown to be most vulnerable is the medium spiny neuron, which projects from the striatum to the globus pallidus and is associated with the inhibitory transmitter γ-aminobutyric acid (GABA). At a cellular level, the mutant protein huntingtin is expressed throughout the body. The highest levels in the brain are found not in the striatum but in the cortex and the cerebellum. Therefore, there appears to be a selective vulnerability of the striatum to this protein, perhaps due to novel interactions of the huntingtin protein with other proteins.

Accuracy of diagnosis in symptomatic individuals, when based on direct genetic testing, is >98% sensitive and >99% specific (Kremer et al. 1994). Although the new mutation rate was once believed to be very low, it is now considered to be 1%–3%. The most common reasons for a negative family history suggesting a new mutation include individuals with late age of onset and nonpaternity.

Studies of at-risk presymptomatic individuals undergoing neurological examination to predict the development of Huntington's disease have not revealed a single constellation of signs or symptoms that reliably predict Huntington's disease. In the largest reported study, Foroud et al. (1995) compared cognitive function in 260 first-degree relatives of persons with Huntington's disease who were not gene carriers and 120 asymptomatic carriers. Performance on the digit symbol and the picture arrangement tests from the Wechsler Adult Intelligence Scale–Revised (WAIS-R) were significantly worse in those with expanded repeats. In the same cohort, asymptomatic gene carriers were found to have slower saccadic velocity and slower movement and visual reaction time.

Descriptive Studies

In North America and Western Europe, the prevalence of Huntington's disease is 5–10 per 100,000 (Northern Ireland study and Olmstead County, Minnesota) while among African blacks, Japanese, Chinese, and Finnish people the prevalence is 10 times lower because of both a lower CAG repeat length and an altered frequency of DNA haplotypes.

There have been only two incidence studies. The first was done in an extended family in Maracaibo, Venezuela (Young et al. 1986). Over a 7-year period from 1981 to 1988, 30 incident cases of Huntington's disease were identified among 171 gene-positive individuals, based on an unequivocal extrapyramidal movement disorder. Over a 3-year period the cumulative incidence among individuals with a normal exam at first visit was 3%; it was 23% for those with mildly abnormal examination and 60% for those with highly abnormal baseline examinations. Abnormalities of saccadic eye movement and slowed rapid alternating movements were the most common abnormalities on exam. The authors suggest that there is a time period of onset, rather than a discrete age of onset. This study, however, was limited to one family

and specific families were prioritized and those who had signs suggestive of early Huntington's disease were more carefully evaluated the following year. The incidence of Huntington's disease was calculated in Olmsted County, Minnesota, from 1950 through 1989 and was found to be 0.4 (0.1–0.8) for women and 0.2 (0.04–0.6) for men per 100,000 person-years (Kokmen et al. 1994).

In another large study of 728 Huntington's disease patients with manifest Huntington's disease and 321 presymptomatic individuals, Brinkman et al. (1997) determined the cumulative probability of being affected with Huntington's disease for a given CAG repeat length. Age of onset was determined retrospectively by chart review and was not defined solely by an extrapyramidal disorder. The average 5-year probability of developing Huntington's disease over a 5-year period was 14% using the Brinkman data. Repeating this study prospectively with a standardized instrument using a uniform definition of onset of Huntington's disease may yield more accurate estimates of the rate of conversion to manifest Huntington's disease.

Analytic Studies

Huntington's disease is an autosomal dominant disease with complete penetrance, yet defining age of onset of the disease has been inconsistent. Definitions of Huntington's disease have varied according to whether an unequivocal extrapyramidal movement disorder is mandatory, whether chorea must be present, and whether cognitive and psychiatric features alone can define the age of onset. Although there is increasing evidence that cognitive and behavioral symptomatology may occur early in Huntington's disease as well as in other neurodegenerative diseases, because these signs are nonspecific, they are rarely used as defining features of the disease. Even when considering the extrapyramidal motor disorder, some investigators have considered certain signs to be definitive (chorea, dystonia, and parkinsonism) while other signs are "soft," such as abnormal eye movements, hyperreflexia, impaired rapid alternating movements, or excessive and inappropriate movements of the limbs during stress. These soft signs were present in about one-third of a cohort at risk for Huntington's disease (Young et al. 1986). These soft signs may be the earliest signs of Huntington's disease, but they have also been seen in individuals who have been gene negative (2%) (false positive). By not including those individuals who have prominent psychiatric or cognitive presentations, specific genetic or environmental modifiers associated with these phenotypes may be missed.

Another important issue is that as in other neurodegenerative diseases such as Alzheimer's disease and amyotrophic lateral sclerosis (ALS), the genes that affect the age of onset may not affect disease progression. This will be particularly relevant in the design of clinical trials. An effective treatment for symptomatic individuals will not necessarily mean that presymptomatic individuals will benefit from this treatment and should not mean that individuals should undergo genetic testing solely for this reason. A trial in known gene-positive individuals will be important before conducting a large-scale trial in presymptomatic individuals who don't know their carrier status.

Genetic Studies. The fact that Huntington's disease is an inherited disorder is indisputable. In 14 studies of monozygotic twins, including 5 in which zygosity was proven, age of onset differed by only a few years. Since 1993, when the gene for Huntington's disease was identified, it has been recognized that, although all individuals who have inherited an allele with greater than 39 CAG repeats will develop Huntington's disease, some, but not all, individuals with 36–39 repeats may manifest the disease, and some individuals with 30–35 repeats will not have Huntington's disease but may pass an expanded repeat to their children. Those with 36–39 repeats would be expected to

have the oldest, and possibly the mildest, presentation (incomplete penetrance). The discovery of the gene has also provided an explanation for genetic anticipation. Intergenerational CAG changes occur in less than 1% of normal chromosomes while they occur in 70% of meioses on Huntington's disease chromosomes. Large expansions occur almost exclusively through paternal transmission, while offspring of mothers with Huntington's disease generally show no change in size of the CAG repeat. This explains why most cases of juvenile Huntington's disease have an affected father and why most sporadic cases of Huntington's disease have a father with a CAG repeat length in the intermediate range (Kremer et al. 1994). In addition to repeat length in the offspring, age of onset and gender of the parent contribute significantly to the variance in age of onset of the offspring (Ranen et al. 1995). There may be genetic modifiers of the age of onset. The range of onset ages for a given repeat length may exceed 30 years for people with age of onset in mid- to late life (Brinkman et al. 1997). In people with age of onset over age 50, variation in repeat length accounted for only 7% of the variation in age of onset, a finding that suggests other genetic or environmental modifiers.

Environmental Modifiers. There are no known environmental risk factors for Huntington's disease. Evidence to suggest the possibility that there may be environmental modifiers of age of onset includes (*1*) animal models and (*2*) the role of environmental factors in other neurodegenerative diseases. Mice transgenic for two different repeat lengths of huntingtin in exon 1 showed delayed disease onset after repeated exposure to novel environments from 4 weeks of age onward. Additionally, changes in feeding regimes and regular behavioral testing led to improvement in behavior and life expectancy. Thus it is possible that environmental enrichment might affect disease onset, progression, and ultimately mortality in transgenic mice.

Prognostic Studies

In a study of 2494 patients with Huntington's disease, patients with juvenile Huntington's disease (age of onset <20) and those with age of onset >50 had a shorter disease duration compared to those between 20 and 49 years of age. The mean disease duration was 21.4 years (1.2–40.8) (Foroud et al. 1999). Compared with age-matched controls, Huntington's disease patients are less likely to have cancer, perhaps due to the apoptotic properties of Huntington's disease. How this affects overall survivorship is unclear.

Future Directions and Conclusions

Huntington's disease provides an unparalleled opportunity for secondary prevention studies because at-risk individuals who have an expanded CAG repeat will definitely develop Huntington's disease. In preparation for the development of clinical trials, two areas deserve further investigation. First, measures for clinical progression in Huntington's disease need to be refined so that the rate of change or "zone of onset" for Huntington's disease can be narrowed. Ideally these measures, which may be cognitive, behavioral, or neuroimaging tools (PET, MR spectroscopy, or fMRI), will define the period during which the intervention should be initiated. The other necessary information for designing a clinical trial is the accurate assessment of when the individual has developed Huntington's disease. Further work toward establishing a consensus diagnosis of Huntington's disease and prospectively assessing the development of Huntington's disease for a given CAG repeat length is imperative. Additional efforts should be directed toward defining factors that influence rate of progression for those with manifest Huntington's disease, which may differ from factors influencing age of onset.

Essential Tremor

Disease Description

The diagnosis of essential tremor, considered to be the most prevalent adult movement disorder (Louis et al. 1998a), with a prevalence of 20 times that of Parkinson's disease (Snow et al. 1989), rests solely on clinical criteria. It has been described as a 4–12 HZ postural tremor and kinetic tremor, yet among 19 prevalence studies published between 1960 and 1995, only 9 specified their criteria for inclusion. Among the remaining 10, the type of tremor (postural alone, action alone, or both), severity of tremor, requirement of a family history of tremor, or duration of tremor for a certain period varied substantially. Ninety-eight movement disorder specialists could not agree on the clinical definition of essential tremor, with 45% requiring postural or kinetic tremor, 26% requiring postural only, 17% requiring kinetic only, and 12% requiring both. In contrast, 81% would diagnose essential tremor in a person with an isolated head tremor (Chouinard et al. 1997).

Postmortem studies have not revealed reproducible pathology (Hassler 1939; Herskovits and Blackwood 1969; LaPresle et al. 1974; Elble 1996), and there are no known biomarkers for essential tremor. Areas of the brain with inherent rhythmicity in the frequency range of essential tremor include thalamic nuclei and the inferior olive. Hypermetabolism of the inferior olive has been demonstrated in patients with essential tremor (Dubinsky and Hallett 1993). Abnormal activation in the cerebellum, red nucleus, and thalamus has also been demonstrated on essential tremor.

Because of the lack of anatomical or biochemical data to define essential tremor, the validity of the diagnosis of essential tremor is impossible to assess. In addition to the specification of either an isolated postural tremor, kinetic tremor, or both, some investigators have characterized essential tremor on the basis of tremor frequency alone, noting an inverse relationship between amplitude size and tremor rate. Larger-amplitude, lower-frequency tremor has been found to be more functionally disabling (Hubble et al. 1989). Investigators have also tried to characterize the body parts affected by essential tremor. Tremor of the hands occurred in 80%–100% of cases (Hubble et al. 1989). Though tremor of the tongue, head or voice can occur in isolation, it is often associated with tremor in the hands. These cross-sectional descriptive studies have not adjusted for duration of illness or severity of tremor. During the course of essential tremor, in addition to worsening severity of tremor, there may be spread to previously unaffected body parts. Therefore it is impossible to say whether these represent subtypes or just a more severe form of essential tremor. Hubble et al. (1997) have reported that women are more likely to have head and voice tremor (OR = 2.6, 95% CI 1.6–4.1) and men had more severe postural tremor. Louis et al. (2001) reported similar, but nonsignificant trends. Koguchi et al. (1995) have suggested that patients with postural tremor alone may be more likely to respond to propranol than those with more complex tremor. There is no accurate data on age of onset of essential tremor. In fact, there is only one incidence study of essential tremor (Rajput et al. 1991b). Although it has been suggested that the familial form of essential tremor has an earlier age of onset than the sporadic form (Larsson et al. 1960; Rautakorpi 1978), this may be solely due to ascertainment bias. Age of onset has not been related to clinical course or response to therapy.

Descriptive Studies

It is generally believed that the prevalence of essential tremor increases with age. In a review by Louis et al. (1998b), estimates of the crude prevalence of essential tremor range from 0.08 to 220 per 1000 persons. Only a few studies provide age-specific prevalence data (Rajput et al 1984; Bharucha et al. 1988; Mohadjer et al. 1990). The prevalence of essential tremor over age 60 in these studies ranges from 13 to 50.5 per 1000, perhaps reflecting differences in case definitions and population studied. There has been only one incidence study of essential tremor (Rajput et al. 1984).

Gender Differences. Essential tremor has been reported throughout the world. In a community-based study in Washington Heights Inwood in northern Manhattan, New York Caucasians had a higher age-specific prevalence 30.5 (17.4–52.5) per 1000 than African Americans 17.9 (9.5–30.6), with Hispanics having an intermediate prevalence 21.5 (13.0–32.7) (Louis et al. 1998a). In the only other study where ethic groups were compared using the same methodology, Haerer et al. (1987) found a trend for higher prevalence of essential tremor in whites than in African Americans.

Methodological Issues in Descriptive Studies. As described above, the most problematic aspect in estimating the prevalence of essential tremor is that there is no gold standard for the diagnosis. Louis et al. (1998a) applied 10 published diagnostic criteria for essential tremor to a well-characterized population-based sample of patients. Liberal criteria that specified the presence of mild action or postural tremor classified many "normal" subjects as having essential tremor. In contrast, those criteria that specified a long duration or a positive family history of tremor would classify many subjects originally classified as essential tremor as being normal. Schrag et al. (2000) described overuse of essential tremor in a review of cases diagnosed by neurologists. Of 50 cases, 25 did not meet one set of published criteria for essential tremor (Bain et al. 2000). Although essential tremor can be arbitrarily physiologically defined, the demarcation between physiologic, enhanced physiologic, and essential tremor is unknown. Because there are so many factors that influence tremor, including anxiety, stimulants (caffeine, nicotine), and numerous medications, the reliability of the measurement of tremor frequency is doubtful. Whether essential tremor requires functional disability is also not defined, and whether that functional disability is subjective or performance based is rarely specified. Estimates of the proportion of people with essential tremor who seek medical attention range from 0.5% (Rautakorpi et al. 1978) to 11.1% (Louis et al. 1998b). This suggests that the vast majority of people with essential tremor either do not recognize it or do not find the condition to be disabling or do not perceive it to be a condition warranting medical attention. Those people who do seek attention may have either more severe or more disabling disease. It is interesting to note that among service-based studies, the dominant arm, which would be more likely to affect function, is more likely to be involved, while in a community-based study it was the nondominant arm. Service-based estimates (Snow et al. 1989) are substantially lower than community-based estimates, again suggesting that only the most clinically severe or disabling cases of essential tremor reach medical attention.

Essential tremor may be particularly difficult to distinguish from Parkinson's disease. Patients with essential tremor may have a rest tremor, and patients with Parkinson's disease may have a prominent action tremor. Studies differ as to whether Parkinson's disease and essential tremor are etiologically related (Jankovic et al. 1993; Koller et al. 1994).

Familial Aggregation of Disease

The existence of familial aggregation in some families with essential tremor has lead some investigators to require a family history of essential tremor to make the diagnosis. An extensive review of the literature (Louis and Ottman 1996) reveals several methodological problems with this assumption. Most of the studies on familial aggregation in essential tremor have been family history studies rather than family studies. The studies have not controlled for family size or years at risk and none have included a control group. The lack of definition of essential tremor in probands is compounded when trying to assess the risk of essential tremor in family members. Most studies have not used structured, reliable, and valid interviews, and even when

a structured interview is used, mild essential tremor may not be recognized by either probands reporting on their relatives or the relatives themselves.

Example 6–5 The validity of family history as reported by a person with essential tremor was investigated in a community-based population (Louis et al. 1999). Forty-six cases with essential tremor were interviewed to determine whether any of their relatives had essential tremor. Two neurologists reviewed videotaped evaluations of 160 of their relatives (and the 46 cases) to determine whether essential tremor was present. Twelve relatives were judged to have essential tremor, but only 2 of these had been reported by interviewing the essential tremor case (sensitivity of 16.7%). One of the unaffected relatives was falsely reported to have essential tremor (specificity of 99.3%.). Better sensitivity was associated with more severe tremor in the informant and in the relative, female informant, higher education, and sibling relationship. Of the 12 relatives with essential tremor, only 6 endorsed their own tremors. The low sensitivity of reporting of family history data for essential tremor necessitates a neurological examination in cases where accurate enumeration of cases of essential tremor is important.

In the Washington Heights–Inwood Genetic Study of Essential Tremor, a population-based family study of ET that enrolled relatives of ET cases and relatives of control subjects, a first-degree relative of an ET cases was 4.7 times more likely to have ET than was a first-degree relative of a control subject. In addition, the magnitude of increased risk in relatives of ET patients versus controls was greater in relatives of ET cases with onset <50 years than in relatives of those with older onset (relative risk [RR] = 10.38 vs. 4.82) (Louis et al. 2001). In a twin study (Tanner et al. 2001), three of five (60%) monozygotic twins were concordant for ET, compared with only three of eight (27%) dizygotic twins. Although concordance in monozygotic twins was approximately two times that in dizygotic twins, the monozygotic concordance was not 100%, suggesting that both genetic and environmental factors are important.

Although it is commonly stated that essential tremor is inherited in 50% of cases, the reporting of a family history of essential tremor is quite variable, ranging from 17.4% to 100% (Louis et al. 1999). To date, linkage to a region on chromosome 2p22–25 has been reported in one large Czech family (Higgins et al. 1997) and to 3q13 in 16 Icelandic families with 75 members (Gulcher et al. 1997), but genes have not been identified. No other loci have been identified in the majority of cases.

Nongenetic Causes

In contrast to other neurodegenerative diseases such as Alzheimer's disease and Parkinson's disease, environmental risk factors have not been studied. Although there are a number of compounds that are tremorogenic in both animals and humans, such as the β-carboline alkaloids (harmaline and harmine), organochlorine pesticides, and lead and manganese, none of these have been compared in case–control studies (Louis 2001).

Prognostic Studies

The development of essential tremor has not been associated with increased mortality. African Americans and Hispanics may have more severe tremor despite similar duration of illness, perhaps reflecting a more rapid disease course (Louis et al 2000). Women were more likely to have head or voice tremor while men had more severe postural hand tremor (Hubble et al. 1997).

Future Directions and Conclusions

The study of essential tremor has been hampered by the lack of consistent definitions employed across studies and the lack of reliable clinical, electrophysiological, and functional measures. Future studies will need to focus on refining the phenotype to perform more meaningful genetic studies. In addition, environmental causes or modifiers of genetic predisposition need to be explored.

References

Abuzzahab FS, Anderson FO. Gilles de la Tourette Syndrome: International Registry. St. Paul, MN: Mason Publishing, 1976.

Almasy L, Bressman S, de Leon D, Risch N. Ethnic variation in the clinical expression of idiopathic torsion dystonia. *Mov Disord* 1997;12:715–721.

Anderson C, Checkoway H, Franklin GM, et al. Dietary factors in Parkinson's disease: the role of food groups and specific foods. *Mov Disord* 1999;14:21–27.

Andrew SE, Goldberg YP, Kremer B, et al. The relationship between trinucleotide (CAG) repeat length and clinical features of Huntington's disease. *Nat Genet* 1993;4:398–403.

Apter A, Pauls D, Bleich A, et al. A population-based epidemiologic study of Gilles de la Tourette syndrome among adolescents in Israel. In: Chase TN, Friedhoff AJ, Cohen DJ, eds. Second International Tourette Syndrome Symposium. New York: Raven Press, 1992.

Apter A, Pauls DL, Bleich A, et al. An epidemiologic study of Gilles de la Tourette's syndrome in Israel. *Arch Gen Psychiatry* 1993; 50:734–738.

Ascherio A, Zhang SM, Hernan MA, et al. Prospective study of caffeine consumption and risk of Parkinson's disease in men and women. *Ann Neurol* 2001;50:56–63.

Autere JM, Moilanen JS, Myllyla VV, Majamaa K. Familial aggregation of Parkinson's disease in a Finnish population. *J Neurol Neurosurg Psychiatry* 2000;69:107–109.

Bai CH, Han-Quin LF. Tourette syndrome: report of 19 cases. *Chin Med J* 1983;96:45–48.

Bain P, Brin M, Deuschl G, et al. Criteria for the diagnosis of essential tremor. *Neuorolgy* 2000;54;(Suppl 4):S7.

Baldereschi M, Di Carlo A, Rocca WA, et al. Parkinson's disease and parkinsonism in a longitudinal study: two-fold higher incidence in men. ILSA Working Group. Italian Longitudinal Study on Aging. *Neurology* 2000; 55:1358–1363.

Benedetti MD, Bower JH, Maraganore DM, et al. Smoking, alcohol, and coffee consumption preceding Parkinson's disease: a case–control study. *Neurology* 2000;55:1350–1358.

Betarbet R, Sherer TB, MacKenzie G, et al. Chronic systemic pesticide exposure reproduces features of Parkinson's disease. *Nat Neurosci* 2000;3:1301–1306.

Bharucha NE, Bharucha EP, Baruch AE, Bhise AV. Prevalence of essential tremor in the

Parsi Community of Bombay, India. *Arch Neurol* 1988;45:907–909.

Biederman J, Newcorn J, Sprich S. Comorbidity of attention deficit hyperactivity disorder with conduct, depressive, anxiety and other disorders. *Am J Psychiatry* 1991;148:564–577.

Bonifati V, Rizzu P, Van baren M, Schaap O, Breedveld G, Krieger E, Dekker M, Squitieri F, Ibanez P, van Dongen JW, Vanacore N, van Swieten JC, Brice A, Meco G, van Duijn CM, Oostra BA, Heutink P. Mutations in the DJ-1 Gene associated with Autosomal Recessive Early Onset Parkinsonism. Sciencexpress/www.sciencexpress.org. Nov 21, 2002.

Bower JH, Maraganore DM, Peterson BJ, et al. Head trauma preceding Parkinson's disease (PD): a case–control study. *Mov Disord* 2002;17:S131.

Brandt J, Bylsma FW, Gross R, et al. Trinucleotide repeat length and clinical progression in Huntington's disease. *Neurology* 1996;46:527–531.

Bressman SB, de Leon D, Brin MF, et al. Idiopathic dystonia among Ashkenazi Jews: evidence for autosomal dominant inheritance. *Ann Neurol* 1989;26:612–620.

Bressman SB. Dystonia update. *Clin Neuropharmacol* 2000;23:239–251.

Brinkman RR, Mezei MM, Theilmann J, et al. The likelihood of being affected with Huntington disease by a particular age, for a specific CAG size. *Am J Hum Genet* 1997;60:1202–1210.

Burd L, Kerbeshian J, Wikenheiser M, Fisher W. Prevalence of Gilles de la Tourette's syndrome in North Dakota children. *J Am Acad Child Adoles Psychiatry* 1986;25:552–553.

Butler AG, Duffey PO, Hawthorne MR, Barnes MP. The socioeconomic implications of dystonia. *Adv Neurol* 1998;78:349–358.

Butterfield PG, Valanis BG, Spencer PS, et al. Environmental antecedents of young-onset Parkinson's disease. *Neurology* 1993;43:1150–1158.

Caine ED, McBride MC, Chiverton P, et al. Tourette's syndrome in Monroe County. *Neurology* 1988;38:472–475.

Chen JF, Xu K, Petzer JP, et al. Neuroprotection by caffeine and A(2A) adenosine receptor inactivation in a model of Parkinson's disease. *J Neurosci* 2001;21:RC143.

Chen R, Hallett M. Focal dystonia and repetitive motion disorders. *Clin Orthop* 1998:102–106.

Chouinard S, Louis ED, Fahn S. Agreement among movement disorder specialists on the clinical diagnosis of essential tremor. *Mov Disord* 1997;12:973–976.

Comings DE, Comings BG. A controlled study of Tourette syndrome. I. Attention-deficit disorder, learning disorders and school problems. *Am J Hum Genet* 1987;41:701–741.

Comings DE, Himes JA, Comings BG. A controlled family history study of Tourette's syndrome. I. Attention-deficit disorder and learning disorder. *J Clin Psychiatry* 1990a;51:275–280.

Comings DE, Himes JA, Comings BG. An epidemiologic study of Tourette's syndrome in a single school district. *J Clin Psychiatry* 1990b;51:463–469.

Corrigan FM, Wienburg CL, Shore RF, et al. Organochlorine insecticides in substantia nigra in Parkinson's disease. *J Toxicol Environ Health A* 2000;59:229–234.

Costello EJ, Angold A, Burns BJ, et al. The Great Smoky Mountains study of youth: goals, design, methods, and the prevalence of DSM-III-R disorders. *Arch Gen Psychiatry* 1996;53:1129–1136.

Defazio G, Berardelli A, Abbruzzese G, et al. Possible risk factors for primary adult onset dystonia: a case–control investigation by the Italian Movement Disorders Study Group. *J Neurol Neurosurg Psychiatry* 1998;64:25–32.

De Stefano AL, Golbe LI, Mark MH, et al. Genome-wide scan for Parkinson's disease: the Gene PD Study. *Neurology* 2001;57:1124–1126.

Doll R, Peto R, Wheatley K, et al. Mortality in relation to smoking: 40 years' observations on male British doctors. *BMJ* 1994;309:901–911.

Duan W, Mattson MP. Dietary restriction and 2-deoxyglucose administration improve behavioral outcome and reduce degeneration of dopaminergic neurons in models of Parkinson's disease. *J Neurosci Res* 1999;57:195–206.

Dubinsky R, Hallet M. Glucose metabolism in the brain of patients with essential tremor. *J Neurol Sci* 1993;114:45–48.

Duffy POF, Butler AG, Hawthorne MR, Barnes MP. The epidemiology of the primary dystonias in the north of England. In: Fahn S, Marsden CD, DeLong M, eds. Advances in Neurology: Dystonia 3. Philadelphia: Lippincott-Raven, 1998, pp 121–125.

Duvoisin RC, Eldridge R, Williams A, Nutt J, Calne D. Twin study of Parkinson disease. *Neurology* 1981;31:77–80.

Duyao M, Ambrose C, Myers R, et al. Trinucleotide repeat length instability and age of onset in Huntington's disease. *Nat Genet* 1993;4:387–392.

Elbaz A, McDonnell SK, Maraganore DM, Schaid DJ, Bower JH, Rocca WA. Validity of family history data on Parkinson's disease:

evidence for a family information bias. *Mov Disord* 2002;17(Suppl 5):S141.

Elble RJ. Central mechanisms of tremor. *J Clini Neurophysiol* 1996;13:133–144.

Epidemiologic Study of Dystonia in Europe Collaborative Group. Sex-related influences on the frequency and age of onset of primary dystonia. *Neurology* 1999;53:1871–1873.

Epidemiologic Study of Dystonia in Europe Collaborative Group. A prevalence study of primary dystonia in eight European countries. *Neurology* 2000;247:787–792.

Erenberg G, Cruse RP, Rothner AD. Tourette syndrome: an analysis of 200 pediatric and adolescent cases. *Cleve Clin Q* 1986;53:127–131.

Factor SA, Weiner WJ. Prior history of head trauma in Parkinson's disease. *Move Disord* 1991;6:225–229.

Fahn S. Concept and classification of dystonia. In: Fahn S, Marsden CD, DeLong MR, eds. Advances in Neurology: Dystonia 2. New York: Raven Press, 1988, pp 1–8.

Fahn S, Bressman SB, Marsden CD. Classification of dystonia. *Adv Neurol* 1998;78:1–10.

Fall PA, Fredrikson M, Axelson O, Granerus AK. Nutritional and occupational factors influencing the risk of Parkinson's disease: a case–control study in southeastern Sweden. *Mov Disord* 1999;14:28–37.

Farrer M, Destee A, Becquet E, et al. Linkage exclusion in French families with probable Parkinson's disease. *Mov Disord* 2000;15:1075–1083.

Farrer M, Gwinn-Hardy K, Muenter M, et al. A chromosome 4p haplotype segregating with Parkinson's disease and postural tremor. *Hum Mol Genet* 1999;8:81–85.

Fearnley JM, Lees AJ. Ageing and Parkinson's disease: substantia nigra regional selectivity. *Brain* 1991;114:2283–2301.

Findley LF, Gresty MA. Tremor. *Br J Hosp Med* 1981;26:16–32.

Fleming L, Mann JB, Bean J, et al. Parkinson's disease and brain levels of organochlorine pesticides. *Ann Neurol* 1994;36:100–103.

Fletcher NA, Harding AE, Marsden CD. The relationship between trauma and idiopathic torsion dystonia. *J Neurol Neurosurg Psychiatry* 1991;54:713–717.

Foroud T, Gray J, Ivashina J, Conneally PM. Differences in duration of Huntington's disease based on age at onset. *J Neurol Neurosurg Psychiatry* 1999;66:52–56.

Foroud T, Siemers E, Kleindorfer D, et al. Cognitive scores in carriers of Huntington's disease gene compared to noncarriers. *Ann Neurol* 1995;37:657–664.

Freeman RD, Fast DK, Burd L, et al. An international perspective on Tourette syndrome: selected findings from 3,500 individuals in 22 countries. *Dev Med Child Neurol* 2000; 42:436–437.

Funayama M, Hasegawa K, Kowa H, Saito M, Tsuji S, Obata F. A new locus for Parkinson's disease (PARK8) maps to chromosome 12p11.2-q13.1. *Ann Neurol* 2002;51:296–301.

Gasser T, Muller-Myhsok B, Wszolek ZK, et al. A susceptibility locus for Parkinson's disease maps to chromosome 2p13. *Nat Genet* 1998;18:262–265.

Gelb DJ, Oliver E, Gilman S. Diagnostic criteria for Parkinson's disease. *Arch Neurol* 1999;56:33–39.

Gibb WR, Lees AJ. Anatomy, pigmentation, ventral and dorsal subpopulations of the substantia nigra, and differential cell death in Parkinson's disease. *J Neurol Neurosurg Psychiatry* 1991;54:388–396.

Goetz CG, Tanner CM, Stebbins GT, et al. Adult tics in Gilles de la Tourette syndrome: description and risk factors. *Neurology* 1992;42:784–788.

Golbe LI, Di Iorio G, Bonavita V, et al. A large kindred with autosomal dominant Parkinson's disease. *Ann Neurol* 1990;27:276–282.

Gorell J, Johnson C, Rybicki B, Peterson E. A population-based case–control study of nutrient intake in Parkinson's disease. *Neurology* 1997;48:A298.

Gorell JM, Johnson CC, Rybicki BA, et al. The risk of Parkinson's disease with exposure to pesticides, farming, well water, and rural living. *Neurology* 1998;50:1346–1350.

Gorell JM, Johnson CC, Rybicki BA, et al. Occupational exposure to manganese, copper, lead, iron, mercury and zinc and the risk of Parkinson's disease. *Neurotoxicology* 1999; 20:239–247.

Gowers WR. Diseases of the Nervous System. Philadelphia: P Blakiston, Son and Company, 1888.

Grandinetti A, Morens DM, Reed D, MacEachern D. Prospective study of cigarette smoking and the risk of developing idiopathic Parkinson's disease. *Am J Epidemiol* 1994; 139:1129–1138.

Gulcher JR, Jonsson P, Kong A, et al. Mapping of a familial essential tremor gene, *FET1,* to chromosome 3q13. *Nat Genet* 1997;17:84–87.

Haerer AF, Anderson DW, Schoenberg BE. Survey of major neurologic disorders in a biracial United States population: the Copiah County study. *South Med J* 1987;80:339–343.

Hassler R. Zur pathologischen Anatomie des senilen und des parkinsonistischen Tremor. *J Psychol Neurol* 1939;49:193–230.

Hattori N, Kitada T, Matsumine H, et al. Molecular genetic analysis of a novel parkin gene in Japanese families with autosomal recessive juvenile parkinsonism: evidence for variable homozygous deletions in the parkin gene in affected individuals. *Ann Neurol* 1998a;44:935–941.

Hellenbrand W, Boeing H, Robra BP, et al. Diet and Parkinson's disease. II: a possible role for the past intake of specific nutrients. Results from a self-administered food-frequency questionnaire in a case–control study. *Neurology* 1996;47:644–650.

Herskovits E, Blackwood W. Essential (familial, hereditary) tremor: a case report. *J Neurol Neurosurg Psychiatry* 1969;32:509–511.

Hicks AA, Petursson H, Jonsson T, Stefansson H, Johannsdottir HS, Sainz J, Frigge ML, Kong A, Gulcher JR, Stefansson K, Sveinbjornsdottir S. A susceptibilty gene for late-onset idiopathic Parkinson's disease. *Ann Neurol* 2002;52:549–555.

Hicks AA, Petursson H, Jonsson T, et al. A susceptibility gene for late-onset idiopathic Parkinson's disease. *Ann Neurol* 2002;52: 549–555.

Higgins JJ, Pho LT, Nee LE. A gene (ETM) for essential tremor maps to chromosome 2p22–p25. *Mov Disord* 1997;12:859–864.

Ho SC, Woo J, Lee CM. Epidemiologic study of Parkinson's disease in Hong Kong. *Neurology* 1989; 39:1314–1318.

Hubble JP, Busenbark KL, Koller WC. Essential tremor. *Clin Neuropharmacol* 1989;12:453–482.

Hubble JP, Busenbark KL, Pahwa R, et al. Clinical expression of essential tremor: effects of gender and age. *Mov Disord* 1997;12:969–972.

Hubble JP, Cao T, Kjelstrom JA, et al. Nocardia species as an etiologic agent in Parkinson's disease: serological testing in a case–control study. *J Clin Microbiol* 1995;33: 2768–2769.

Hughes AJ, Daniel SE, Blankson S, Lees AJ. A clinicopathologic study of 100 cases of Parkinson's disease. *Arch Neurol* 1993;50: 140–148.

Huntington Disease Collaborative Research Group. A novel gene containing a trinucleotide repeat that is expanded and unstable on Huntington's disease chromosomes. *Cell* 1993;72:971–983.

Illarioshkin SN, Igarashi S, Onodera O, et al. Trinucleotide repeat length and rate of progression of Huntington's disease. *Ann Neurol* 1994;36:630–635.

Jankovic J. Post-traumatic movement disorders: central and peripheral mechanisms. *Neurology* 1994;44:2006–2014.

Jankovic J. Can peripheral trauma induce dystonia and other movement disorders? Yes! *Mov Disord* 2001;16:7–12.

Jankovic J, Contant C, Perlmutter J. Essential tremor and PD. *Neurology* 1993;43:1447–1449.

Janson AM, Moller A. Chronic nicotine treatment counteracts nigral cell loss induced by a partial mesodiencephalic hemitransection: an analysis of the total number and mean volume of neurons and glia in substantia nigra of the male rat. *Neuroscience* 1993;57: 931–941.

Kadesjo B, Gillberg C. Tourette's disorder: epidemiology and cormorbidity in primary school children. *J Am Acad Child Adolesc Psychiatry* 2000;39:548–555.

Kieburtz K, MacDonald M, Shih C, et al. Trinucleotide repeat length and progression of illness in Huntington's disease. *J Med Genet* 1994;31:872–874.

Kitada T, Asakawa S, Hattori N, et al. Mutations in the parkin gene cause autosomal recessive juvenile parkinsonism. *Nature* 1998; 392:605–608.

Klein C, Ozelius LJ. Dystonia: clinical features, genetics, and treatment. *Curr Opin Neurol* 2002;15:491–497.

Koguchi Y, Nakajima M, Kawamura M, Hirayama K. Clinical subtypes of essential tremor and their electrophysiological and pharmacological differences [in Japanese]. *Rinsho Shinkeigaku* 1995;35:132–136.

Kohbata S, Beaman BL. L-dopa-responsive movement disorder caused by Nocardia asteroids localized in the brains of mice. *Infect Immun* 1991:59:181–191.

Kokmen E, Ozekmekci FS, Beard CM, et al. Incidence and prevalence of Huntington's disease in Olmsted County, Minnesota (1950 through 1989). *Arch Neurol* 1994;51:696–698.

Koller WC, Busenbark K, Miner K. The relationship of essential tremor to other movement disorders: report on 678 patients. Essential Tremor Study Group. *Ann Neurol* 1994;35:717–723.

Konkiewitz EC, Trender-Gerhard I, Kamm C, et al. Service-based survey of dystonia in Munich. *Neuroepidemiology* 2002;21:202–206.

Korczyn AD, Kahana E, Zilber N, et al. Torsion dystonia in Israel. *Ann Neurol* 1980;8:387–391.

Kremer B, Goldberg P, Andrew SE, et al. A worldwide study of the Huntington's disease mutation. The sensitivity and specificity of measuring CAG repeats. *N Engl J Med* 1994; 330:1401–1406.

Kruger R, Kuhn W, Muller T, et al. Ala30Pro mutation in the gene encoding alpha-synuclein in Parkinson's disease. *Nature Genet* 1998;18:106–108.

Kuopio AM, Marttila RJ, Helenius H, Rinne UK. Changing epidemiology of Parkinson's disease in southwestern Finland. *Neurology* 1999;52:302–308.

Kuopio A, Marttila RJ, Helenius H, Rinne UK. Familial occurrence of Parkinson's disease in a community-based case–control study. *Parkinsonism Relat Disord* 2001;7:297–303.

Kurlan R, Behr J, Medved L, et al. Familial Tourette's syndrome: report of a large pedigree and potential for linkage analysis. *Neurology* 1986;36:772–776.

Kurlan R. McDermott MP, Deeley C, et al. Prevalence of tics in schoolchildren and association with placement in special education. *Neurology* 2001;57:1383–1388.

Landgren M, Petterson R, Kjellman B, Gillberg C. ADHD, DAMP, and other neurodevelopmental/psychiatric disorders in 6-year-old children: epidemiology and co-morbidity. *Dev Med Child Neurol* 1996;38:891–906.

Langston JW. The etiology of Parkinson's disease with emphasis on the MPTP story. *Neurology* 1996;47:S153–S160.

Langston JW, Ballard PA, Tetrud JW, Irwin I. Chronic parkinsonism in humans due to a product of meperidine analog synthesis. *Science* 1983;219:979–980.

Lapouse R, Monk MA. Behavior deviations in a representative sample of children: variation by sex, age, race, social class and family size. *Am J Orthopsychiatry* 1964;34:436–446.

LaPresle J, Rondot P, Said G. Tremblement idiopathique de repos, d'attitude et d'action. Étude anatomo-clinique d'une observation. *Rev Neurol* 1974;130:343–348.

Larsson T, Sjogren T. Essential tremor: a clinical and genetic population study. *Acta Psychiatry Neurol Scand* 1960;36(144):1–176.

Lees AJ, Robertson M, Trimble MR, Murray NMF. A clinical study of Gilles de la Tourette syndrome in the United Kingdom. *J Neurol Neurosurg Psychiatry* 1984;47:1–8.

Leroy E, Boyer R, Auburger G, et al. The ubiquitin pathway in Parkinson's disease. *Nature* 1998;395:451–452.

Li S, Schoenberg B, Wang C, et al. A prevalence survey of Parkinson's disease and other movement disorders in the People's Republic of China. *Arch Neurol* 1985;42:655–657.

Lieh Mak F, Chung SY, Lee P, Chen S. Tourette syndrome in the Chinese: a follow-up of 15 cases. In: Friedhoff AJ, Chase TN, eds. Gilles de la Tourette Syndrome. New York: Raven Press, 1982, pp 281–284.

Liou HH, Tsai MC, Chen CJ, et al. Environmental risk factors and Parkinson's disease: a case–control study in Taiwan. *Neurology* 1997;48:1583–1588.

Logroscino G, Marder K, Cote L, et al. Dietary lipids and antioxidants in Parkinson's disease: a population-based, case–control study. *Ann Neurol* 1996;39:89–94.

Louis ED. Etiology of essential tremor: should we be searching for environmental causes? *Mov Disord* 2001;16:822–829.

Louis ED, Ford B, Frucht S, et al. Risk of tremor and impairment from tremor in relatives of patients with essential tremor: a community-based family study. *Ann Neurol* 2001;49:761–769.

Louis ED, Ford B, Lee H, et al. Diagnostic criteria for essential tremor: a population perspective. *Arch Neurol* 1998a;55:823–828.

Louis ED, Ford B, Wendt K, Ottman R. Validity of family history data on essential tremor. *Mov Disord* 1999;14:456–461.

Louis ED, Marder K, Cote L, et al. Differences in the prevalence of essential tremor among elderly African Americans, whites, and Hispanics in northern Manhattan, NY. *Arch Neurol* 1995;52:1201–1205.

Louis ED, Ottman R. How familial is familial tremor? The genetic epidemiology of essential tremor. *Neurology* 1996;46:1200–1205.

Louis ED, Ottman R, Hauser WA. How common is the most common adult movement disorder? Estimates of the prevalence of essential tremor throughout the world. *Mov Disord* 1998b;13:5–10.

Lücking CB, Abbas N, Dürr A, et al. Homozygous deletions in parkin gene in European and North African families with autosomal recessive juvenile parkinsonism. *Lancet* 1998;352:1355–1356.

MacDonald ME, Vonsattel JP, Shrinidhi J, et al. Evidence for the GluR6 gene associated with younger onset age of Huntington's disease. *Neurology* 1999;53:1330–1332.

Marder K, Tang M, Mejia H, et al. Risk of Parkinson's disease among first-degree relatives: a community-based study. *Neurology* 1996;47:155–160.

Marder K, Logroscino G, Alfaro B, et al. Environmental risk factors for Parkinson's disease in an urban multiethnic community. *Neurology* 1998;50:279–281.

Marras C, Tanner CM. The epidemiology of Parkinson's disease. In: Watts RL, Koller WC, eds. Movement Disorders Neurologic Principles and Practice, 2nd ed. New York: McGraw Hill, 2002.

Marsden CD. Twins and Parkinson's disease. *J Neurol Neurosurg Psychiatry* 1987;50:105–106.

Marsden CD, Obeso J, Rothwell JC. Benign essential tremor is not a single entity. In: Yarh

MD, ed. Current Concepts in Parkinson's Disease. Amsterdam: Excerpta Medica, 1983, pp 31–46.

Marttila RJ, Kaprio J, Koshewvuo M, Rinne UK. Parkinson's disease in a nation-wide twin cohort. *Neurology* 1988;38:1217–1219.

Marttila RF, Rinne UK. Epidemiology of Parkinson's disease in Finland. *Acta Neurol Scand* 1976;53:81–102.

Mason A, Banerjee S, Eapen V, et al. The Prevalence of Tourette syndrome in a mainstream school. *Dev Med Child Neurol* 1998;40: 292–296.

Mayeux R, Marder K, Cote LJ, et al. The frequency of idiopathic Parkinson's disease by age, ethnic group and sex in northern Manhattan, 1988–1993. *Am J Epidemiol* 1995; 142:820–827.

McCann SJ, LeCouteur DG, Green AC, et al. The epidemiology of Parkinson's disease in an Australian population. *Neuroepidemiology* 1998;17:310–317.

McCormack AL, Thiruchelvam M, Manning-Bog AB. Environmental risk factors and Parkinson's disease: selective degeneration of nigral dopaminergic neurons caused by the herbicide paraquat. *Neurobiol Dis* 2002;10: 119–127.

McGeer P, Itagaki S, Akiyama H, McGeer E. Rate of cell death in parkinsonism indicates active neuropathological process. *Ann Neurol* 1988;24:574–576.

Meara J, Bhowmick BK, Hobson P. Accuracy of diagnosis in patients with presumed Parkinson's disease. *Age Ageing* 1999;28:335–336.

Melcon MO, Anderson DW, Vergara RH, Rocca WA. Prevalence of Parkinson's disease in Junin, Buenos Aires Province, Argentina. *Mov Disord* 1997;12:197–205.

Menza M. The personality associated with Parkinson's disease. *Curr Psychiatry Rep* 2000;2:421–426.

Mohadjer M. Goerke H, Milios E, et al. Long-term results of stereotaxy in the treatment of essential tremor. *Stereotact Funct Neurosurg* 1990;54–55:125–129.

Morano A, Jimenez-Jimenez FJ, Molina JA, Antolin MA. Risk-factors for Parkinson's disease: case–control study in the province of Caceres, Spain. *Acta Neurol Scand* 1994;89: 164–170.

Morens DM, Davis JW, Grandinetti A, et al. Epidemiologic observations on Parkinson's disease: incidence and mortality in a prospective study of middle-aged men. *Neurology* 1996;46:1044–1050.

Muller J, Kiechl S, Wenning GK, et al. The prevalence of primary dystonia in the general community. *Neurology* 2002;59:941–943.

Mutch WJ, Dingwall-Fordyce I, Downie AW, et al. Parkinson's disease in a Scottish city. *BMJ* 1986;292:534–536.

Nakashima K, Kusumi M, Inoue Y, Takahashi K. Prevalence of focal dystonias in the western area of Tottori Prefecture in Japan. *Mov Disord* 1995;10:440–443.

Nolan EE, Sverd J, Gadow KD, et al. Associated psychopathology in children with both ADHD and chronic tic disorder. *J Am Acad Child Adolesc Psychiatry* 1996;35:1622–1629.

Nomura Y, Segawa M. Tourette syndrome in oriental children: clinical and pathophysiological considerations. In: Friedhoff AJ, Chase TN, eds. Gilles de la Tourette Syndrome. New York: Raven Press, 1982, pp 277–280.

Noshirvani HF, Kasvikis Y, Marks IM, et al. Gender-divergent aetiological factors in obsessive-compulsive disorder. *Br J Psychiatry* 1991;158:260–263.

Ozelius LJ, Hewett JW, Page CE, et al. The early-onset torsion dystonia gene (DYT1) encodes an ATP-binding protein. *Nat Genet* 1997;17:40–48.

Paganini-Hill A. Risk factors for parkinson's disease: the leisure world cohort study. *Neuroepidemiology* 2001;20:118–124.

Panas M, Avramopoulos D, Karadima G, et al. Apolipoprotein E and presenilin-1 genotypes in Huntington's disease. *J Neurol* 1999; 246:574–577.

Papadimitriou A, Veletza V, Hadjigeorgiou GM, et al. Mutated α-synuclein gene in two Greek kindreds with familial PD: incomplete penetrance? *Neurology* 1999;52:651–654.

Park S, Como PG, Cui L, Kurlan R. The early course of the Tourette's syndrome clinical spectrum. *Neurology* 1993;43:1712–1715.

Parkinson J. An Essay on the Shaking Palsy. London: Sherwood, Neely and Jones, 1817.

Pauls, DL, Leckman JF. The inheritance of Gilles de la Tourette's syndrome and associated behaviors. *N Engl J Med* 1986;315:993–997.

Pauls DL, Raymond CL, Stevenson JM, Leckman JF: A family study of Gilles de la Tourette syndrome. *Am J Hum Genet* 1991; 48:154–163.

Payami H, Larsen K, Bernard S, Nutt H. Increased risk of Parkinson s disease in parents and siblings of patients. *Ann Neurol* 1994; 36:659–661.

Polymeropoulos MH, Lavedan C, Leroy E, et al. Mutation in the α-synuclein gene identified in families with Parkinson's disease. *Science* 1997;276:2045–2047.

Prasad C, Ikegami H, Shimizu I, Onaivi ES. Chronic nicotine intake decelerates aging of nigrostriatal dopaminergic neurons. *Life Sci* 1994;54:1169–1184.

Priyadarshi A, Khuder SA, Schaub EA, Shrivastava S. A meta-analysis of Parkinson's disease and exposure to pesticides. *Neurotoxicology* 2000;21:435–440.

Rajput AH, Offord KP, Beard CM, Kurland LT. Essential tremor in Rochester, Minnesota: a 45-year study. *J Neurol Neurogurg Psychiatry* 1984;47:466–470.

Rajput AH, Rozdilsky B, Ang L, Rajput A. Clinicopathological observations in essential tremor: report of six cases. *Neurology* 1991b; 41:1422–1424.

Rajput AH, Rozdilsky B, Rajput A. Accuracy of clinical diagnosis in parkinsonism—a prospective study. *Can J Neurol Sci* 1991a;18: 275–278.

Ranen NG, Stine OC, Abbott MH, et al. Anticipation and instability of IT-15 (CAG)n repeats in parent–offspring pairs with Huntington disease. *Am J Hum Genet* 1995;57:593–602.

Rautakorpi I. Essential tremor: an epidemiological, clinical, and genetic study [academic dissertation]. University of Turku, Turku, Finland, 1978.

Riggs JE. The nonenvironmental basis for rising mortality from Parkinson's disease. *Arch Neurol* 1993;50:653–656.

Risch N, de Leon D, Ozelius L, et al. Genetic analysis of idiopathic torsion dystonia in Ashkenazi Jews and their recent descent from a small founder population. *Nat Genet* 1995;9:152–9.

Robertson MM, Trimble MR. Gilles de la Tourette syndrome in the Middle East. *Br J Psychiatry* 1991;158:416–419.

Rocca WA, Bower JH, McDonnell SK, et al. Time trends in the incidence of parkinsonism in Olmsted County, Minnesota. *Neurology* 2001;57:462–467.

Ross GW, Abbott RD, Petrovitch H, et al. Association of coffee and caffeine intake with the risk of Parkinson disease. *JAMA* 2000; 283:2674–2679.

Rutter M, Hemming M. Individual items of deviant behavior. Their prevalence and clinical significance. In: Rutter M, Tizard J, Whitmore K, eds. Education, Health, and Behavior. London: Longman, 1970, pp 2020–2032.

Rybicki BA, Johnson CC, Peterson EL, et al. A family history of Parkinson's disease and its effect on other PD risk factors. *Neuroepidemiology* 1999;18:270–278.

Saunders-Pullman RJ, Wendt JJ, Parides MK, et al. Environmental modifiers of genetic dystonia: possible role of infection. *Neurology* 2000;54:A198.

Schrag A, Munchau A, Bhatia KP, et al. Essential tremor: an overdiagnosed condition? *J Neurol* 2000;247:955–959.

Schulte PA, Burnett CA, Boeniger MF, Johnson J. Neurodegenerative diseases: occupational occurrence and potential risk factors, 1982 through 1991. *Am J Public Health* 1996; 86:1281–1288.

Scott WK, Nance MA, Watts RL, et al. Complete genomic screen in Parkinson's disease: evidence for multiple genes. *JAMA* 2001; 286:2239–2244.

Seidler A, Hellenbrand W, Robra BP, et al. Possible environmental, occupational, and other etiologic factors for Parkinson's disease: a case–control study in Germany. *Neurology* 1996;46:1275–1284.

Semchuk KM, Love EJ, Lee RG. Parkinson's disease and exposure to agricultural work and pesticide chemicals. *Neurology* 1992;42: 1328–1335.

Shapiro AK, Shapiro ES, Bruun RD, Sweet RD. Gilles de la Tourette Syndrome. New York: Raven Press, 1978.

Snow B, Wiens M, Hertzman C, Calne D. A community survey of Parkinson's disease. *Can Med Assoc J* 1989;141:418–424.

Spencer T, Biederman J, Harding M, et al. The relationship between tic disorders and Tourette's syndrome revisited. *J Am Acad Child Adolesc Psychiatry* 1995;34:1133–1139.

Stern M, Dulaney E, Gruber SB, et al. The epidemiology of Parkinson's disease. A case–control study of young-onset and old-onset patients. *Arch Neurol* 1991;48:903–907.

Stine OC, Pleasant N, Franz ML, et al. Correlation between the onset age of Huntington's disease and length of the trinucleotide repeat in IT-15. *Hum Mol Genet* 1993;2:1547–1549.

Sugita M, Izuno T, Tatemichi M, Otahara Y. Meta-analysis for epidemiologic studies on the relationship between smoking and Parkinson's disease. *J Epidemiol* 2001;11: 87–94.

Sveinbjornsoottir S, Hicks A, Jonsson T, et al. Familial aggregation of Parkinson's disease in Iceland. *N Engl J Med* 2000;343:1765–1770.

Swedo SE, Leonard HL. Pediatric autoimmune neuropsychiatric disorders associated with streptococcal infections: clinical description of the first 50 cases. *Am J Psychiatry* 1998;155:264–271.

Tanner CM. Epidemiology of movement disorders. In: Anderson D, ed. Neuroepidemiology: A Memorial to Bruce Schoenberg. Boca Raton: CRC Press, 1991, pp 193–216.

Tanner CM, Aston DA. Epidemiology of Parkinson's disease and akinetic syndromes. *Curr Opin Neurol* 2000;13:427–430.

Tanner CM, Ben-Shlomo Y. Epidemiology of Parkinson's disease. *Adv Neurol* 1999;80: 153–159.

Tanner CM, Goldman SM. Epidemiology of movement disorders. *Curr Opin Neurol* 1994; 7:340–345.

Tanner CM, Goldman SM. Epidemiology of Parkinson's disease. *Neurol Clin* 1996;14: 317–335.

Tanner CM, Goldman SM, Lyons KE, Aston DA, Tetrud JW, Welsh MD, Langston JW, Koller WC. Essential tremor in twins: an assessment of genetic vs environmental determinants of etiology. *Neurology* 2001;57: 1389–1391.

Tanner CM, Ottman R, Goldman SM, et al. Parkinson's disease in twins: an etiologic study. *JAMA* 1999;281:341–346.

Taylor CA, Saint-Hilaire MH, Cupples LA, et al. Environmental, medical, and family history risk factors for Parkinson's disease: a New England–based case control study. *Am J Med Genet* 1999;88:742–749.

Thiruchelvam M, Brockel BJ, Richfield EK, et al. Potentiated and preferential effects of combined paraquat and maneb on nigrostriatal dopamine systems: environmental risk factors for Parkinson's disease? *Brain Res* 2000;873:225–234.

Tsui JK, Calne DB, Wang Y, et al. Occupational risk factors in Parkinson's disease. *Can J Public Health* 1999;90:334–347.

Valente EM, Bentivoglio AR, Dixon PH, et al. Localization of a novel locus for autosomal recessive early-onset parkinsonism, PARK6, on human chromosome 1p35-p36. *Am J Hum Genet* 2001;68:895–900.

Valente EM, Brancati F, Ferraris A, et al. PARK6-linked parkinsonism occurs in several European families. *Ann Neurol* 2002; 51:14–18.

Van den Eeden SK, Tanner CM, Bernstein AL, et al. Incidence of idiopathic Parkinson's disease (PD) in a health maintenance organization: variations by age, gender and race/ethnicity. *Am J Epidemiol* 2003;157:1015–1022.

Van Duijn CM, Dekker MC, et al. Park7, a novel locus for autosomal recessive early-onset parkinsonism, on chromosome 1p36. *Am J Hum Genet* 2001;69:629–634.

Verhulst FC, Van der Ende J, Ferdinand RF, Kasius M. The prevalence of DSM-III-R diagnoses in a national sample of Dutch adolescents. *Arch Gen Psychiatry* 1997;54:329–336.

Vieregge P, Schiffke KA, Friedrich, et al. Parkinson s disease in twins. *Neurology* 1992;42: 1453–1461.

Walkup JT, LaBuda MC, Singer HS, et al. Family study and segregation analysis of Tourette syndrome: evidence for a mixed model of inheritance. *Am J Hum Genet* 1996;59:684–693.

Ward CD, Duvoisin RC, Ince SE, et al. Parkinson's disease in 65 pairs of twins and in a set of quadruplets. *Neurology* 1983;33:815–824.

Willems-Giesbergen P, de Rijk M, van Swieten J, et al. Smoking, alcohol, and coffee consumption and the risk of PD: results from the Rotterdam Study. *Neurology* 2000;54: A347.

Wszolek ZK, Pfeiffer RF, Fulgham JR, et al. Western Nebraska family (family D) with autosomal dominant parkinsonism. *Neurology* 1995;45:502–505.

Young AB, Shoulson I, Penney JB, et al. Huntington's disease in Venezuela: neurologic features and functional decline. *Neurology* 1986;36:244–249.

Zhang ZX, Roman GC: Worldwide occurrence of Parkinson's disease: an updated review. *Neuroepidemiology* 1993;12:195–208.

7

Amyotrophic Lateral Sclerosis

CARMEL ARMON

Amyotrophic lateral sclerosis (ALS), also known as Lou Gehrig's disease or Charcot's disease, is the most common motor neuron disease. The pathologic hallmark of ALS is the gradual, progressive, and selective death of (*a*) motor neurons in the spinal cord and brain stem (known as "lower motor neurons" [LMN]) that innervate skeletal and bulbar muscles; and (b) motor neurons in the precentral gyrus of the cerebral cortex (known as "upper motor neurons" [UMN]) that innervate the lower motor neurons. The clinical results are muscle wasting and spasticity, which cause progressive weakness, motor dysfunction, and paralysis, until the affected individual dies, usually of ventilatory failure. Sometimes, higher-order, prefrontal motor neurons become involved, resulting in a unique pattern of cognitive changes that have some similarities to changes seen in the frontotemporal dementias (Ludolph et al. 1992).

Inroads have been made over the past 10 years into understanding the Mendelian forms of ALS, which account for 5%–10% of the cases, and of other diseases of the mo-

tor neuron. Six loci and two genes have been identified for familial ALS (Siddique et al. 1991, 1997; Al-Chalabi et al. 1998; Hentati et al. 1998; Hadano et al. 2001; Yang et al. 2001; Hand and Rouleau 2002) and the genes for the spinal muscular atrophies have also been identified (Harding 1993). Although the molecular mechanisms by which the affected genes cause ALS have not been elucidated, the discovery of these genetic variants has led to considerable progress in animal and laboratory research. The excitement in identifying the genetic basis of some Mendelian forms of the disease notwithstanding, the relevance of these discoveries to understanding the nonfamilial (sporadic) forms has yet to be shown, and the causes of sporadic ALS remain unknown.

Classification of the Diseases of Motor Neurons

Clinical and Pathological Classification

Chronic diseases of the motor neuron include a group of system degeneration diseases known as the motor neuron diseases

(MNDs) (Armon 1994), the late sequelae of poliomyelitis (LSP) (Dalakas 1995), and multifocal motor mononeuropathy (MMM), an immune-mediated treatable condition. The principal forms of MND are amyotrophic lateral sclerosis (ALS), progressive bulbar palsy (PBP), progressive muscular atrophy (PMA), primary lateral sclerosis (PLS), and the spinal muscular atrophies (SMAs) (Armon 1994). Late sequelae of poliomyelitis and MMM will not be considered further in this chapter. Since over 90% of patients with MNDs have ALS, the terms motor neuron disease (MND, singular form) and ALS are sometimes used interchangeably, particularly in the British neurological community (Rowland 1991; Williams and Windebank 1991).

The term ALS should be reserved for patients who have clinical involvement of both upper and lower motor neurons. World Federation of Neurology (WFN) criteria require the presence, evolution, and progression of UMN and LMN dysfunction at multiple levels (bulbar, cervical, thoracic, or lumbosacral) for the clinical diagnosis of ALS (Brooks 1994; Brooks et al. 1998). Pure lower motor neuron syndromes include the SMAs and PMA. Spinal muscular atrophies can be diagnosed on genetic grounds, distinguishing them from PMA. *Progressive bulbar palsy* involves only bulbar-innervated muscles; symptoms include dysarthria (slurred speech) and dysphagia (difficulty swallowing). Although 70% of patients with ALS have signs of both upper and lower motor neuron involvement at multiple levels at initial presentation, ALS may present initially with pure LMN involvement, appearing to be PMA (10% of patients), or pure bulbar involvement, appearing to be PBP (20% of patients). The disease declares itself as ALS in most of these cases as it progresses. There is no practical distinction between the course of patients with PMA and that of ALS, once look-alikes have been excluded. The individual rate of disease progression, rather than the diagnostic term, determines survival (Armon et al. 2000).

Primary lateral sclerosis is a form of MND with pure UMN involvement (Younger et al. 1988; Pringle et al. 1992). Primary lateral sclerosis is usually not included in epidemiologic studies under the classification ALS. Estimates of the prevalence of PLS are hard to find, but may be less than 1% that of ALS (Pringle et al. 1992; Armon 2000). Although the course of PLS is considerably slower than that of ALS, it may be just as disabling in its late stages. For patients presenting with pure UMN disease, a period of observation of 3–5 years has been recommended before one can be reasonably confident that the disease will not progress to have significant LMN involvement and that the disease can be classified as PLS (Armon 2000).

With rare exceptions, most past epidemiologic studies of ALS, and particularly those depending on the International Statistical Classification of Disease (ICD) codes, have not distinguished between ALS and the other motor neuron diseases. In particular, ICD-9 has no subdivision for the major forms of motor neuron disease, all of which are coded as 335.2. More recently, epidemiologic studies initiated by researchers familiar with the WFN criteria have been able to establish patients' diagnosis of ALS based on these criteria. The results are consequently more specific for patients with ALS and may serve for comparison with similarly diagnosed patients in the future. However, caution should be exercised when making comparisons with earlier studies, because most non-ALS cases included under ICD–9 code 335.2 have a younger age at onset and a slower rate of disease progression than those for patients with ALS.

Epidemiologic Classification of Forms of Amyotrophic Lateral Sclerosis

Three major forms of ALS have been identified on the basis of epidemiologic and genetic features: (1) the sporadic form of ALS, (2) the familial or hereditary form of ALS, and (3) the western Pacific (Mariana Islands) form. The latter form was first described among the indigenous population (Chamorros) of Guam, often in association with another progressive and fatal disorder—a parkinsonism–dementia complex (PDC) (Hirano et al. 1961a, 1961b). The ALS/PDC was subsequently recognized also in two villages on the Kii Peninsula of Japan (Kimula et al. 1963; Shiraki 1969) and among the Auyu and Jakai people of Irian Jaya (western New Guinea) (Gajdusek and Salazar 1982). The excess occurrence of ALS/PDC in the western Pacific makes it the largest and best–known cluster, or geographic isolate, of ALS (Kurland 1978) (Fig. 7–1).

An Etiological Hypothesis of Amyotrophic Lateral Sclerosis

One of the most interesting clinical features of ALS is that it usually starts in one anatomical location and spreads (Armon 1999; 2003a,b). Weakness first spreads within the initially affected limb, then frequently crosses to the contralateral limb at the same spinal level, and then proceeds to affect spinal levels contiguous to those in which it began. The ALS pathology also spreads up and down the motor neuron system of the neuroaxis, involving first-, second-, and third-order motor neurons. This behavior is similar to that of a malignancy that has metastasized, except that subcellular components, rather than entire cells, are involved in the spread of the malignancy. The biochemical trigger(s) that sets off the processes that lead to motor neuron loss can be conceptualized as a malignant biochemical transformation (Fig. 7–2). A structural or conformational change may occur in a protein that is involved in cellular function or intercellular communication. Instead of causing uninhibited cellu-

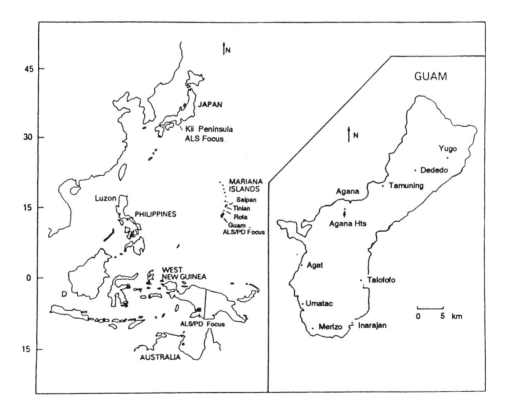

Figure 7–1 Western Pacific and the island of Guam (from the U.S. Census of Guam, 1960–1990). (Reprinted with permission from Armon C, Kurland CT, Smith GE, Steele JC. Sporadic and western pacific amyotrophic lateral sclerosis epidemiologic implications. In: Smith RA, ed. Handbook of ALS. New York: Marcel Dekker, 1992, pp 93–131.)

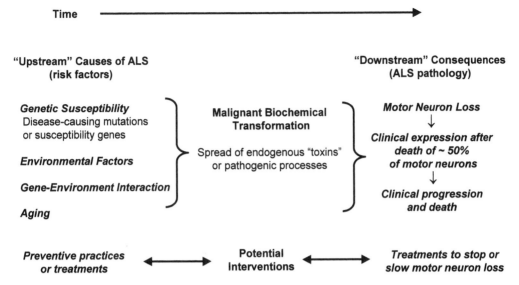

Figure 7–2 The malignant biochemical transformation hypothesis. Under this hypothesis, genetic, environmental, and time- and age-dependent factors operate upstream from a biochemical change or trigger that sets off an inexorable chain of events that results in the clinical condition amyotrophic lateral sclerosis (ALS). There may be more than one way for this to occur. The trigger results in the production of "malignant" molecules, or endogenous toxins, that spread locally and metastasize, in a way analogous to a cellular malignancy, except that this process occurs at a subcellular level. See text for further discussion.

lar proliferation (as is the case in the usual malignancies), the abnormal protein (or abnormally conformed protein) interacts abnormally with other proteins and interferes with normal cell function or intercellular communication. The change might occur at the level of the protein or at the level of the nucleic acids that program its structure or synthesis. This malignant biochemical transformation is a hypothetical concept, because the nature of the biochemical trigger (or triggers) in ALS remains elusive.

The etiologic framework presented in Figure 7–2 permits us to think of processes that precede the malignant transformation ("upstream") and processes that are consequences of this transformation ("downstream"). It is worthwhile to distinguish between upstream factors that make the occurrence of the transformation more likely to happen and those that actually mediate the transformation. Factors that increase the likelihood of the transformation happening are termed "risk factors" for the disease; these include susceptibility genes, environmental factors and their interactions (e.g., gene–gene and gene–environment interactions). The factors which mediate the transformation are unknown. The direct biological "causes" of motor neuron loss are the biochemical processes that develop after the transformation and convert normally functioning cells into abnormally functioning neurons. The pathological mechanisms that mediate these effects are likely to include glutamate excitotoxicity, oxidative stress, mitochondrial dysfunction, and aggregation of neurofilament proteins. After approximately 50% of motor neurons have been lost, the clinical symptoms of muscle weakness and atrophy are expressed. The extent to which the analogy to carcinogenesis is relevant to the pathogenesis of some forms of ALS remains to be seen. The biochemical steps connecting the risk factors, biochemical causes, and consequences of ALS have yet to be elucidated, even for the most well-defined forms of ALS, the Mendelian forms. Epidemiologic and genetic studies of ALS are critical for identifying the "upstream" risk factors of sporadic ALS (Fox et al. 1970). A greater understanding of these factors may point to likely pathogenic mechanisms and ultimately lead to strategies for disease prevention, arrest of disease progression, or cure.

Special Methodological Considerations in Amyotrophic Lateral Sclerosis Research

Epidemiologic inferences are only as good as the data on which they are based. Several methodologic concerns arise when conducting epidemiologic research on ALS, some that are unique to the study of ALS and some that are shared with other neurodegenerative or chronic diseases (Armon 1994).

Case Definition

Correct classification of subjects with ALS is crucial to the epidemiologic study of ALS. The term *case definition* refers to the diagnostic criteria used for epidemiologic or study purposes (Chapter 1). The development of a universally accepted and universally applicable case definition for ALS was the subject of two major consensus conferences convened by the WFN ALS Research Subcommittee. The first conference was held at El Escorial, Spain, and resulted in clinically based criteria for "definite," "probable," and "possible" ALS (Brooks 1994). These criteria were refined at a subsequent conference, held at Airlie House, Virginia, to include laboratory test–based criteria (Brooks et al. 1998). Based on the work of Ross et al. (1998), a diagnosis of "laboratory–supported" probable ALS can be made based on electromyographically confirmed characteristic patterns of denervation in two limbs at one level and UMN findings at or above that level, if other causes have been excluded. In an individual who carries a gene for familial ALS, progressive LMN signs alone, even if only in one limb, can be accepted for diagnosing definite ALS if other causes have been excluded (Brooks et al. 1998). In practice, many clinicians avoid the conundrum generated by the qualifiers "definite," "probable," and "possible," and state that a patient either has or does not have the disease. They rely on a combination of the clinical findings of progressive upper and lower motor neuron dysfunction, electromyographic evidence of widespread muscle de-nervation, and the absence of identifiable structural or reversible biochemical abnormalities. There remain rare patients, who might be classified as having possible ALS by WFN criteria, in whom ALS cannot be diagnosed definitively initially. Over time, only a small minority of patients remains in this diagnostic limbo, probably 1%–2% of patients. Unfortunately for the patient, the inexorable progression of the disease usually resolves the dilemma, if ALS is the correct ultimate diagnosis. Death certificates also do not allow for qualification of the diagnosis of ALS—usually the correct diagnosis, if it has taken the patient's life. For a diagnosis of classic ALS, literal application of the WFN criteria (Brooks 1994; Brooks et al. 1998) requires the absence of clinically significant involvement of additional systems; if other systems are affected, patients should be classified as ALS variants. This guarantees exclusion from clinical trials or from epidemiologic studies, patients with known variants, such as those in whom ALS was diagnosed several years after having a diagnosis of L-dopa–responsive Parkinson's disease, or patients with Guamanian ALS (ALS/PDC). The need for, or benefit of, making this distinction under other circumstances is uncertain. When patients with "classic" ALS have been studied more intensively (Tandan and Bradley 1985a, 1985b; Sasaki et al. 1992), some patients have been shown to have central, peripheral, or autonomic nervous system involvement, in addition to upper and lower motor neuron dysfunction, including a unique form of frontal cognitive impairment (ALS/fronto–temporal dementia) (Ben

Hamida et al. 1987, Armon et al. 1991a; Ludolph et al. 1992).

Case Ascertainment

Case ascertainment refers to the methods of finding potential patients for inclusion in epidemiologic series or studies. At least five recognizable factors have contributed to improved ascertainment of ALS over the past 20 years: (*a*) increased public awareness of the disease, including that generated by the major clinical trials launched in the 1990s; (*b*) increased awareness by the aging population that progressive weakness is not a normal part of aging; (*c*) an increase in the number of neurologists per capita; (*d*) the increased availability of electrodiagnostic and radiologic diagnostic techniques; and (*e*) the enactment of the Medicare Act in 1965, which guaranteed improved access to health care for the elderly.

Accompanying this increase in awareness of ALS is the recognition that some individuals, particularly family members of patients with ALS, may have a MND that remains undiagnosed during their lifetime.

> *Example 7–1* In a case–control study of patients with ALS (Armon et al. 1991b), 1.2% of the relatives of the controls who lived to be over 60 were reported to have developed a painless, progressive, weakening and wasting illness in their later life, comprising a potential pool of individuals who in past generations may have died of undiagnosed ALS. The number is six times higher than the U.S. death ratio for ALS: approximately 1/500 of those reaching adulthood. Thus, if improved ascertainment resulted in a positive diagnosis of ALS in only 15% of such individuals, the crude rates of ALS would appear to double, without a true increase in incidence having occurred.

Referral bias is another example of the impact of ascertainment or, in this case, underascertainment, on descriptive data obtained from ALS patients who have been referred to or sought care at specialized clinics or tertiary care centers. Older or more rapidly progressing patients are less likely to be referred to such centers. Consequently, studies conducted in referral centers consistently report a mean age of onset 10 years younger and survival longer than that reported in well-ascertained population-based series (see below).

Impact of Earlier Diagnosis and Supportive Treatment

Improved ascertainment of ALS cases and earlier diagnosis of patients may appear to increase the duration of disease, if survival is dated from the time of diagnosis. However, shorter average survival may result if earlier diagnosis results in ascertainment and inclusion of older patients with rapidly progressive disease who in the past would not have been diagnosed with ALS before they died. In addition, variability in how the date of diagnosis is defined may make it difficult to interpret data regarding survival from onset or regarding onset-to-diagnosis latency (Armon 2003b). Survival from the time of disease onset may be a better measure of the natural history of ALS, but it may be difficult for patients and their doctors to establish the precise date of disease onset. As patients reflect on the period that preceded what they initially considered the date of onset of their disease, a progressively earlier date of onset tends to emerge. As neurologists become experienced in early diagnosis of ALS/MND, they may concurrently be able to determine earlier dates of disease onset. The average onset-to-diagnosis latency will then appear unchanged, but patient survival from onset and from diagnosis will appear to have increased without any actual change in the biology of the disease or the longevity of patients. These factors suggest that caution is needed when drawing conclusions about changes in the natural history of the disease and that the efficacy of current interventions cannot be established by making comparisons to historical controls (Armon 2002; 2003b). Direct comparison of the survival of historical cohorts and contemporary cohorts of ALS patients requires even greater caution because current survival may be extended by the availability of more aggressive supportive treatments, such as noninvasive ventilatory support and percutaneous enteral feeding (Miller et al. 1999).

Descriptive Studies

Incidence and Mortality Data, and Patient Characteristics

Incidence studies of ALS or MND conducted in the United States that have achieved near-complete case ascertainment (and excluding the Western Pacific foci) report rates that are fairly constant geographically, approximately 2 per 100,000 per year (Yoshida et al. 1986; Kurtzke 1989; Lilienfeld and Perl 1993; McGuire et al. 1996; Sorenson et al. 2002). Incidence rates reported from other countries have ranged from 0.86 to 2.4 per 100,000 per year (Armon and Kurland 1989; Christensen et al. 1990; Armon et al. 1992; Traynor et al. 1999; Seljeseth et al. 2000; Maasilta et al. 2001; Piemonte and Valle d'Aosta Register 2001). With an average duration of 3 years, the prevalence of ALS is approximately three times the incidence rate, or about 6 per 100,000 (see Chapter 2). Mortality rates for ALS would be expected to parallel incidence rates fairly closely, as almost all patients with ALS die of their disease. However, several factors impact the reporting of ALS on death certificates, including patients' socioeconomic status and profession (Armon 2003a). Overall, ALS is underreported on death certificates. For example, the reported mortality rates for ALS in the United States during recent decades was under 1.5 per 100,000 per year for all ages combined, a figure that is lower than the average ALS incidence of 2 per 100,000 per year. Most ALS or MND incidence and mortality data show higher rates in recent years than were previously reported in the industrialized nations (Ludolph et al. 1992; Lilienfeld and Perl 1993; Seljeseth et al. 2000; Maasilta et al. 2001). This increase in absolute rates may be accounted for without implicating

the operation of any new etiologic agents. At least four factors to consider are (*a*) the aging of the population (see below); (*b*) loss of competing causes of mortality in a susceptible cohort (Gompertz 1825; Riggs 1990; Nielson et al. 1992; Riggs and Schochet 1992); (*c*) improved diagnosis and ascertainment; and (*d*) better reporting of ALS on death certificates.

In population-based series, average (and median) age at clinical onset is 65 years, and median disease duration from onset to death is approximately 3 years (Sorenson et al. 2002; del Aguila et al. 2003). In referral series patients, including most reported clinical trials, mean age at onset has been younger (e.g., 55 years old), and median survival has varied but is usually reported as greater than 3 years. In clinical trials, ALS onset often has been defined as onset of clinical weakness.

Example 7–2 The relationship between age at onset and incidence rates in several studies (DeDomenico et al. 1988; Lopez-Vega et al. 1988; Scarpa et al. 1988; Salemi et al. 1989) illustrates the potential effect of referral bias and ascertainment bias, since a higher incidence rate was associated with a higher mean age at onset and with a shorter survival. This observation suggests that improved diagnosis and ascertainment may identify patients with a disease course shorter than the previously considered median of 3 years, and with an older age at onset. This finding is consistent with observations that older age of onset is associated with a shorter disease course (Brooks et al. 1991; Munsat et al. 1991).

Incidence and Mortality Rates: Effects of Gender, Age, and Race

The incidence of sporadic ALS in men is greater than that in women (1.2:1 to 1.6:1) (Armon et al. 1994; McGuire et al. 1996). In this context it is worth considering that Kennedy's disease, a LMN disease caused by a trinucleotide repeat expansion on chromosome X, affects male but not female carriers of the repeat (Buchanan and Malamud 1973), and that a gene for familial ALS has been identified on the X chromosome. This suggests that there could be also a susceptibility gene for sporadic ALS on the X chromosome, which may be the same as or adjacent to the genes for Kennedy's disease or for X-linked familial ALS, but with lesser penetrance.

Age-specific incidence rates have been shown to increase with age in population-based series (Yoshida et al. 1986; Christensen et al. 1990; McGuire et al. 1996; Seljeseth et al. 2000; Maasilta et al. 2001; Sorenson et al. 2002) (Fig. 7–3), rather than peaking at 55–60 years, as occurred in referral-based case series (Gunnarsson et al. 1991; Kurtzke 1991). Consequently, aging of the population is expected to result in an increase in the incidence of ALS.

Information regarding the incidence of ALS in racial or ethnic groups other than Caucasians is lacking. Several death certificate studies have reported race-specific mortality rates for ALS, but only one incidence study in the United States has estimated ALS incidence for non-Caucasian groups.

Example 7–3 A study in Harris County, Texas, reported an overall annual incidence rate of 1.5 per 100,000 per year for all racial and ethnic groups combined (Annegers et al. 1991). The authors noted that annual ALS incidence did not appear to vary substantially among racial/ethnic groups (Caucasians, African Americans, and Hispanics). However, the authors acknowledged that case ascertainment for Hispanics and African Americans was poor and may have resulted in underestimates of ALS incidence in these groups. This study encountered the challenges that any geographically based study of rare neurologic conditions faces: the difficulty of achieving near-complete case ascertainment. Furthermore, because of the diversity of healthcare systems and of access to these systems, the degree of underascertainment may have varied among the racial/ethnic groups in the area. Thus, existing data are insufficient to permit comparisons of ALS incidence rates on the basis of race/ethnicity.

In contrast, earlier mortality studies using death certificate ascertainment of ALS cases had shown racial and ethnic differ-

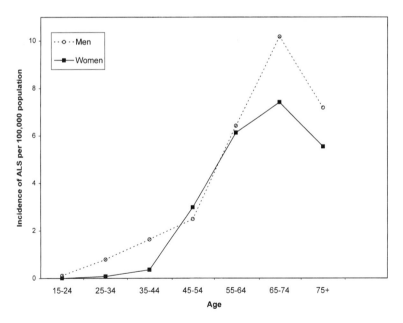

Figure 7–3 Age-specific incidence of amyotrophic lateral sclerosis (ALS) in men and women for western Washington State from April 1990 to March 1995). (Reprinted with permission from McGuire VN, Longstreth WT, Jr., Koepsell TD, van Belle G. Incidence of amyotrophic lateral sclerosis in three counties in western Washington State. Neurology 1996;47:571–573.)

ences in death rates from ALS in the United States. Mortality studies for the years 1959–1961 found that the rates for whites exceeded those for non-whites by 1.7 to 1 (Kurland et al. 1973; Kurtzke 1991). Subsequent studies of the mortality rates for 1971 and 1973–1978 and 1962–1984 continued to show lower rates among non-whites, particularly those older than 60 years and especially among women (Kurtzke 1991). The ALS mortality rates among U.S. African Americans were reported in one study to be lower than mortality rates of U.S. Caucasians (Leone et al. 1987). While these differences may be real, it is more likely that they represented selective underascertainment of ALS in populations with limited access to health care or among groups who may have been less likely to have ALS listed on their death certificates as a contributing cause of death. Given the potential of bias due to selective under-ascertainment of ALS cases when using death certificate data, it is difficult to draw any conclusions from mortality data with regard to the effect of race on the true incidence of ALS. While this methodological point has been made using race-specific United States national or regional data, it also applies to inferring regional variations within the United States or other countries, and to international comparisons.

Western Pacific Amyotrophic Lateral Sclerosis

The Western Pacific form of ALS has aroused interest since its identification in the mid-1950s, because ALS incidence, prevalence, and mortality rates when first identified were 50–100 times those of the sporadic form that occurs in the continental United States (Kurland and Mulder 1954, 1955). Clusters of ALS were noted in three distinct geographic isolates (Kurland 1978): in the southern Mariana Islands, in two villages of the Kii Peninsula of Japan, and among the Auyu and Jakai people in a small area of Irian Jaya (western New Guinea). From the standpoint of epidemiological research, the distinction between these investigator-identified geographic isolates and apparent clusters reported from the community is important. Western Pacific ALS had unique clinical characteristics because it was associated frequently with a parkinsonism/dementia complex (PDC), the male/female ratio approximated 2 to 1, and the median age at onset was 44 years. The extreme excess of occurrence (initially 100-fold, rather than just a few–fold greater than the expected number) and the persistence of the excess over time (Lavine et al. 1991) confirm that this is a true excess. The incidence of ALS/PDC is not due to methodologic problems resulting from the way it was defined or ascertained, or to the operation of chance alone. Consequently, there can be no question that an underlying etiologic cause is present in the Western Pacific foci.

Familial aggregation of ALS/PDC on Guam was recognized in the first published reports from Guam (Koerner 1952; Arnold et al. 1953; Kurland and Mulder 1954). This pattern has persisted to date, with the result that some families have been considered "afflicted," and their members perceived as less than ideal candidates for marriage. The putative inheritance within "afflicted" families has not followed simple Mendelian patterns; therefore, disease clustering in families may reflect common exposure to an environmental agent rather than a genetic cause. Plato et al. (2002) examined the incidence and prevalence of ALS/PDC on Guam over the 40 years since 1960. They found that the rates of ALS and PD among relatives of ALS/PDC cases were significantly higher than the rates in the Guamanian population as a whole, particularly among siblings but also among wives (but not husbands) of patients with ALS, and among the offspring of patients with PDC. Since the excess was observed among wives and siblings (more than other first degree relatives) of ALS/PDC patients, the authors concluded that the clustering observed in family members could be the result of a shared environment rather than shared genes and that there was little support for the hypothesis that ALS/PDC is a Mendelian genetic disorder. However, the certainty in this conclusion might be diminished if there were a fair amount of consanguinity among spouses. A more recent report, of separate familial clustering of ALS and PDC on Guam, suggests again that a genetic etiology should be considered, this time in terms of a two-gene model, with environmental interaction (McGeer et al. 1997). The authors reported a shift in age of onset by 16 years for ALS and 13 years for PDC, and speculated that environmental (dietary) changes may have had a beneficial effect in a genetically susceptible population (McGeer et al. 1997).

The prevalence of neurofibrillary tangles in asymptomatic Chamorros (Galasko et al. 2002; Perl et al. 2003), which may suggest a predisposition to neurodegenerative disorders or subclinical disease in asymptomatic individuals, is also a possible clue to the etiology of ALS/PDC. In addition to patterns of familial aggregation, three factors suggest that genetics alone does not account for Western Pacific ALS. They are (1) involvement of three apparently different ethnic populations; (2) the apparent excess of ALS or PDC among Filipinos who have settled in Guam as young adults (Garruto et al. 1981); and (3) the increasing age of onset of ALS and PDC in the southern villages of Guam over the past 30 years (Lavine et al. 1991, McGeer et al. 1997).

Two primary environmental hypotheses have been proposed to account for Western Pacific ALS/PDC. One suggested that ALS/PDC was due to a deficiency or an excess of essential minerals; low levels of calcium and magnesium in the soil were proposed as causes (Yase 1978; Gajdusek et al. 1980). This hypothesis was weakened when subsequent studies on Guam showed an adequate calcium and magnesium content of water and foods grown in the soil of areas such as Umatac, where ALS and PDC were particularly prevalent (Zolon and Ellis-Neill 1986; Armon et al. 1992).

The most widely held hypothesis about the cause of ALS/PDS is that there is a toxic environmental agent common to the three affected areas. The postulated exposure to this toxin peaked during World War II and declined, but did not disappear. According to this hypothesis, individuals exposed to higher doses of toxin developed ALS at a relatively early age, with or without associated PDC, and individuals exposed to a lesser dose developed, at a later date, ALS with or without PDC, PDC alone, or dementia alone. In field studies, Marjorie Whiting (1963) identified the seed of the false sago palm, *Cycas circinalis*, and its products as a potential cause. The most immediately active toxin of *Cycas circinalis* is cycasin, a glycoside component with hepatotoxic and carcinogenic effects but only minimal neurotoxic effects. This toxin is usually removed by the soaking process, which is used in the preparation of the cycad for consumption. A single animal experiment by Dastur (1964) described production of muscle weakness and degeneration of anterior horn cells in a young rhesus monkey fed washed cycad in which cycasin was not detected using the methods of assay available at the time. This finding appeared to be an isolated observation, and support for the cycad hypothesis declined. However, it was kept alive by Kurland (Kurland and Molgaard 1982; Kurland and Mulder 1987) and received new impetus from Spencer and Schaumberg (1983). They suspected that there might be parallels between the neurotoxicity of β-N-oxalylamino-L-alanine (BOAA), the compound responsible for lathyrism, and β-N-methylamino-L-alanine (BMAA), which is present in the cycad, both of which have structures similar to glutamic acid. Using a purified L-isomer of BMAA, Spencer was able to produce in monkeys an illness with features of human ALS and possible Parkinson's disease (Spencer et al. 1986, Spencer 1987). Spencer reported use of unwashed cycad as a medicinal in both other foci of Western Pacific ALS, namely, the Irian Jaya focus in western New Guinea (as a poultice) and the Kii Peninsula of Japan (as a "tonic" made from dried seeds of *Cycas revoluta*) (Spencer et al. 1987a, 1987b). However, the results of Spencer's feeding experiment in monkeys were not replicated (Garruto et al. 1988). The chief difference between the course of disease in humans (ALS/PDC) and in animals exposed to exogenous toxins is the lack of progression of the disease among animals (Spencer et al. 1991; Duncan 1991). Recognizing the limitations of the neurotoxicity hypothesis, Spencer currently favors methylazoxymethanol (the aglycone of cycasin), a potent alkylating agent, as the primary mechanism for the long-latency induction of Western Pacific ALS (Esclaire et al. 1999; Kisby et al. 1999). He postulates that methylazoxymethanol may produce postmitotic DNA damage and interfere with DNA repair, up-regulate the expression of tau mRNA by itself or in conjunction with an endogenous excitotoxic agent (the neurotransmitter glutamate), and thus promote the accumulation of tau protein and neuronal degeneration in Western Pacific ALS/PDC. The primary neurotoxicity hypothesis remains alive, however, with current focus on a new group of non–water soluble neurotoxic agents, which may be found in washed cycad: three sterol β-D-glucosides (Khabazian et al. 2002; Wilson et al. 2002). They appear to have distinct effects on NMDA receptor activation, and NMDA antagonists can block their various actions in vitro. Their acute mode of action results in induction of release of glutamate and lactate dehydrogenase. It remains to be shown whether these neurotoxins can produce chronic, progressive neurodegenerative disease, possibly at a time remote from the time of their consumption, even though other neurotoxins affecting the motor and cognitive systems have not been shown to do so. A recent contribution to the discussion of how a toxic product originating in the cycad may be transmitted to humans, bypassing the detoxification process that usually precedes human consumption of cycad-derived products, has been a hypothesis that consumption of bats, which feed on cycad, may place humans at risk for ALS/PDC (Cox and Sacks 2002a). As part

of this hypothesis, it is postulated also that a process of biomagnification of the toxic effect may occur, by concentrating the putative cycad-derived toxin in the body of the bat. This hypothesis has been debated (Chen et al. 2002; Cox and Sacks 2002b) but adds a tantalizing twist to the route by which cycad may cause Western Pacific ALS/PDC. It is exciting and gratifying that specific epidemiological observations made over 40 years ago (Whiting 1963) continue to drive the etiologic investigations of Western Pacific ALS/PDC.

The Role of Clusters in the Study of Sporadic Amyotrophic Lateral Sclerosis

The basic principle of epidemiology is that disease does not occur by chance alone, but through the operation of underlying causes (Fox et al. 1970). Where disease clusters exist, underlying causal agents may also aggregate, offering clues to etiology. When large numbers of affected cases appear at once in a small geographic area, as in infectious disease epidemics, the etiologic agent is often isolated rapidly. Even small clusters can lead to etiologically important discoveries if the disease is newly recognized (for example, Legionnaires' disease and AIDS) or if the disease is extremely rare in a particular population. Examples of the latter include the occurrence of vaginal cancer in young women associated with DES use by their mothers during pregnancy (Herbst et al. 1971), and the occurrence of MPTP-induced parkinsonism in young intravenous drug abusers (Langston et al. 1983).

Unfortunately, clusters of patients with relatively common chronic diseases, including ALS, have so far yielded no causal clues (Armon et al. 1991a). The etiologic significance even of the best-documented and most persistent clusters of ALS, those in the Western Pacific foci, has remained elusive. Clusters based on smaller numbers of cases, smaller increases in relative incidence or mortality rates, and with less persistence in time are less likely to be informative. Moreover, very few suspected clusters that have arisen from community reports have been confirmed as true excesses of disease once rigorous criteria have been applied. These include meticulous attention to case definition, identification of an appropriate population size (denominator) and period of observation to derive incidence rates, and choice of an appropriate reference control population with equal ascertainment of cases. It is also important to take into consideration the role of the multiple comparisons implicit in the production of these apparent clusters, as chance alone, rather than the operation of an underlying etiologic agent, may have produced the findings (Armon et al. 1991a). Several approaches have been suggested to compensate for the effect of chance in assessing the potential significance of clusters arising from the community (Kurtzke 1966; Armon et al. 1991a). For example, we have proposed to increase the value for the ratio of observed to expected cases that may be considered of potential epidemiologic significance (Armon et al. 1991a). Case ascertainment and field investigations would be reserved only for those reports that, if confirmed, would represent a cluster that could not be accounted for on the basis of chance alone (Armon et al. 1991a).

A recent epidemiologic investigation followed the observation of an apparent cluster of patients with ALS associated with former work at Kelly Air Force Base in San Antonio, Texas (Mundt et al. 2002). This investigation was a benchmark for collaboration between federal and state agencies, patients and patient interest groups, and external scientific advisors. The guiding principles for this collaboration were the choice of an appropriate study design; the identification of a suitable cohort; assessment of ALS mortality in the context of overall mortality and other disease-specific mortality data; performance of the mortality study itself by an independent epidemiology research company; and publication of the results in an appropriate, peer-reviewed journal prior to their release to the public. The report of the investigators indicated that, for now, there is no evidence for excess mortality from ALS in the Kelly Air Force Base civilian worker cohort (Mundt et al. 2002). The recognized limitations of a mortality study done when most of the affected population is alive do not detract from its strengths in providing a scientifically sound platform for the identification of any large, early excess of cases, if such an excess had been evident.

Genetic Risk Factors

Familial Amyotrophic Lateral Sclerosis

In most series, familial cases comprise only 5%–10% of patients with ALS (Mulder et al. 1986; Yoshida et al. 1986; Li et al. 1988; Williams et al. 1988; Williams and Windebank 1991; Swash and Leigh 1992). The word *familial* refers to the fact that an ALS patient has one or more other affected family members with ALS, and includes patients who have a Mendelian pattern of disease inheritance (e.g., autosomal dominant or autosomal recessive) as well as patients with no apparent Mendelian inheritance pattern. Mendelian ALS is usually inherited in an autosomal dominant pattern, and more rarely follows an autosomal recessive, or X–linked recessive pattern (Kurland and Mulder 1954; Hirano et al. 1967; Husquinet and Frank 1980; Emery and Holloway 1982; Mulder et al. 1986; Sobue et al. 1989; Ben Hamida et al. 1990; Veltema et al. 1990; Siddique et al. 1991, 1997; Appelbaum et al. 1992; Swash and Leigh 1992; Al-Chalabi et al. 1998; Hentati et al. 1998; Hadano et al. 2001; Yang et al. 2001; Hand and Rouleau 2002).

Twenty percent of familial cases are due to mutations at the *SOD1* gene on chromosome 21 (Siddique et al. 1991), with over 100 alleles now identified. Most result in an autosomal dominant pattern of inheritance, except one (Al-Chalabi et al. 1988), which results in autosomal recessive inheritance. Additional chromosomes implicated in autosomal recessive ALS are chromosomes 15 (Hentati et al. 1998) and 2 (Siddique et al. 1997), and an X–linked gene has also been identified.

The mean age of onset for familial ALS is approximately 15 to 20 years earlier than the mean age of onset for the sporadic form. With regard to age of onset and duration of disease, variability within families is smaller than variability between families. This observation extends to allelic variants of transgenic mouse models of familial ALS. There is variable penetrance (approximately 80%) among individuals carrying a gene for an autosomal dominant form of the disease. Since not all carriers of the gene will develop ALS, even if they live longer than relatives who developed ALS, additional factors must be at work in determining which carriers will develop disease.

Recent reviews of familial ALS provide additional details of these and other genes for Mendelian ALS (Brown and Robberecht 2001; Hand and Rouleau 2002). The other genes have been implicated in just a few families, and the phenotype has often differed from that of classic ALS. There has been evidence for phenotypic and genotypic variability of familial ALS (Horton et al. 1976; Chio et al. 1987). At least half of patients will have, in addition to anterior horn cell degeneration, clinically silent involvement of spinocerebellar tracts, posterior columns, and the columns of Clarke. Some patients with familial ALS lack UMN signs or evidence of UMN involvement on autopsy (Cudkowicz et al. 1998). Some of the distinguishing features of familial ALS may be the result of selective recognition of stronger familial aggregation among cases with an early average age of onset (Williams et al. 1988).

Genetic factors are hypothesized to have a role in the production of "sporadic" ALS, by determining the degree of individual genetic susceptibility to environmental risk factors. The earliest candidate susceptibility genes evaluated have been those involved in the development of the spinal muscular atrophies, *SMN* (survival motor neuron) and *NAIP* (neuronal apoptosis inhibitory protein). In a transgenic animal model of *SOD1* ALS, a modifier gene has been mapped to a region that includes the *SMN* and *NAIP* genes (Kunst et al. 2000). The *SMN1* gene has been shown to impact prognosis of individuals with sporadic ALS and the number of *SMN1* copies has been linked to the appearance of an ALS phenotype in a family with individuals having either SMA or ALS (Corcia et al. 2002a, 2002b). Homozygous deletion of the *SMN2* gene has been shown to be a prognostic factor in sporadic ALS (Veldink et al. 2001). Another series showed that deletions causing spinal muscular atrophy do not predispose to ALS (Parboosingh et al. 1999). Collection of material for genetic analysis performed concurrently with future epidemiologic studies may permit a search for genes that make individuals susceptible to particular exposures.

Analytic Studies

ALS risk factor research has evolved in the past decade, with a shift in focus away from isolated antecedent events toward lifelong exposures or behaviors. This shift has been driven in part by biologic plausibility and in part by evidence that free radicals and excitotoxins may play a part in the progression of ALS after it has been initiated. The reasoning behind the latter was that there might be similarity between the mechanisms leading to disease initiation and those involved in its progression (Fig. 7–4). It remains to be seen whether that is the case. On average, about 12 months elapse between the onset of the first clinical symptom of ALS and its diagnosis (Granieri et al. 1983; Yoshida et al. 1986; Christensen et al. 1990; Armon et al. 1991b; Gunnarsson et al. 1992; McGuire et al. 1996; Sorenson et al. 2002). However, the onset of first clinical symptoms undoubtedly occurs some time after the disease has been biologically active, because muscle weakness in ALS accrues in a gradual, cumulative manner. If progression from clinical onset of first symptom to death averages 3 years, when approximately 90% of the anterior horn cells at affected levels have degenerated, and if clinical disease can be recog-

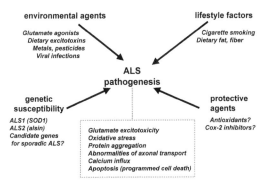

Figure 7–4 A general model for the pathogenesis of amyotrophic lateral sclerosis (ALS).

nized when one-half the motor neurons are affected, then it has been argued that biological onset might predate clinical onset by as much as 3 years (Armon and Kurland 1989). Identifying risk factors for ALS is complicated by this lag because the relevant exposures would likely have taken place more than 3 years prior to the recognized clinical onset of ALS. For case–control studies, this may affect the choice of reference date, that is, the date after which information related to etiologic factors is not assessed because of the presence of the disease. One strategy is to exclude the time period 1–5 years prior to diagnosis from consideration when evaluating risk factors, since this period likely encompassed a preclinical period when the disease pathology was present but had not come to medical attention. Many earlier analytic studies of risk factors for ALS are of limited value because they failed to exclude these periods from consideration.

Types of Analytic Studies: Strengths and Limitations

Three major types of analytical study designs can be used to identify potential risk factors for ALS: cross-sectional or prevalence studies, cohort (prospective or retrospective) studies, and case–control studies (see Chapter 2). Because of the relatively low incidence of ALS, prospective cohort studies have been considered impractical as a means of identifying risk factors, and cross-sectional studies of prevalent cases are affected by prevalence-incidence bias (see Chapters 1 and 2). The case–control design is most useful to evaluate hypotheses generated contemporarily. A retrospective cohort study may be used to follow up on hypotheses generated by a case–control study, provided that an appropriate cohort exists. Although occupational/mortality studies are not subject to recall bias, they are susceptible to biases due to the variability in diagnosis and registration of ALS on death certificates, which may depend on profession and socioeconomic status, and variability in registration of profession on death certificates (Armon 2003a). Consequently, results based on small numbers of cases cannot be relied on.

Special Methodologic Considerations in Case–Control Studies of Amyotrophic Lateral Sclerosis. The six major considerations in designing and assessing the significance of published case–control studies are patient homogeneity, choice of controls, recall bias, quantification of activities or exposures, testing of multiple hypotheses, and statistical power, which depends on sample size and the magnitude of the expected difference between patients and controls (Armon et al. 1992). The chief limitations of case–control studies are the multiple sources of biases to which they are susceptible (Schlesselman 1982). Furthermore, testing multiple hypotheses (a "fishing expedition") is likely to cause some associations to attain statistical significance by chance alone. The effect of chance alone should be suspected particularly when the increased odds ratio is based on a small number of cases. The potential etiologic significance of risk factors identified in only a small number of cases may also be limited.

The past 10 years have seen an evolution in the standards for design of case–control studies, resulting in increased rigor in more recent studies. According to these emerging standards, an important limitation of previous studies was reliance on small numbers of prevalent ALS cases from referral centers. Three population-based case–control studies of patients with ALS have been conducted: in Scotland (Chancellor et al. 1993), in Washington State (McGuire et al. 1996), and in New England (Kamel et al. 1999, 2002). The study from Scotland was limited, however, because a sizable portion of incident ALS cases (39 of 103) in the registry were deceased prior to the initiation of the case–control study and proxy respondents were not sought. The New England study relied on a subgroup of referred cases, with population-based controls. The study in Washington State (McGuire et al. 1996) used incident ALS cases and was larger than all but one previous case–control study. All other published case–control studies to date have used prevalent cases. A concern is that some risk factors might be underrepresented in patients if these risk factors caused rapidly progressing disease, because patients with rapidly progressing disease are less likely to be referred to tertiary centers or to be included in studies based on prevalent patients. Moreover, when long-lived cases are over represented, identifying risk factors that preceded ALS becomes difficult, as does distinguishing factors associated with prognosis from those with etiologic significance. A second concern is that ALS case–control studies conducted in secondary study bases, such as hospitals, referral centers, or ALS societies, may not be representative of ALS patients in the general population in ways that are unknown. A third limitation of many previous studies is sample size and statistical power—only a few studies included more than 100 ALS cases. Additional limitations are inappropriate choice of control subjects, recall bias, and the testing of multiple hypotheses. Furthermore, publication bias, whereby a positive finding is more likely to be published than the lack of a finding (Koren and Klein 1991; Dickersin et al. 1992), may have favored the identification of spurious risk factors. Insufficient statistical power (Hennekens and Buring 1987) may result in failure to identify associations or in failure of associations to attain statistical significance. The variability of patient selection criteria and study methodologies in past case–control studies of ALS precludes using meta-analysis to overcome this shortcoming. However, in future, if data are gathered using uniform methods at multiple centers, it may be possible to combine them to achieve greater statistical power for addressing hypotheses.

In summary, methodologic limitations often make it difficult to draw inferences from the findings of many of the published studies. Positive findings may be the result of bias or of multiple comparisons. Negative findings in some studies may be the result of low statistical power.

An evidence–based medicine (EBM) approach may be applied to the analysis of risk factors for sporadic ALS (Armon 2003a, 2003b) by defining an explicit method of rating articles according to their "evidence-worthiness" and translating the evidence into conclusions. It may be appropriate to assign importance to conclusions that attain various levels of certainty according to their potential impact on the general public. This approach considers the percent of the patient population affected and the degree to which risk factors are modifiable. This chapter presents a summary of risk factors for ALS according to the traditional approach, followed by a summary resulting from application of the evidence-based medicine approach. Greater detail is found elsewhere (Armon 2003a, 2003b).

Risk Factors for Sporadic Amyotrophic Lateral Sclerosis: Traditional Approach

Because of the methodological limitations noted above, case–control studies have yielded conflicting results and very few definitive conclusions about risk factors are possible. A brief summary of the epidemiologic evidence regarding risk factors is presented here; more extensive reviews are available from other sources (Williams and Windebank, 1991).

Skeletal Trauma. One of the most controversial purported risk factors for ALS has been mechanical trauma (Kurtzke 1991; Kurland et al. 1992). A recently reported population-based case–control study of risk factors for ALS showed no association of ALS with skeletal trauma (Cruz et al. 1999) and an earlier cohort study failed to show an increased risk of ALS among patients who had suffered head injuries during life.

> *Example 7–4* A retrospective cohort study of ALS (Williams et al. 1991) showed no increased incidence of ALS in survivors of head trauma. However, due to the fairly low lifetime cumulative risk of ALS (approximately 1/500) of those attaining adulthood, even a large cohort, such as that assembled by Williams et al. (1991), which included 821 patients, might not show a modest increase in risk. Conversely, a chance occurrence of ALS in one or two extra people might have resulted in a statistically significant elevation in the attributed risk.

Environmental Toxicants. Eight epidemiologic studies have been conducted to investigate the association of heavy metal exposure and ALS. Several investigations have reported elevated risk associated with exposure to lead (Felmus et al. 1976; Armon et al. 1991c; Chancellor et al. 1993; Kamel 2002). All but two previous studies (Armon et al. 1991c; Chancellor et al. 1993) used spouses, relatives, friends, and/or coworkers as control subjects, raising the possibility that cases and controls were overmatched with respect to exposure opportunity for the metals of interest. Despite the possibility of overmatching, all studies except two (Deapen and Henderson 1986; Gresham et al. 1986) found a significant increased risk associated with exposure to lead, mercury, or other heavy metals as a class with odds ratios ranging from 2.0 to 6.0. Only two studies obtained information on the duration of lead exposure. One of these studies identified increased risk of ALS among men associated with greater than 200 lifetime cumulative hours of lead exposure (OR = 5.5; 95% CI 1.4–21) (Armon et al. 1991c). In the other, greater than 12 months of employment in occupations in-

volving lead exposures resulted in increased risk for ALS (OR = 5.7; 95% CI 1.6–30.0) (Chancellor et al. 1993). A limitation of these studies is that they were based on self-report, which is susceptible to recall bias. Either the cases are more likely to remember and report certain exposures or control subjects may underreport exposures (Kurland et al. 1992).

Case–control studies have also identified associations of ALS with occupations that involve exposure to heavy metals, such as electrical work and welding (Deapen et al. 1986; Armon et al. 1991c; Gunnarsson et al. 1992). The Washington State population-based case–control study showed no associations for exposures to metals and solvents when relying on assessment by a panel of industrial hygienists evaluating job histories, blinded to participant status, though such associations were found when relying on self-report (McGuire et al. 1997).

Several other lines of investigation have linked ALS to heavy metal exposure, including studies finding increased metal content in tissues of ALS patients (Kurlander and Patten 1979; Mitchell et al. 1986). However, such studies cannot determine whether increased metal content in tissues is the cause or the effect of ALS. Only two previous studies have attempted to obtain measures of bone lead among ALS cases. An early study examined lead concentration in bone specimens obtained from the iliac crest from 25 ALS cases and from 17 autopsy controls (Campbell et al. 1970). No significant difference in bone lead concentration was found. More recently, Kamel et al. (2002) conducted a case–control study of ALS among 109 ALS cases and 256 population-based controls in New England between 1993 and 1996. Self-reported occupational exposure to lead was associated with a nearly twofold increased risk of ALS (OR = 1.9; 95% CI 1.1–3.3), and a dose-response trend was observed for lifetime days of lead exposure. Blood and bone lead measurements were taken in 107 cases and a subset of 41 controls. The ALS cases had significantly higher blood lead values than controls, and measures of lead concentration in bone (tibia and patella) were somewhat higher among ALS cases than controls, suggesting that exposure to lead may be associated with ALS. A possible source of bias in this study is possible self-selective participation of patients exposed to lead and self-exclusion of unexposed controls. Although no single study has provided definitive proof that lead is a risk factor for ALS, the evidence warrants continued investigation of the possibility that lead or other heavy metals may contribute to the risk of developing ALS.

An increased risk of ALS has been observed among farm workers (Granieri et al. 1988; Gunnarsson et al. 1991); however, methodologic limitations of occupational mortality studies limit the ability to draw inferences from these observations. Associations with pesticides have not been observed, except in a recent population-based study from western Washington State (McGuire et al. 1997). An increased risk of ALS was observed among men who were exposed to agricultural chemicals (OR = 2.8; 95% CI 1.3–6.1) and a dose–response relationship with lifetime years of chemical exposure was observed. The association was reported for pesticides, specifically insecticides, and for fertilizers. This study is the first to identify pesticide exposure as a possible risk factor for ALS.

Electrical Occupations, Electrical Shock, and Electromagnetic Field Exposure. Electrical shocks came under scrutiny as risk factors for ALS due to *post hoc ergo propter hoc* reasoning in cases when clinical disease onset was related to an immediately antecedent electric shock. In addition to factors such as selective reporting and recall bias, this reasoning was facilitated by failure to recognize that ALS is biologically active up to several years before it is evident clinically and, consequently, that an apparent risk factor that occurs after disease onset cannot be a true risk factor. The conflicting data have been discussed elsewhere (Armon et al. 1991a). Case–control studies continue to inquire about the role of electric

shocks (Cruz et al. 1999). Electromagnetic field (EMF) exposure became the next focus and has been the subject of several epidemiologic investigations of ALS (Davanipour et al. 1997; Johansen and Olsen 1998; Savitz et al. 1998; Noonan et al. 2002). In a retrospective cohort study conducted in Finland, Johansen and Olsen (1998) reported a twofold increase in mortality from ALS among men employed in utility companies and hypothesized that the association may reflect repeated exposures to electrical shocks among electrical workers. In another cohort study, Savitz et al. (1998) reported that employment as an electrical worker for 20 years or longer was associated with a threefold increase in the risk of ALS (RR = 3.1, 95% CI 1.1–9.8). Noonan et al. (2002) conducted a case–control study in Colorado using death certificate identification of ALS cases for the years 1987 through 1996. No association was observed according to mean magnetic field indices obtained from a job-exposure matrix; however, individuals with a history of work in electrical occupations had a greater than twofold increased risk of ALS (OR = 2.3, 95% CI 1.3–4.1). All of these studies have significant methodological shortcomings, including those related to differential ascertainment of ALS and reporting of occupation and ALS diagnosis on death certificates in various occupations, and no definitive conclusions can be drawn (Armon 2003a, 2003b).

Lifestyle Factors. To date, very few studies have investigated the association of ALS with lifestyle factors such as diet, cigarette smoking, and alcohol consumption.

Diet. If *SOD1* mutations and free radical–induced damage are important in motor neuron death, then it can be hypothesized that individuals with relatively low dietary intake of exogenous antioxidants might be at greater risk for ALS due to low oxidative reserves. It should be recognized that in familial ALS, the *SOD1* mutations cause ALS through a gain of function (rather than oxidative stress caused by a deficiency in *SOD1* function); further, even if free radical–induced damage might be one of the mechanisms of cell death in active ALS, that does not mean that it is involved in initiating ALS. A study using comprehensive methods to assess diet was undertaken.

Example 7–5   Nelson et al. (2000a) conducted a population-based case–control study of ALS in three counties in western Washington State. Incident ALS cases were identified ($n = 161$) and matched individually on age and gender to population-based controls recruited by means of random-digit dialing and Medicare lists ($n = 321$). Diet was assessed by a self-administered food frequency questionnaire. After adjusting for education, smoking, fiber intake, and total energy intake, dietary fat intake (>93 grams per day compared with <42 grams per day) was associated with a nearly threefold increase risk of ALS (OR = 2.7, 95% CI 0.9–8.0; *p* for trend = 0.06). Polyunsaturated fat, saturated fat, and linoleic acid contributed to this positive association. Dietary fiber intake (>18 grams per day compared with <10 grams per day) was associated with a 70% decrease in risk (fat-adjusted OR = 0.3, 95% CI 0.1–0.7; *p* for trend = 0.02). The investigators also evaluated the intake of certain amino acids and found that glutamate intake (>15 grams per day compared with <8.6 grams per day) increased the risk for ALS (OR = 3.2, 95% CI 1.2–8.0; *p* for trend <0.02). Antioxidant vitamin consumption was not associated with the risk of ALS. The positive association with glutamate intake is consistent with those etiologic theories that suggest that glutamate excitotoxicity has a role in causing ALS. However, the dietary history was obtained for the year prior to onset of symptoms when the disease was biologically active; hence the dietary survey cannot be construed directly as a risk factor assessment, unless one postulates that patients' diet during the year prior to clinical onset is representative of lifelong dietary habits. It is possible that the findings may reflect dietary adjustments made in response to preclinical disease.

Physical activity. Several epidemiologic studies had suggested that vigorous physical activity at work and during leisure time was associated with ALS (Kurtzke 1991; reviewed in Longstreth et al. 1991), although two case–control studies did not report such an association (Armon et al. 1991b; Longstreth et al. 1998). This notion was strengthened by the well-publicized instances of ALS in prominent professional athletes, including Lou Gehrig. The hypothesis was that physical activity may modify the effects of a neurotoxin (e.g., the spraying of pesticides on the playing fields) or that exposure to a neurotoxin selective for motor neurons occurred at the time of the exercise (Longstreth et al. 1991). In a population-based case–control study of ALS conducted in western Washington State, the investigators obtained detailed information on lifetime physical activity both at work and at leisure from incident cases ($n = 174$) and population-based controls ($n = 348$) (Longstreth et al. 1998). For physical activity at work, subjects estimated the percent of time spent at each of five levels of physical activity ranging from sedentary activities to doing heavy physical work. For leisure time activity, a value was assigned to each activity that reflected an estimate of the rate of energy expended by the individual. In addition, the investigators examined physical activity in terms of indoor–outdoor and field–nonfield sports. No associations between physical activity and risk of ALS were reported for overall physical activity or for vigorous activity, either in workplace or leisure settings. Compared with previous studies, this study was population based, recruited a relatively large number of newly diagnosed cases of ALS, and obtained very detailed, quantitative information on lifetime physical activity from cases and their age- and sex-matched population-based controls subjects. While findings from a single study cannot be considered on their own as absolutely conclusive, the results from this study cast considerable doubt on the likelihood that vigorous physical activity is a risk factor for ALS.

Cigarette smoking and alcohol consumption. Despite the hypothesis of a possible environmental exposure contributing to the development of ALS, only a few studies have investigated the role of cigarette smoking or alcohol use (Kondo and Tsubaki 1981; Granieri et al. 1988; Savettieri et al. 1991; Gunnarsson et al. 1992; Chancellor et al. 1993; Mitchell et al. 1995; Kamel et al. 1999; Nelson et al. 2000b). The New England study (Kamel et al. 1999) showed an increased risk of ALS associated with smoking, and a dose–response trend was demonstrated with number of cigarettes per day as the measure. Approximately 12% of cases and 4% of controls had stopped smoking within the 5 years before the interview date. This likely reflects a case where the consequences of the disease interfered with continued exposure to the risk factor (Kamel et al. 1999). In the Washington State study, ever having smoked cigarettes was associated with a twofold increase in risk of ALS (alcohol-adjusted OR = 2.0; 95% CI 1.3–3.2). A greater than threefold increase was observed among current smokers (alcohol-adjusted OR = 3.5; 95% CI 1.9–6.4). A dose–response trend with increasing pack years of smoking was demonstrated (Nelson et al. 2000b).

Risk Factors for Sporadic Amyotrophic Lateral Sclerosis: Summary of an Evidence-Based Medicine Approach

Details of using an evidence-based medicine approach to evaluate the findings of ALS case–control studies are available elsewhere (Armon 2003a, 2003b). Smoking is the only risk factor that merits a rating as a probable ("more likely than not") risk factor for ALS. There are two studies providing fairly reliable evidence to support this conclusion (Kamel et al. 1999; Nelson et al. 2000b). This risk factor warrants a high ranking of importance because it is modifiable, it has no redeeming features, and it affects a relatively large segment of the population. It is intriguing to speculate that some of the reduction of the male/female

preponderance of ALS in more recent epidemiologic studies is due to the rise in prevalence of smoking among women in the latter part of the last century. Previously, smoking was not considered in the context of environmental risk factors. Thus, the significance of the two recent studies identifying smoking as a risk factor may not have struck the scientific and patient community with the same force as would have even one study of equal quality implicating an external risk factor. Trauma (Cruz et al. 1999), physical activity (Longstreth et al. 1998), residence in rural areas (Cruz et al. 1999), alcohol consumption (Nelson et al. 2000b), and antecedent medical conditions (Armon et al. 1991c) are probably ("more likely than not") not risk factors for ALS. Currently, there are no conflicting data of equal or higher reliability as evidence. Evidence-based medicine methodology does not permit assignment of estimates of the type I or type II errors inherent in drawing such conclusion. These conclusions may be revised if conflicting, high-quality data become available in the future (Armon 2003a, 2003b).

Future Directions and Conclusions

The epidemiologic study of ALS has come of age, giving hope that the application of contemporary methodology will provide better understanding of genetic, behavioral, and environmental risk factors for this condition. Epidemiology has contributed to ALS research by identifying the familial, Western Pacific, and sporadic forms of the disease. Each has been the subject of separate research using the appropriate scientific tools, as they become available. Epidemiology has provided the conceptual basis for requiring accuracy in case definition. Epidemiology provides the frame of reference to complement the statistical tools used in evaluating the outcomes and significance of clinical trials (Armon et al. 2002), and in investigating clusters reported from the community. The methodologic rigor of the better-designed population-based case–control epidemiologic studies has called into question many commonly held beliefs about the etiology of ALS, at the same time identifying new associations and raising new hypotheses. Introduction of an evidence-based medicine approach to the evaluation of epidemiologic literature and the planning of future epidemiologic research may provide additional focus and leverage to epidemiologic contributions to elucidating the etiology of ALS (Armon 2003, 2003b, 2003c).

Future case–control studies should attempt to avoid the methodologic limitations of previous studies by (1) conducting studies in large study populations that provide a well-defined study base for the selection of ALS cases and control subjects; (2) seeking incident rather than prevalent cases, so that identification of factors of potential etiologic significance is not clouded by the inclusion of prevalent cases; (3) augmenting statistical power by including more than 200 ALS cases and/or by recruiting more than one control for every ALS case; (4) including individuals from non-Caucasian racial and ethnic groups; (5) assessing exposures to environmental toxicants with the most rigorous and objective methods possible, including blinded exposure assessments and biological measures when possible; and (6) collecting and storing genomic DNA for both ALS cases and controls for the future evaluation of candidate susceptibility genes.

The epidemiologic study of ALS will also benefit from identifying existing large cohort studies that have accumulated enough person-years of observation to be able to generate a large enough number of ALS patients for epidemiologic study. Cohort studies avoid the issues of recall bias that can affect case–control studies because information on the etiologic factors of interest is collected in the cohort prior to the development of disease. However, they permit the study of only those risk factors for which information was gathered as the cohort was followed. Prospective cohort studies may permit gathering quality information based on hypotheses specified a priori,

and it is necessary to accept that their outcomes may not become available for some time. Acquisition of material for genetic study, concurrently with the performance of epidemiological studies, may accelerate the identification of susceptibility genes for sporadic ALS. It is expected that susceptibility genes, the genes conferring susceptibility to environmental etiologic factors, will more likely be present in individuals with ALS who were exposed to that environmental risk factor, but not in people exposed to the same risk factor who did not develop disease.

As we begin a new century, patients with ALS are better off than they were 10 years ago (Armon 1998), primarily because of the availability of knowledgeable professionals interested in treating them. Changes in the way society supports patients with ALS and facilitates their access to care, rather than new scientific developments, may be the next realistic step that can be taken to improve the lives of patients with ALS in the short run. Research into the causes of the disease offers the hope of its ultimate eradication, even if only future generations may realize the fulfillment of this hope.

ACKNOWLEDGMENTS

I would like to acknowledge with gratitude the contributions of colleagues, not only through the published literature and interactions in open conferences but also within recent conferences and meetings coordinated by the ALS Association, California, USA, including a recent workshop on Environmental Factors and Genetic Susceptibility in Amyotrophic Lateral Sclerosis held in May 29–31, 2002, in Keystone, Colorado (ALS Association 2002).

References

Al-Chalabi A, Anderson PM, Chioza B, et al. Recessive amyotrophic lateral sclerosis families with the D90A SOD1 mutation share a common founder: evidence for a linked protective factor. *Hum Mol Genet* 1998;7: 2045–2050.

ALS Association. Workshop on Environmental Factors and Genetic Susceptibility in Amyotrophic Lateral Sclerosis. May 29–31, 2002, Keystone, Colorado. http://www.alsa.org/research/workshops1.cfm.

Annegers JF, Appel S, Lee JR, Perkins P. Incidence and prevalence of amyotrophic lateral sclerosis in Harris County, Texas, 1985–1988. *Arch Neurol* 1991;48:589–593.

Appelbaum JS, Roos RP, Salazar-Grueso EG, et al. Intrafamilial heterogeneity in hereditary motor neuron disease. *Neurology* 1992;42:1488–1492.

Armon C. Motor neuron disease. In: Gorelick PB, Alter M, eds. Handbook of Neuroempidemiology. New York: Marcel Dekker, 1994, pp 407–456.

Armon C. Are patients with ALS better off today than they were 10 years ago? Presented at American Academy of Neurology Annual Meeting Dinner Seminar April 26, 1998.

Armon C. ALS: Clinical and epidemiologic clues to pathogenesis. In: Neurobiology of ALS. Course Syllabus, 51st Annual Meeting, American Academy of Neurology, 1999.

Armon C. Linear estimates of disease progression predict survival in patients with ALS. *Muscle Nerve* 2000;23:874–882.

Armon C. Environmental risk factors for amyotrophic lateral sclerosis. *Neuroepidemiology*; 2001;20:2–6.

Armon C. An evidence-based medicine approach to the evaluation of the role of exogenous risk factors in sporadic amyotrophic lateral sclerosis. Invited editorial. *Neuroepidemiology* 2003a;22:217–228.

Armon C. Epidemiology of ALS/MND. In: Shaw P, Strong M, eds. Motor Neuron Disorders. St. Louis: Elsevier Science, 2003b.

Armon C. Epidemiology of amyotrophic lateral sclerosis: risk factors and clusters. In: Causes of Sporadic ALS. Course Syllabus, 55st Annual Meeting, American Academy of Neurology, 2003c

Armon C, Daube JR, O'Brien PC, et al. When is an apparent excess of neurologic cases epidemiologically significant? *Neurology* 1991a;41:1713–1718.

Armon C, Guillof R Bedlack R. Limitations of inferences from observational databases: all that glitters is not gold. *Amyotroph Lateral Scler Other Motor Neuron Disord* 2002;3:109–112.

Armon C, Kurland LT. Classic and Western Pacific amyotrophic lateral sclerosis: epidemiologic comparisons. In: Hudson AJ, ed. Amyotrophic Lateral Sclerosis: Concepts in Pathogenesis and Etiology. Toronto: University of Toronto Press, 1989, pp 144–165.

Armon C, Kurland LT, Daube JR, O'Brien PC. Epidemiologic correlates of sporadic amyotrophic lateral sclerosis. *Neurology* 1991b;41:1077–1084.

Armon C, Kurland LT, O'Brien PC, Mulder DW.

Antecedent medical diseases in patients with amyotrophic lateral sclerosis: a population-based case-controlled study in Rochester, Minnesota, 1925–1987. *Arch Neurol* 1991c;48:283–286.

Armon C, Kurland LT, Smith GE, Steele JC. Sporadic and western pacific amyotrophic lateral sclerosis epidemiological implications. In: Smith RA, ed. Handbook of ALS. New York: Marcel Dekker, 1992, pp 93–131.

Arnold A, Edgren DC, Palladino VS. Amyotrophic lateral sclerosis: fifty cases observed on Guam. *J Nerv Ment Dis* 1953;117:135–139.

Ben Hamida M, Hentati F, Ben Hamida C. Hereditary motor system diseases (chronic juvenile amyotrophic lateral sclerosis). Conditions combining a bilateral pyramidal syndrome with limb and bulbar amyotrophy. *Brain* 1990;113:347–363.

Ben Hamida M, Letaief F, Hentati F, Ben Hamida C. Morphometric study of the sensory nerve in classical (or Charcot disease) and juvenile amyotrophic lateral sclerosis. *J Neurol Sci* 1987;78:313–329.

Brooks BR. El Escorial World Federation of Neurology criteria for the diagnosis of amyotrophic lateral sclerosis. Subcommittee on Motor Neuron Diseases/Amyotrophic Lateral Sclerosis of the World Federation of Neurology Research Group on Neuromuscular Diseases and the El Escorial "Clinical Limits of Amyotrophic Lateral Sclerosis" workshop contributors. *J Neurol Sci* 1994;124:96–107.

Brooks BR, Miller RG, Swash M, Munsat TL. El Escorial Revisited: revised criteria for the diagnosis of amyotrophic lateral sclerosis. A consensus conference held at Airlie House, Warrenton, VA April 2–4, 1998.

Brooks BR, Sufit RL, Depaul R, et al. Design of clinical therapeutic trials in amyotrophic lateral sclerosis. In: Rowland LP, ed. Advances in Neurology, Vol 56: Amyotrophic Lateral Sclerosis and Other Motor Neuron Diseases. New York: Raven Press, 1991, pp 521–546.

Brown RH Jr, Robberecht W. Amyotrophic lateral sclerosis: pathogenesis. *Semin Neurol* 2001;21:131–139.

Buchanan DS, Malamud N. Motor neuron disease with renal cell carcinoma and postoperative neurologic remission. A clinicopathologic report. *Neurology* 1973;23:891–894.

Campbell AM, Williams ER, Barltrop D. Motor neurone disease and exposure to lead. *J Neurol Neurosurg Psychiatry* 1970;33:877–885.

Chancellor AM, Slattery JM, Fraser H, Warlow

CP. Risk factors for motor neuron disease: a case–control study based on patients from the Scottish Motor Neuron Disease Register. *J Neurol Neurosurg Psychiatry* 1993;56: 1200–1206.

Chen KM, Craig UK, Lee CT, Haddock R. Cycad neurotoxin, consumption of flying foxes, and ALS/PDC disease in Guam. *Neurology* 2002;59:1664.

Chio A, Brignolio F, Meineri P, Schiffer D. Phenotypic and genotypic heterogeneity of dominantly inherited amyotrophic lateral sclerosis. *Acta Neurol Scand* 1987;75:277–282.

Christensen PB, Hojer-Pedersen E, Jensen NB. Survival of patients with amyotrophic lateral sclerosis in two Danish counties. *Neurology* 1990;40:600–604.

Corcia P, Khoris J, Couratier P, et al. *SMN1* gene study in three families in which ALS and spinal muscular atrophy co-exist. *Neurology.* 2002a;59:1464–1466.

Corcia P, Mayeux-Portas V, Khoris J, et al. Abnormal *SMN1* gene copy number is a susceptibility factor for amyotrophic lateral sclerosis. *Ann Neurol* 2002b;51:243–246.

Cox PA, Sacks OW. Cycad neurotoxins, consumption of flying foxes, and ALS-PDC disease in Guam. *Neurology* 2002a;58:956–959.

Cox PA, Sacks OW. Cycad neurotoxin, consumption of flying foxes, and ALS/PDC disease in Guam. *Neurology* 2002b;59:1664–1665 (reply from the authors).

Cruz DC, Nelson LM, McGuire V, Longstreth WT Jr. Physical trauma and family history of neurodegenerative diseases in amyotrophic lateral sclerosis: a population-based case–control study. *Neuroepidemiology* 1999; 18:101–110.

Cudkowicz ME, McKenna-Yasek D, et al. Limited corticospinal tract involvement in sclerosis subjects with the A4V mutation in the copper/zinc superoxide dismutase gene. *Ann Neurol* 1998;43:703–710.

Dalakas MC. The post-polio syndrome as an evolved clinical entity. Definition and clinical description. *Ann N Y Acad Sci* 1995; 753:68–80.

Dastur DK. Cycad toxicity in monkeys: clinical, pathological, and biochemical aspects. *Fed Proc* 1964;23:1368–1369.

Davanipour Z, Sobel E, Bowman JD, et al. Amyotrophic lateral sclerosis and occupational exposure to electromagnetic fields. *Bioelectromagnetics* 1997;18:28–35.

Deapcn DM, Henderson BE. A case–control study of amyotrophic lateral sclerosis. *Am J Epidemiol* 1986;123:790–799.

DeDomenico P, Malara CE, Marabello L, et al. Amyotrophic lateral sclerosis: an epidemiologic study in the province of Messina, Italy, 1976–1985. *Neuroepidemiology* 1988;7: 152–158.

Del Aguila MA, Longstreth WT Jr, McGuire V, et al. Prognosis in amyotrophic lateral sclerosis: a population-based study. *Neurology* 2003;60:813–819.

Dickersin K, Min YI, Meinert CL. Factors influencing publication of research results. Follow-up of applications submitted to two institutional review boards. *JAMA* 1992;267: 374–378

Duncan MW. Role of the cycad neurotoxin BMAA in the amyotrophic lateral sclerosis–parkinsonism dementia complex of the western Pacific. *Adv Neurol* 1991;56:301–310.

Emery AEH, Holloway S. Familial motor neuron diseases. In: Rowland LP, ed. Human Motor Neuron Diseases. New York: Raven Press, 1982, pp 139–147.

Esclaire F, Kisby G, Spencer P, et al. The Guam cycad toxin methylazoxymethanol damages neuronal DNA and modulates tau mRNA expression and excitotoxicity. *Exp Neurol* 1999;155:11–21.

Felmus MT, Patten BM, Swanke L. Antecedent events in amyotrophic lateral sclerosis. *Neurology* 1976;26:167–172.

Fox JP, Hall CE, Elveback LR. Epidemiology: Man and Disease. London: Macmillan, 1970.

Gajdusek DC, Garruto RM, Salazar AM. Ecology of high incidence foci of motor neuron disease in eastern Asia and western Pacific and the frequent occurrence of other chronic degenerative neurological diseases in these foci. In: Tenth International Congress on Tropical Medicine and Malaria, Manila, Philippines, Nov 9–15, 1980, p 382.

Gajdusek DC, Salazar AM. Amyotrophic lateral sclerosis and parkinsonian syndromes in high incidence among the Auyu and Jakai people of West New Guinea. *Neurology* 1982;32:107–126.

Galasko D, Salmon DP, CraigUK, et al. Clinical features and changing patterns of neurodegenerative disorders on Guam, 1997–2000. *Neurology* 2002;58:90–97.

Garruto RM, Gajdusek DC, Chen K-M. Amyotrophic lateral sclerosis and parkinsonism-dementia among Filipino migrants of Guam. *Ann Neurol* 1981;10:341–350.

Garruto RM, Yanagihara R, Gajdusek DC. Cycads and amyotrophic lateral sclerosis/parkinsonism dementia. *Lancet* 1988;2:1079.

Gompertz B. On the nature of the function expressive of the law of human mortality. *Phil Trans R Soc Lond* 1825;115:513–585.

Granieri E, Carreras M, Tola R, et al. Motor

neuron disease in the province of Ferrara, Italy in 1964–1982. *Neurology* 1988;38:1604–1608.

Granieri E, Murgia SB, Rosati G, et al. The frequency of amyotrophic lateral sclerosis among workers in Sardinia. *IRCS Med Sci* 1983;11:898.

Gresham LS, Molgaard CA, Golbeck AL, Smith R. Amyotrophic lateral sclerosis and occupational heavy metal exposure: a case–control study. *Neuroepidemiology* 1986;5:29–38.

Gunnarsson LG, Bodin L, Soderfeldt B, Axelson O. A case–control study of motor neuron disease: its relation to heritability, and occupational exposures, particularly to solvents. *Br J Ind Med* 1992;49:791–798.

Gunnarsson L-G, Lindberg G, Soderfeldt B, Axelson O. Amyotrophic lateral sclerosis in Sweden in relation to occupation. *Acta Neurol Scand* 1991;83:394–398.

Hadano S, Hand CK, Osuga H, et al. A gene encoding a putative GTPase regulator is mutated in familial amyotrophic lateral sclerosis. *Nat Genet* 2001;29:166–173.

Hand CK, Rouleau GA. Familial amyotrophic lateral sclerosis. *Muscle Nerve* 2002;25:135–159.

Harding AE. Inherited neuronal athophy and degeneration predominantly of lower motor neurons. In: Dyck PJ, Thomas PK, eds. Peripheral Neuropathy. Philadelphia: WB Saunders, 1993, pp 1051–1064.

Hennekens CH, Buring JE. Epidemiology in Medicine. Boston/Toronto: Little, Brown and Company, 1987.

Hentati A, Oahchi K, Pericak-Vance MA, et al. Linkage of a commoner form of recessive amyotrophic lateral sclerosis to chromosome 15q15–122 markers. *Neurogenetics* 1998;2:55–60.

Herbst AL, Ulfelder H, Poskanzer DC. Adenocarcinoma of the vagina. Association of maternal steilbestrol therapy with tumor appearance in young women. *N Engl J Med* 1971;285:390–392.

Hirano A, Kurland LT, Krooth RS, Lessell S. Parkinsonism-dementia complex, an endemic disease on the island of Guam. I. Clinical features. *Brain* 1961a;84:642–661.

Hirano A, Kurland LT, Sayre GP. Familial amyotrophic lateral sclerosis: a subgroup characterized by posterior and spinocerebellar tract involvement and hyaline inclusions in the anterior horn cells. *Arch Neurol* 1967;16:232–243.

Hirano A, Malamud N, Kurland LT. Parkinsonism-dementia complex, an endemic disease on the island of Guam. II. Pathological features. *Brain* 1961b;84:662–679.

Horton WA, Eldridge R, Brody JA. Familial motor neuron disease. *Neurology* 1976;26:460–465.

Husquinet H, Franck G. Hereditary ALS transmitted for five generations. *Clin Genet* 1980;18:109–115.

Johansen C, Olsen JH. Mortality from amyotrophic lateral sclerosis, other chronic disorders, and electric shocks among utility workers. *Am J Epidemiol* 1998;15;148:362–368.

Kamel F, Umbach DM, Munsat TL, et al. Association of cigarette smoking with amyotrophic lateral sclerosis. *Neuroepidemiology* 1999;18:194–202.

Kamel F, Umbach DM, Munsat TL, et al. Lead exposure and amyotrophic lateral sclerosis. *Epidemiology* 2002;13:311–319.

Khabazian I, Bains JS, Williams DE, et al. Isolation of various forms of sterol beta-D-glucoside from the seed of *Cycas circinalis*: neurotoxicity and implications for ALS–parkinsonism dementia complex. *J Neurochem* 2002;82:516–528.

Kimula K, Yase Y, Higashi Y, et al. Epidemiological and geomedical studies on amyotrophic lateral sclerosis. *Dis Nerv Syst* 1963;24:155–159.

Kisby GE, Kabel H, Hugon J, Spencer P. Damage and repair of nerve cell DNA in toxic stress. *Drug Metab Rev* 1999;31:589–618.

Koerner DR. Amyotrophic lateral sclerosis on Guam: a clinical study and review of the literature. *Ann Intern Med* 1952;37:1204–1220.

Kondo K, Tsubaki T. Case–control studies of motor neuron disease. Association with mechanical injuries. *Arch Neurol* 1981;38:220–226.

Koren G, Klein N. Bias against negative studies in newspaper reports of medical research. *JAMA* 1991;266:1824–1826.

Kunst CB, Messer L, Gordon J, et al. Genetic mapping of a mouse modifier gene that can prevent ALS onset. *Genomics* 2000 70:181–189.

Kurland LT. Geographic isolates: their role in neuroepidemiology. *Adv Neurol* 1978;19:69–82.

Kurland LT, Kurtzke JF, Goldberg ID, Choi NW. Amyotrophic lateral sclerosis and other motor neuron disease. In: Kurland LT, Kurtzke JF, Goldberg ID, eds. Epidemiology of Neurologic and Sense Organ Disorders (Vital and Health Statistics Monograph, American Public Health Association). Cambridge, MA: Harvard University Press, 1973, pp. 108–127.

Kurland LT, Molgaard CA. Guamaniam ALS: hereditary or acquired? In: Rowland LP, ed.

Human Motor Neuron Diseases. New York: Raven Press, 1982, pp 165–171.

Kurland LT, Mulder DW. Epidemiologic investigations of amyotrophic lateral sclerosis: 1. Preliminary report on geographic distribution, with special reference to the Mariana Islands, including clinical and pathologic observations. *Neurology* 1954;4:355–378.

Kurland LT, Mulder DW. Epidemiologic investigations of amyotrophic lateral sclerosis. 2. Familial aggregations indicative of dominant inheritance. *Neurology* 1955;5:182–258.

Kurland LT, Mulder DW. Overview of motor neurone disease. In: Gourie-Devi M, ed. Motor Neuron Disease: Global Clinical Patterns and International Research. New Delhi: Oxford and IBH, 1987, pp 31–44.

Kurland LT, Radhakrishnan K, Smith GE, et al. Mechanical trauma as a risk factor in classic amyotrophic lateral sclerosis: lack of epidemiologic evidence. *J Neurol Sci* 1992;113:133–143.

Kurlander HM, Patten BM. Metals in spinal cord tissue of patients dying of motor neuron disease. *Ann Neurol* 1979;6:21–24.

Kurtzke JF. On statistical testing of prevalence studies. *J Chron Dis* 1966;19:909–922.

Kurtzke JF. Which "neurodegenerative diseases" are on the rise? *Health Environ Digest* 1989;3:3–8.

Kurtzke JF. Risk factors in amyotrophic lateral sclerosis. *Adv Neurol* 1991;56:245–270.

Langston JW, Ballard PA, Tetrud JW, Irwin I. Chronic parkinsonism in humans due to a product of meripine-analog synthesis. *Science* 1983;219:979–980.

Lavine L, Steele JC, Wolf N, et al. Amyotrophic lateral sclerosis/parkinsonism dementia complex in southern Guam. Is it disappearing? *Adv Neurol* 1991;271–285.

Leone M, Chandra V, Schoenberg BS. Motor neuron disease in the United States, 1971 and 1973–1978: patterns of mortality and associated conditions at the time of death. *Neurology* 1987;37:1339–1343.

Li TM, Alberman E, Swash M. Comparison of sporadic and familial disease amongst 580 cases of motor neuron disease. *J Neurosurg Psychiatry* 1988;51:778–784.

Lilienfeld DE, Perl DP. Projected neurodegenerative disease mortality in the United States, 1990–2040. *Neuroepidemiology* 1993;12(4):219–228.

Longstreth WT Jr, McGuire V, Koepsell TD, et al. Risk of amyotrophic lateral sclerosis and history of physical activity: a population-based case–control study. *Arch Neurol* 1998;55:201–206.

Longstreth WT Jr, Nelson LM, Koepsell TD, van Belle G. Hypotheses to explain the as-

sociation between vigorous physical activity and amyotrophic lateral sclerosis. *Med Hypotheses* 1991;34:144–148.

Lopez-Vega JM, Calleja J, Combarros O, et al. Motor neuron disease in Cantabria. *Acta Neurol Scand* 1988;77:1–5.

Ludolph AC, Langen KJ, Regard M, et al. Frontal lobe function in amyotrophic lateral sclerosis: a neuropsychologic and positron emission tomography study. *Acta Neurol Scand* 1992;85:81–89.

Maasilta P, Jokelainen M, Loytonen M, et al. Mortality from amyotrophic lateral sclerosis in Finland, 1986–1995. *Acta Neurol Scand* 2001;104:232–235.

McGeer PL, Schwab C, McGeer EG, et al. Familial nature and continuing morbidity of the amyotrophic lateral sclerosis–parkinsonism dementia complex of Guam. *Neurology* 1997;49:400–409.

McGuire V, Longstreth WT Jr, Koepsell TD, van Belle G. Incidence of amyotrophic lateral sclerosis in three counties in western Washington State. *Neurology* 1996;47:571–573.

McGuire V, Longstreth WT Jr, Nelson LM, et al. Occupational exposures and amyotrophic lateral sclerosis. A population-based case–control study. *Am J Epidemiol* 1997;145:1076–1088.

Miller RG, Rosenberg JA, Gelinas DF, et al. Practice parameter: the care of the patient with amyotrophic lateral sclerosis (an evidence-based review): report of the Quality Standards Subcommittee of the American Academy of Neurology: ALS Practice Parameters Task Force. *Neurology* 1999;52:1311–1323.

Mitchell JD, Davies RB, al-Hamad A, et al. MND risk factors: an epidemiological study in the north west of England. *J Neurol Sci* 1995;129(Suppl):61–64.

Mitchell JD, East BW, Harris IA, et al. Trace elements in the spinal cord and other tissues in motor neuron disease. *J Neurol Neurosurg Psychiatry* 1986;49:211–215.

Mulder DW, Kurland LT, Offord KP, Beard CM. Familial adult motor neuron disease: amyotrophic lateral sclerosis. *Neurology* 1986;36:511–517.

Mundt DJ, Dell LD, Luippold RS, et al. Cause-specific mortality among Kelly Air Force Base civilian employees, 1981–2001. *J Occup Environ Med* 2002;44:989–996.

Munsat TL, Hollander D, Andres P, Finison L. Clinical trials in ALS: measurement and natural history. *Adv Neurol* 1991;56:515–519

Nelson LM, Matkin C, Longstreth WT Jr, McGuire V. Population-based case–control study of amyotrophic lateral sclerosis in western Washington State. II. Diet. *Am J Epidemiol* 2000a;151:164–173.

Nelson LM, McGuire V, Longstreth WT Jr, Matkin C. Population-based case–control study of amyotrophic lateral sclerosis in western Washington State. I. Cigarette smoking and alcohol consumption. *Am J Epidemiol* 2000b;151:156–163.

Nielson S, Robinson I, Hunter M. Longitudinal Gompertzian analysis of ALS mortality in England and Wales, 1963–1989: estimates of susceptibility in the general population. *Mech Ageing Dev* 1992;64:210–216.

Noonan CW, Reif JS, Yost M, Touchstone J. Occupational exposure to magnetic fields in case–referent studies of neurodegenerative diseases. *Scand J Work Environ Health* 2002; 28:42–48.

Parboosingh JS, Meininger V, McKenna-Yasek D, et al. Deletions causing spinal muscular atrophy do not predispose to amyotrophic lateral sclerosis. *Arch Neurol* 1999;56:710–712

Perl DP, Hof PR, Purohit DP, et al. Hippocampal and entorhinal cortex neurofibrillary tangle in Guamanian Chamorros free of overt neurologic dysfunction. *J Neuropathol Exp Neurol* 2003;62:381–386.

Piemonte and Valle d'Aosta Register for Amyotrophic Lateral Sclerosis (PARALS). Incidence of ALS in Italy: evidence for a uniform frequency in Western countries. *Neurology* 2001;56:239–244.

Plato CC, Galasko D, Garruto RM, et al. ALS and PDC of Guam. Forty year follow-up. *Neurology* 2002;58:765–773.

Pringle CE, Hudson AJ, Munoz DG, et al. Primary lateral sclerosis: clinical features, neuropathology and diagnostic criteria. *Brain* 1992;115:495–520.

Riggs JE. Longitudian Gompertzian analysis of amyotrophic lateral sclerosis mortality in the U.S., 1977–1986: evidence for an inherently susceptible population subset. *Mech Ageing Dev* 1990;55:207–220.

Riggs JE, Schochet S Jr. Rising mortality due to parkinson's disease and amyotrophic lateral sclerosis: a manifestation of the competitive nature of human mortality. *J Clin Epidemiol* 1992;45:1007–1012.

Ross MA, Miller RG, Berchert L, et al. Toward earlier diagnosis of amyotrophic lateral sclerosis: revised criteria. rhCNTF ALS Study Group. *Neurology* 1998;50:768–772.

Rowland LP, ed. Advances in Neurology (Vol. 56): Amyotrophic Lateral Sclerosis and Other Motor Neuron Diseases. New York: Raven Press, 1991.

Salemi G, Fierro B, Arcara A, et al. Amyotrophic lateral sclerosis in Palermo, Italy: an epidemiologic study. *Ital J Neurol Sci* 1989;10:505–509.

Sasaki S, Tsutsumi Y, Yamane K, et al. Sporadic amyotrophic lateral sclerosis with extensive neurological involvement. *Acta Neuropathol* 1992;84:211–215.

Savettieri G, Salemi G, Arcara A, et al. A case–control study of amyotrophic lateral sclerosis. *Neuroepidemiology* 1991;10:242–245.

Savitz DA, Checkoway H, Loomis DP. Magnetic field exposure and neurodegenerative disease mortality among electric utility workers. *Epidemiology* 1998;9:398–404

Scarpa M, Colombo A, Panzetti P, Sorgato P. Epidemiology of amyotrophic lateral sclerosis in the province of Modena, Italy. Influence of environmental exposure to lead. *Acta Neurol Scand* 1988;77:456–460.

Schlesselman JJ. Case–Control Studies Design, Conduct, Analysis. New York: Oxford University Press, 1982.

Seljeseth YM, Vollset SE, Tysnes OB. Increasing mortality from amyotrophic lateral sclerosis in Norway? *Neurology* 2000;55:1262–1266.

Shiraki H. The neuropathology of amyotrophic lateral sclerosis (ALS) in the Kii Peninsula and other areas of Japan. In: Norris FH Jr, Kurland LT, eds. Motor Neuron Diseases: Research on Amyotrophic Lateral Sclerosis and Related Disorders. New York: Grune & Stratton, 1969, pp 80–84.

Siddique T, Figlewicz DA, Pericak-Vance MA, et al. Linkage of a gene causing familial amyotrophic lateral sclerosis to chromosome 21 and evidence of genetic-locus heterogeneity. *N Engl J Med* 1991;324:1381–1384.

Siddique T, Nijhawan D, Hentati A. Familial amyotrophic lateral sclerosis. *J Neural Transm Suppl* 1997;49:219–233.

Sobue G, Hashizume Y, Mukai E, et al. X-linked recessive bulbospinal neuronopathy: a clinicopathological study. *Brain* 1989;112:209–232.

Sorenson EJ, Stalker AP, Kurland LT, Windebank AJ. Amyotrophic lateral sclerosis in Olmsted County, Minnesota, 1925 to 1998. *Neurology* 2002;59:280–282.

Spencer PS. Guam ALS/Parkinsonism–dementia: a long-latency neurotoxic disorder caused by "slow toxin(s)" in food? *Can J Neurol Sci* 1987;14:347–357.

Spencer PS, Allen CN, Kisby GE, et al. Lathyrism and western Pacific amyotrophic lateral sclerosis: etiology of short and long latency motor system disorders. *Adv Neurol* 1991;287–299.

Spencer PS, Nunn PB, Hugon J, et al. Motor neuron disease on Guam: possible role of a food toxin. *Lancet* 1986;1:965.

Spencer PS, Ohta M, Palmer VS. Cycad use and

motor neurone disease in the Kii Peninsula of Japan. *Lancet* 1987a;2:1462–1463.

Spencer PS, Palmer VS, Herman A, Asmedi A. Cycad use and motor neurone disease in Irian Jaya. *Lancet* 1987b;2:1273–1274.

Spencer PS, Schaumburg HH. Lathyrism: a neurotoxic disease. *Neurobehav Toxical Teratol* 1983;5:625–629.

Swash M, Leigh N. Criteria for diagnosis of familial amyotrophic lateral sclerosis. *Neuromuscul Disord* 1992;2:7–9.

Tandan R, Bradley WG. Amyotrophic lateral sclerosis: Part 1. Clinical features, pathology, and ethical issues in management. *Ann Neurol* 1985a;18:271–280.

Tandan R, Bradley WG. Amyotrophic lateral sclerosis: Part 2: Etiopathogenesis. *Ann Neurol* 1985b;18:419–431.

Traynor BJ, Codd MB, Corr B, Forde C, Frost E, Hardiman O. Incidence and prevalence of ALS in Ireland, 1995–1997: a population-based study. *Neurology* 1999;52:504–509.

U.S. Bureau of Census. U.S. Census Population, Guam. Washington, DC: U.S. Governement Printing Office 1960, 1970, 1980, 1990.

Veldink JH, van den Berg LH, Cobben JM, et al. Homozygous deletion of the survival motor neuron 2 gene is a prognostic factor in sporadic ALS. *Neurology* 2001;56:749–752.

Veltema AN, Roos RAC, Bruyn GW. Autosomal dominant adult amyotrophic lateral sclerosis: a six generation Dutch family. *J Neurol Sci* 1990;97:93–115.

Whiting MG. Toxicity of cycads. *Econ Bot* 1963;17:271–302.

Williams DB, Annegers JF, Kokmen E, et al. Brain injury and neurological sequelae: a cohort study of dementia, parkinsonism and amyotrophic lateral sclerosis. *Neurology* 1991;41:1554–1557.

Williams DB, Floate DA, Leicester J. Familial motor neuron disease: differing penetrance in large pedigrees. *J Neurol Sci* 1988;86:215–230.

Williams DB, Windebank AJ. Motor neuron disease (amyotrophic lateral sclerosis). *Mayo Clin Proc* 1991;66:54–82.

Wilson JM, Khabazian I, Wong MC, et al. Behavioral and neurological correlates of ALS–parkinsonism dementia complex in adult mice fed washed cycad flour. *Neuromol Med* 2002;1:207–221.

Yang Y, Hentati A, Deng HX, et al. The gene encoding alsin, a protein with three guanine-nucleotide exchange factor domains, is mutated in a form of recessive amyotrophic lateral sclerosis. *Nat Genet* 2001;29:160–165.

Yase Y. [Motor neuron disease] *Nippon Rinsho* 1978;35 (Suppl):1716–1717.

Yoshida S, Mulder DW, Kurland LT, et al. Follow-up study on amyotrophic lateral sclerosis in Rochester, Minnesota, 1925–1984. *Neuroepidemiology* 1986;5:61–70.

Younger DS, Chou S, Hays JP, Lange DJ, Emerson R, Brin M, et al. Primary lateral sclerosis: a clinical diagnosis reemerges. *Arch Neurol* 1988;45:1304–1307.

Zolon WJ, Ellis–Neill L. University of Guam Technical Report No. 64, 1986.

8

Multiple Sclerosis

ALBERTO ASCHERIO AND KASSANDRA MUNGER

Multiple sclerosis (MS) is the most common disabling neurological disease in young adults in North America and Europe. Although treatment may modify the course of the disease, there is no cure. Substantial progress has been made in understanding the pathogenesis of MS, and there is compelling evidence of strong genetic and environmental determinants of risk, but neither has been conclusively identified.

Disease Description

Clinical and Pathological Features

Multiple sclerosis is a chronic inflammatory disease of the central nervous system characterized by large multiple focal areas of demyelination. The lesions, or plaques, are of varying age and are distributed from the cerebrum through the spinal cord. This "scattering in time and place" was recognized by Jean-Martin Charcot (1825–1893) in 1865 as a key feature of the disease. The optic nerves, periventricular areas, corpus callosum, brain stem, and cervical spinal cord are among the commonly affected areas. Micro-

scopically, plaques represent an inflammatory reaction with infiltration of T cells and macrophages, loss of myelin, and reactive glial scar formation. Axons are only relatively spared, and axonal injury in actively demyelinating lesions can lead to the accumulation of irreversible neurological deficit. The symptoms and signs of MS are variable, reflecting the location and severity of the demyelinating lesions. Common initial symptoms include one or more of the following: weakness in one or more limbs, visual problems (blurring, diplopia), sensory loss or paraesthesiae, and impaired balance. Repeated magnetic resonance image (MRI) scans in MS patients enrolled in clinical trials have revealed that the early course of MS in most patients is more active than suspected from clinical signs, as most lesions seen on MRI scans are asymptomatic (Jacobs et al. 1986; Ormerod et al. 1987; O'Riordan et al. 1998).

The clinical course of MS is extremely variable, both between patients and within a given patient over time (Fig. 8–1). The clinical course of MS has been traditionally described as relapsing-remitting, secondary progressive, or primary progressive (Ebers 1998). Not all patients fall neatly into these categories, however, and "transition" forms have been described, as presented schematically in Figure 8–1 (Lublin and Reingold 1996). Most patients experience discrete attacks at the onset of the disease, with complete or partial recovery between attacks (relapsing-remitting MS). About 80% of patients recover from

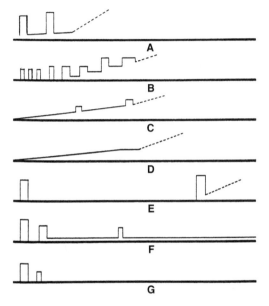

Figure 8–1 Clinical patterns of multiple sclerosis (MS). Each panel corresponds to different patterns of occurrence of MS symptoms over time. *A:* Relapsing–remitting with residual deficits after relapses and subsequent progressive course. *B:* Relapsing-remitting with full recovery followed by relapsing-remitting with residual deficits and subsequent progressive course. *C:* Chronic progressive with superimposed relapses. *D:* Chronic progressive from onset. *E:* Relapsing-remitting with full recovery, long periods of remission, subsequent relapses, and subsequent progressive course. *F:* Relapsing-remitting with initial full recovery, long periods of remission, and subsequent relapses with residual neurologic deficits. *G:* Benign MS with relapsing-remitting, with full recovery and subsequent full remission. (Reprinted with permission from Lublin FD, Reingold RC. Defining the clinical course of multiple sclerosis: results of an international survey. *Neurology* 1996;46:906–911.)

the first attack and remain asymptomatic for variable periods of time (Matthews 1998b). Discrete attacks tend to become less frequent over time and the disease may enter a progressive phase (secondary progressive MS). In about 10% of patients the disease is progressive from onset without recognizable attacks (primary progressive MS); it has been suggested that this form may be a pathologically and etiologically distinct disease.

The spectrum of MS severity ranges from benign disease, with minimal or no disability accumulated even after many years (Thompson et al. 1986), to rapidly fatal massive cerebral demyelination (Marburg's variant of acute MS). Rare, atypical forms of MS may occur (neuromyelitis optica or Devic's disease; Balo's concentric sclerosis) that may or may not have the same etiology as the most typical forms. The MS lesions in a given individual appear to conform to one of four distinct types (Lassmann et al. 2001), suggesting that what we call MS could be in fact the aggregate of four distinct disorders. Although these four types of lesions were defined by histological examination of brain tissue, subsets of MS patients may in the future become identifiable using MRI and magnetic imaging spectroscopy, with important implications for epidemiologic research.

Accuracy of Clinical Diagnosis

The diversity of symptoms and signs and the unpredictable clinical course make the differential diagnosis of MS complex. A large number of conditions can be confused with MS, but most of these are rare, especially in young adults. A detailed account on the differential diagnosis of MS can be found in classical textbooks (Matthews 1998a). As MS is rarely fatal, there is only limited pathological validation of clinical diagnoses. Moreover, autopsy is usually performed selectively and may not provide a good estimate of the predictive value of clinical diagnoses in population-based studies. The largest pathological series is probably that reported by Engell (1988). This author used the Danish MS Registry to identify all patients with a clinical diagnosis of definite MS who died during the period of 1965–86 and had a postmortem examination. The diagnosis of MS was confirmed in 485 (94%) of 518 cases, while it was found erroneous in 33, including 9 with brain tumors, 18 with other neurological diseases, and 6 with miscellaneous conditions. Conversely, clinically silent cases of MS discovered unexpectedly at autopsy have also been described.

Case Definition Criteria

No single clinical feature or diagnostic test is sufficient for the diagnosis of MS. Several case definition criteria have been proposed to verify dissemination in time and space of lesions typical of MS and to exclude other explanations of the clinical features. The criteria most commonly used in recent studies are those of the Poser committee (Poser et al. 1983), which were introduced in 1983 (Table 8–1). The four groups defined by these criteria allow some flexibility for investigators in need of definitions with differing degrees of sensitivity and specificity in epidemiological studies. More recently a new classification has been proposed by the international panel on the Diagnosis of Multiple Sclerosis (McDonald et al. 2001), who integrated MRI into the diagnostic scheme, added criteria for the diagnosis of primary progressive disease, and specified that the outcome of a diagnostic evaluation should be one of the following: MS, possible MS, or not MS (see Table 8–2).

The widespread use of MRI has greatly reduced the time from first onset of neurological symptoms to diagnosis and is also likely to decrease the proportion of cases that remain undiagnosed. Gadolinium enhancement identifies putative areas of active inflammatory process (McDonald 1998) and the appearance of new enhancing lesions is considered a clear sign of disease activity. Concern has been expressed, however, that excessive reliance on MRI can lead to overdiagnosis (Kurtzke 1988, Herndon 1994), because current MRI techniques are not specific for demyelination. Until MRI techniques are improved, epidemiologists should classify patients on the basis of both MRI-independent and MRI-dependent criteria: Poser's criteria to facilitate comparisons with earlier studies and the new recommendations of the International Panel to incorporate the more rigorous MRI results.

Descriptive Epidemiology

Multiple sclerosis is primarily a disease of young adults and is more common in

Table 8–1 Poser et al.'s Diagnostic Criteria for Multiple Sclerosis

Category	Attacks	Clinical evidence		Paraclinical evidence	CSF OB/IgG
A. Clinically defined					
CDMS A1	2	2			
CDMS A2	2	1	*and*	1	
B. Laboratory supported definite					
LSDMS B1	2	1	*or*	1	+
LSDMS B2	1	2			+
LSDMS B3	1	1	*and*	1	+
C. Clinically probable					
CPMS C1	2	1			
CPMS C2	1	2			
CPMS C3	1	1	*and*	1	
D. Laboratory supported probable					
LSPMS D1	2				+

CSF, cerebrospinal fluid; OB/IgG, oligoclonal bands *or* increased immunoglobulin G (IgG); CDMS, clinically definite MS; LS-DMS, laboratory-supported definite MS; CPMS, clinically probable MS; LSPMS, laboratory-supported probable MS.

Reprinted with permission from Poser S, Ritter C, Bauer HJ, et al. New diagnostic criteria for multiple sclerosis: guidelines for research protocols. *Ann Neurol* 1983;13:227–231.

Table 8–2 Diagnostic Criteria for Multiple Sclerosis from the International Panel on Multiple Sclerosis Diagnosis

Dissemination in time	DISSEMINATION IN NEUROANATOMICAL SPACE		
	Clinical presentation	Laboratory evidence	
Two or more attacks	Objective clinical evidence of two or more lesions	Neither MRI nor CSF negative*	
Two or more attacks	Objective clinical evidence of one or more lesions	Dissemination in space demonstrated by MRI† or two or more MRI-detected lesions consistent with MS and positive CSF‡ or await further clinical attack implicating a different site	
One attack or dissemination in time demonstrated by MRI** or a second clinical attack	Objective clinical evidence of two or more lesions		
Dissemination in time demonstrated by MRI** or second clinical attack	Objective clinical evidence of one lesion (monosymptomatic presentation)	Dissemination in space demonstrated by MRI† or two or more MRI-detected lesions consistent with MS plus positive CSF‡	
Insidious neurological progression suggestive of MS. Dissemination in time demonstrated by MRI** or continued clinical progression of disability for 1 year	No better clinical explanation	Evidence of inflammation and immune abnormality is essential. Abnormal CSF‡ finding and dissemination in space demonstrated by MRI or abnormal VEP***	

If criteria in table are fulfilled, the diagnosis is multiple sclerosis (MS). If the criteria are not completely met, the diagnosis is "possible MS." If the criteria are fully explored and not met, the diagnosis is "not MS".

*No additional tests are required; however, if tests (magnetic resonance imaging [MRI]; cerebral spinal fluid [CSF]) are undertaken and are negative, extreme caution should be taken before making a diagnosis of MS. Alternative diagnoses must be considered. There must be no better explanation for the clinical picture.

†MRI demonstration of space dissemination must fulfill several criteria listed in Table 1 of McDonald et al. (2001).

‡Positive CSF determined by oligoclonal bands detected by established methods; see McDonald et al. (2001).

**MRI demonstration of time dissemination must fulfill several criteria listed in Table 2 of McDonald et al. (2001).

***Abnormal visual evoked potential (VEP) in addition to MRI demonstration of space dissemination; criteria listed in Table 3 of McDonald et al. (2001).

Source: McDonald WI, Compstona A, Edan G, et al. Recommended diagnostic criteria for multiple sclerosis: guidelines from the Internal Panel on the Diagnosis of Multiple Sclerosis. *Ann Neurol* 2001;50:121–127

women than men; the F:M ratio is about two in most populations. Incidence peaks late in the third decade of life and the disease is rare in children and older adults. The observation of a latitude gradient in the distribution of MS, marked by increasing rates farther from the equator, has intrigued epidemiologists for decades and provides important etiological clues. The vast literature on this topic must be interpreted with caution, however, as rate estimates are not always comparable between studies. This section highlights the methodological problems encountered in describing the distribution of MS, provides an overview of the worldwide prevalence, and focuses on selected regions and studies that are particularly informative.

Methodological Issues

Estimating Multiple Sclerosis Incidence and Prevalence. The incidence rates of MS in most high-risk areas range from 1 to 10 cases per 100,000. Not surprisingly, most studies are based on cross-sectional surveys, from which investigators have often derived both prevalence and incidence rates of MS; prospective incidence studies would require the follow-up of large cohorts for long periods of time. An important exception is the MS registry that has been operating in Denmark since 1948 and has provided a valuable source for monitoring trends in MS incidence over time (Koch-Henriksen and Hyllested 1988).

Geographical surveys attempt to identify and confirm all the cases of MS among residents in an area for which demographic data are available at a defined point of time, usually from a census. The first step in case identification is a systematic search of hospitals, outpatient clinics, individual physicians, health insurance organizations, MS societies, and other institutions that provide care for or otherwise may hold information on individuals with MS. The success of this search depends on the probability that an individual with MS is diagnosed and the probability that a diagnosed individual is identified by the search, which is determined in part by the completeness and accessibility of the provider lists (Nelson et al. 1986; Rosati 1994).

The diagnosis of MS is influenced by the standards of medical care, including coverage and quality, the level of MS awareness in the community, and the sensitivity of the diagnostic criteria applied. When these are lacking, the lag time between onset of symptoms and diagnosis is long, the prevalence of undiagnosed cases is high, and MS prevalence is underestimated. Incidence will also be underestimated, as some cases will die before being diagnosed. Surveying small populations can help overcome this problem because intensive efforts can be made to identify and thoroughly review all possible sources of information.

Example 8–1 An example is a study of the prevalence of MS in Northern Colorado (Nelson et al., 1986) where the investigators used a variety of methods, including the direct review of records from all neurologists, to strive for near-complete case ascertainment of MS patients in the region. The estimates of MS prevalence from this study were approximately 40% higher than prevalence estimates for the same latitude derived from a survey of randomly selected hospitals and physicians in the United States (Baum and Rothschild 1981). Unlike the Colorado study, this national study did not survey MS service organizations nor audit the case records of practicing neurologists. The estimates from the national survey can be considered an average rate whereas the Colorado study yielded an observed rate for a specific period of time.

Because of improvements in medical care, increased MS awareness, and widespread use of MRI, the lag time between onset of symptoms and diagnosis is decreasing. Faster diagnoses may spuriously increase incidence rates for recent time periods, so some investigators have relied exclusively on clinical criteria to define MS cases when studying time trends (Wynn et al. 1990).

Example 8–2 The medical records should also be searched for conditions that present with clinical features similar to those of MS and records that may include misclassified MS cases. For example, in a study in Israel, the investigators reviewed the medical records of all hospitals, referral clinics, and chronic care facilities for the period 1955 through 1959 for the following diagnoses: MS, primary lateral sclerosis, nontraumatic paraplegia, optic or retrobulbar neuritis, cerebellar ataxia, and myelopathy (Alter et al. 1962). After review of the medical records, they accepted 193 cases as probable MS and 89 cases as possible MS, of which 11 and 25, respectively, were found under different diagnostic labels.

Capture–recapture methods have been used in some surveys to assess the completeness of case ascertainment (Forbes and Swingler 1999). These methods should be applied with caution, as the assumptions required to estimate prevalence are often not satisfied (Hook and Regal 1995); however, a comparison of the proportion of cases identified by different sources can provide some sense of the overall level of under-ascertainment.

The second critical step in case ascertainment is the diagnostic confirmation of the cases detected in the first phase of the survey. Methods have ranged from accepting the hospital or physician diagnoses without further documentation (Svenson et al. 1994) to one or more of the investigators conducting the clinical examination themselves (Alter et al. 1962; Hammond et al. 1988). The impact on the results is important. In the study conducted in the early 1960s in Israel (Alter et al. 1962), for example, the authors personally examined 520 presumed MS cases identified from a medical record review. Of these, only 193 (37%) were accepted as probable and 89 (17%) as possible MS. Even investigations that rely on direct examination of all suspected cases of MS may not be comparable if different diagnostic criteria are used (see Compston 1998a for a comparison of

U.K. surveys that used different diagnostic criteria).

Finally, it is important to estimate accurately the denominators of the prevalence and incidence rates and to age-adjust to a common standard for comparison. All of the rates that we will directly compare in this chapter are age–adjusted, unless otherwise stated.

Fortunately, the difficulties of comparing incidence or prevalence rates from different studies were recognized early in the history of MS epidemiology, and efforts have been made to survey different geographical areas with similar methods and diagnostic criteria. Examples include the investigations that established the existence of a strong latitude gradient in Australia (Hammond et al. 1988) and New Zealand (Skegg et al. 1987) and the 10-fold difference in MS prevalence in Sicily (Dean et al. 1979) as compared with that in Malta (Vassallo et al. 1979).

Age at onset. The MS literature is replete with comparisons of age at onset between different populations or groups within a population. Almost universally these are crude comparisons, sometimes of groups with very different age structures. These comparisons are meaningless and should be ignored, except when the age structure of the compared populations is similar or can otherwise be taken into account.

Temporal changes in multiple sclerosis frequency. Time trends in the incidence and prevalence of MS can be estimated in certain populations that have been repeatedly and consistently surveyed. Information on time trends in MS incidence in the United States is sparse. The best information, from the Rochester Epidemiology Project, a longitudinal study in Olmsted County, Minnesota, shows that the incidence of MS increased in this century from 1.2 per 100,000 (95% CI 0.0–2.5) in 1905–1914 to 6.5/100,000 (5.5 to 7.5) in 1975–84 (Wynn et al. 1990). The veracity of this increase is supported by the fact that

92% of the cases had clinically definite MS; MRI results, which were not available for the earlier time period, were disregarded. In more recent years, surveys in some areas of southern Europe have provided much higher estimates of prevalence than studies from earlier time periods (Rosati 1994). In the United Kingdom, prevalence in the southern part of England has been steadily rising but has remained stable in northeast Scotland (Compston 1998a). Whether these findings represent true changes or simply reflect better ascertainment of cases is a matter of controversy (Rosati 1994; Compston 1998a).

Scandinavia is one of the most intensively studied regions for MS frequency because of the region's stable and relatively homogeneous population, high standards of medical care, free universal access to health services, and high level of education and MS awareness, as well as the existence of some MS registries. In spite of these advantages and decades of repeated surveys, the findings regarding time trends in MS prevalence are still controversial. The emerging pattern is that of inconsistent fluctuations across the region (Koch-Henriksen 1995). Incidence rates have apparently increased between the 1950s and 1980s in Norway (Grønning et al. 1991; Midgard et al. 1991, 1996) but have decreased or remained stable over the same period in Gotenburg, Sweden (Svenningsson et al. 1990). In Denmark, the incidence was highest in 1950, declined to a minimum in 1967, and then increased again, but without reaching the 1950 level (Koch-Henriksen 1995). The existence of a well-established registry in Denmark and the application of uniform diagnostic criteria make the Danish fluctuations difficult to explain by bias. The investigators suggested that they reflect changes in environmental factors, but skepticism about this explanation remains (Compston 1998a).

Geography and Multiple Sclerosis

The interest in the geographic distribution of MS is motivated by the hope of finding etiological clues. In this context, the main question is whether there are regional variations in the incidence of MS that cannot be explained by genetic differences and may thus provide a clue to an environmental cause.

Because of the scarcity of incidence data, worldwide maps of MS distribution are based mostly on prevalence (Rosati 2001; Pugliatti et al. 2002). Early studies of MS prevalence established a latitude gradient, with prevalence increasing with increasing distance from the equator in both hemispheres. The few studies conducted close to the equator consistently reported a low prevalence of MS (subtropical part of Australia, South Africa, and Israel) (Kurtzke 1995). Kurtzke (1995) created a simplified map based on areas of high (over 30/100,000), medium (5–29/100,000), and low MS prevalence (<5/100,000). In spite of the methodological difficulties in comparing prevalence of MS in different countries, few epidemiologists question the existence of a latitude gradient, as this is quite strong, it has been consistently found in independent studies in the United States, and it was shown in Australia and New Zealand after repeated rigorous surveys conducted with similar methods.

In the United States, a north–south gradient in MS distribution was noted in the 1920s and was originally attributed to the higher proportion of individuals of Scandinavian ancestry in the northern states (Davenport 1921). Since then, several studies have independently demonstrated that MS incidence and prevalence have been substantially higher in the northern part of the United States (Visscher et al., 1977; Kurtzke et al. 1979; Baum and Rothschild 1981; Hernán et al. 1999) and in Canada (Kurland et al. 1952; Stazio et al. 1967) than in the southern United States (Fig. 8–2a). Although any one of these studies is subject to scrutiny because of methodological difficulties in comparing MS rates among different regions, taken together, these studies provide solid

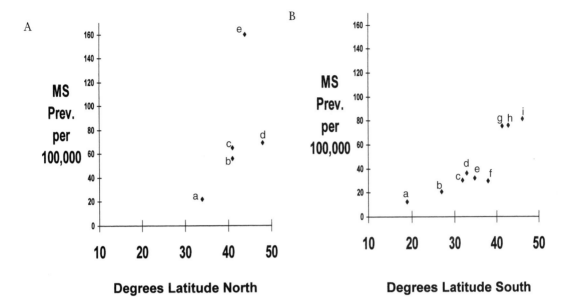

Degrees Latitude North **Degrees Latitude South**

Figure 8–2 **A:** Multiple sclerosis (MS) prevalence and latitude for surveys conducted between 1965 and 1985, north of the equator (North America). *a:* MS prevalence for year 1970, Los Angeles, CA (Visscher et al. 1977). *b:* MS prevalence for year 1965, Rochester, MN (Kurland et al. 1965). *c:* MS prevalence for year 1976, for regions above the 37th parallel (Baum et al. 1981). *d:* MS prevalence for year 1970, Seattle, WA (Visscher et al. 1977). *e:* MS prevalence for year 1982, northern Colorado (Nelson et al. 1986). **B:** Multiple sclerosis prevalence and latitude for surveys conducted between 1981 and 1983 that use similar methodology, south of the equator (Australia, New Zealand). Surveys: (*a*) tropical Queensland, Australia; (*b*) subtropical Queensland, Australia; (*c*) Perth, Australia; (*d*) Newcastle, Australia (*e*) Adelaide, Australia; (*f*) Waskato, New Zealand; (*g*) Wellington, New Zealand (*h*) Hobart, Australia; (*i*) Otago Southland, New Zealand. (Reprinted with permission from Miller DH, Hammond SR, McCleod JG, et al. Multiple sclerosis in Australia and New Zealand: are the determinants genetic or environmental? *J Neurol Psychiatry* 1990;53:903–905.)

evidence of an MS latitude gradient in North America.

Example 8–3 The first study that provided strong evidence for a gradient in the *incidence* of MS was the landmark investigation of U.S. Army veterans (Kurtzke et al. 1979). The study population comprised 5305 veterans with a diagnosis of MS occurring before 1969 and an equal number of matched controls. Since veterans with MS occurring during service or within 7 years from discharge were eligible for recompensation, the degree of case ascertainment was likely to be very high. A review of the clinical records of a random sample of the cases found that 96% met the criteria for definite MS (Kurtzke et al. 1979). The relative incidence of MS was 2.7 among veterans who entered the service in

the northern United States (states generally north of 41°–42° north latitude) as compared with those who entered the service in the southern United States (states lying south of 37° north latitude); incidence for the middle states was in between.

Studies from the Southern Hemisphere (New Zealand, Australia) have been methodologically similar and close in time, providing clarity about the nature of the geographic gradient and the possible role of genetic factors in explaining the gradient. A combined analysis of the data from Australia and New Zealand revealed a sevenfold gradient in MS prevalence between Queensland in tropical Australia (12.4 per 100,000) and Otago in southern New Zealand (81.7 per 100,000) (Miller et al. 1990). It may be noted that although these data display a strong linear correlation with latitude (Fig. 8–2b), they are more consistent with low, intermediate, and high prevalence zones.

When considered together, the studies from both hemispheres support the interpretation that the frequency of MS increases as distance from the equator increases. Epidemiologists have been searching for factors that might explain this striking geographic distribution. We focus here on selected studies that allow a separation of genetic from environmental factors, and include information from migrant studies as they are critical for this purpose.

Is the Gradient an Effect of Genetics?

Many studies have examined the role of ethnicity or ancestral background as a surrogate measure of a possible genetic explanation for the geographic gradient. Data from the U.S. Army veterans study (Kurtzke et al. 1979) were used to assess the role of genetic factors in the MS latitude gradient in the United States (Bulman and Ebers 1992). Strong correlations were found between the case/control ratios and the proportion of the population in each state with Scandinavian or northern European ancestry, and the authors suggested that genetic susceptibility may explain the distribution of the disease in the United States. An independent analysis of the same data, however, challenged this conclusion, showing that latitude explained 66.5% of the variance in MS risk, whereas Swedish ancestry, the strongest predictor after latitude, explained only 9% (Page et al. 1993). The contributions of other ancestries were small (3.9% for French, positive, and 2.3% for Dutch, negative correlation; other ancestries not significant). These results, although consistent with a contribution of genes to the distribution of MS in the United States, strongly suggest a predominance of environmental factors.

Genetic explanations of geographical variations have also been proposed for New Zealand and Australia. For example, New Zealand has a higher proportion of people of Scottish ancestry, who are believed to have a genetically determined higher risk, in the south (Miller et al. 1990). Subsequent studies, however, revealed that variations in the proportion of people with Scottish ancestry had only a modest impact on MS rates in New Zealand, and that variations in MS frequency in Australia and New Zealand cannot be explained by genetic factors (Swingler and Compston 1986; Hammond et al. 1988; Robertson and Compston 1995).

Migrant Studies

Early investigators thought that migrant studies might help elucidate the contribution of geography to MS risk, primarily by tracking migrant populations who moved from high-risk regions to low-risk regions. The results of these studies and related methodological issues are thoroughly reviewed elsewhere (Gale and Martyn 1995). Migrants often differ in socioeconomic status and education from non-migrants, may have a different genetic constitution, and are usually less likely to have a chronic illness (that is both a disincentive to migrate and at times a barrier to immigration as the host countries may impose restrictions on people with disabilities). There is often scarcity of data on the frequency of MS in the country of origin, availability of medical care may differ between country of origin and that of destination, and migrants may differ from the host population in their use of health services and probability of being diagnosed (Gale and Martyn 1995). Denominators are often uncertain, as up-to-date figures may not be available and illegal immigrants are not included in the statistics. Despite these limitations, migrant studies have provided compelling evidence on the role of environmental factors and have shown convincingly that migration from a high- to a low-risk zone is associated with a reduction in risk. Two points that remain unclear are whether this reduction in risk benefits only those who migrate in childhood and whether migration in the opposite direction (low risk to high risk) is associated with an increased risk.

Migration from High- to Low-Risk Areas. Several studies have considered changes in MS risk in immigrants who migrate from European countries to lower-risk areas of Israel, South Africa, and Australia, and in people who migrate from northern to southern areas of the United States (Table 8–3a). In general, these studies have supported the hypothesis that migration from a high- to a low-risk area in childhood decreases the risk of MS, but they are equivocal as to whether migration as an adult confers any benefit. This pattern is consistent with an environmental risk factor, possibly one that operates in childhood.

Because of its large immigrant population and good access to health care, Israel provides an interesting setting for the investigation of migration and MS. A nationwide survey of MS completed in 1961 revealed that the prevalence of MS among European immigrants to Israel was over six times higher than that among Afro-Asian immigrants (Alter et al. 1962) and that the incidence rate ratios comparing European with Afro-Asian immigrants were 1.7 for those who immigrated before age 15, 8.9 for those who immigrated between age 15 and 29 years, and 5.4 for those who immigrated between age 30 and 44 years (Alter et al. 1966, 1978). Despite the small number of cases among immigrants below age 15 (four among Europeans and four among Afro-Asians), this result adds to the evidence that immigration in childhood from high- to low-risk areas reduces the risk of MS. The effects of migration in adulthood cannot be determined from these data, as comparable rates in the country of origin of the migrants are not available.

One of the most influential studies concerning the importance of age at migration was conducted in South Africa (Dean 1967). The estimated age-adjusted incidence rates of MS were 0.4 per 100,000 among South African–born whites and 2.8 among immigrants from the United Kingdom, which is similar to that of their country of origin. The observation that people of similar British stock had quite different rates of disease depending on their place of birth provides further evidence of the importance of environmental factors. Noting that white children born in South Africa are more likely to be exposed early in life to several infections than those born in the United Kingdom, Dean interpreted these data as supportive of the "poliomyelitis hypothesis," i.e., a virus that increases the risk of MS if acquired after infancy or in early childhood (Poskanzer et al. 1976). Consistent with this interpretation was the higher rate of poliomyelitis among immigrant children than that in South-African born whites. This survey was updated in 1968 to study the effects of age at immigration on risk of MS (Kurtzke et al. 1970). The number of cases of MS among individuals who were 15 or younger at migration was about 3 to 4 times lower than expected under the hypothesis that age at immigration was irrelevant. In spite of some uncertainty concerning the indirect calculations of the expected number of cases, these results support a stronger effect of migration in childhood than later in life. The number of cases was too small to determine whether there is a specific age at which this benefit is lost. Most importantly, since it is not known what the rates of MS among these immigrants would have been if they had remained in their countries of origin, the overall effect of migration on risk of MS cannot be reliably estimated from these data.

Compelling evidence for the predominantly environmental origin of the MS gradient in the United States is provided by the U.S. Army veterans study. The case/control ratio for veterans born in the north tier decreased from 1.48 if they remained in the northern tier to 0.74 (0.47 to 1.14) if they entered service in the southern tier (Kurtzke et al. 1985). One U.S. study (Detels et al. 1978) found that the benefit of migration from a high- to a low-risk area declined with age, but was still present for migration between 15 and 19 years of age. A

Table 8-3a Migration Studies of Multiple Sclerosis Frequency: Migration from High-risk to Low-risk Areas

Reference	Migration route	Results	Age at migration effects
Dean 1967; Kurtzke et al. 1970	United Kingdom to South Africa	Sevenfold higher MS prevalence in U.K. immigrants than in South African–born whites	Three- to fourfold lower MS prevalence than expected for U.K. immigrants who were ≤15 years old at migration
Alter et al. 1962; 1966; 1978	Europe to Israel	Sixfold higher MS prevalence in European immigrants to Israel than in Afro-Asian immigrants to Israel	Only 1.7-fold higher in European immigrants who were ≤15 years old at migration
Detels et al. 1978	Northern United States (42° latitude) to King and Pierce Counties, WA or to Los Angeles, CA	Lower MS prevalence for those moving from northern U.S. to Los Angeles, CA, than for those moving to King and Pierce, WA	Fivefold lower MS prevalence for migration to Los Angeles, CA, for those ≤9 years old at migration; threefold lower for ages 10–14; twofold lower for ages 15–19 years
Kurtzke et al. 1985	Northern to Southern United States	Decrease in risk of MS among white U.S. veterans born in the north and entering into active duty in the south	N/A
Hammond et al. 2000a	United Kingdom to Australia	Risk of MS was low in U.K. immigrants who migrated to an area of Australia where MS is rare	None—reduced MS risk seen at all ages

study from Australia (Hammond et al. 2000a) found both adults and children who migrated from the United Kingdom to Australia were protected, suggesting an environmental factor operating also during adult life and not only in childhood.

Migration from Low- to High-Risk Areas. The effect of migration from low- to high-risk areas is controversial. In general, studies suggest that migrants tend to retain their low-risk level, but results are mixed. Some studies suggest that subsequent generations have increased risk (Table 8–3b).

In the U.S. veterans study, migration from the southern to northern United States was associated with a nonsignificant increase in risk of MS (Kurtzke et al. 1985); however, the period of follow-up may have been too short (9 to 10 years) for a complete expression of the increased risk associated with migration (Kurtzke et al. 1998). In the same study, case/control ratios increased from 1.0 to 1.4 (1.1 to 1.8) among those veterans who were born in the middle tier and entered service in the north tier. Investigations conducted among immigrants to the United Kingdom suggested that migration from low- to high-risk areas does not increase the risk of MS (Dean et al. 1976, 1977). The interpretation of these data is difficult, however, because most immigrants from low-risk areas had been in the United Kingdom for less than 5 years, which may not have been sufficient time for the effect of migration to become manifest (Kurtzke 1976). A later study in the United Kingdom confirmed the scarcity of deaths attributed to MS among Asian immigrants (6 vs. 82 expected) or immigrants born in the West Indies (12 vs. 59 expected) (Elian and Dean 1993). The data above could of course reflect a lower genetic susceptibility to MS among Asians and other immigrants. However, U.K.-born children of these immigrants were later found to have rates of MS substantially higher than those of their parents and similar to those in the general population in England and Ireland, a finding confirm-

ing their susceptibility to MS (Elian and Dean 1987; Elian et al. 1990).

Similarly, the low rates of MS in Asian and African immigrants to Israel have been cited to support the hypothesis that the move from low- to high-risk areas is not associated with an increased risk of MS (Gale and Martyn 1995). Risk does appear to increase in ensuing generations, however; prevalence of MS among Israelis whose fathers were born in Africa or Asia was 1.4 to 1.8 times higher than among African and Asian immigrants (Gale and Martyn 1995).

With the exception of the U.S. veterans study, none of the investigations described in this section provides a direct comparison of risk in migrants from low- to high-risk areas with that for people of the same ancestral origin who remained in their country of origin, although they do suggest that any increase in risk of MS caused by migration from a low- to a high-risk area is modest compared to the high risk that migrants would have experienced had they been born in the host country. Even this conclusion is uncertain because comparisons are made between different generations that may have different risks of MS independently from migration.

Multiple Sclerosis Clusters

The Faroes are a group of islands in the North Atlantic Ocean that have been a semi-independent unit of the Kingdom of Denmark since 1948 (Kurtzke and Heltberg 2001). Intensive efforts to ascertain all cases of MS among Faroese from 1900 to 1983 started in the 1940s and 32 cases of MS were identified among native resident Faroese (Fog and Kyllested 1966, Kurtzke and Hyllested 1979, Kurtzke 1986). The absence of cases with onset before 1943, and the clustering of cases with onset between 1943 and 1949, was interpreted as supporting the occurrence of an epidemic of MS. The observation that the beginning of the epidemic started soon after the British occupation of the islands (April 1940 to 1944) and the strong and highly

Table 8–3b. Migration Studies of Multiple Sclerosis Frequency: Migration from Low-risk to High-risk Areas

Reference	Migration route	Results	Next generation effects
Kurtzke et al. 1985	Southern to northern United States	Nonsignificant increase in risk of MS	N/A
Kurtzke et al. 1998	North Africa to France	1.5-fold higher MS prevalence among North African migrants than among general French population	N/A
Kahana et al. 1994; Gale and Martyn 1995	Asian and African immigrants to Israel	Maintained low MS risk of country of origin	1.4- to 1.8-fold higher risk of MS in second-generation Afro-Asian immigrants than in first-generation immigrants
Dean et al. 1976, 1977	India, Pakistan, and the West Indies to Greater London	Low rates of hospital admission for MS among immigrants; rates high for immigrants from high-risk areas	N/A
Elian and Dean 1987, 1993	Asia or West Indies to United Kingdom	Fewer MS deaths than expected in immigrants	U.K.-born children of immigrants had higher rates of MS than parents and similar rates to native English and Irish

N/A, not applicable.

significant association between troop location and parishes of residence (Kurtzke and Heltberg 2001) led the authors to conclude that the epidemic was caused by some agent introduced by the British troops. On the basis of further analyses of the time course of the epidemic, it was concluded that this agent was a widespread, specific, persistent infection, probably asymptomatic (Kurtzke and Heltberg 2001). Critics questioned whether an epidemic had occurred at all (Dean 1988; Poser and Hibberd 1988; Poser et al. 1988), noting that the date of onset of illness is irrelevant, as the disease is supposedly acquired between the ages of 5 and 15 years (Poser et al. 1988). In our view, this is a rather weak objection, because the proposed narrow range of susceptibility is hypothetical; further, the introduction of a new infectious agent in a nonimmune population may result in a different pattern of age susceptibility than what is typical in populations where the infection is endemic. Other criticisms, including suggestions that case exclusions were arbitrary (Poser et al. 1988) and that case ascertainment was incomplete, seem unlikely to account for the sudden excess of cases seen in the 1940s, and the claim of an epidemic occurrence of MS in the Faroes seems well founded. The detailed interpretation offered by the investigators remains more speculative, but overall the Faroese experience supports the play of environmental factors in MS incidence.

Genetic Epidemiology

Familial Studies

Population-based twin studies of MS have consistently shown a higher concordance rate among monozygotic (MZ) than dizygotic (DZ) pairs. As shown in Table 8–4, these rates ranged from 26% to 31% for MZ pairs, and from 0% to 5% for DZ pairs (Bobowick et al. 1978; Heltberg and Holm 1982; Ebers et al. 1986; Kinnunen et al. 1988; Sadovnick et al. 1993; Mumford et al. 1994). The risk in non-twin siblings of an MS proband was similar to that of DZ twins. These results clearly indicate the importance of genetic factors in determining the susceptibility to MS, as the degree to which MZ and DZ pairs share the same environment should be similar, and DZ twins are as genetically similar to each other as non-twin siblings. Further, the large difference in risk between MZ and DZ twins and other siblings provides strong evidence against the existence of a single disease susceptibility locus, as this would imply approximately a twofold gradient in risk between MZ and DZ twins (Risch 1990). Age-adjusted recurrence risks in first-degree relatives of MS probands are elevated and appear to vary by the nature of the relationship (e.g., child or sibling) (Sadovnick et al. 1993; Robertson et al. 1996; Carton et al. 1997). Second- and third-degree relatives also had substantially higher risk of MS than expected from gen-

Table 8–4 Percent Concordance for Multiple Sclerosis Among Monozygotic and Dizygotic Twins

	MONOZYGOTIC PAIRS		DIZYGOTIC PAIRS	
Reference	n	% Concordance	n	% Concordance
Bobowick et al. (1978)	5	20	4[†]	0
Heltberg and Holm (1982)	19	21	28[†]	4
Ebers et al. (1986)	27	26	43	2
Kinnunen et al. (1988)	7	29	6[†]	0
Sadovnick et al. (1993)	19	26	23	0
Sadovnick et al. (1993)*	26	31	43	5
Mumford et al. (1994)	44	25	61	3

*Adapted from Ebers et al. 1986, with permission; one case from original series did not have MS and one dizygotic pair became concordant.

†Same-sex twins.

eral population rates (Robertson et al. 1996). Since these relatives are less likely to share a common environment, this further supports the importance of genetic factors.

As members of the same family share a common environment and lifestyle, non-genetic factors could contribute to familial aggregation.

Example 8–4 Studies of half-siblings, children adopted by individuals with MS, and parents who adopted a child who developed MS were conducted to address this possibility. From a population-based sample of 15,000 individuals with MS in Canada (Ebers et al. 1995), investigators selected Caucasian adoptees with MS who were adopted as infants and determined the occurrence of MS among their nonbiologic relatives, including 470 parents, 345 siblings, and 386 children. In each group, the age-adjusted risk was similar to that expected in the general population and significantly less than predicted from the biological risk data. These results provide strong evidence for a genetic cause for familial aggregation. In a separate study, the risk of MS was compared between full-sibs and half-sibs of the cases. The age-adjusted MS risk was 1.32% in 1839 half-sibs and 3.46% in 1395 full-sibs ($p < 0.001$). There were no significant differences in risk for half-sibs raised together or apart from the index case (1.17% vs. 1.47%) or for maternal versus paternal half-sibs (1.42% vs. 1.19%) (Sadovnick et al. 1996). This last finding, and the fact that children of an affected father have similar risk to that of children of an affected mother, suggests that the impact of maternal effects, such as imprinting, mitochondrial inheritance, intrauterine factors, or breast feeding, must be modest (Sadovnick et al. 1997). Further analyses revealed a low prevalence of conjugal MS and a high risk of MS in offspring of MS parents (Ebers et al. 2000), comparable to the risk of MZ twins of affected individuals. This high rate is consistent with a role of recessive alleles that are shared among unrelated individuals with the disease. The small number of cases and concerns over the appropriateness of age adjustment (which does not take into account that children with both affected parents may have an earlier age at MS onset than average) dictate some caution in interpreting this provocative result (Ebers et al. 2000).

A high risk of MS among children of conjugal pairs was also suggested in a U.K. study (Robertson et al. 1997). Five of 86 offspring from conjugal pairs in which both parents had MS met the criteria for clinically definite MS, and a further 5 had either characteristic MRI abnormalities or clinical symptoms consistent with demyelination, but did not meet criteria for clinically definite disease.

In summary, the results of familial studies indicate that aggregation of MS within families is due to shared genes rather than environment, that more than one gene contributes to MS susceptibility, and that there is little or no role of maternal factors in the inheritance of MS.

Candidate Genes

Whereas evidence for a strong genetic component in MS is undisputable, progress in identifying the responsible genes has been disappointing. If inheritance of MS susceptibility is polygenic, each of the involved genes may by itself only provide a modest increase in risk and could be difficult to identify. A detailed review of the genetic epidemiology of MS has been published (Compston 1998b). Only selected findings will be discussed below.

HLA Region. The only region that appears certain to contain a gene that confers susceptibility to MS is the major histocompatibility complex (MHC), or HLA encoded on chromosome 6q21.1–21.3 (Compston 1998b). Within this region, the most consistent association is with the class II alleles defined in serological tests as HLA-DR15 and DQ6 (DR15 is a split of the serological specificity previously identified as DR2). The serological specificity DR15 is the expression of the genotype DRB1*1501, DRB5*0101 (DRB1 and

DRB5 are two different loci both encoding the β chain of the HLA class II molecule in the DR region; the numbers after the asterisk denote specific alleles), whereas DQ6 is the expression of DQA1*0102, DQB1*0602 (DQA1 is the locus encoding the α chain, and DQB1 is the locus encoding the β chain of the class II molecule in the DQ region). Because of strong linkage disequilibrium, the individual contributions of DR and DQ polymorphisms have been difficult to separate. Previously reported associations with class I alleles (A3 and B7) appear to be due to linkage disequilibrium with DR15 and DQ6. The association with DR15 has been found in most but not all populations. A notable exception is Sardinia, where the strongest association is with DR4. In a recent case–control study of 159 patients with definite relapsing-remitting MS and 273 control subjects, investigators reported an association between an allele in a microsatellite marker telomeric to the HLA class II region and the risk of developing relapsing-remitting MS (OR = 2.0, 95% CI 1.2–3.1; $p = 0.004$). This allele is encoded within an ancestral haplotype that is highly linked to HLA-DR3. The joint effect of this ancestral haplotype and HLA-DR2 on the risk of developing relapsing-remitting MS was 8.7 (95% CI 2.7–29; $p < 0.0001$). This result suggests that within the HLA region, other loci besides HLA-DR2 haplotype modulate susceptibility for relapsing-remitting MS (de Jong et al. 2002). Kalman and Lublin (1999) and Giordano et al. (2002) have recently reviewed the associations of HLA and MS. Overall, the associations with DR15 or other HLA class II alleles are too weak to explain most of the genetic variability of MS, which suggests that other important loci may exist.

Other Candidate Genes. Several other genes have been explored as candidates for MS susceptibility (Compston 1998b). Because of the associations with the HLA class II alleles reported above, logical candidates are other polymorphic genes in the same region on chromosome 6. These include the peptide transporter genes *TAP1* and *TAP2,* the heat-shock protein, genes involved in the alternate pathway of the complement cascade, and the genes encoding tumor necrosis factors (TNF) α and β. TNF-α is particularly interesting because of its role in oligodendrocyte injury. Some studies (Sandberg-Wollheim et al. 1995; Epplen et al. 1997; Kirk et al. 1997) but not others (Fugger et al. 1990a; Roth et al. 1994; He et al. 1995; Wingerchuk et al. 1997) support an association between TNF-α alleles and risk of MS. Also on chromosome 6 is the gene for myelin oligodendrocyte glycoprotein (MOG), but no consistent associations have been reported with alleles in this region (Hilton et al. 1995; Roth et al. 1995; Rodriguez et al. 1997). Other cytokines and their receptors not encoded in the HLA region have also been investigated as potential candidates, but findings have again been inconsistent (Compston 1998b). Among the genes that could interact with the HLA class II alleles in increasing the risk of MS, the most appealing would include the alleles encoding the T-cell receptors that recognize antigens presented by the class II molecules. A strong interaction between an α-chain T-cell receptor allele (encoded on chromosome 14) and DR2 was reported in one study (Sherritt et al. 1992) but was not confirmed by others (Hashimoto et al. 1992; Hillert et al. 1992; Eoli et al. 1994). The role of polymorphisms of the β-chain remains controversial (Oksenberg et al. 1988; Beall et al. 1989; Fugger et al. 1990b; Hillert et al. 1991; Martinez-Naves et al. 1993). Another locus that could be important is the immunoglobulin heavy-chain gene on chromosome 14q. Most evidence does not appear to support a role of mitochondrial genes or genes encoding structural myelin proteins (Compston 1998b).

Genome Screening

Complete genomic screens are an alternative to the candidate gene approach. The evidence of a strong genetic component in MS contrasts with the relatively weak associations identified thus far, suggesting that there are unknown genes with stronger effects on MS susceptibility. Genome screens are conducted among families with more than one member affected by MS (multiplex family) to identify both the regions that are more likely to harbor disease susceptibility genes and those that are very unlikely to harbor disease susceptibility genes. Four large, full genome screens have been conducted among Caucasians in the United States, Canada, the United Kingdom, and Scandinavia (Ebers et al. 1996; Haines et al. 1996; Sawcer et al. 1996; Akesson et al. 2002); smaller genome-wide screens have been conducted in Finland, Sardinia, and Italy (Kuokkanen et al. 1997; Coraddu et al. 2001; Broadley et al. 2001). No locus with overwhelming evidence of linkage emerged in any of the studies. A meta-analysis of the pooled data from three of these studies (Ebers et al. 1996; Haines et al. 1996; Sawcer et al. 1996) confirmed that no region could be clearly identified as the prime candidate for harboring a strong susceptibility gene (The American Group 2001). The strongest statistical association was on chromosome 17q11; this region encodes many potential candidates, including the gene for neurofibromatosis I (NF1), a gene that had been previously proposed as related to MS (Ferner et al. 1995). A different region of chromosome 17 (q22–q24) previously identified in the Finnish screening has been recently fine mapped using a dense set of 31 markers. This study, carried out in 22 Finnish multiplex MS families, restricted the original linkage to a region of approximately 4 centimorgan (cM) flanked by the markers D17S1792 and ATA43A10; linkage in this region was identified in 17 of the families (77.3%) (Saarela et al. 2002). The multipoint linkage analyses provided further evidence for the same 4 cM region, with a maximal multipoint NPL score of 5.98 ($p < 0.0002$). This region includes several functional candidate genes.

Overall, the results of genome screens support the view that heritable MS susceptibility is determined by multiple interacting genes. Stratification of the analyses by HLA-DR haplotype, refinement of the genotyping using more dense microsatellite markers as described above, and screening of regions of interest in association studies may soon lead to important discoveries.

Infection and Multiple Sclerosis

An association between infection and MS was proposed in 1883 by Pierre Marie, and an infectious cause is still being pursued, though no specific organism has been conclusively linked to MS. Two distinct theories underlie epidemiological research on infection and MS. These theories both posit that a widespread microbe, rather than a rare pathogen, causes the disease, but they differ in other aspects, as outlined below.

The first theory, based on the investigation of the Faroe Islands epidemic (Kurtzke 1993), postulates that MS is caused by a pathogen that is more common in regions of high MS incidence. According to this theory, there is a widespread transmissible agent that causes an asymptomatic persistent infection or "primary MS affection (PMSA)"; rarely, and years after the primary infection, this agent would cause neurological symptoms (MS). The second theory is the polio hypothesis (Poskanzer et al. 1963; Brody 1972), which posits that the microbe causing MS is ubiquitous and transmitted early in life in populations with low MS incidence and that being infected with this microbe after childhood increases risk of MS.

Both theories provide a reasonable explanation of the geographical distribution of MS, and could account for the reduction in risk in individuals who migrate in early childhood from high- to low-risk areas (reduced risk of exposure according to the PMSA hypothesis, infection before adolescence according to the polio hypothesis). The two theories would predict different outcomes for migration from low- to high-risk areas—the PMSA hypothesis would predict an increase in risk, whereas the polio hypothesis would predict no increase unless the migration occurred before a child was infected—but the data on migration from low- to high-risk areas are too inconsistent to distinguish between the two theories.

If the PMSA hypothesis is true and there is a specific infectious agent that is more common in areas of high MS frequency, then some degree of space–time clustering of cases would be expected. Although several investigators have failed to find space–time clustering during childhood and adolescence among individuals in the same community who developed MS (Neutel et al. 1977; Isager et al. 1980; Larsen et al. 1985a; Riise et al. 1991; Riise 1997), the PMSA agent might be so ubiquitous that almost everyone is infected or it might be difficult to transmit among siblings. Another alternative is that clustering at the time of disease onset might be masked because of the restricted age of susceptibility, the hypothetically long asymptomatic period (at least 6 years according to Kurtzke and Hyllested 1987), and the fact that individuals with MS may no longer be infectious.

Although it has been criticized (Nathanson and Miller 1978), the polio theory retains substantial appeal (Detels et al. 1972; Alvord et al. 1987; Riise et al. 1991). Among the supportive findings are the positive association of MS with socioeconomic status (Beebe et al. 1967; Russell 1971; Kurtzke and Page 1997), the later age at infection with childhood viruses in MS cases than in controls (Granieri and Casetta 1997), and the increased risk of MS among individuals with a history of infectious mononucleosis (Operskalski et al. 1989; Lindberg et al. 1991; Martyn et al. 1993; Haahr et al. 1997; Marrie et al. 2000).

An alternative but related hypothesis is that MS is an autoimmune reaction triggered in susceptible individuals in response to infection by multiple pathogens; exposure to several infectious agents early in life

would be protective, as in the polio model, but there would not be a specific agent responsible.

Whether a single specific agent or multiple microbes are involved, the prevailing view is that MS is a reaction to common pathogens that could initiate autoimmunity with or without residing in the central nervous system (CNS) (Hafler 1999; Hunter and Hafler 2000).

Candidate viruses that have been proposed as causative agents in MS include measles, rubella, mumps, herpes viruses I and II, herpes zoster, Epstein-Barr virus (EBV), cytomegalovirus, human herpes virus 6 (HHV-6), canine distemper virus, and many others (Cook et al. 1995). Most of these hypotheses originated from the finding of elevated levels of antibodies in sera from MS patients as compared with that in controls. A major limitation of this approach is that differences between cases and controls may represent a consequence of an abnormal immune response in MS patients and be of little etiological relevance (Granieri and Casetta 1997). Our view is that the data provide strong evidence, though not conclusive proof, of a causal[1] association between EBV and MS.

Epstein-Barr Virus

A causal association between EBV and MS was originally suggested 20 years ago (Warner and Carp 1981), primarily because of the similarities in the epidemiology of infectious mononucleosis (IM) and MS. Both diseases affect mostly young adults, follow a latitude gradient (Brodsky and Heath 1972; Hallee et al. 1974; Kurtzke 1995), are rare among populations where children are infected with EBV at an early age (Kurtzke 1995; Niederman and Evans 1997), occur at an earlier age in women

---

[1]By "causal" we mean that prevention of EBV infection, for example, by a suitable vaccine, would substantially reduce the risk of MS. This does not exclude a possible role of other microbes or noninfectious factors, nor does it imply that EBV is infecting oligodendrocytes or other cells in the CNS.

than in men (Martyn 1991; Niederman and Evans 1997), are more frequent in individuals with high socioeconomic status (Beebe et al. 1967; Russell 1971; Nye 1973; Carvalho et al. 1981; Hesse et al. 1983; Kurtzke and Page 1997), are less frequent in blacks (Brodsky and Heath 1972; Heath et al. 1972; Kurtzke et al. 1979) and Asians (Chang et al. 1979) than in whites, and occur rarely among Eskimos (Chan 1977; Melbye et al. 1984). Further, the risk of MS is significantly increased among individuals with a history of IM (Operskalski et al. 1989, Lindberg et al. 1991; Martyn et al. 1993; Haahr et al. 1997; Marrie et al. 2000; Hernán et al. 2001b).

Epstein-Barr virus is a herpesvirus that establishes a persistent latent infection in B lymphocytes (Rickinson and Kieff 1996). Antibodies against the EBV antigens persist at stable levels throughout life, and it is thus possible to determine serologically whether an individual is or is not infected with EBV. Titers of these antibodies have been found to be elevated in MS patients (Larsen et al. 1985b; Shirodaria et al. 1987) but could reflect immune disregulation in MS. Despite a high prevalence of EBV infection in most populations (typically over 90% in adults), a recent meta-analysis showed that the risk of MS is more than 10 times higher among EBV-positive than among EBV-negative subjects (Table 8–5) (Ascherio and Munch 2000). Since primary EBV infection is rare among patients with MS (Munch et al. 1998; Wandinger et al. 2000), this finding suggests that EBV itself increases the risk of MS. An important limitation of the data presented in Table 8–5 is the potential bias from control selection, as controls were not randomly sampled from the population that generated the cases. Nevertheless, the consistency of the association across studies conducted in different countries and with different control groups makes bias an unlikely explanation. Moreover, these results have now been confirmed by two more studies (Wandinger et al. 2000; Ascherio et al. 2001a), one of which (Ascherio et al. 2001a) was nested within a cohort

and thus not prone to selection bias. Further evidence supporting a causal role of EBV in MS is provided by the recent report that active viral replication occurs more commonly in MS patients during exacerbations than in patients with stable disease (Wandinger et al. 2000) and by the finding in two separate studies that elevations of anti-EBV antibody titers among cases of MS precede the onset of the disease by several years (Ascherio et al. 2001a; Levin et al. 2003). In the largest of these investigations (Levin et al. 2003), the risk of developing MS was 30-fold higher among individuals in the highest category of serum IgG antibodies against the EBV nuclear antigen (EBNA) as compared with those in the lowest.

The failure to demonstrate EBV in MS plaques by in situ hybridization (Hilton et al. 1994) or polymerase chain reaction (PCR) (Morré et al. 2001) suggests that direct CNS infection is not involved. Rather, EBV could trigger an autoimmune reaction (Wucherpfennig and Strominger 1995; Vaughan et al. 1996), since infection with EBV elicits a strong, persistent, cytotoxic response. Autoimmunity could occur if some of these T cells recognized myelin epitopes.

Other Viruses

Comparisons of antibody titers for most other viruses between MS cases and controls have produced inconsistent results. Null results have been published for herpes viruses I and II (Cremer et al. 1980; Myhr et al. 1998), herpes zoster (Cremer et al. 1980; Myhr et al. 1998), cytomegalovirus (Cremer et al. 1980; Myhr et al. 1998), rubella (Cremer et al. 1980), measles (Poskanzer et al. 1980), and mumps (Cremer et al. 1980). Most importantly, a causal role of many of these viruses would not by itself explain the epidemiology of MS. For example, the lack of a decline in MS incidence following massive immunization against measles (Bansil et al. 1990) makes a primary etiological role of this virus unlikely. Human herpes virus 6, a β-

Table 8-5 Epstein-Barr Seropositivity among Patients with Multiple Sclerosis Compared with Controls by Study

Reference	Cases	Controls	OR	95% CI
Sumaya et al. 1980	157 cases with clinically definite MS	81 subjects including spouses, other household members, and laboratory personnel	5.1	0.8–54.3
Bray et al. 1983	313 cases with clinical diagnosis of MS and oliglonal bands in CSF	406 normal blood donors and patients with other nondemyelinating neurological diseases	9.2	3.2–35.4
Larsen et al. 1985b	100 cases with definite MS	100 healthy hospital staff or blood donors	Undefined	
Sumaya et al. 1985	104 cases with clinically definite MS	104 healthy subjects, unrelated to the cases	Undefined	
Shirodaria et al. 1987	26 cases with clinically definite MS	26 healthy blood donors	Undefined	
Ferrante et al. 1987	30 cases with definite MS	51 subjects with other diseases	10.3	1.3–45.8
Munch et al. 1997	138 cases	138 normal controls	15.5	2.3–65.8
Myhr et al. 1998	144 cases (130 definite MS; 10 probable MS; 4 possible MS)	170 hospital subjects admitted for trauma or minor surgery	Undefined	
Ascherio and Munch 2000	1005 cases from the 8 case–control studies listed above	1060 control from the 8 case–control studies listed above	13.5*	6.3–31.4

CI, confidence intervals; CSF, cerebrospinal fluid; OR, odds ratio.
*Mantel-Haenszel odds ratio.
Source: Reprinted with permission from Ascherio A, Munch M. Epstein-Barr virus and multiple sclerosis. *Epidemiology* 2000;11:1–5.

herpesvirus that exists in two variants, A and B, has been associated with MS (Wilborn et al. 1994, Soldan et al. 1997); however, other investigators could not confirm these findings (Martin et al. 1997; Fillet et al. 1998; Mayne et al. 1998; Goldberg et al. 1999; Taus et al. 2000). Recently, an association has been reported between variant A of the human herpesvirus (HHV-6) and MS (Akhyani et al. 2000; Knox et al. 2000; Soldan et al. 2000). Unlike the HHV-6 variant B, variant A may infect EBV-positive B-cell lines and activate the latent EBV genome (Cuomo et al. 1995; Flamand and Menezes 1996). These observations suggest that interactions between herpesviruses may contribute to the pathogenesis of MS.

Chlamydia pneumoniae. An association between chlamydial infections and risk of MS was first suggested in French MS literature in the 1960s (Le Gac 1960; Jadin 1962), but the hypothesis remained relatively obscure until the recent report of a patient with rapidly progressive MS and positive cerebrospinal fluid (CSF) culture for *C. pneumoniae* who improved markedly after antibiotic treatment (Sriram et al. 1998). This observation was followed by a systematic study of 37 patients with MS and 27 controls with other neurological diseases (Sriram et al. 1999). *C. pneumoniae* was cultured from the CSF in 64% of cases and 11% of controls; moreover, 97% of the cases were positive for the presence of *C. pneumoniae* DNA by PCR, compared to 18% of the controls. These findings renewed the interest in Chlamydia as a possible cause of MS and several groups of investigators have attempted to reproduce them, though most have been unsuccessful (Boman et al. 2000; Hammerschlag et al. 2000; Li et al. 2000; Morré et al. 2000; Poland and Rice 2000; Pucci et al. 2000; Gieffers et al. 2001). Results of serological analyses are also conflicting (Boman et al. 2000; Krametter et al. 2001; Munger et al. 2003). The lack of consensus among *C. pneumoniae*–MS association studies may be due in part to the lack of standardized laboratory procedures for detection and isolation of *C. pneumoniae* (Peeling et al. 2000; Tompkins et al. 2000), small sample sizes, and use of different control groups.

Lifestyle and Other Factors

Cigarette Smoking

Several reports have described an aggravation of MS symptoms after smoking (Franklin and Brickner 1947; Spillane 1955; Anonymous 1964; Perkin et al. 1975; Perkin and Rose 1976; Emre and de Decker 1987, 1992), and a positive association between cigarette smoking before age of onset and risk of MS was found in a case–control study in Israel (Antonovsky et al. 1965) and in one in Canada (Ghadirian et al. 2001), although not in others (Warren et al. 1982). Most notably, a positive association was found in each of the three cohort studies that have addressed this question. Two studies in the United Kingdom reported relative risks (RR) of 1.8 (95% CI 0.8–3.6) [(Villard-Mackintosh and Vessey 1993) and 1.4 (95% CI 0.9–2.2) (Thorogood and Hannaford 1998)] among women smoking 15 or more cigarettes per day as compared with never-smokers. In the third study, conducted among U.S. nurses, the RR was 1.7 (95% CI 1.2–2.4; $p < 0.01$) for women who smoked 25 or more pack-years as compared with never-smokers (Hernán et al. 2001a); this association was not explained by latitude or ancestry. The combined evidence from these studies and the lack of alternative explanations suggest that smoking could increase the risk of MS. This potential effect could be due to the neurotoxic (Smith et al. 1963) or immunomodulatory (Francus et al. 1988; Sopori and Kozak 1998) effects of components of cigarette smoke. These mechanisms are indirectly supported by the association of cigarette smoking with optic neuropathy (Cuba Neuropathy Field Investigation Team 1995) and autoimmune diseases such as systemic lupus erythematosus (Hardy et al. 1998) and rheumatoid arthritis (Vessey et al. 1987; Hernandez Avila et al. 1990; Heliovaara et al. 1993; Voigt et al. 1994; Silman et al. 1996). Finally, cigarette smoke increases the frequency and duration of respiratory infections (Graham 1990) that may contribute to the etiology of MS. If these findings are confirmed, cigarette smoking may emerge as the first modifiable risk factor for MS. Further, differences in smoking habits across populations could explain some of the variation in MS incidence, and particularly variation in the sex ratio, because of the wide range of smoking prevalence in men and women in different countries and periods.

Diet

Example 8–5 The observation in Norway of a lower prevalence of MS in coastal fishing communities, where the diet is richer in polyunsaturated fish oils, than in agricultural inland communities, where meat and dairy provide most of the fat, suggests that animal fat or saturated fat may increase the risk of MS (Swank et al. 1952). This hypothesis was supported by a significant positive correlation between consumption of calories from animal sources and prevalence of MS in a comparative study of 22 countries (Alter et al. 1974). The pooled results of three randomized trials suggested that high amounts of polyunsaturated fat may modestly reduce the severity and duration of relapses (Dworkin et al. 1984), but a 0.5 gram n-3 polyunsaturated fat supplement was not shown to be beneficial after 2 years (Bates et al. 1989). Consumption of meat (Lauer 1989a, 1989b, 1991) or milk (Agranoff and Goldberg 1974) has also been related to risk of MS in ecological investigations but not in case–control studies (Antonovsky et al. 1965; Cendrowski et al. 1969; Poskanzer et al. 1980; Butcher 1986). No significant associations were found between intake of total fat, cholesterol, specific fatty acids, dairy products, seafood, poultry, or red meats and risk of MS in a large prospective study (Zhang et al. 2000). An increase in 1% of energy from linolenic acid was associated with a lower risk (RR = 0.3,

95% CI 0.1–1.1), but this association was of borderline significance and needs confirmation (Zhang et al. 2000).

It has also been suggested that low concentrations of antioxidant enzymes leave the white matter vulnerable to oxygen free radicals and lipid peroxidation, which could be involved in the etiology of MS (Mickel 1975; Hunter et al. 1985; Clausen et al. 1988; Langemann et al. 1992). Epidemiological data on intake of antioxidants and MS are sparse. In a case–control study, intake of vitamin C was associated with a lower risk of MS, but no associations were found with vitamin E or carotene (Ghadirian et al. 1998). Intake of fruits and vegetables, which are rich in carotenoids and other dietary antioxidants, was not associated with risk of MS in several case–control studies (Antonovsky et al. 1965; Warren et al. 1982; Berr et al. 1989; Gusev et al. 1996; Ghadirian et al. 1998). In the only prospective investigation, no associations were found between intake of vitamin E, vitamin C, or specific carotenoids and risk of MS (Zhang et al. 2001).

A protective role of vitamin D has also been proposed, and could explain in part the latitude gradient, but support for this hypothesis is so far limited to experimental animal data (Hayes 2000). Because of the consistent contribution of dietary intake and sunlight to vitamin D status, the potential protective effect of this vitamin will be better assessed in prospective serological studies. Diet could also be important because of specific antigenic stimulation rather than the effect of specific nutrients. In an experiment in rodents, the immune response to a cow milk protein, butyrophilin, led to encephalitis through antigenic mimicry with MOG (Stefferl et al. 2000; Winer et al. 2001). These studies suggest a mechanism by which consumption of milk products could affect the risk of MS, but, as discussed above, epidemiological evidence supporting this association is weak.

In summary, a role of diet in the etiology of MS remains unproven but cannot be excluded, as most reported investigations were retrospective and prone to several sources of bias (Willett 1998). A potential beneficial effect of linolenic acid and vitamin D should be further addressed in larger prospective investigations.

Hormonal Factors

Sex hormones modulate the immune response and could thus influence the onset and progression of MS (Grossman 1985; Whitacre et al. 1999, 2001). Low levels of estrogens seem to favor a pro-inflammatory type 1 response in T cells, whereas high levels of estrogens and progesterone favor a type 2 response. In animals, exogenous estrogens suppress experimental autoimmune encephalomyelitis (Kim et al. 1999; Bebo et al. 2001). Relapses of MS are rare during pregnancy, when levels of circulating estrogens are high, but increase in frequency during the puerperium, so that overall there seems to be little impact of pregnancy on the progression of the disease (Confavreux et al. 1998). Also, there is no evidence in prospective studies that parity or age at first birth affects the risk of MS (Vessey et al. 1976; Thorogood and Hannaford 1998; Hernán et al. 2000). The effect of use of oral contraceptives on risk of MS was also investigated in the same cohorts, but no significant associations were found (Vessey et al. 1976; Thorogood and Hannaford 1998; Hernán et al. 2000). The largest of these investigations comprised over 200,000 women followed for up to 18 years and among whom 315 cases of definite or probable MS were documented. The RR of MS among women who used oral contraceptives for 8 years or more as compared with never-users was 1.2 (95% CI 0.8–1.2) (Hernán et al. 2000). Therefore, a protective effect of oral contraceptives seems unlikely.

Other Factors

It has been proposed that trauma could increase the risk of MS by disrupting the blood–brain barrier (Poser 1987), but overall little evidence supports this hypothesis

(Compston 1998a). Recently, concerns were raised about the possibility that administration of the hepatitis B vaccine may increase the risk of MS (Marshall 1998; Touze et al. 2000), but no associations between the vaccine and risk of MS (Ascherio et al. 2001a) or MS relapses (Confavreux et al. 2001) were found in prospective studies. Other environmental factors investigated in relation to MS include exposures to heavy metals, solvents, and other contaminants (Eastman et al. 1973; Stein et al. 1987; Irvine et al. 1988; Ingalls 1989; Landtblom 1997); their roles remain uncertain.

Prognostic Studies

Since MS is a chronic and often progressive disease with a variable course, the investigation of factors that may modify the course of the illness and its effects on the quality of life is of great importance. Randomized trials typically include selected groups of patients, and the follow-up rarely extends beyond a few years. Thus, complementary information from large, long-term, prospective studies is important.

Prognostic Factors

Factors predictive of shorter survival after the onset of MS include late age at onset (Riise et al. 1988; Poser et al. 1989; Midgard et al. 1995; Wallin et al. 2000), male gender (McAlpine 1961; Poser et al. 1986; Wynn et al. 1990; Wallin et al. 2000), an initial progressive course (Poser et al. 1986; Phadke 1987; Riise et al. 1988; Midgard et al. 1995), and absence of sensory symptoms at onset (Midgard et al. 1995). The shorter life expectancy observed among males and those with an older age at MS onset may in part reflect general population trends. Among U.S. Army veterans, there was a significant difference in survival rates between men and women with MS, but this difference was similar to that found among U.S. Army personnel without MS (Wallin et al. 2000). In Olmsted County, Minnesota, however, MS was associated with higher mortality in men, but not in women (Wynn et al. 1990).

There is some disagreement as to whether early age at onset and female gender are prognostic for a favorable disability outcome independent of initial disease course (McAlpine 1961; Leibowitz and Alter 1970; Kurtzke et al. 1977; Confavreux et al. 1980; Clark et al. 1982; Detels et al. 1982; Poser et al. 1982; Verjans et al. 1983; Visscher et al. 1984; Thompson et al. 1986; Lauer and Firnhaber 1987; Phadke 1990; Weinshenker et al. 1991; Riise et al. 1992; Runmarker and Andersen 1993; Amato et al. 1999; Hammond et al. 2000b; Liguori et al. 2000). In some studies, gender was not a significant predictor of disability outcome after adjustment for type of MS, onset symptoms, and disease duration, whereas age at onset remained significant (Weinshenker et al. 1991a; Hammond et al. 2000b). In others, neither gender nor age at onset was a significant predictor of disability after controlling for type of MS and symptoms (Amato et al. 1999). Onset with motor symptoms has been associated with a poor MS course as compared with onset with sensory symptoms (Clark et al. 1982; Visscher et al. 1984; Sanders et al. 1986; Phadke 1990; Amato et al. 1999) or optic neuritis (McAlpine 1961; Poser et al. 1982; Sanders et al. 1986; Optic Neuritis Study Group 1997). These differences remained significant after adjustment for gender, age at onset, and disease course (Weinshenker et al. 1991; Amato et al. 1999; Hammond et al. 2000b). Some studies, however, have found no predictive value of onset symptoms (Kurtzke et al. 1977; Confavreux et al. 1980; Lauer and Firnhaber 1987) and one study reported a favorable prognosis with motor symptoms at onset (Leibowitz and Alter 1970). The HLA-DR2 genotype has also been associated with a more severe disease course in some studies (Jersild et al. 1973; Engell et al. 1982; Duquette et al. 1985) but not in others (Poser et al. 1981; Madigand et al. 1982; Dejaegher et al. 1983). A recent prospective study in The Netherlands assessed whether systemic in-fections contributed to the natural course of exacerbations (Buljevac et al. 2002). The investigators observed 167 infections and 145 exacerbations in 73 patients with relapsing-remitting MS during 6466 patient weeks. Exacerbations increased twofold during a predefined period of 2 weeks before until 5 weeks after onset of a clinical infection (mainly upper airway infections). Systemic infections may lead to more sustained damage than other exacerbations. Other factors found predictive of a favorable disability outcome include monoregional onset symptoms (Runmarker and Andersen 1993), complete recovery from relapses (Runmarker and Andersen 1993), and longer interval between early relapses (Confavreux et al. 1980; Thompson et al. 1986; Phadke 1990; Amato et al. 1999; Myhr et al. 2001).

Future Directions and Conclusions

Epidemiological studies support the existence of a strong but still unidentified environmental determinant(s) of MS. Less certain is whether this is an infectious or a noninfectious agent. Several aspects in the epidemiology of MS are consistent with the hypothesis that MS is an autoimmune reaction to infection with one or more microbes, and there is strong, albeit nonconclusive, evidence that EBV alone or in combination with other viruses is involved in the etiology of MS. This hypothesis does not exclude a role of noninfectious factors, such as cigarette smoking and diet.

Familial studies indicate that the aggregation of MS within families is clearly due to genetic and not to environmental factors. The risk of MS among genetically predisposed individuals appears to be over 100-fold higher than in the general population, yet the responsible genes have not been identified. It is now recognized that two or more genes interact in increasing the risk of MS; only large investigations and pooling of data from different studies will provide the power needed to detect these epistatic effects. Advances in both genome-screening techniques and statistical methods will be critical to this search, but its success will also depend on the complexity of nature, as genetic heterogeneity and poligenicity could present formidable obstacles. The research on environmental and genetic determinants will probably converge and spur each other, as interactions are most likely to exist between genes and environment.

References

Agranoff BW, Goldberg D. Diet and the geographical distribution of multiple sclerosis. *Lancet* 1974;2:1061–1066.

Akesson E, Oturai A, Berg J, et al. A genome-wide screen for linkage in Nordic sib-pairs with multiple sclerosis. *Genes Immun* 2002; 3:279–285.

Akhyani N, Berti R, Brennan MB, et al. Tissue distribution and variant characterization of human herpesvirus (HHV)-6: increased prevalence of HHV-6A in patients with multiple sclerosis. *J Infect Dis* 2000;182:1321–1325.

Alter M, Halpern L, Kurland LT, et al. Multiple sclerosis in Israel. *Arch Neurol* 1962;7:253–263.

Alter M, Kahana E, Loewenson R. Migration and risk of multiple sclerosis. *Neurology* 1978;28:1089–1093.

Alter M, Leibowitz U, Speer J. Risk of multiple sclerosis related to age at immigration to Israel. *Arch Neurol* 1966;15:234–237.

Alter M, Yamoor M, Harshe M. Multiple sclerosis and nutrition. *Arch Neurol* 1974;31:267–272.

Alvord EC Jr, Jahnke U, Fischer EH, et al. The multiple causes of multiple sclerosis: the importance of age of infections in childhood. *J Child Neurol* 1987;2:313–321.

Amato MP, Ponziani G, Bartolozzi ML, Siracusa G. A prospective study on the natural history of multiple sclerosis: clues to the conduct and interpretation of clinical trials. *J Neurol Sci* 1999;168:96–106.

American Group. A meta-analysis of genomic screens in multiple sclerosis. *Mult Scler* 2001;7:3–11.

Anonymous. Smoking and multiple sclerosis. *BMJ* 1964;1:773.

Antonovsky A, Leibowitz U, Smith HA, et al. Epidemiologic study of multiple sclerosis in Israel. *Arch Neurol* 1965;13:183–193.

Ascherio A, Munger KL, Lennette ET, et al. Epstein-Barr virus antibodies and risk of multiple sclerosis: a prospective study. *JAMA* 2001a;286:3083–3088.

Ascherio A, Munch M. Epstein-Barr virus and multiple sclerosis. *Epidemiology* 2000;11:1–5.

Ascherio A, Zhang SM, Hernán MA, et al. Hepatitis B vaccination and the risk of multiple sclerosis. *N Engl J Med* 2001b;344:327–332.

Bansil S, Troiano R, Dowling PC, Cook SD. Measles vaccination does not prevent multiple sclerosis. *Neuroepidemiology* 1990;9:248–254.

Bates D, Cartlidge NEF, French JM, et al. A double-blind controlled trial of long chain n-3 polyunsaturated fatty acids in the treatment of multiple sclerosis. *J Neurol Neurosurg Psychiatry* 1989;52:18–22.

Baum HM, Rothschild BB. The incidence and prevalence of reported multiple sclerosis. *Ann Neurol* 1981;10:420–428.

Beall SS, Concannon P, Charmley P, et al. The germline repertoire of T cell receptor β-chain genes in patients with chronic progressive multiple sclerosis. *J Neuroimmunol* 1989;21:59–66.

Bebo BF Jr, Fyfe-Johnson A, Adlard K, et al. Low-dose estrogen therapy ameliorates experimental autoimmune encephalomyelitis in two different inbred mouse strains. *J Immunol* 2001;166:2080–2089.

Beebe G, Kurtzke JF, Kurland LT, et al. Studies on the natural history of multiple sclerosis. 3. Epidemiologic analysis of the Army experience in World War II. *Neurology* 1967;17:1–17.

Berr C, Puel J, Clanet M, et al. Risk factors in multiple sclerosis: a population-based case–control study in Hautes-Pyrenees, France. *Acta Neurol Scand* 1989;80:46–50.

Bobowick AR, Kurtzke JF, Brody JA, et al. Twin study of multiple sclerosis: an epidemiologic inquiry. *Neurology* 1978;28:978–987.

Boman J, Roblin PM, Sundstrom P, et al. Failure to detect *Chlamydia pneumoniae* in the central nervous system of patients with MS. *Neurology* 2000;54:265.

Bray PF, Bloomer LC, Salmon VC, et al. Epstein-Barr virus infection and antibody synthesis in patients with multiple sclerosis. *Arch Neurol* 1983;40:406–408.

Broadley S, Sawcer S, D'Alfonso S, et al. A genome screen for multiple sclerosis in Italian families. *Genes Immun* 2001;2:205–210.

Brodsky AL, Heath CW Jr. Infectious mononucleosis: epidemiologic patterns at United States colleges and universities. *Am J Epidemiol* 1972;96:87–93.

Brody JA. Epidemiology of multiple sclerosis and a possible virus aetiology. *Lancet* 1972;2:173–176.

Buljevac D, Flach HZ, Hop WCJ, et al. Prospective study on the relationship between infections and multiple sclerosis exacerbations. *Brain* 2002;125:952–960.

Bulman DE, Ebers GC. The geography of multiple sclerosis reflects genetic susceptibility. *J Tropic Geograph Neurol* 1992;2:66–72.

Butcher PJ. Milk consumption and multiple sclerosis—an etiological hypothesis. *Med Hypothes* 1986;19:169–178.

Carton H, Vlietinck R, Debruyne J, et al. Risks of multiple sclerosis in relatives of patients in Flanders, Belgium. *J Neurol Neurosurg Psychiatry* 1997;62:329–333.

Carvalho RP, Evans AS, Pannuti CS, et al. EBV infections in Brazil. III—Infectious mononucleosis. *Rev Inst Med Trop Sao Paulo* 1981;23:167–172.

Cendrowski W, Wender M, Dominik W, et al. Epidemiological study of multiple sclerosis in Western Poland. *Eur Neurol* 1969;2:90–108.

Chan WW. Eskimos and multiple sclerosis. *Lancet* 1977;1:1370.

Chang RS, Char DFB, Jones JH, Halstead SB. Incidence of infectious mononucleosis at the Universities of California and Hawaii. *J Infect Dis* 1979;140:479–486.

Clark VA, Detels R, Visscher BR, et al. Factors associated with a malignant or benign course of multiple sclerosis. *JAMA* 1982;248:8568–8560.

Clausen J, Jensen GE, Nielsen SA. Selenium in chronic neurologic diseases. *Biol Trace Element Res* 1988;15:179–203.

Compston A. Distribution of multiple sclerosis. In: Compston A, ed. McAlpine's Multiple Sclerosis, 3rd edition. New York: Churchill Livingstone, 1998a, pp 63–100.

Compston A. Genetic susceptibility to multiple sclerosis. In: Compston A, ed. McAlpine's Multiple Sclerosis, 3rd edition. New York: Churchill Livingstone, 1998b, pp 101–142.

Confavreux C, Aimard G, Devic M. Course and prognosis of multiple sclerosis assessed by the computerized data processing of 349 patients. *Brain* 1980;103:281–300.

Confavreux C, Hutchinson M, Hours MM, et al. Rate of pregnancy-related relapse in multiple sclerosis. Pregnancy in multiple sclerosis group. *N Engl J Med* 1998;339:285–291.

Confavreux C, Suissa S, Saddier P, et al. Vaccinations and the risk of relapse in multiple sclerosis. Vaccines in Multiple Sclerosis Study Group. *N Engl J Med* 2001;344:319–326.

Cook SD, Rohowsky-Kochan C, Bansil S, Dowling PC. Evidence for multiple sclerosis as an infectious disease. *Acta Neurol Scand* 1995;161(Suppl):34–42.

Coraddu F, Sawcer S, D'Alfonso S, et al. A genome screen for multiple sclerosis in Sardinian multiplex families. *Eur J Hum Genet* 2001;9:621–626.

Cremer NE, Johnson KP, Fein G, Likosky WH. Comprehensive viral immunology of multiple sclerosis. II. Analysis of serum and CSF antibodies by standard serologic methods. *Arch Neurol* 1980;37:610–615.

Cuba Neuropathy Field Investigation Team. Epidemic optic neuropathy in Cuba—clinical characterization and risk factors. The Cuba Neuropathy Field Investigation Team. *N Engl J Med* 1995;333:1176–1182.

Cuomo L, Angeloni A, Zompetta C, et al. Human herpesvirus 6 variant A, but not variant B, infects EBV-positive B lymphoid cells, activating the latent EBV genome through a BZLF-1-dependent mechanism. *AIDS Res Hum Retroviruses* 1995;11:1241–1245.

Davenport CB. Multiple sclerosis from the standpoint of geographic distribution and race. *Arch Neurol Psychiatry* 1922;8:51–58.

Dean G. Annual incidence, prevalence, and mortality of multiple sclerosis in white South-African-born and in white immigrants to South Africa. *BMJ* 1967;2:724–730.

Dean G. Was there an epidemic of multiple sclerosis in the Faroe Islands? *Neuroepidemiology* 1988;7:165–167.

Dean G, Brady R, McLoughlin H, et al. Motor neurone disease and multiple sclerosis among immigrants to Britain. *Br J Prev Soc Med* 1977;31:141–147.

Dean G, Grimaldi G, Kelly R, Karhausen L. Multiple sclerosis in southern Europe. I: Prevalence in Sicily in 1975. *J Epidemiol Community Health* 1979;33:107–110.

Dean G, McLoughlin H, Brady R, et al. Multiple sclerosis among immigrants in Greater London. *BMJ* 1976;1:861–864.

Dejaegher L, de Bruyere M, Ketelaer P, Carton H. HLA antigens and progression of multiple sclerosis. Part II. *J Neurol* 1983;229:167–174.

de Jong BA, Huizinga TWJ, Zanelli E et al. Evidence for additional genetic risk indicators of relapse-onset MS within the HLA region. *Neurology* 2002;59:549–555.

Detels R, Brody JA, Edgar AH. Multiple sclerosis among American, Japanese and Chinese immigrants to California and Washington. *J Chron Dis* 1972;25:3–10.

Detels R, Clark VA, Valdiviezo NL, et al. Factors associated with a rapid course of multiple sclerosis. *Arch Neurol* 1982;39:337–341.

Detels R, Visscher BR, Haile RW, et al. Multiple sclerosis and age at migration. *Am J Epidemiol* 1978;108:386–393.

Duquette P, Decary F, Pleines J, et al. Clinical sub-groups of multiple sclerosis in relation to HLA: DR alleles as possible markers of disease progression. *Can J Neurol Sci* 1985; 12:106–110.

Dworkin RH, Bates D, Paty DW. Linoleic acid and multiple sclerosis. *Neurology* 1984;34: 1141–1445.

Eastman R, Sheridan J, Poskanzer DC. Multiple sclerosis clustering in a small Massachusetts community, with possible common exposure 23 years before onset. *N Engl J Med* 1973; 289:793–794.

Ebers G. Natural history of multiple sclerosis. In: Compston A, ed. McAlpine's Multiple Sclerosis, 3rd edition. New York: Churchill Livingstone, 1998, pp 191–221.

Ebers GC, Bulman DE, Sadovnick AD, et al. A population-based study of multiple sclerosis in twins. *N Engl J Med* 1986;315:1638–1642.

Ebers GC, Kukay K, Bulman DE, et al. A full genome search in multiple sclerosis. *Nat Genet* 1996;13:472–476.

Ebers GC, Sadovnick AD, Risch NJ. A genetic basis for familial aggregation in multiple sclerosis. Canadian Collaborative Study Group. *Nature* 1995;377:150–151.

Ebers GC, Yee IM, Sadovnick AD, Duquette P. Conjugal multiple sclerosis: population-based prevalence and recurrence risks in offspring. Canadian Collaborative Study Group. *Ann Neurol* 2000;48:927–931.

Elian M, Dean G. Multiple sclerosis among the United Kingdom–born children of immigrants from the West Indies. *J Neurol Neurosurg Psychiatry* 1987;50:327–332.

Elian M, Dean G. Motor neuron disease and multiple sclerosis among immigrants to England from the Indian subcontinent, the Caribbean, and East and West Africa. *J Neurol Neurosurg Psychiatry* 1993;56: 454–457.

Elian M, Nightingale S, Dean G. Multiple sclerosis among United Kingdom–born children of immigrants from the Indian subcontinent, Africa and the West Indies. *J Neurol Neurosurg Psychiatry* 1990;53:906–911.

Emre M, de Decker C. Nicotine and CNS. *Neurology* 1987;37:1887–1888.

Emre M, de Decker C. Effects of cigarette smoking on motor functions in patients with multiple sclerosis. *Arch Neurol* 1992;49:1243–1247.

Engell T. A clinico-pathoanatomical study of multiple sclerosis diagnosis. *Acta Neurol Scand* 1988;78:39–44.

Engell T, Raun NE, Thomsen M, Platz P. HLA and heterogeneity of multiple sclerosis. *Neurology* 1982;32:1043–1046.

Eoli M, Wood NW, Kellar-Wood HF, et al. No linkage between multiple sclerosis and the T cell receptor alpha chain locus. *J Neurol Sci* 1994;124:32–37.

Epplen C, Jäckel S, Santos EJM, et al. Genetic predisposition to multiple sclerosis as revealed by immunoprinting. *Ann Neurol* 1997;41:341–352.

Ferner RE, Hughes RA, Johnson MR. Neurofibromatosis 1 and multiple sclerosis. *J Neurol Neurosurg Psychiatry* 1995;58:582–585.

Ferrante P, Castellani P, Barbi M, Bergamini F. The Italian Cooperative Multiple Sclerosis case–control study: preliminary results on viral antibodies. *Ital J Neurol Sci* 1987;Suppl 6:45–50.

Fillet A-M, Lozeron P, Agut H, et al. HHV-6 and multiple sclerosis. *Nat Med* 1998;4:537.

Flamand L, Menezes J. Cyclic AMP–responsive element-dependent activation of Epstein-Barr virus zebra promoter by human herpesvirus 6. *J Virol* 1996;70:1784–1791.

Fog M, Kyllested K. Prevalence of disseminated sclerosis in the Faroes, the Orkneys and Shetland. *Acta Neurol Scand* 1966;42(Suppl 19):9–11.

Forbes RB, Swingler RJ. An epidemiologic study of multiple sclerosis in Northern Ireland. *Neurology* 1999;52:215–216.

Francus T, Klein RF, Staiano-Coico L, et al. Effects of tobacco glycoprotein (TGP) on the immune system. II. TGP stimulates the proliferation of human T cells and the differentiation of human B cells into Ig secreting cells. *J Immunol* 1988;140:1823–1829.

Franklin CR, Brickner RM. Vasospasm associated with multiple sclerosis. *Arch Nerurol Psychiatry* 1947;58:125–162.

Fugger L, Morling N, Sandberg-Wollheim M, et al. Tumor necrosis factor alpha gene polymorphism in multiple sclerosis and optic neuritis. *J Neuroimmunol* 1990a;27:85–88.

Fugger L, Sandberg-Wollheim M, Morling N, et al. The germline repertoire of T-cell receptor beta chain genes in patients with relapsing/remitting multiple sclerosis or optic neuritis. *Immunogenetics* 1990b;31:278–280.

Gale CR, Martyn CN. Migrant studies in multiple sclerosis. *Prog Neurobiol* 1995;47:425–448.

Ghadirian P, Dadgostar B, Azani R, Maisonneuve P. A case–control study of the association between sociodemographic, lifestyle and medical history factors and multiple sclerosis. *Can J Public Health* 2001;92:281–285.

Ghadirian P, Jain M, Ducic S, et al. Nutritional factors in the aetiology of multiple sclerosis: a case–control study in Montreal, Canada. *Int J Epidemiol* 1998;27:845–852.

Gieffers J, Pohl D, Treib J, et al. Presence of *Chlamydia pneumoniae* DNA in the cerebral spinal fluid is a common phenomenon in a variety of neurological diseases and not restricted to multiple sclerosis. *Ann Neurol* 2001;49:585–589.

Giordano M, D'Alfonso S, Momigliano-Richiardi P. Genetics of multiple sclerosis: linkage and association studies. *Am J Pharmacogenomics* 2002;2:37–58.

Goldberg SH, Albright AV, Lisak RP, González-Scarano F. Polymerase chain reaction analysis of human herpesvirus-6 sequences in the sera and cerebrospinal fluid of patients with multiple sclerosis. *J Neurovirol* 1999;5:134–139.

Graham NM. The epidemiology of acute respiratory infections in children and adults: a global perspective. *Epidemiol Rev* 1990;12: 149–178.

Granieri E, Casetta I. Part III: selected reviews. Common childhood and adolescent infections and multiple sclerosis. *Neurology* 1997;49(Suppl 2):S42–S54.

Grønning M, Riise T, Kvale G, et al. Incidence of multiple sclerosis in Hordaland, western Norway: a fluctuating pattern. *Neuroepidemiology* 1991;10:53–61.

Grossman CJ. Interactions between the gonadal steroids and the immune system. *Science* 1985;227:257–261.

Gusev E, Boiko A, Lauer K, et al.. Environmental risk factors in MS: a case–control study in Moscow. *Acta Neurol Scand* 1996; 94:386–394.

Haahr S, Koch-Henriksen N, Moeller-Larsen A, et al. Increased risk of multiple sclerosis after late Epstein-Barr virus infection. *Acta Neurol Scand* 1997;169(Suppl):70–75.

Hafler DA. The distinction blurs between an autoimmune versus microbial hypothesis in multiple sclerosis. *J Clin Invest* 1999;104: 527–529.

Haines JL, Ter-Minassian M, Bazyk A, et al. A complete genomic screen for multiple sclerosis underscores a role for the major histocompatability complex. The Multiple Sclerosis Genetics Group. *Nat Genet* 1996;13: 469–471.

Hallee TJ, Evans AS, Niederman JC, et al. Infectious mononucleosis at the United States Military Academy. A prospective study of a single class over four years. *Yale J Biol Med* 1974;3:182–195.

Hammerschlag MR, Ke Z, Lu F, et al. Is chlamydia pneumoniae present in brain lesions of patients with multiple sclerosis? *J Clin Microbiol* 2000;38:4274–4276.

Hammond SR, English DR, McLeod JG. The age-range of risk of developing multiple sclerosis: evidence from a migrant population in Australia. *Brain* 2000a;123:968–974.

Hammond SR, McLeod JG, Macaskill P, English DR. Multiple sclerosis in Australia: prognostic factors. *J Clin Neurosci* 2000b;7: 16–19.

Hammond SR, McLeod JG, Millingen KS, et al. The epidemiology of multiple sclerosis in three Australian cities: Perth, Newcastle and Hobart. *Brain* 1988;111:1–25.

Hardy CJ, Palmer BP, Muir KR, et al. Smoking history, alcohol consumption, and systemic lupus erythematosus: a case–control study. *Ann Rheum Dis* 1998;57:451–455.

Hashimoto LL, Mak TW, Ebers GC. T cell receptor alpha chain polymorphisms in multiple sclerosis. *J Neuroimmunol* 1992;40:41–48.

Hayes CE. Vitamin D: a natural inhibitor of multiple sclerosis. *Proc Nutr Soc* 2000;59: 531–535.

He B, Navikas V, Lundahl J, et al. Tumor necrosis factor alpha-308 alleles in multiple sclerosis and optic neuritis. *J Neuroimmunol* 1995;63:143–147.

Heath CW Jr., Brodsky AL, Potolsky AI. Infectious mononucleosis in a general population. *Am J Epidemiol* 1972;95:46–52.

Heliovaara M, Aho K, Aromaa A, Knekt P, Reunanen A. Smoking and risk of rheumatoid arthritis. *J Rheumatol* 1993;20:1830–1835.

Heltberg A, Holm NV. Concordance in Twins and Recurrence in Sibships in Multiple Sclerosis. London: Lancet, 1982.

Hernán M, Hohol M, Olek M, et al. Oral contraceptives and the incidence of multiple sclerosis. *Neurology* 2000;55:848–854.

Hernán MA, Olek MJ, Ascherio A. Geographic variation of MS incidence in two prospective studies of US women. *Neurology* 1999;53: 1711–1718.

Hernán M, Olek M, Ascherio A. Cigarette smoking and incidence of multiple sclerosis. *Am J Epidemiol* 2001a;154:69–74.

Hernán M, Zhang SM, Lipworth L, et al. Multiple sclerosis and age at infection with common viruses. *Epidemiology* 2001b;12:301–306.

Hernandez Avila M, Liang MH, Willett WC, et al. Reproductive factors, smoking, and the risk for rheumatoid arthritis. *Epidemiology* 1990;1:285–291.

Herndon RM. The changing pattern of misdiagnosis in multiple sclerosis. In: Hernson RM, Seil FS, eds. Multiple Sclerosis: Current Status of Research and Treatment. New York: Demos, 1994, pp 149–155.

Hesse J, Ibsen KK, Krabbe S, Uldall P. Prevalence of antibodies to Epstein-Barr Virus (EBV) in childhood and adolescence in Denmark. *Scand J Infect Dis* 1983;15:335–338.

Hillert J, Leng C, Olerup O. No association with germline T cell receptor beta-chain gene alleles or haplotypes in Swedish patients with multiple sclerosis. *J Neuroimmunol* 1991;32: 141–147.

Hillert J, Leng C, Olerup O. T-cell receptor alpha chain germline gene polymorphisms in multiple sclerosis. *Neurology* 1992;42:80–84.

Hilton AA, Slavin AJ, Hilton DJ, Bernard CC. Characterization of cDNA and genomic clones encoding human myelin oligodendrocyte glycoprotein. *J Neurochem* 1995;65: 309–318.

Hilton DA, Love S, Fletcher A, Pringle JH. Absence of Epstein-Barr virus RNA in multiple sclerosis as assessed by in situ hybridisation. *J Neurol Neurosurg Psychiatry* 1994;57: 975–976.

Hook EB, Regal RR. Capture–recapture methods in epidemiology: methods and limitations. *Epidemiol Rev* 1995;17:243–264.

Hunter MIS, Nlemadim BC, Davidson DLW. Lipid peroxidation products and antioxidant proteins in plasma and cerebrospinal fluid from multiple sclerosis patients. *Neurochem Res* 1985;10:1645–1652.

Hunter SF, Hafler DA. Ubiquitous pathogens: links between infection and autoimmunity in MS? *Neurology* 2000;55:164–165.

Ingalls TH. Clustering of multiple sclerosis in Galion, Ohio, 1982–1985. *Am J Forensic Med Pathol* 1989;10:213–215.

Irvine DG, Schiefer HB, Hader WJ. Geotoxicology of multiple sclerosis: the Henribourg, Saskatchewan, cluster focus. II. The soil. *Sci Total Environ* 1988;77:175–188.

Isager H, Larsen S, Hyllested K. School contact between patients with multiple sclerosis. *Int J Epidemiol* 1980;9:145–147.

Jacobs L, Salazar AM, Herndon RM, et al. Multicentre double-blind study of effect of intrathecally administered natural human fibroblast interferon on exacerbations of multiple sclerosis. *Lancet* 1986;2:1411–1413.

Jadin J. Rickettsial diseases and multiple sclerosis. *Ann Soc Belge Med Trop* 1962;42:321–345.

Jersild C, Fog T, Hansen GS, et al. Histocompatibility determinants in multiple sclerosis, with special reference to clinical course. *Lancet* 1973;2:1221–1225.

Kahana E, Zilber N, Abramson JH, et al. Multiple sclerosis: genetic versus environmental aetiology: epidemiology in Israel updated. *Neurology* 1994;241:341–346.

Kalman B, Lublin FD. The genetics of multiple sclerosis. A review. *Biomed Pharmacother* 1999;53:358–370.

Kim S, Liva SM, Dalal MA, et al. Estriol ameliorates autoimmune demyelinating disease: implications for multiple sclerosis. *Neurology* 1999;52:1230–1238.

Kinnunen E, Juntunen J, Ketonen L, et al. Genetic susceptibility to multiple sclerosis. A co-twin study of a nationwide series. *Arch Neurol* 1988;45:1108–1111.

Kirk CW, Droogan AG, Hawkins SA, et al. Tumour necrosis factor microsatellites show association with multiple sclerosis. *J Neurol Sci* 1997;47:21–25.

Knox KK, Brewer JH, Henry JM, et al. Human herpesvirus 6 and multiple sclerosis: systemic active infections in patients with early disease. *Clin Infect Dis* 2000;31:894–903.

Koch-Henriksen N. Multiple sclerosis in Scandinavia and Finland. *Acta Neurol Scand* 1995;161:55–59.

Koch-Henriksen N, Hyllested K. Epidemiology of multiple sclerosis: incidence and prevalence rates in Denmark 1948–64 based on the Danish Multiple Sclerosis Registry. *Acta Neurol Scand* 1988;78:369–380.

Krametter D, Niederwieser G, Berghold A, et al. *Chlamydia pneumoniae* in multiple sclerosis: humoral immune responses in serum and cerebrospinal fluid and correlation with disease activity marker. *Mult Scler* 2001;7:13–18.

Kuokkanen S, Gschwend M, Rioux JD, et al. Genomewide scan of multiple sclerosis in Finnish multiplex families. *Am J Hum Genet* 1997;61:1379–1387.

Kurland LT. The frequency and geographic distribution of multiple sclerosis as indicated by mortality statistics and morbidity surveys in the United States and Canada. *Am J Hyg* 1952;55:457–476.

Kurland LT, Stasio A, Reed D. An appraisal of population studies of multiple sclerosis. *Ann NY Acad Sci* 1965;122:520–541.

Kurtzke JF. Multiple sclerosis among immigrants. *BMJ* 1976;1:1527–1528.

Kurtzke JF. Multiple sclerosis in the Faroe Islands. II. Clinical update, transmission, and the nature of MS. *Neurology* 1986;36:307–328.

Kurtzke JF. Multiple sclerosis: what's in a name? *Neurology* 1988;38:309–316.

Kurtzke JF. Epidemiologic evidence for multiple sclerosis as an infection. *Clin Microbiol Rev* 1993;6:382–427.

Kurtzke JF. MS epidemiology worldwide. One view of current status. *Acta Neurol Scand* 1995;161(Suppl):23–33.

Kurtzke JF, Beebe GW, Nagler B, et al. Studies on the natural history of multiple sclerosis—8. Early prognostic features of the later course of the illness. *J Chron Dis* 1977;30: 819–830.

Kurtzke JF, Beebe GW, Norman JE. Epidemiology of multiple sclerosis in U.S. veterans: 1. Race, sex, and geographic distribution. *Neurology* 1979;29:1228–1235.

Kurtzke JF, Beebe GW, Norman JE. Epidemiology of multiple sclerosis in US veterans: III. Migration and the risk of MS. *Neurology* 1985;35:672–678.

Kurtzke JF, Dean G, Botha DPJ. A method for estimating the age at immigration of white immigrants to South Africa, with an example of its importance. *S Afr Med J* 1970;44:663–669.

Kurtzke JF, Delasnerie-Laupretre N, Wallin MT. Multiple sclerosis in North African migrants to France. *Acta Neurol Scand* 1998;98:302–309.

Kurtzke JF, Heltberg A. Multiple sclerosis in the Faroe Islands: an epitome. *J Clin Epidemiol* 2001;54:1–22.

Kurtzke JF, Hyllested K. Multiple sclerosis in the Faroe Islands. I. Clinical and epidemiological features. *Ann Neurol* 1979;5:6–21.

Kurtzke JF, Hyllested K. Multiple sclerosis in the Faroe Islands. III. An alternative assessment of the three epidemics. *Acta Neurol Scand* 1987;76:317–339.

Kurtzke JF, Page WF. Epidemiology of multiple sclerosis in US veterans: VII. Risk factors for MS. *Neurology* 1997;48:204–213.

Landtblom AM. Exposure to organic solvents and multiple sclerosis. *Neurology* 1997;49:S70–S74.

Langemann H, Kabiersch A, Newcombe J. Measurement of low-molecular-weight antioxidants, uric acid, tyrosine and tryptophan in plaques and white matter from patients with multiple sclerosis. *Eur Neurol* 1992;32:248–252.

Larsen JP, Riise T, Nyland H, et al. Clustering of multiple sclerosis in the county of Hordaland, Western Norway. *Acta Neurol Scand* 1985a;71:390–395.

Larsen PD, Bloomer LC, Bray PF. Epstein-Barr nuclear antigen and viral capsid antigen antibody titers in multiple sclerosis. *Neurology* 1985b;35:435–438.

Lassmann H, Bruck W, Lucchinetti C. Heterogeneity of multiple sclerosis pathogenesis: implications for diagnosis and therapy. *Trends Mol Med* 2001;7:115–121.

Lauer K. Dietary changes in temporal relation to multiple sclerosis in the Faroe Islands: an evaluation of literary sources. *Neuroepidemiology* 1989a;8:200–206.

Lauer K. Multiple sclerosis in relation to meat preservation in France and Switzerland. *Neuroepidemiology* 1989b;8:308–315.

Lauer K. The food pattern in geographical relation to the risk of multiple sclerosis in the Mediterranean and Near East region. *J Epidemiol Community Health* 1991;45:251–252.

Lauer K, Firnhaber W. Epidemiological investigations into multiple sclerosis in Southern Hesse. V. Course and prognosis. *Acta Neurol Scand* 1987;76:12–17.

Le Gac P. The treatment of multiple sclerosis caused by rickettsia and neorickettsia. *J Med Bordeaux* 1960;137:577–589.

Leibowitz U, Alter M. Clinical factors associated with increased disability in multiple sclerosis. *Acta Neurol Scand* 1970;46:53–70.

Li W, Cook S, Blumberg B, Dowling P. *Chlamydia pneumoniae* sequence frequently present in both MS and control spinal fluid. *Neurology* 2000:A165.

Liguori M, Marrosu MG, Pugliatti M, et al. Age at onset in multiple sclerosis. *Neurol Sci* 2000;21:S825–S829.

Lindberg C, Andersen O, Vahlne A, et al. Epidemiological investigation of the association between infectious mononucleosis and multiple sclerosis. *Neuroepidemiology* 1991;10:62–65.

Lublin FD, Reingold SC. Defining the clinical course of multiple sclerosis: results of an international survey. National Multiple Sclerosis Society (USA) Advisory Committee on Clinical Trials of New Agents in Multiple Sclerosis. *Neurology* 1996;46:907–911.

Madigand M, Oger JJ, Fauchet R, et al. HLA profiles in multiple sclerosis suggest two forms of disease and the existence of protective haplotypes. *J Neurol Sci* 1982;53:519–529.

Marrie RA, Wolfson C, Sturkenboom MC, et al. Multiple sclerosis and antecedent infections: a case–control study. *Neurology* 2000;54:2307–2310.

Marshall E. A shadow falls on hepatitis B vaccination effort. *Science* 1998;281:630–631.

Martin C, Enbom M, Soderstrom M, et al. Absence of seven human herpesviruses, including HHV-6, by polymerase chain reaction in CSF and blood from patients with multiple sclerosis and optic neuritis. *Acta Neurol Scand* 1997;95:280–283.

Martinez-Naves E, Victoria-Gutierrez M, Uria DF, Lopez-Larrea C. The germline repertoire of T cell receptor β-chain genes in multiple sclerosis patients from Spain. *J Neuroimmunol* 1993;47:9–13.

Martyn CN. The epidemiology of multiple sclerosis. In: Matthews WB, Compston A, Allen IV, Martyn CN, eds. McAlpine's Multiple Sclerosis. Edinburgh: Churchill-Livingstone, 1991, pp 2–40.

Martyn CN, Cruddas M, Compston DAS. Symptomatic Epstein-Barr virus infection and multiple sclerosis. *J Neurol Neurosurg Psychiatry* 1993;56:167–168.

Matthews B. Differential diagnosis of multiple sclerosis and related disorders. In: Compston

A, ed. McAlpine's Multiple Sclerosis, 3rd edition. New York: Churchill Livingstone, 1998a, p. 223–250.

Matthews B. Symptoms and signs of multiple sclerosis. In: Compston A, ed. McAlpine's Multiple Sclerosis, 3rd edition. New York: Churchill Livingstone, 1998b, pp 145–190.

Mayne M, Krishnan J, Metz L, et al. Infrequent detection of human herpesvirus 6 DNA in peripheral blood mononuclear cells from multiple sclerosis patients. *Ann Neurol* 1998;44:391–394.

McAlpine D. The benign form of MS. A study based on 241 cases seen within three years of onset and followed up until the tenth year or more of the disease. *Brain* 1961;84:186–203.

McDonald I. Diagnostic methods and investigation in multiple sclerosis. In: Compston A, ed. McAlpine's Multiple Sclerosis, 3rd edition. New York: Churchill Livingstone, 1998, pp 251–279.

McDonald WI, Compston A, Edan G, et al. Recommended diagnostic criteria for multiple sclerosis: guidelines from the International Panel on the Diagnosis of Multiple Sclerosis. *Ann Neurol* 2001;50:121–127.

Melbye M, Ebbesen P, Bennike T. Infectious mononucleosis in Greenland: a disease of the non-indigenous population. *Scand J Infect Dis* 1984;16:9–15.

Mickel HS. Multiple sclerosis: a new hypothesis. *Perspect Biol Med* 1975;18:363–374.

Midgard R, Albrektsen G, Riise T, et al. Prognostic factors for survival in multiple sclerosis: a longitudinal, population based study in More and Romsdal, Norway. *J Neurol Neurosurg Psychiatry* 1995;58:417–421.

Midgard R, Riise T, Nyland H. Epidemiologic trends in multiple sclerosis in More and Romsdal, Norway: a prevalence/incidence study in a stable population. *Neurology* 1991;41:887–892.

Midgard R, Riise T, Svanes C, et al. Incidence of multiple sclerosis in More and Romsdal, Norway from 1950 to 1991. An age-period-cohort analysis. *Brain* 1996;119:203–211.

Miller DH, Hammond SR, McLeod JG, et al. Multiple sclerosis in Australia and New Zealand: are the determinants genetic or environmental? *J Neurol Neurosurg Psychiatry* 1990;53:903–905.

Morré SA, De Groot CJ, Killestein J, et al. Is *Chlamydia pneumoniae* present in the central nervous system of multiple sclerosis patients? *Ann Neurol* 2000;48:399.

Morré SA, van Beek J, De Groot CJ, et al. Is Epstein-Barr virus present in the CNS of patients with MS? *Neurology* 2001;56:692.

Mumford CJ, Wood NW, Kellar-Wood H, et al. The British Isles survey of multiple sclerosis in twins. *Neurology* 1994;44:11–15.

Munch M, Møoller-Larsen A, Christensen T, et al. Production of retrovirus and Epstein-Barr virus in cell lines from multiple sclerosis patients. *Acta Neurol Scand* 1997;169(Suppl): 65–69.

Munch M, Riisom K, Christensen T, et al. The significance of Epstein-Barr virus seropositivity in multiple sclerosis patients? *Acta Neurol Scand* 1998;97:171–174.

Munger KL, Peeling RW, Hernán M, et al. Infection with *Chlamydia pneumoniae* and risk of multiple sclerosis. *Epidemiology* 2003;14: 141–147.

Myhr K-M, Riise T, Barrett-Connor E, et al. Altered antibody pattern to Epstein-Barr virus but not to other herpesviruses in multiple sclerosis: a population-based case–control study from western Norway. *J Neurol Neurosurg Psychiatry* 1998;64:539–542.

Myhr KM, Riise T, Vedeler C, et al. Disability and prognosis in multiple sclerosis: demographic and clinical variables important for the ability to walk and awarding of disability pension. *Mult Scler* 2001;7:59–65.

Nathanson N, Miller A. Epidemiology of multiple sclerosis: critique of the evidence for a viral etiology. *Am J Epidemiol* 1978;107: 451–461.

Nelson LM, Hamman RF, Thompson DS, et al. Higher than expected prevalence of multiple sclerosis in northern Colorado: dependence on methodologic issues. *Neuroepidemiology* 1986;5:17–28.

Neutel CI, Walter SD, Mousseau G. Clustering during childhood of multiple sclerosis patients. *J Chron Dis* 1977;30:217–224.

Niederman JC, Evans AS. Epstein-Barr virus. In: Evans AS, Kaslow RA, eds. Viral Infections of Humans: Epidemiology and Control. New York: Plenum Medical Book Company, 1997, pp 253–283.

Nye FJ. Social class and infectious mononucleosis. *J Hyg* 1973;71:145–149.

Oksenberg JR, Gaiser CN, Cavalli-Sforza LL, Steinman L. Polymorphic markers of human T-cell receptor alpha and beta genes. Family studies and comparison of frequencies in healthy individuals and patients with multiple sclerosis and myasthenia gravis. *Hum Immunol* 1988;22:111–121.

Operskalski EA, Visscher BR, Malmgren RM, Detels R. A case–control study of multiple sclerosis. *Neurology* 1989;39:825–829.

Optic Neuritis Study Group. The 5-year risk of MS after optic neuritis: experience of the optic neuritis treatment trial. *Neurology* 1997; 49:1404–1413.

O'Riordan JI, Losseff NA, Phatouros C, et al.

Asymptomatic spinal cord lesions in clinically isolated optic nerve, brain stem, and spinal cord syndromes suggestive of demyelination. *J Neurol Neurosurg Psychiatry* 1998;64:353–357.

Ormerod IE, Miller DH, McDonald WI, et al. The role of NMR imaging in the assessment of multiple sclerosis and isolated neurological lesions. A quantitative study. *Brain* 1987; 110:1579–616.

Page WF, Kurtzke JF, Murphy FM, Norman JE Jr. Epidemiology of multiple sclerosis in U.S. veterans: V. Ancestry and the risk of multiple sclerosis. *Ann Neurol* 1993;33:632–639.

Peeling RW, Wang SP, Grayston JT, et al. *Chlamydia pneumoniae* serology: interlaboratory variation in microimmunofluorescence assay results. *J Infect Dis* 2000; 181(Suppl 3):S426–S429.

Perkin GD, Bowden P, Rose FC. Smoking and optic neuritis. *Postgrad Med J* 1975;51: 382–385.

Perkin GD, Rose FC. Uhthoff's syndrome. *Br J Ophthalmol* 1976;60:60–63.

Phadke JG. Survival pattern and cause of death in patients with multiple sclerosis: results from an epidemiological survey in north east Scotland. *J Neurol Neurosurg Psychiatry* 1987;50:523–531.

Phadke JG. Clinical aspects of multiple sclerosis in north-east Scotland with particular reference to its course and prognosis. *Brain* 1990;113:1597–1628.

Poland SD, Rice GPA. *Chlamydiae pneumonia* and Multiple sclerosis. *Neurology* 2000: 56:A165.

Poser CM. Trauma and multiple sclerosis. An hypothesis. *J Neurol* 1987;234:155–159.

Poser CM, Hibberd PL. Analysis of the 'epidemic' of multiple sclerosis in the Faroe Islands. II. Biostatistical aspects. *Neuroepidemiology* 1988;7:181–189.

Poser CM, Paty DW, Scheinberg L, et al. New diagnostic criteria for multiple sclerosis: guidelines for research protocols. *Ann Neurol* 1983;13:227–231.

Poser S, Kurtzke JF, Poser W, Schlaf G. Survival in multiple sclerosis. *J Clin Epidemiol* 1989; 42:159–168.

Poser S, Poser W, Schlaf G, et al. Prognostic indicators in multiple sclerosis. *Acta Neurol Scand* 1986;74:387–392.

Poser S, Raun NE, Poser W. Age at onset, initial symptomatology and the course of multiple sclerosis. *Acta Neurol Scand* 1982; 66:355–362.

Poser S, Ritter G, Bauer HJ, et al. HLA-antigens and the prognosis of multiple sclerosis. *J Neurol* 1981;225:219–221.

Poskanzer DC, Schapira K, Miller H. Multiple sclerosis and poliomyelitis. *Lancet* 1963;2: 917–921.

Poskanzer DC, Sever JL, Sheridan JL, Prenney LB. Multiple sclerosis in the Orkney and Shetland Islands: IV. Viral antibody titres and viral infections. *J Epidemiol Community Health* 1980;34:258–264.

Poskanzer DC, Walker AM, Yonkondy J, Sheridan JL. Studies in the epidemiology of multiple sclerosis in the Orkney and Shetland Islands. *Neurology* 1976;Part 2:14–17.

Pucci E, Taus C, Cartechini E, et al. Lack of Chlamydia infection of the central nervous system in multiple sclerosis. *Ann Neurol* 2000;48:399–400.

Pugliatti M, Sotgiu S, Rosati G. The worldwide prevalence of multiple sclerosis. *Clin Nerol Neurosurg* 2002;104:182–191.

Rickinson AB, Kieff E. Epstein-Barr virus. In: Fields BN, Knipe DM, Howley PM, eds. Fields Virology. Philadelphia: Lippincott-Raven, 1996, pp 2397–2446.

Riise T. Cluster studies in multiple sclerosis. *Neurology* 1997;49(Suppl 2):S27–S32.

Riise T, Gronning M, Aarli JA, et al. Prognostic factors for life expectancy in multiple sclerosis analysed by Cox-models. *J Clin Epidemiol* 1988;41:1031–1036.

Riise T, Gronning M, Fernandez O, et al. Early prognostic factors for disability in multiple sclerosis, a European multicenter study. *Acta Neurol Scand* 1992;85:212–218.

Riise T, Grønning M, Klauber MR, et al. Clustering of residence of multiple sclerosis patients at age 13 to 20 years in Hordaland, Norway. *Am J Epidemiol* 1991;133:932–939.

Risch N. Linkage strategies for genetically complex traits. I. Multilocus models. *Am J Hum Genet* 1990;46:222–228.

Robertson N, Compston A. Surveying multiple sclerosis in the United Kingdom. *J Neurol Neurosurg Psychiatry* 1995;58:2–6.

Robertson NP, Fraser M, Deans J, et al. Age-adjusted recurrence risks for relatives of patients with multiple sclerosis. *Brain* 1996; 119:449–455.

Robertson NP, O'Riordan JI, Chataway J, et al. Offspring recurrence rates and clinical characteristics of conjugal multiple sclerosis. *Lancet* 1997;349:1587–1590.

Rodriguez D, Della Gaspera B, Zalc B, et al. Identification of a Val I45 Ile substitution in the human myelin oligodendrocyte glycoprotein: lack of association with multiple sclerosis. The Reseau de Recherche Clinique INSERM sur la Susceptibilite Genetique a la Sclerose en Plaques. *Mult Scler* 1997;3: 377–381.

Rosati G. Descriptive epidemiology of multiple

sclerosis in Europe in the 1980s: a critical overview. *Ann Neurol* 1994;36(S2):S164–S174.

Rosati G. The prevalence of multiple sclerosis in the world: an update. *Neurol Sci* 2001; 22:117–139.

Roth MP, Dolbois L, Borot N, et al. Myelin oligodendrocyte glycoprotein (MOG) gene polymorphisms and multiple sclerosis: no evidence of disease association with MOG. *J Neuroimmunol* 1995;61:117–122.

Roth MP, Nogueira L, Coppin H, et al. Tumor necrosis factor polymorphism in multiple sclerosis: no additional association independent of HLA. *J Neuroimmunol* 1994;51: 93–99.

Runmarker B, Andersen O. Prognostic factors in a multiple sclerosis incidence cohort with twenty-five years of follow-up. *Brain* 1993; 116:117–134.

Russell WR. Multiple sclerosis: occupation and social group at onset. *Lancet* 1971;2:832–834.

Saarela J, Schoenberg Fejzo MS, Chen D, et al. Fine mapping of a multiple sclerosis locus to 2.5 Mb on chromosome 17q22–q24. *Hum Mol Genet* 2002;11:2257–2267.

Sadovnick AD, Armstrong H, Rice GP, et al. A population-based study of multiple sclerosis in twins: update. *Ann Neurol* 1993;33:281–285.

Sadovnick AD, Baird PA, Ward RH. Multiple sclerosis: updated risks for relatives. *Am J Med Genet* 1988;29:533–541.

Sadovnick AD, Dyment D, Ebers GC. Genetic epidemiology of multiple sclerosis. *Epidemiol Rev* 1997;19:99–106.

Sadovnick AD, Ebers GC, Dyment DA, Risch NJ. Evidence for genetic basis of multiple sclerosis. The Canadian Collaborative Study Group. *Lancet* 1996;347:1728–1730.

Sandberg-Wollheim M, Ciusani E, Salmaggi A, Pociot F. An evaluation of tumor necrosis factor microsatellite alleles in genetic susceptibility to multiple sclerosis. *Mult Scler* 1995;1:181–185.

Sanders EA, Bollen EL, van der Velde EA. Presenting signs and symptoms in multiple sclerosis. *Acta Neurol Scand* 1986;73:269–272.

Sawcer S, Jones HB, Feakes R, et al. A genome screen in multiple sclerosis reveals susceptibility loci on chromosome 6p21 and 17q22. *Nat Genet* 1996;13:464–468.

Sherritt MA, Oksenberg J, de Rosbo NK, Bernard CC. Influence of HLA-DR2, HLA-DPw4, and T cell receptor alpha chain genes on the susceptibility to multiple sclerosis. *Int Immunol* 1992;4:177–181.

Shirodaria PV, Haire M, Fleming E, et al. Viral antibody titers. Comparison in patients with multiple sclerosis and rheumatoid arthritis. *Arch Neurol* 1987;44:1237–1241.

Silman AJ, Newman J, MacGregor AJ. Cigarette smoking increases the risk of rheumatoid arthritis. Results from a nationwide study of disease-discordant twins. *Arthritis Rheum* 1996;39:732–735.

Skegg DC, Corwin PA, Crave RS, et al. Occurrence of multiple sclerosis in the north and south of New Zealand. *J Neurol Neurosurg Psychiatry* 1987;50:134–139.

Smith ADM, Duckett S, Waters AH. Neuropathological changes in chronic cyanide intoxication. *Nature* 1963;200:179–181.

Soldan SS, Berti R, Salem N, et al. Association of human herpes virus 6 (HHV-6) with multiple sclerosis: increased IgM response to HHV-6 early antigen and detection of serum HHV-6 DNA. *Nat Med* 1997;3:1394–1397.

Soldan SS, Leist TP, Juhng KN, et al. Increased lymphoproliferative response to human herpesvirus type 6A variant in multiple sclerosis patients. *Ann Neurol* 2000;47:306–313.

Sopori ML, Kozak W. Immunomodulatory effects of cigarette smoke. *J Neuroimmunol* 1998;83:148–156.

Spillane J. The effect of nicotine on spinocerebellar ataxia. *BMJ* 1955;2:1345–1351.

Sriram S, Mitchell W, Stratton C. Multiple sclerosis associated with *Chlamydia pneumoniae* infection of the CNS. *Neurology* 1998;50: 571–572.

Sriram S, Stratton CW, Yao S, et al. *Chlamydia pneumonaie* infection of the central nervous system in multiple sclerosis. *Ann Neurol* 1999;46:6–14.

Stazio A, Paddison RM, Kurland LT. Multiple sclerosis in New Orleans, Louisiana, and Winnipeg, Manitoba, Canada: follow-up of a previous survey in New Orleans, and comparison between the patient populations in the two communities. *J Chron Dis* 1967;20: 311–332.

Stefferl A, Schubart A, Storch M, et al. Butyrophilin, a milk protein, modulates the encephalitogenic T cell response to myelin oligodendrocyte glycoprotein in experimental autoimmune encephalomyelitis. *J Immunol* 2000;165:2859–2865.

Stein EC, Schiffer RB, Hall WJ, Young N. Multiple sclerosis and the workplace: report of an industry-based cluster. *Neurology* 1987; 37:1672–1677.

Sumaya CV, Myers LW, Ellison GW. Epstein-Barr virus antibodies in multiple sclerosis. *Arch Neurol* 1980;37:94–96.

Sumaya CV, Myers LW, Ellison GW, Ench Y. Increased prevalence and titer of Epstein-Barr virus antibodies in patients with multiple sclerosis. *Ann Neurol* 1985;17:371–377.

Svenningsson A, Runmarker B, Lycke J, Andersen O. Incidence of MS during two fifteen-year periods in the Gothenburg region of Sweden. *Acta Neurol Scand* 1990;82:161–168.

Svenson LW, Woodhead SE, Platt GH. Regional variations in the prevalence rates of multiple sclerosis in the province of Alberta, Canada. *Neuroepidemiology* 1994;13:8–13.

Swank RL, Lerstad O, Strom A, Backer J. Multiple sclerosis in rural Norway. *N Engl J Med* 1952;246:721–728.

Swingler RJ, Compston D. The distribution of multiple sclerosis in the United Kingdom. *J Neurol Neurosurg Psychiatry* 1986;49:1115–1124.

Taus C, Pucci E, Cartechini E, et al. Absence of HHV-6 and HHV-7 in cerebrospinal fluid in relapsing-remitting multiple sclerosis. *Acta Neurol Scand* 2000;101:224–228.

Thompson AJ, Hutchinson M, Brazil J, et al. A clinical and laboratory study of benign multiple sclerosis. *Q J Med* 1986;58:69–80.

Thorogood M, Hannaford PC. The influence of oral contraceptives on the risk of mulitple sclerosis. *Br J Obstet Gynaecol* 1998;105:1296–1299.

Tompkins LS, Schachter J, Boman J, et al. Collaborative multidisciplinary workshop report: detection, culture, serology, and antimicrobial susceptibility testing of *Chlamydia pneumoniae*. *J Infect Dis* 2000;181(Suppl 3):S460–S461.

Touze E, Gout O, Verdier-Taillefer MH, et al. The first episode of central nervous system demyelinization and hepatitis B virus vaccination. *Rev Neurol (Paris)* 2000;156:242–246.

Vassallo L, Elian M, Dean G. Multiple sclerosis in southern Europe. II: Prevalence in Malta in 1978. *J Epidemiol Community Health* 1979;33:111–113.

Vaughan JH, Riise T, Rhodes GH, et al. An Epstein-Barr virus–related cross reactive autoimmune response in multiple sclerosis in Norway. *J Neuroimmunol* 1996;69:95–102.

Verjans E, Theys P, Delmotte P, Carton H. Clinical parameters and intrathecal IgG synthesis as prognostic features in multiple sclerosis. Part I. *J Neurol* 1983;229:155–165.

Vessey M, Doll R, Peto R, et al. A long-term follow-up study of women using different methods of contraception—an interim report. *J Biosoc Sci* 1976;8:373–427.

Vessey MP, Villard-Mackintosh L, Yeates D. Oral contraceptives, cigarette smoking and other factors in relation to arthritis. *Contraception* 1987;35:457–464.

Villard-Mackintosh L, Vessey MP. Oral contraceptives and reproductive factors in multiple sclerosis incidence. *Contraception* 1993;47:161–168.

Visscher BR, Detels R, Coulson AH, et al. Latitude, migration, and the prevalence of multiple sclerosis. *Am J Epidemiol* 1977;106:470–475.

Visscher BR, Liu KS, Clark VA, Detels R, et al. Onset symptoms as predictors of mortality and disability in multiple sclerosis. *Acta Neurol Scand* 1984;70:321–328.

Voigt LF, Koepsell TD, Nelson JL, et al. Smoking, obesity, alcohol consumption, and the risk of rheumatoid arthritis. *Epidemiology* 1994;5:525–532.

Wallin MT, Page WF, Kurtzke JF. Epidemiology of multiple sclerosis in US veterans. VIII. Long-term survival after onset of multiple sclerosis. *Brain* 2000;123:1677–1687.

Wandinger K, Jabs W, Siekhaus A, et al. Association between clinical disease activity and Epstein-Barr virus reactivation in MS. *Neurology* 2000;55:178–184.

Warner HB, Carp RI. Multiple sclerosis and Epstein-Barr virus. *Lancet* 1981;2:1290.

Warren SA, Warren KG, Greenhill S, Paterson M. How multiple sclerosis is related to animal illness, stress and diabetes. *Can Med Assoc J* 1982;126:377–385.

Weinshenker BG, Rice GP, Noseworthy JH, et al. The natural history of multiple sclerosis: a geographically based study. 3. Multivariate analysis of predictive factors and models of outcome. *Brain* 1991;114:1045–1056.

Whitacre CC. Sex differences in autoimmune disease: focus on multiple sclerosis. *Nat Immunol* 2001;2:777–780.

Whitacre CC, Reingold SC, O'Looney PA. A gender gap in autoimmunity. *Science* 1999;283:1277–1278.

Wilborn F, Schmidt CA, Brinkmann V, et al. A potential role for human herpesvirus type 6 in nervous sytem disease. *J Neuroimmunol* 1994;49:213–214.

Willett WC. Nutritional Epidemiology, 2nd edition. New York: Oxford University Press, 1998.

Winer S, Astsaturov I, Cheung RK, et al. T cells of multiple sclerosis patients target a common environmental peptide that causes encephalitis in mice. *J Immunol* 2001;166:4751–4756.

Wingerchuk D, Liu Q, Sobell J, et al. A population-based case–control study of the tumor necrosis factor alpha-308 polymorphism in multiple sclerosis. *Neurology* 1997;49:626–628.

Wucherpfennig KW, Strominger JL. Molecular mimicry in T cell-mediated autoimmunity: viral peptides activate human T cell clones specific for myelin basic protein. *Cell* 1995; 80:695–705.

Wynn DR, Rodriguez M, O'Fallon WM, Kurland LT. A reappraisal of the epidemiology of multiple sclerosis in Olmsted County, Minnesota. *Neurology* 1990;40:780–786.

Zhang S, Hernán M, Olek M, et al. Intakes of carotenoids, vitamin C, and vitamin E and MS risk among two large cohorts of women. *Neurology* 2001;57:75–80.

Zhang SM, Willett WC, Hernan MA, et al. Dietary fat in relation to risk of multiple sclerosis among two large cohorts of women. *Am J Epidemiol* 2000;152:1056–1064.

9

Stroke

BERNADETTE BODEN-ALBALA AND RALPH L. SACCO

For many years stroke has been recognized as a leading cause of disability and mortality in the United States and other industrialized countries (Murray and Lopez 1997; World Health Organization 1997; American Heart Association 1999). Stroke is more disabling than fatal: the estimated annual cost of stroke-related health care is between 20 and 40 billion dollars measured in both health-care dollars and lost productivity (American Heart Association 1999).

Awareness of the importance of this disease has led to a vast and accumulating literature on stroke risk factors, stroke etiology, and stroke outcome. Stroke risk factors have been elucidated and clinical trials have indicated the benefits of treatment for persons with hypertension, atrial fibrillation, hypercholesterolemia, and asymptomatic carotid disease. During the past several years, the first approved treatment for acute stroke, recombinant tissue plasminogen activator (rtPA), has become available. Additionally, the pharmaceutical industry continues to actively pursue the development of "neuroprotective" agents to be used acutely for enhanced recovery from this disabling disease. As we enter the twenty-first century, technological advancements in the field of brain imaging, genotyping, and medical information systems will help facilitate epidemiological study designs that will elucidate stroke risk markers at the molecular level and risk factors at the subclinical level. Such advancements will provide neuroepidemiologists with more precision in stroke diagnosis and classification, including documentation and timing of events through the use of diffusion-weighted brain imaging techniques.

While improved technology has increased the precision and generalizablility of data on stroke, epidemiologists who study stroke still struggle with a number of critical issues. Despite recognition of and treatment modalities for modifiable stroke risk factors such as hypertension and cardiac disease, stroke incidence appears to be rising (Broderick et al. 1989, 1998). Overall stroke mortality may be declining, but differentials in stroke mortality continue to be reported between whites and other racial/ethnic groups including African Americans, Hispanics, and Asian Pacific Islanders. Over the next three decades, the public health impact of stroke is likely to increase, as the proportion of our population over age 65 is expected to grow rapidly. The aging of the population and the changing racial/ethnic composition of certain nations could lead to an increased absolute number of strokes per year, resulting in greater incidence, mortality, morbidity, and cost.

Clinical Definition of Stroke

A stroke is a focal neurologic deficit caused by a local disturbance in cerebral circulation—predominantly either an obstruction of cerebral blood (ischemic stroke) or a rupture to a vessel wall supplying blood to either the brain or spinal cord (intracebral hemorrhage or subarachnoid hemorrhage, respectively). These three distinct etiological groups—ischemic stroke (IS), intracerebral hemorrhage (ICH), and subarachnoid hemorrhage (SAH)—comprise 75%–85%, 15%–20%, and about 6%, respectively, of all strokes annually (American Heart Association 1999).

From an epidemiological perspective, the establishment of standardized practical diagnostic criteria for defining stroke is critical. Agreement on a definition for stroke enables comparison of incidence and prevalence rates in studies throughout the world. A number of large prospective studies have adopted a uniform definition of stroke: patients with a "neurological deficit lasting 24 hours or longer, or a defined lesion on imaging associated with presenting symptoms"(World Health Organization 1997). These criteria have been used since the late 1960s when study subjects from Framingham began to be evaluated neurologically in the hospital at the time of stroke (Wolf et al. 1992). A neurological deficit lasting less than 24 hours is called a transient isch-

emic attack (TIA). Categorizing stroke by time is becoming antiquated with the increased ability to image lesions with deficits lasting only a few hours.

The universal application of computed tomography (CT) brain imaging to confirm the presence of a lesion has been critical for early recognition and diagnosis of stroke. Epidemiological studies report the use of CT in between 90% and 99% of stroke cases (Wolf et al. 1992). Indeed, the universal practice of CT for stroke differential may have added to the initial increase in stroke incidence reported in the early 1980s.

Burden of Stroke: Mortality and Incidence

The burden of stroke remains significant: recent figures from the American Heart Association reported 161,000 deaths in the United States from stroke annually (American Heart Association 1999). Stroke mortality estimates are typically derived from national or local vital statistics data. Stroke data are obtained from sources that have used standardized classification systems such as the eighth or ninth versions of the International Code of Diseases (ICD; American Medical Association 1998). Stroke mortality has been on the decline in the United States and worldwide. A 60% decline in stroke mortality between 1960 and 1990 has been reported (American Heart Association 1999), although 1-year stroke mortality rates still approach 25% (American Heart Association 1999). Although ischemic stroke accounts for the greatest public health impact because it occurs more frequently, ICH and SAH are more fatal and thus also contribute significantly to the burden of stroke. Mortality rates range from 30% to 70% for ICH and 25% to 50% for SAH (McGovern et al. 1993).

Stroke mortality rates differ by country and geographic region. Greater 28-day mortality rates were reported in Yugoslavia, Poland, Lithuania, Finland, and the Russian Federation than in Sweden,

Denmark, Italy, and Germany (Feigin et al. 1995b). The Seven Countries Study, which provides multinational comparisons of stroke mortality over 25 years, reported lower age-adjusted death rates in North America and northern Europe (35–50 per 1000) than in southern Europe, Serbia, Croatia, and Japan (83–107 per 1000) (Menotti et al. 1996).

Over the last 20 years, a number of important studies have attempted to enumerate the incidence of stroke cases in the United States and other countries each year. Incidence estimates have been indirectly calculated, using figures from smaller community samples to project national figures.

Example 9-1 The more recent systematic collection of incidence data has contributed much to our knowledge about stroke incidence and trends in stroke occurrence. The World Health Organization MONItoring CArdiovascular Disease (WHO MONICA) project is an important ongoing international collaboration that monitors stroke occurrence in 17 centers among 10 countries including China, Denmark, Finland, Italy, Poland, Russia, Sweden, and Yugoslavia. The strength of this project lies in the uniformity of data collection, allowing comparison of stroke occurrence across diverse populations. Use of death certificates, hospital admission and discharge data, and non-hospital sources linked to prior medical information provides the foundation for identification of stroke cases. This study has been collecting information about stroke since 1980 and has provided important information on global stroke trends. Age-standardized stroke attack rates are provided in Figure 9-1. While the MONICA Project reported an overall decline in the stroke attack rate, a number of countries, including Lithuania and Poland, did not exhibit this downward trend; Novosibirsk, Russia, had one of the greatest age- and sex-adjusted annual stroke incidence rates at 232 per 100,000 in 1992 (Feigin et al. 1995a, 1995b).

In the United States, several population-based studies from Framingham, Massachusetts (Wolf et al 1992), Rochester, Minnesota (Brown et al. 1996), and the Lehigh Valley, Pennsylvania/New Jersey (Friday et al. 1989) have contributed significantly to our knowledge about stroke trends, subtypes, risk factors, and incidence rates in men and women. Extensive stroke surveillance systems were used to ascertain all incident stroke cases within a defined geographical area. The Olmsted County study reported a decline in stroke incidence from 205 per 100,000 between 1955 and 1959 to 128 per 100,000 between 1975 and 1979 and has recently reported an increase in incidence to approximately 150 per 100,000 (Brown et al. 1996; Menghini et al. 1998). Early incidence figures came from the Framingham Study, a large epidemiological study initiated in 1950 that is following 5000 men and women who were initially free of cardiovascular disease. This study indicated differences in stroke incidence by gender, with greater incidence rates among men than among women (Wolf et al. 1992) (Fig. 9-1).

Stroke incidence is 25% to 66% higher for men than women (Ricci et al. 1991; Hu et al. 1992; Jerntorp and Berglund 1992; Sacco 1997). Women have a higher stroke prevalence, however, because they have a longer life expectancy and are more likely to survive a stroke.

Despite the important contributions of these primarily white cohorts, these findings may not be generalizable to multiethnic populations. Studies have begun to report differences in stroke incidence between racial/ethnic groups, especially stroke incidence rates among blacks. The greater Cincinnati/North Kentucky study estimated 730,000 new or recurrent strokes per year, with incidence rates of 288 per 100,000 among African Americans, compared to 179 per 100,000 among whites from Rochester, Minnesota (Broderick et al. 1998).

Example 9-2 Multiethnic population-based studies compare rates in different groups or populations. The community-based Northern Manhattan Stroke Study

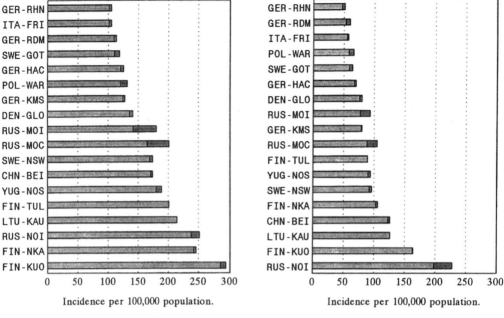

Incidence per 100,000 population.   Incidence per 100,000 population.

▨ Definite first stroke ■ Order unknown

Figure 9–1 Charts showing age-standardized annual incidence rates of definite stroke among men (**left**) and women (**right**) aged 35–64 years, divided according to WHO Monitoring Trends and Determinants in Cardiovascular Disease Project (MONICA). CHN-BEI, Beijing, China; DEN-GLO, Glostrup, Denmark; FIN-KUO, Kuopio Province, Finland; FIN-NKA, North Karelia, Finland; FIN-TUL, Turku/Loimaa, Finland; GER-HAC, Halle County, Germany; GER-KMS, Karl-Marx-Stadt County, Germany; GER-RDM, Rest of DDR MONICA: Germany; GER-RHN, Rhein-Neckar Region, Germany; ITA-FRI, Friuli, Italy; LTU-KAU, Kaunas, Lithuania; POL-WAR, Warsaw, Poland; RUS-MOC, Moscow Control, Russia; RUS-MOI, Moscow Intervention, Russia; RUS-NOI, Novosibirsk Intervention, Russia; SWE-GOT, Gothenurg, Sweden; SWE-NSW, Northern Sweden, Sweden; YUG-NOS, Novi Sad, Yugoslavia. (Reprinted with permission from Thorvaldsen P, Asplund K, Kuulasmaa K, et al. Stroke incidence, case fatality, and mortality in the WHO MONICA project. *Stroke* 1995;26: 361–367.)

(NOMASS) used a comprehensive surveillance system to document all incident strokes in a defined geographical area, over a defined time period, including both hospitalized and non-hospitalized cases. The NOMASS reported a 2.4-fold higher rate of first stroke among African Americans and a twofold higher incidence of stroke among Hispanics than that for whites (Sacco et al. 1998a). Knowledge about incidence differences in different racial/ethnic groups may allow for the development of more effective targeted stroke prevention programs.

A number of epidemiological issues arise in the enumeration of stroke cases in inci-

dence and prevalence studies. Diagnostic criteria for stroke and sensitivity of the diagnosis may differ from study to study. Indeed, early increases in stroke incidence may be attributed to the transition to universal use of CT imaging. Prior to the general use of CT imaging to confirm strokes, underdiagnosis or misclassification of stroke was more likely to occur. Difficulty obtaining death certificates and inaccuracy of the diagnosis on death certificates may contribute to underreporting of stroke. Assessment of population data such as census data may not be accurate for underserved or minority populations such as blacks or Hispanics because undercounting is considerable. Studies have reported stroke rates for nonhospitalized cases as between 5% and 20%. This variability in stroke admissions has lead to difficulties in obtaining accurate incidence rates using hospital-based cohorts or stroke registries because of underreporting of mild or non-hospitalized cases of stroke.

Ischemic Stroke

Racial/ethnic disparities in stroke mortality and morbidity, and in the recognition and treatment of underlying stroke etiologies, underscore the need for further classification and subtyping of ischemic stroke. Few stroke studies that report cerebral infarction incidence rates have provided detailed data on infarct subtypes and those that have included a classification system came from data banks or hospital-based studies. Ischemic stroke subtypes have generally been classified on the basis of the mechanism of the ischemia (embolic or hemodynamic) and the pathology of the vascular lesion: atherosclerotic lacunar, cardioembolic, or cryptogenic (of undetermined etiology) (Foulkes et al. 1988; Adams et al. 1993). The distribution of these subtypes varies depending on the geographical region of the study, the sample from which the cases are drawn (hospital or community or population-based), the demographic and risk factor profile of the cohort, the completeness of the stroke work-up, and the framework within which diagnostic decisions are made. Generally, cardioembolic stroke accounts for between 15% and 30% of ischemic stroke cases, atherosclerotic infarction ranges from 14% to 40%, and lacunar accounts for 15%–30% of cases. Stroke of undetermined etiology or cryptogenic strokes may account for as many as 40% of infarct cases (Sacco et al. 1989a).

There are many illustrations of controversies regarding classification, reliability, and validity. For example, the inclusion of a cryptogenic category as an infarct subtype alters the distribution of infarct subtypes, putatively making subtype categories more homogeneous. Exclusion of this category forces the epidemiologist to choose a definite subtype often without reasonable certainty. This may lead to misclassification bias. For example, the distribution of infarct subtypes in the Stroke Data Bank was compared with those in Rochester, Minnesota. The prevalence of lacune stroke was higher in the Stroke Data Bank than in Rochester (27% vs. 16%) whereas the distribution of cardioembolic strokes was lower (19% vs. 29%) (Sacco et al. 1989b).

Ischemic strokes are difficult to classify by infarct subtype on clinical grounds alone. Reliance on presenting clinical syndromes may be preferable in large community cohorts where confirmatory laboratory data are difficult to ascertain. The clinical description is also useful in distinguishing subtypes; for example, the presentation of fractional arm weakness may be more common with atherosclerotic subtype (Timsit et al. 1992). However, clinical features reported at stroke onset may not provide enough reliable information to confirm a definite subtype. A subtype classification system that incorporates both presenting clinical syndrome with other lab findings will allow for the most precise subtype grouping.

Finally, accuracy of diagnostic subtyping depends on the extent of diagnostic work-up and evaluation. If appropriate testing is performed, the timing of the specific test may impact the subtype groupings. Continued use of a wide range of diagnostic tests including CT, noninvasive Doppler ultrasonography, magnetic resonance imaging (MRI) and angiography, transesophageal echo, and hematological tests may help to redistribute those who would otherwise be grouped as crypotgenic.

Ischemic stroke subtype may differ among racial/ethnic groups, and these differences may result in disparities in mortality. In the Cincinnati study, stroke incidence subtypes among African Americans were found to be greatest for the cryptogenic group (103 per 100,000), followed by cardioembolic (56 per 100,000), small vessel infarct (52 per 100,000), and large vessel infarct (17 per 100,000) (Broderick et al. 1998). In the Northern Manhattan Stroke Study a disproportionate increase in atherosclerotic and small vessel infarcts was reported among African Americans and Hispanics (Sacco et al. 2001a). These differences may help to explain the increased stroke mortality of African Americans. Further, these differences may reflect possible genetic or environmental factors. Continued investigation in larger prospective cohorts with emphasis on racial/ethnic differences in subtype classification needs to be undertaken.

Ischemic Stroke Risk Factors

In recent years, great strides have been made in understanding the pathophysiology of ischemic stroke and in developing treatments that reduce morbidity and mortality after stroke. The most effective way to reduce the burden of stroke, however, is through prevention. Stroke prevention strategies can occur at multiple stages: in the healthy, stroke-free population (primary prevention), among those who have developed recognizable risk factors and may have subclinical disease (late primary or early secondary prevention), and after the development of neurological symptoms of stroke or TIA (late secondary or tertiary prevention).

Classification and Determination of Stroke Risk Factors

An understanding of stroke risk factors is essential for effective stroke prevention. Some factors are not modifiable and may be better characterized as risk markers, while others are amenable to behavioral, medical, or surgical modification. Risk markers may include age, gender, race/ethnicity, or heredity. Modifiable risk factors may include environmental or even genetic exposures that, when modified, lead to reductions in the risk of stroke. Factors that may have both environmental and genetic links include hypertension and hyperlipidemia.

Stroke risk factors have been identified through both case–control and cohort studies. In case–control studies, selection bias may lead to a collection of cases that do not adequately reflect all individuals with stroke and controls that are not representative of the general population. One solution is to use population-based study designs in which all the cases of stroke within a specific area are included and controls are randomly derived from the same community.

In cohort studies, the attributable risk or etiologic fraction—a measure of the proportion of cases explained or attributed to the exposure—can be readily calculated. Prospective cohorts usually require systematic, lengthy follow-up after a baseline assessment. The clear advantage to cohort studies is the measurement of the exposure pre-stroke and the ability to determine the prevalence of the exposure in the general population; however, these studies are time consuming and expensive and require large numbers of subjects.

Experimental epidemiological studies such as the randomized, controlled clinical trial are the mainstay of demonstrating that modification of a risk factor can lead to a reduction in stroke risk. Subjects who exhibit the risk factor of interest are randomly assigned to an intervention or not and then followed for the occurrence of a specific outcome such as stroke. Randomization is used to help ensure that the groups are balanced for known and unknown confounders. While these studies can also be expensive and require large numbers of patients, they are essential to the development of evidence-based guidelines for stroke prevention. Before the fall of 2001, for example, it was a common practice to prescribe warfarin for secondary stroke prevention in patients whose stroke etiology was thought to be cryptogentic or of non-cardioembolic origin. Results of the large National Institutes of Health (NIH)-funded multicenter Warfarin-Aspirin Recurrent Stroke Study (WARSS) found no significant difference between aspirin use and warfarin use in the prevention of recurrent stroke. Now the use of warfarin for noncardioembolic stroke is slowly declining (Mohr et al. 2001).

Nonmodifiable Risk Markers for Ischemic Stroke

Age. Age is one of the strongest determinants of ischemic stroke. Stroke incidence rises with age—nearly doubling every decade after age 55—and most strokes occur in persons older than 65 (Sacco et al. 1997a). The predicted increase in the number of strokes occurring each year is largely due to the aging of populations.

Gender. As discussed above, men consistently exhibit a greater stroke incidence (Sacco et al. 1998a). The male-to-female ratio has been estimated to be 1.3 to 1 and differs by stroke subtype. Since women are more likely to survive a stroke, the prevalence and morbidity rates and the impact of stroke disability are greater among women than among men (Brown et al. 1996). These differentials may reflect differences in hormonal risk factors, such as estrogen and oral contraceptive use. For example, the results from the Women's Health Initiative (WHI) randomized clinical trial of some 16,608 postmenopausal women followed for a mean of 5.2 years showed a 41% increase in stroke for women who were assigned to the estrogen-plus-progestin group compared with women who were not assigned to take the hormones (29 vs. 21 per 100,000 person-years) (Writing Group for the Women's Health Initiative Investigators 2002). The elevated risk occurred in nonfatal strokes, with a twofold increase in risk for thromboembolic disease.

Race or Ethnicity. Despite the reported decline in overall stroke mortality, a twofold higher stroke mortality persists in African Americans compared to that in whites (Brown et al. 1996). Few studies have adequate numbers of patients from different racial/ethnic groups to compare stroke incidence by race/ethnicity. Various studies have found that blacks have a greater stroke incidence and prevalence than whites of comparable age, gender, and residence (Caplan et al. 1986; Schoenberg et al. 1986; Gillum 1988; Broderick et al. 1998; Sacco et al. 1998a). In the National Health and Nutrition Survey, the relative risk of stroke for African Americans was higher than for whites even after adjustment for age, hypertension, and diabetes (Kittner et al. 1990). In northern Manhattan (Fig. 9–2), the overall age-adjusted 1-year stroke incidence rate for African Americans was 2.4 times that of whites in a population-based stroke incidence study among white, African American, and Hispanic residents (Sacco et al. 1998a).

Hispanics have rarely been identified separately in epidemiologic studies of stroke (Kattapong et al. 1993; Bruno et al. 1996; Morgenstern and Spears 1997; Staub and Morgenstern 2000). In northern Manhattan, Hispanics, predominately from the Dominican Republic, had an overall age-adjusted 1-year stroke incidence rate two times that of whites (Sacco et al. 1998a). Asians, particularly Chinese and Japanese, have exceedingly high stroke incidence rates, which seem to be decreased among those who have migrated to Hawaii and California.

Increased stroke mortality in different racial/ethnic groups may be directly explained by increased incidence. Different groups may demonstrate a unique burden of stroke risk factors after controlling for differences in socioeconomic status and other demographic variables (Sacco et al. 2001a). By calculating the attributable risk or etiologic fraction (EF) of the risk factor, one can gauge the differential burdens in stroke risk across different groups. Identification of differences in risk factor profiles across racial/ethnic groups will allow more targeted and better justified therapeutic or preventative interventions.

Example 9–3 In the Northern Manhattan Stroke Study, the prevalence, odds ra-

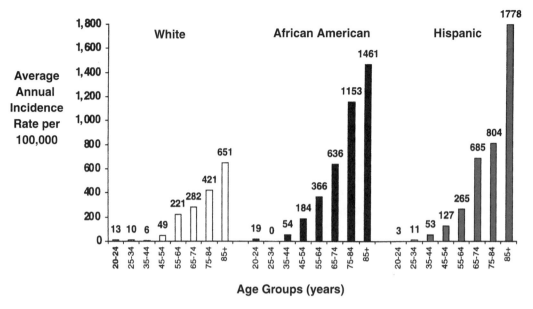

Figure 9–2 Average annual age-specific incidence rates of stroke (per 100,000 population) among whites, African-Americans, and Hispanics aged ≥20 years in northern Manhattan, July 1, 1993 to June 30, 1996 (Sacco et al. 1998a). (Reprinted with permission.)

tios (OR), and EF for stroke risk factors vary by race/ethnicity (Sacco et al. 2001a) (Table 9–1). Hypertension was an independent risk factor for stroke for whites (OR 1.8, EF 25%), African Americans (OR 2.0, EF 37%), and Caribbean Hispanics (OR 2.1, EF 32%), but greater prevalence of hypertension in African Americans and Caribbean Hispanics led to an elevated EF for these groups. Greater prevalence rates of diabetes increased the stroke risk in African Americans (OR 1.8, EF 14%) and Caribbean Hispanics (OR 2.1, $p < 0.05$, EF 10%) compared to that in whites (OR 1.0, EF 0%), while atrial fibrillation had a greater

prevalence and EF for whites (OR 4.4, EF 20%) than for African Americans (OR 1.7, EF 3%) and Caribbean Hispanics (OR 3.0, EF 2%). Prevalence of physical inactivity was greater among Caribbean Hispanics, but elevated EF was found in all groups. These differences are crucial to the etiology of stroke, as well as to the design and implementation of stroke prevention programs (Sacco et al. 2001a).

Heredity. The heritability or genetic risk of cerebrovascular disease has been underemphasized. Stroke may be caused by several different genes whose individual effects are determined by certain environmental

Table 9–1 Etiologic Fractions and 95% Confidence Intervals for Stroke Risk Factors among Whites, African-Americans, and Hispanics for Northern Manhattan Stroke Study

Risk factor	Whites	African Americans	Hispanics
	EF (95% CI)	EF (95% CI)	EF (95% CI)
Hypertension	0.25 (0.01–0.45)	0.37 (0.16–0.57)	0.32 (0.15–0.43)
Diabetes	0 (−0.08–0.10)	0.14 (0.04–0.25)	0.10 (0.04–0.15)
Atrial fibrillation	0.20 (0.06–0.39)	0.03 (−0.02–0.08)*	0.02 (0.00–0.04)*
Coronary artery disease	0.16 (−0.008–0.35)	0.02 (−0.06–0.13)	0.06 (0.001–0.14)
Physical activity	0.18 (0.07–0.36)	0.29 (0.19–0.44)	0.38 (0.24–0.44)

*Significantly different etiologic fractions (EFs) were attributed to atrial fibrillation in whites, compared to EFs for African Americans and Hispancics.

Reprinted with permission from Sacco RL, Boden-Albala B, Abel G, et al. Race-ethnic disparities in the impact of stroke risk factors: the Northern Manhattan Stroke Study. *Stroke* 2001a;32:1725–1731.

triggers in a complex gene–environmental interaction model. Twin studies have shown a significantly greater concordance of stroke in monozygotic than in dizygotic twins (Brass et al. 1992). Cohort studies in different populations have demonstrated an association between parental stroke death and an increased risk of stroke in offspring (Kiely et al. 1993). Variations in the incidence of ischemic stroke in racial groups support the notion of a genetic component (Rubattu et al. 2000). Relatives of people with ischemic stroke often share the same risk factors, making it difficult to separate genetic factors from shared environment.

The familial effect is thought to represent indirect genetic influences that operate through well-documented risk factors such as hypertension, diabetes mellitus, cardiac diseases, and abnormal lipid states. Each of these risk factors remains under genetic influences that may or may not interact with environmental factors, and this observation argues against the notion that any single gene is a sufficient or necessary cause of stroke. Knowledge of these possible indirect genetic causes of stroke is incomplete. Potential genetic stroke risk factors include apolipoprotein E and lipoprotein (a), as well as genetic markers of thrombosis such as factor V Leiden and fibrinogen (Rubattu et al. 2000).

The identification of genetic determinants for stroke would allow early identification of persons with increased risk of stroke through genetic screening. At present, genetic screening is not available for atherosclerosis and stroke. In the future it may be possible to alter genes with molecular biological techniques and modify the risk of stroke. Prior to these advances, the detection of a genetic factor could lead to more intensive environmental risk factor modification.

Modifiable Risk Factors

Major reductions in stroke morbidity and mortality are more likely to arise from identification and control of modifiable factors in the stroke-prone individual. Modifiable stroke risk factors include hypertension, cardiac disease (particularly atrial fibrillation), diabetes, dyslipidemia, cigarette use, alcohol abuse, physical inactivity, diet, asymptomatic carotid stenosis, and TIAs (see Table 9–2).

Hypertension. Hypertension is the most powerful and potentially modifiable stroke risk factor. It is prevalent in both men and women, and is of even greater significance in African Americans. Stroke risk rises proportionately with increasing blood pressure. Isolated systolic hypertension is increasingly prevalent with age and increases the risk of stroke by 2 to 4, even after controlling for age and diastolic blood pressure (Davis et al. 1987; MacMahon and Rodgers 1994; Kurl et al. 2001).

Reduction of both systolic and diastolic pressure in hypertensive individuals substantially decreases stroke risk. A large multicenter hypertension detection and follow-up program trial in which standardized stepped care was compared with routine care showed a 35% reduction in total strokes and 44% reduction in fatal strokes over a 5-year period (Hypertension, Detec-

Table 9–2 Modifiable Risks Factors for Stroke

Risk factor	Estimated relative risk	Estimated prevalence (%)
Hypertension	2.0–4.0	25–50
Cardiac disease	2.0–4.0	10–20
Atrial fibrillation	4.0–18.0	1–2
Diabetes mellitus/insulin resistance	1.5–3.0	4–8
Smoking	1.5–2.5	20–40
Carotid stenosis	1.5–3.0	1–10
Hyperlipidemia	1.0–1.5	20–50
Heavy alcohol use	1.0–3.0	2–15
No physical activity	1.8–3.5	10–25

tion and Follow-up Cooperative Group 1982). Reduction of isolated systolic hypertension to <140 mmHg in elderly individuals is clearly beneficial (Dahlof et al. 1991; SHEP Cooperative Research Group 1991; MRC Working Party 1992). Meta-analyses of prospective randomized controlled trials indicated that a decrease in diastolic blood pressure of 5 to 6 mmHg reduced the risk for stroke by 42% with similar magnitudes of risk reduction for men, women, and subjects of all ages (Collins et al. 1990; Hebert et al. 1993; Staessen et al. 1997). The Syst-Eur trial demonstrated that treatment of older patients with isolated systolic hypertension led to a 42% reduction in stroke risk with no significant decline in overall mortality (Staessen et al. 1997).

Current guidelines for treatment of hypertension have been published by the Joint National Committee on Prevention, Detection, Evaluation, and Treatment of High Blood Pressure (Sixth Report of the Joint National Committee on Prevention, Detection, Evaluation and Treatment of High Blood Pressure 1997). Definitions of hypertension have been broadened to include individuals who were once considered borderline hypertensive. Since the attributable stroke risk for hypertension (proportion of strokes explained by hypertension) ranges from 35% to 50% depending on age, even a slight improvement in the control of hypertension could translate into a substantial reduction in stroke frequency (MacMahon and Rodgers 1994). The National Stroke Association guidelines to decrease risk for first stroke include (1) blood pressure control in patients with hypertension who are most likely to develop stroke, (2) physician check of blood pressure in all patients at every visit, and (3) patient self-monitoring of blood pressure at home.

Cardiac Diseases. Various cardiac conditions have been clearly associated with an increase in the risk of ischemic stroke. Since certain stroke risk factors, such as hypertension, may also be determinants of cardiac disease, some cardiac conditions may be viewed as intervening events in the causal chain for stroke. Cardiac factors that independently increase the risk of stroke include atrial fibrillation (AF), valvular heart disease, myocardial infarction, coronary artery disease, congestive heart failure, and electrocardiographic evidence of left ventricular hypertrophy. Improved cardiac imaging has led to the increased detection of potential stroke risk factors such as mitral annular calcification, patent foramen ovale (PFO), aortic arch atherosclerotic disease, atrial septal aneurysms, spontaneous echo contrast (a smoke-like appearance in the left cardiac chambers visualized on transesophageal echocardiography), and valvular strands.

Nonvalvular AF is a potent predictor of stroke, increasing the relative risk of stroke nearly fivefold (Wolf et al. 1991). Atrial fibrillation affects more than 2 million Americans and becomes more frequent with age, ranking as the leading cardiac arrhythmia in the elderly. The overall prevalence of AF is approximately 1%, but the prevalence among those ≥65 years is close to 6% (Wolf et al. 1991).

Clinical trials have demonstrated conclusive evidence of the efficacy of oral anticoagulation for stroke prevention among individuals with nonvalvular AF (Stroke Prevention in Atrial Fibrillation Study 1991). Aspirin may also have some efficacy among lower-risk groups or those who have relative contraindications to anticoagulation. For example, the Stroke Prevention in Atrial Fibrillation III (SPAF III) study demonstrated that warfarin with an international normalized ratio (INR) of 2–3 was far superior to ASA and minidose warfarin with an INR <1.5 in the prevention of stroke among high-risk patients with nonvalvular AF (Stroke Prevention in Atrial Fibrillation III 1996)

The recommendation from the Fifth American College of Chest Physicians Consensus Conference on Antithrombotic Therapy was that long-term oral warfarin therapy (INR 2.0–3.0, target 2.5) be used in patients with AF who are eligible for anticoagulation (Laupacis et al. 1998). It has been estimated that for every 1000 patients with nonvalvular AF treated with warfarin for 1 year, 35 thromboembolic events can be prevented at a cost of one major bleed.

Stroke risk nearly doubles in those with antecedent coronary artery disease, triples with left ventricular hypertrophy, and quadruples in subjects with cardiac failure (Di Tullio et al. 1998). Acute myocardial infarction has been associated with stroke. Even uncomplicated angina, non–Q wave infarction, and silent myocardial infarction were found to be stroke risk factors in the Framingham Study cohort (Benjamin et al. 1995). The attributable risk of stroke for coronary heart disease was approximately 12% and ranged from 2.3% to 6.0% for cardiac failure depending on age.

Mitral stenosis, endocarditis, and prosthetic heart valves are some of the valvular diseases that can increase the risk of stroke. After adjusting for other risk factors in the Framingham cohort, the presence of mitral annular calcification (MAC) was associated with a relative risk of stroke of 2.1 (Benjamin et al. 1992). Recent studies with more stringent diagnostic criteria for mitral valve prolapse have failed to demonstrate a convincing independent increase in stroke risk.

Atrial septal aneurysm (ASA) is another important cardiac factor associated with increased stroke risk. Case series have demonstrated a higher prevalence of ASA in patients with ischemic stroke of unknown cause (Lucas et al. 1999). Patients with ASA were younger and more likely to have a PFO or a cryptogenic stroke. In one study, the prevalence of ASA was 8% in controls, 28% in all stroke cases, and 39% in those with cryptogenic stroke (OR 4.3, 95% CI 1.3–14.6) (Labovitz et al. 1993). A strong association was found between ASA and PFO, with evidence of a synergistic effect for cryptogenic stroke (OR 33.3 for both, 3.0 for PFO, 2.1 for ASA). Paradoxical embolism through a PFO has long

been recognized as a potential cause of stroke (Lechat et al. 1988). This paradoxical embolism is defined as the arrival of a thrombus originating in the venous system into the systemic circulation through a right-to-left shunt (Lippmann and Rafferty 1993). Numerous case series reported finding this abnormality usually in young persons with cryptogenic stroke (Biller and Adams 1986; Hust et al. 1995). Case–control studies showed a PFO prevalence of between 26% and 40% in the event group compared to 3.2% and 15% in controls (Sacco et al. 1993). Another study classified ischemic stroke cases according to Stroke Data Bank criteria into those with defined cause of stroke and those with cryptogenic stroke. A PFO was more frequent in patients with cryptogenic stroke (42%) than in patients with stroke of determined origin (7%). The odds ratio for PFO and cryptogenic stroke diagnosis was 9.8 for the entire group, 20.9 for patients under 55, and 7.1 for the older subgroup (Di Tullio et al. 1992). Factors that may modify probability of stroke include PFO size, presence of a hypercoagulable state, and existence of a source of venous thrombus (Di Tullio et al. 1992).

Diabetes Mellitus and Insulin Resistance. Diabetes is a determinant of atherosclerosis and microangiopathy of the coronary, peripheral, and cerebral arteries. Death from cerebrovascular disease is greatly increased among subjects with elevated blood glucose values (Balkau et al. 1998). Cohort studies have demonstrated an independent effect of diabetes on stroke risk after controlling for other risk factors, with relative risks ranging from 1.5 to 3.0 (Barrett-Connor and Khaw 1988). Some studies suggest that the effect of diabetes on stroke risk is modified by gender (Davis et al. 1987). A Swedish study showed a sixfold rise in the risk of stroke in diabetic males compared to a 13-fold rise in females (Lindegard et al. 1987). Among Hawaiian men of Japanese descent, diabetics had twice the risk of thromboembolic stroke independent of other risk factors (Burchfiel et al. 1994). In the Framingham Study, the incidence of atherothrombotic infarction among diabetics was almost twice that of nondiabetics (Wolf et al. 1992). Insulin resistance is emerging as an important stroke risk factor as well (Adachi et al. 2001).

In Western Europe, insulin-dependent or type 1 diabetes accounts for about 10%–20% of all diabetic patients. Worldwide, type 2 diabetes is increasing, from an estimated 124 million at present to a predicted 221 million by the year 2010 (Watkins and Thomas 1998). In a multiethnic community, the prevalence of diabetes is 22% and 20% among elderly African Americans and Hispanics, with corresponding etiologic factors of 13% and 20% (Sacco et al. 2001a).

Intensive treatment of both type 1 and type 2 diabetes, aimed at maintaining near-normal levels of blood glucose, can substantially reduce the risk of microvascular complications such as retinopathy, nephropathy, and neuropathy, but has not been conclusively shown to reduce macrovascular complications including stroke (Diabetes Control and Complications Trial Research Group 1993). However, the U.K. Prospective Diabetes Study Group (1998) reported that aggressive treatment of blood pressure (<150/85 mmHg) among type 2 diabetics helped reduce the risk of stroke by 44%. Guidelines for management of diabetes have lowered the target fasting blood glucose level to 126 mg/dl (American Diabetes Association 1998). The National Stroke Association (NSA) recommends rigorous comprehensive control of blood sugar levels for adherent patients with type 1 diabetes and type 2 diabetes to prevent microvascular complications.

Dyslipidemias. Abnormalities of serum lipids (triglyceride, cholesterol, low-density lipoprotein [LDL], high-density lipoprotein [HDL]) are clear risk factors for atherosclerotic disease, particularly coronary disease. Recent studies have helped clarify the relationship between lipids and stroke risk.

Studies utilizing ultrasound technology have established that total cholesterol or LDL cholesterol is directly associated and HDL cholesterol is inversely associated with extracranial carotid atherosclerosis and intima-media plaque thickness (Heiss et al. 1991; O'Leary et al. 1992; Fine-Edelstein et al. 1994; Ansell 2000). Case–control studies have found the concentration of HDL to be lower in stroke cases after controlling for other risk factors (Qizilbash et al. 1991; Sacco et al. 2001b). Many prospective studies have found no association between serum cholesterol and cerebral infarction (Benfante et al. 1994). However, in the Multiple Risk Factor Intervention Trial, mortality from ischemic stroke was greater among men with high cholesterol (Iso et al. 1989). The Honolulu Heart Program demonstrated a continuous and progressive increase in both coronary heart disease and thromboembolic stroke rates with increasing levels of cholesterol, with a relative risk of 1.4 when comparing highest and lowest quartiles (Burchfiel et al. 1994).

Meta-analyses of prospective studies have found either no or only a minimally increased relative risk of stroke due to elevated total cholesterol (Qizilbash et al. 1991; Prospective Studies Collaboration 1995). The absence of a consistent significant relationship between cholesterol and stroke may be partially explained by the recognition that not all stroke subtypes are attributable to atherosclerosis. Additionally, most prospective studies were done among younger populations and focused on cardiac outcomes, and lipoprotein fractions were not always evaluated separately from total cholesterol.

Clinical trials analyzing the efficacy of lipid-lowering strategies with statins have demonstrated impressive reductions in stroke risk in various high-risk populations with cardiac disease. In these studies, stroke was either a secondary end point or a nonspecified end point determined on the basis of post-hoc analyses (Scandinavian Simvastatin Survival Study Group 1994,

Hebert et al. 1997). Meta-analyses of some of these trials have found significant reductions in stroke risk, with a 29% reduced risk of stroke and a 22% reduction in overall mortality (Blauw et al. 1997; Hebert et al. 1997). Secondary prevention trials showed a 32% stroke risk reduction and primary trials demonstrated a 20% reduction. Two large trials in which stroke was prespecified as a secondary end point have also shown significant reductions with pravastatin use among subjects with coronary artery disease and normal to only modest elevations of cholesterol (Sacks et al. 1996; LIPID Group 1998).

Using serial carotid ultrasound measurements, some clinical trials have also demonstrated carotid plaque regression with statins (Blakenhorn et al. 1993; Furberg et al. 1994; Crouse et al. 1995; Salonen et al. 1995; Hodis et al. 1996). There is mounting support for the role of lipoproteins as precursors of carotid atherosclerosis and ischemic stroke and for the benefits of cholesterol lowering in stroke reduction. Individuals with cholesterol levels above 200 mg/dl and cardiovascular risk factors should have a complete lipid analysis (total cholesterol, LDL, HDL, triglycerides) and most likely would benefit from cholesterol-lowering regimens including statins (Expert Panel in Detection, Evaluation, and Treatment of High Blood Cholesterol in Adults 1993).

Cigarette Smoking. Despite the clear evidence that cigarette smoking is an independent determinant of stroke and other diseases, it remains a major modifiable public health threat in every nation (Higa and Davanipour 1991). In case–control studies the effect of cigarette smoking remained significant after adjustment for other factors, and a dose–response relationship was apparent (Gorelick et al. 1989). Prospective studies have confirmed these findings in both men and women (Abbott et al. 1986; Colditz et al. 1988).

Example 9–4 The Honolulu Heart Study is a large prospective cohort study of Japanese men followed up to document cardiovascular outcomes and stroke. This study demonstrated that smoking was an independent predictor of ischemic stroke, with adjusted relative risks of 2.5 for men and 3.1 for women, respectively. A meta-analysis of 32 studies found a summary relative risk of stroke for smokers of 1.5 (95% CI 1.4–1.6) (Shinton and Beevers 1989). The risk decreased with age and was slightly higher for women than for men. Stroke risk was increased twofold in heavy smokers (>40 cigarettes per day) compared with that for light smokers (<10 cigarettes per day). The stroke risk attributed to cigarette smoking was greatest for subarachnoid hemorrhage, intermediate for cerebral infarction, and lowest for cerebral hemorrhage. Even the effects of passive cigarette smoking exposure have been found to increase the risk of progression of atherosclerosis (Howard et al. 1998).

Cigarette smoking is an independent determinant of carotid artery plaque thickness and the strongest predictor of severe extracranial carotid artery atherosclerosis (O'Leary et al. 1992; Sacco et al. 1997b; Mast et al. 1998). Other biological mechanisms by which cigarettes may predispose to stroke include increased coagulability, blood viscosity, and fibrinogen levels, enhanced platelet aggregation, and elevated blood pressure. Secondhand smoke or passive smoking may also contribute to increased stroke risk (Denson 2000).

No randomized clinical trial has been performed to support the benefits of cigarette smoking cessation; however, there is ample evidence from observational epidemiologic studies that smoking cessation leads to a reduction in stroke risk. The Nurses' Health Study and the Framingham Study both showed that the risk of ischemic stroke is reduced to that of nonsmokers after 2 and 5 years, respectively (Wolf et al. 1988; Kamachi et al. 1993). It has been estimated that elimination of cigarette smoking in the United States could reduce the number of strokes occurring each year by 61,500, saving 3.08 billion stroke-related health-care dollars (Gorelick 1997).

The NSA recommends the cessation of smoking as a stroke prevention measure, in accordance with guidelines by the Agency for Health Care Policy and Research that address various topics, including screening for tobacco use, advice to quit, interventions, smoking cessation pharmacotherapy, motivation to quit, and relapse prevention.

Alcohol Use. Early case–control studies failed to identify a significant association between alcohol and ischemic stroke (Ben-Shlomo et al. 1992; Beghi et al. 1995; Gorelick 1997). In northern Manhattan, however, a J-shaped relationship between alcohol and stroke was found—an elevated stroke risk for heavy alcohol consumption and a protective effect in light to moderate drinkers (2 or fewer drinks per day) when compared with nondrinkers (Sacco et al. 1999) (Fig. 9–3). The protective effect of alcohol was documented among young women (Malarcher et al. 2001). Methodological problems in a case–control approach to study alcohol and stroke have been well summarized (Camargo 1989,

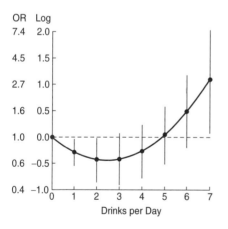

Figure 9–3 Relationship between alcohol use and ischemic stroke. Reference group is those not drinking during past year. Analysis is matched for age, gender, and race/ethnicity and adjusted for hypertension, diabetes mellitus, cardiac disease, current cigarette smoking use, and education. OR, odds ratio; vertical lines indicate 95% confidence intervals. (Reprinted with permission from Sacco et al. 1999.)

1996). One study, for example, demonstrated that the odds ratio for stroke ranged from 0.73 (protective) to 1.93 (deleterious) depending upon whether controls were selected from a general hospital population, a population without potential alcohol-related diagnoses, or the community (Camargo 1996).

Prospective cohort studies, conducted in predominantly white populations, addressing the relationship of stroke to alcohol intake have found evidence of a protective effect of mild alcohol intake (Stampfer et al. 1998; Truelson et al. 1998; Klatsky et al. 2001). The Nurses' Health Study found a protective effect of mild alcohol consumption, up to 1.2 drinks per day in women, for ischemic stroke (Stampfer et al. 1998). Several studies looking specifically at ischemic stroke in Japanese subjects failed to show any protective effect of alcohol, suggesting that alcohol's effect as a stroke risk factor may vary by race/ethnicity.

The various mechanisms through which alcohol may increase the risk of stroke include hypertension, hypercoagulable states, cardiac arrhythmias, and cerebral blood flow reductions. There is also evidence that light to moderate drinking can increase HDL cholesterol, reduce the risk of coronary artery disease, and increase endogenous tissue plasminogen activator. The combination of deleterious and beneficial effects of alcohol is consistent with the observation of a dose-dependent relationship between alcohol and stroke. Elimination of heavy drinking can reduce the incidence of stroke. Since some ingestion of alcohol, perhaps up to 2 drinks per day, may actually help reduce the risk of stroke, drinking in moderation should not be discouraged for most of the public.

Physical Activity. The cardiovascular benefits of physical activity have been broadcast by numerous organizations, including the Centers for Disease Control and Prevention, the National Institutes of Health, and the American Heart Association, based on accumulating data about the effects of physical activity in reducing the risk of heart disease and premature death. Previous studies have shown beneficial effects for physical activity predominantly among white populations, with greater effects in men than in women and in younger than older adults (Abbott et al. 1994; Kiely et al. 1994; Gillum et al. 1996; Sacco et al. 1998b; Lee et al. 1999; Hu et al. 2000). The Honolulu Heart Program, which investigated older middle-aged men of Japanese ancestry, showed a protective effect of habitual physical activity from thromboembolic stroke only among the non-smoking group (Abbott et al. 1994). The Framingham Study demonstrated the benefits of combined leisure and work physical activities for men, but not for women (Kiely et al. 1994). In the Oslo Study, among younger men, increased leisure physical activity was related to a reduced stroke incidence (Haheim et al. 1993). The Nurses' Health Study showed an inverse association between level of physical activity and the incidence of any stroke in women (Hu et al. 2000). Finally, in the Northern Manhattan Stroke Study, the benefits of leisure-time physical activity were noted for all age, gender, and racial/ethnic subgroups (Sacco et al. 1999).

The optimal amount of exercise needed to prevent stroke is unclear, particularly for the elderly. Recent vigorous exercise may be no more protective than walking. In the Framingham Study, the strongest protection was detected in the medium-tertile physical activity subgroup, with no benefit gained from additional activity (Kiely et al. 1994). The protective effect of physical activity may be partly mediated through its role in controlling various risk factors such as hypertension, diabetes, and obesity. Other than control of risk factors, biological mechanisms such as increased HDL and reduced homocysteine level may also be responsible for the effect of physical activity (Nygard et al. 1995; Lee et al. 1999).

Physical activity is a modifiable behavior that requires greater emphasis in stroke prevention campaigns. The 1994 Behavioral Risk Factor Surveillance Survey found that 60% of adults do not achieve the recommended amount of physical activity and people with the lowest incomes and less than 12th grade education are more likely to be sedentary. Moreover, 70% to 80% of older women report levels less than the recommended amount of physical activity (U.S. Department of Health and Human Services 1996). Public health goals are to increase the proportion of people who engage in regular physical activity and to reduce the proportion of those who engage in no leisure-time physical activity, particularly among people aged 65 and older (U.S. Department of Health and Human Services 2000). Leisure-time physical activity could translate into a cost-effective means of decreasing the public health burden of stroke and other cardiovascular diseases among rapidly aging populations.

Dietary Factors. While data have suggested that diet may play an important role in stroke risk, few studies have been able to clarify this relationship because of the complex issues associated with dietary intake and nutritional status. Large ecological studies have suggested that excess fat intake associated with migration may lead to increased risk of both coronary heart disease and stroke. High daily dietary intake of fat is associated with obesity and may act independently or may affect risk factors such as hypertension, diabetes, hyperlipidemia, and cardiac disease. A conflicting report from the Framingham Study demonstrated an inverse association between dietary fat and ischemic stroke (Gillman et al. 1997). Dietary sodium may also be associated with increased stroke risk through hypertension.

Another important dietary component is homocysteine (Goldstein 2000). Case–control studies have demonstrated an association between moderately elevated homocysteine and vascular disease including stroke (Boushey et al. 1995). Genetic and environmental causes of increased serum homocysteine have been implicated as modifiable determinants of cardiovascular and cerebrovascular events (Giles et al. 1998). In the Framingham Study, deficiencies in folate, B_{12} levels, and pyridoxine accounted for most of the elevated homocysteine levels in the study cohort (Selhub et al. 1995). Evidence from case–control studies has suggested that increased dietary and supplemental intake of vitamin B_6 may decrease stroke risk (Spence et al. 2001).

Dietary intake of fruits and vegetables may reduce the risk of stroke and contribute to stroke protection by antioxidant mechanisms or by elevating potassium levels (Khaw and Barrett-Connor 1987; Gey et al. 1993; Gillman et al. 1995; Boden-Albala and Sacco 2000; Leppala et al. 2000). Dietary antioxidants, including vitamin C, vitamin E, and β-carotene, belong to a group of antioxidants called *flavonoids* that are found in fruits and vegetables. These scavengers of free radicals are thought to be associated with stroke risk reduction through the free-radical oxidation of LDL, which inhibits the formation of atherosclerotic plaques (Diaz et al. 1997). The Western Electric cohort found a moderate decrease in stroke risk associated with a higher intake of both β-carotene and vitamin C (Orencia et al. 1996). Other dietary factors associated with a reduced risk of stroke include intake of milk and calcium and of fish oils (Morris et al. 1995; Abbott et al. 1996, Orenica et al. 1996).

Extracranial Carotid Stenosis. Carotid stenosis is an important predictor of TIA and stroke. The occurrence of symptoms may depend on the severity and progression of the stenosis, the adequacy of collateral circulation, the character of the atherosclerotic plaque, and the propensity to form thrombus at the site of the stenosis. In patients with symptomatic disease, the 2-year risk of stroke approaches 26% among medically treated patients with TIA/minor stroke and ipsilateral carotid stenosis >70% (North American Symptomatic Carotid Endarterectomy Trial 1991).

In asymptomatic carotid artery disease, the annual stroke risk is lower (1.3%) in those with stenosis <75%, and 3.3% in those with stenosis >75%, with ipsilateral stroke risk of 2.5% (Norris et al. 1991; North American Symptomatic Carotid Endarterectomy Trial 1991; Barnett et al. 1998). The combined TIA and stroke risk was 10.5% per year in those with >75% carotid stenosis. Asymptomatic carotid disease increases with age, occurring in 53.6% of subjects 65 to 94 years of age (Pujia et al. 1992).

The efficacy of carotid endarterectomy in asymptomatic carotid stenosis has been evaluated in clinical trials including the Asymptomatic Carotid Artery Surgery Study (ACASS) (Executive Committee for the Asymptomatic Carotid Atherosclerosis Study 1995). Patients eligible for the ACASS were under age 80 and had asymptomatic carotid stenosis >60% and no unstable cardiac disease. Overall, the 30-day ipsilateral stroke or death rate in surgically treated patients was 2.3%. The trial found a 5-year ipsilateral stroke risk of 10.5% among the medical group and 4.8% in the surgical group. A 55% risk reduction of ipsilateral stroke was associated with carotid endarterectomy. The benefit for men was greater than for women (risk reduction 69% vs. 16%) (Executive Committee for the Asymptomatic Carotid Atherosclerosis Study 1995). Given the right circumstances based on the degree of the stenosis, other comorbid conditions, and the expertise of the surgeon, endarterectomy may be beneficial in certain asymptomatic persons.

Transient Ischemic Attacks. Transient ischemic attacks are a strong predictor of subsequent stroke, with annual stroke risks of 1% to 15%. The first year following a TIA is associated with the greatest stroke risk. In hospital-referred patients, the average annual risk of stroke, myocardial infarction, or death was 7.5% after TIA (Hankey et al. 1991). Recommendations for the treatment of TIA include identification of the underlying etiology of the TIA, targeted risk factor prevention strategies, and the use of antithrombotic medications (Albers et al. 1998).

Subclinical Markers of Cerebrovascular Disease. Identification of subclinical disease may be important in early detection of stroke risk factors. Important subclinical markers include carotid intima-medial plaque thickness, aortic arch atheroma, lower extremity arterial disease, and white matter disease. Detection of markers include measurement of intimal-medial thickness (IMT) through carotid ultrasound, aortic arch atheroma identification through the use of transesophageal echogardiography, and ankle/brachial blood pressure measurement to assess lower extremity arterial disease and cerebral magnetic resonance imaging to assess white matter disease.

Carotid ultrasound imaging has emerged as a useful noninvasive method of evaluating subclinical atherosclerosis according to both observational epidemiological studies and clinical trials. Ultrasound measures of carotid artery IMT correlate well with pathologically defined atherosclerosis and are highly reproducible (Pignoli et al. 1986; O'Leary et al. 1999). Carotid plaque thickness and morphology have been found to be strongly associated with prevalence and incidence of clinical cardiovascular disease. In the Cardiovascular Health Study, a 1 standard deviation (SD) increment in carotid IMT (0.20 mm CCA) resulted in a 36% increased risk of stroke or myocardial infarction after adjustment for age, gender, and other risk factors (O'Leary et al. 1992). Further, the Atherosclerosis Risk in Communities (ARIC) study, a prospective study of vascular risk factors that was conducted in multiple communities throughout the United States. ARIC found that every 0.19 mm increment in the mean IMT was associated with a statistically significant adjusted 38% increase for women and 17% increase for men in the risk of a coronary ischemic event (Burke et al. 1995).

The presence of protruding or ulcerated atheromas in the ascending aorta and the aortic arch is associated with an increased frequency of peripheral or cerebral embolic events. Protruding aortic arch atheromas may be a risk factor for ischemic stroke because of their potential for embolization to the cerebral circulation (Davila-Roman et al. 1994). A prospective study using transesophageal echocardiography detected a significantly greater frequency of cerebral or peripheral embolic events in 42 patients with protruding aortic atheromas compared to 42 matching controls (33% vs. 7%). Transesophageal echocardiography has also shown a high frequency of protruding aortic atheromas in patients with cryptogenic stroke and confirmed the role of aortic atheromas as an independent risk factor for stroke (Tunick et al. 1994; Di Tullio et al. 2000). In a large autopsy series, Amarenco et al. (1992) detected a much greater frequency of ulcerated aortic atheromas in patients who had died from a stroke than in patients who had died from other neurological diseases (26% vs. 5%; OR 4.0). Moreover, the highest frequency of ulcerated atheromas was found in patients with unexplained cryptogenic stroke subtype (Amarenco et al. 1992).

Ischemic white matter disease was first detected on CT scans from stroke patients in the population-based Framingham Heart Study. Subsequently, MRI-imaged infarcts were associated with stroke in the Cardiovascular Health Study (Manolio et al. 1994; Longstreth et al. 1996). These white matter lesions have been related to previous strokes and are associated with other risk factors and dementia (Hebert et al. 2000).

Other Potential Ischemic Stroke Risk Factors. Other potential stroke risk factors have been identified in some studies but need confirmation and clarification through further epidemiologic investigations. A growing literature suggests that infection and inflammation may be important stroke risk factors (Elkind et al. 2000). Included among the potential genetic markers for lipids are lipoprotein (a) and apolipoprotein E [Apo(e)] (Weir et al.

2001). Markers of hypercoagulable states may be independent stroke risk factors and include antiphospholipid antibodies, lupus anticoagulant, factor V Leiden, and free protein S. The possibility of hormone use being a stroke risk factor is under investigation in the Heart and Estrogen/progestin Replacement Study (HERS) (Simon et al. 2001). Results from the WHI randomized clinical trial showed a twofold increase in risk for nonfatal stroke for postmenopausal women who were randomized to take estrogen plus progestin compared with women who did not receive hormones (Writing Group for the Women's Health Initiative Investigators 2002). The trial continues to follow the women who were randomized to receive estrogen alone to assess their risk for stroke and other diseases. A meta-analysis of observational and case–control studies also indicated a 20% increase in risk for nonfatal thromboembolic stroke in women who had ever used estrogen or estrogen plus progestin compared with women who had never used these hormones (Nelson et al. 2002).

Hemorrhagic Stroke

Subtype and Risk Factors for Intracerebral Hemorrhage

It is estimated that ICH accounts for between 15% and 20% of all stroke with annual incidence figures being close to 75,000 in the United States each year (American Heart Association 1999). Intracerebral hemorrhage is associated with high mortality rates and inadequate methods of treatment and prevention. Incidence rates varied markedly prior to use of CT and even today, distinguishing among primary intracerebral hemorrhages, hemorrhagic infarction, and primary subarachnoid hemorrhages with parenchymal extension remains problematic. The most common ICH subtypes include hypertensive arteriolar disease, amyloid deposition, and vascular malformations. Classification of ICH subtypes is difficult without confirmatory diagnostic laboratory data; therefore many cases of spontaneous ICH could be classified as unknown etiology. Treatment for ICH has been largely restricted to rehabilitation and hypertension control. Patients with ICH in lobar locations such as the frontal, parietal, temporal, and occipital cortices have been found to have hypertension less frequently (Sacco et al. 1991). The identification of risk factors for ICH continues to be elusive because of the relatively low incidence of disease.

Risk Markers for Intracerebral Hemorrhage—Age, Gender, and Race/Ethnicity. Intracerebral hemorrhage is associated with increasing age and has been reported to be greater among men (Bruno et al. 1996). A number of studies have confirmed differences in the incidence of ICH among racial/ethnic groups. In a study comparing ICH and SAH incidence in African Americans and whites, the risk of ICH among African Americans under 75 years was 2.3 (95% CI 1.5–3.6) times greater than that for whites (Broderick et al. 1992). Authors of the National Health and Nutrition Examination Survey (NHANES) I reported an age- and gender-adjusted relative risk for ICH of 1.9 (95% CI 1.1–3.2) when comparing African Americans with whites (Qureshi et al. 1999). Similarly, findings from the Northern Manhattan Stroke Study indicate greater age-adjusted relative risks for ICH among both African Americans and Hispanics than among whites (Sacco et al. 1999). Higher rates of ICH have also been reported in Asian populations compared with Western populations. For example, a retrospective chart review of ICH cases in Bernalillo County, New Mexico, indicated a significantly greater age and gender-adjusted incidence rate of spontaneous ICH cases among Hispanic residents than that for white residents (Bruno et al. 1996). Incidence rates among Hispanic men were greater than those among African American men (RR 2.9). African American women had higher rates of ICH than white women (RR 3.2) and Hispanic women (RR 2.0).

Hypertension. Hypertension remains the most important and most modifiable risk factor associated with primary ICH. The risk of ICH is 2–6 times greater among those with hypertension than among those with no hypertension (Kagan et al. 1985; Ruiz-Sandoval et al. 1999). Data from Rochester, Minnesota, found that either severe short-term hypertension or chronic long-term hypertension is associated with increased risk of hemorrhage (Furlan et al. 1979). The Hiroshima and Nagasaki Cohort demonstrated a dose–response relationship between risk of ICH and systolic blood pressure among Japanese (Okada et al. 1976) and a 3.48 risk of ICH for hypertensive individuals older than 31 years. In a smaller case series, small spontaneous hemorrhages were more frequently associated with small chronic hemorrhage, ischemic lesions, and hypertension, leading the authors to conclude that hypertensive ICH may be associated with the same underlying pathology as that for lacunar infarctions (Tanaka et al. 1999).

Amyloid Deposition in Cerebral Vessels. Cerebral amyloid angiopathy (CAA), also known as cerebral congophilic angiopathy and cerebral amyloidosis, is an important cause of lobar intracerebral hemorrhage (Vinters 1998). The pathology consists of the infiltration of medium-sized cortical vessels by amyloid β-protein, a hyaline eosinophilic substance found in the aging brain and an important component of the senile plaques described with Alzheimer's disease. The clinical syndrome is characterized by lobar ICH with no other definite cause of brain hemorrhage in someone usually over the age of 60 who may have some antecedent memory loss. Although sporadic cases far outnumber those with a family history, a genetic etiology for CAA-ICH seems likely. Family studies from The Netherlands and Iceland have demonstrated the familial aggregation of CAA-ICH and have attributed the disease to autosomal dominant mutations of the amyloid precursor protein on chromosome 21

(Bornebroek et al. 1996). A genetic mechanism has also been suggested by the findings of an association of apolipoprotein E polymorphism (e4 or e2) and the occurrence of CAA-ICH (Greenberg et al. 1995, 1998). The ApoE4 allele has been associated with Alzheimer's disease and multi-infarct dementia (Mayeux et al. 1998). Some investigators have reported that antiplatelet or anticoagulant medication use, hypertension, and minor head trauma were more frequent antecedents among patients with CAA-ICH who were ApoE2 carriers, a finding suggesting possible genetic–environmental interactions (McCarron et al. 1999). Links between amyloid, apolipoprotein E, and the clinical phenotypes of Alzheimer's disease and CAA-ICH suggest shared molecular genetic mechanisms whereby neuronal and microvascular degeneration in the brain may be the end result. A better understanding of the etiology of CAA-ICH will undoubtedly lead to candidate agents to interfere with the generation, deposition, and pathological effects of cerebral amyloid.

Alcohol. The role of alcohol as a risk factor for ICH is controversial and differs by dosage as well as stroke subtype (Gorelick et al. 1989). Almost all studies have shown an increased risk of hemorrhagic stroke associated with increasing alcohol consumption in a dose-dependent fashion (Donahue et al. 1986). A recent case–control study from Australia found that heavy drinking increased the risk of ICH by 3.4 (95% CI 1.4–8.4) (Thrift et al. 1999). A significant increase in the risk of ICH was noted among hypertensive individuals who engaged in heavy alcohol intake in the Hisayama Study, which suggests a synergistic relationship between these two risk factors (Kiyohara et al. 1995).

Anticoagulants. The increased use of anticoagulants for atrial fibrillation, treatment of TIA, and stroke recurrence has resulted in an additional risk of ICH. Early use of high-dose anticoagulants may have resulted in a risk as great as 11-fold for ICH (Furlan et al. 1979). Randomized studies, however, have suggested that the use of warfarin for atrial fibrillation is associated with a lower risk of ICH (Albers et al. 1991). Intracerebral hemorrhage resulting from anticoagulant therapy should continue to be monitored.

Prior Cerebral Infarction. Another potential risk factor for ICH is a history of prior cerebral infarction. The association of these two distinct pathological conditions results from shared risk factors, including hypertension. One study found that 39% of patients with first ICH had a history of either stroke or silent prior infarct on CT (Brott et al. 1986). The hemorrhage may occur early post-infarct, resulting in a hemorrhagic transformation. In a prospective CT study among 65 older patients, evidence of hemorrhagic transformation was seen in 43% of the cases (Hornig et al. 1986).

Cholesterol. Low cholesterol may be a risk factor for ICH, but the evidence is speculative. Three cohort studies reported no significant differences in mean cholesterol between individuals with and without ICH but found an increased risk of between 2.5 and 3 among those whose cholesterol was defined by the lowest quartile of the cohort in the range of 160 to 189 mg/dl (Iso et al. 1989). In a case–control study in Boston, low cholesterol increased the odds for hemorrhage by 2.5 (95% CI 1.0–4.5) (Segal et al. 1999). In the Kaiser Permanente Medical Care program, an association between low serum cholesterol and ICH was found but was confined to men over 65 years of age (RR 2.7, 95% CI 1.4–5.0) (Iribarren et al. 1996).

Subarachnoid Hemorrhage

Subarachnoid hemorrhage accounts for over 6% of all strokes, with an estimated incidence of 30,000 per year (American Heart Association 1999). The most common causes of spontaneous SAH include

aneurysms and arteriovenous malformations. Despite improvement in treatment of SAH, case-fatality rates of between 25% and 50% underscore the importance of identifying risk factors for SAH prevention. There are relatively few studies that have been able to elucidate risk factors for SAH (Longstreth et al. 1993; Inagawa et al. 1995; Ingall et al. 2000). Difficulty in identifying risk factors for SAH stems from the small sample size and poor diagnostic criteria associated with many studies. Poor diagnostic criteria, for example, may lead to misclassification of ICH into SAH groups.

Risk Markers—Age Gender and Race/ethnicity. Age may be a less important risk factor for SAH then for ICH (Broderick et al. 1995). The risk of SAH is greater for women than for men, although the reason for this is unclear (Bruno et al. 1997). In Cincinnati, African Americans had 2.1 (95% CI 1.3–3.6) times the risk of SAH compared to whites (Broderick et al. 1995). A greater SAH incidence rate was found in African American men (RR 5.3, 95% CI 1.0–30.0) in northern Manhattan; however, the small sample size in the SAH group precluded any meaningful conclusion (Sacco et al. 1998a).

Hypertension. The role of hypertension as a risk factor for SAH remains controversial. Retrospective studies have failed to demonstrate a relationship between hypertension and SAH (Bonita 1986; Canhao et al. 1994), but a number of prospective studies have a two- to threefold increased risk of SAH due to hypertension (Knekt et al. 1991; Adamson et al. 1994). Hypertension may lead to aneurysm formation and rupture only in susceptible individuals.

Cigarette Smoking. Cigarette smoking is one of the most important risk factors for SAH (Longstreth et al. 1992). This relationship has been demonstrated in a number of retrospective and prospective studies. A dose–response relationship was documented in the King County Study, with an elevated risk of 11.1 for SAH among those smoking more than one pack a day, compared to a risk of 4.1 among those who reported smoking less than 1 pack per day (Longstreth et al. 1992).

Alcohol Use. Studies disagree on the relationship between alcohol use and risk for SAH. Risk is most often associated with increased use of alcohol; however, this association is less when controlling for smoking (Longstreth 1991). In a meta-analysis, the relative risk of SAH for drinking <150 g/week was 2.8 and for drinking ≥150 g/week was 4.7 (Teunissen et al. 1996).

Hormones. Hormone use has long been thought to account for the greater prevalence of SAH among women. Early studies indicated that use of any oral contraceptives increased risk of SAH (Longstreth and Swanson 1984). Results from a Swedish study suggest, however, that higher doses of oral therapy are more likely to be associated with increased risk of SAH (Lindegard and Hillbom 1987). Oral contraceptives and postmenopausal hormone replacement therapy have been associated with a reduced risk of stroke including SAH (Schwartz et al. 1998; Nelson et al. 2002; Writing Group for the Women Health Initiative Investigators 2002). A pooled study of two population-based case–control studies found that the use of low-dose oral contraceptives was not a predictor of hemorrhagic stroke (OR 1.0, 95 % CI 0.29–1.47), and a trend toward a protective effect against ischemic stroke was associated with use of low-dose oral contraceptives (RR 0.66, 95% CI 0.29–1.47). Low-dose oral contraceptive use was not associated with stroke type among women who were older than 35 years, were cigarette smokers, were obese, and used antihypertensives, but was associated with history of migraine (Schwartz et al. 1998). Other potential risk factors for SAH include hypercholesterolemia and physical inactivity (Abbott et al. 1994).

Outcomes

Both stroke subtype and comorbid conditions influence outcome. Important outcome measures for stroke include mortality, recurrence, functional disability, and quality of life. Death is the most important early outcome of stroke. Mortality is usually measured at 30 days, and then annually. Overall, 30-day mortality is highest in ICH and SAH subtypes, with rates lower for infarct cases. Stroke mortality is classified as vascular or nonvascular. Vascular etiology is more likely to contribute to early mortality. In the Northern Manhattan Stroke Study, 72% of 30-day mortality was attributed to underlying vascular causes as opposed to 43% of deaths at 1 year (Sacco et al. 1994; Hartmann et al. 2001).

Two factors related to early mortality are stroke severity and stroke subtype. Markers of more severe strokes include depressed consciousness, size of infarction, severity of the neurologic deficit, and characteristics of the admitting syndrome. In ischemic stroke, worse outcomes were associated with a major hemispheric or basilar syndrome. Cardioembolic stroke has been shown to be associated with a 15% 30-day mortality whereas those with lacunar syndrome have a better prognosis (Sacco et al. 1994).

Intracerebral hemorrhage is the most lethal of all stroke subtypes. Recent studies have documented lower case-fatality rates for ICH (40%–55%) (Giroud et al. 1991). Despite high mortality rates, little attention has been given to risk factors associated with poor outcomes. Predictors of death after ICH include size of the hemorrhage, degree of impairment of consciousness on admission, Glasgow Coma Scale (GCS) results, presence of intraventricular hemorrhage, and pulse pressure (Juvela et al. 1992; Longstreth et al. 1993; Broderick et al. 1994). Using the admitting Glasgow Coma Score, size of the initial hematoma, and pulse pressure, the 30-day survival for patients with ICH can be estimated with a model developed from the Stroke Data

Bank (Mayer et al. 1994). Hypertension history was a risk factor for early death in an Asian hospital-based cohort (Wong 1999). Significantly greater mean admission blood pressure was associated with early fatal outcomes in those with putaminal and thalamic hemorrhage among the 1701 ICH patients enrolled in the Keio Cooperative Stroke Study (Terayama et al. 1997). Predictors of ICH case fatality in a large German study included ventricular extension, increasing age, surgical treatment localization in basal ganglia, and hypertension as the underlying etiology (Rosenow et al. 1997).

Population studies focusing on prognostic indicators following SAH remain sparse. The King County Study assessed short-term outcomes post-SAH, finding that one-third of patients were dead at 1 month, one-third had neurologic deficits, and one-third were better (Longstreth et al. 1993). A higher score on the admission GCS and absence of blood on the first CT were independent predictors of better recovery. Patients with SAH are often younger at the time of their stroke and present with more life-threatening situations than those with cerebral infarction. Thirty-day SAH case fatality rates range from 25% to 55% (Philips et al. 1980; Sacco et al. 1984; Bonita and Thompson et al. 1985). In the Framingham Study, coma at onset was associated with a case fatality rate of 83%, compared to 56% for those with focal deficits and 13% for those with no focal deficits (Kassel and Torner 1983). There is a direct relationship between the clinical grade at presentation and mortality. In the Rochester study, the 30-day case fatality rates were 30% for grade 1–2 patients, 65% for grade 3, and 85% for grade 4–5 (Drury et al. 1984). Fatality rates are associated with age, intracranial hematoma, alcohol use, and hypertension (Sacco et al. 1984; Juvela 1992, Mayer et al. 1994). Surgical success may vary depending on the timing of the intervention, with success favoring earlier intervention. There is a definite risk of rebleeding among ruptured aneurysms; it may be as high as 50% over the first 60 days, with the greatest risk of rebleeding within the first 24 hours and a persistent 3% risk per year after 6 months (Kassel and Torner 1989).

Example 9–5 Population-based studies often provide information that is generalizible to other populations. Data from the population-based study of SAH in King County, Washington, was used to calculate a simple prognostic score based on admission Glasgow Coma Score, age, and presence or absence of subarachnoid blood on initial CT. A prognostic score makes use of important information and provides clinicians with better estimates for patient outcomes (Longstreth et al. 1993).

Few studies have focused on the long-term outcome after SAH, but data indicate that survival will approach that of the general population for those who survive the early period (Olafsson et al. 1997). Survival is worse among those with significant neurological deficits. Recurrence of SAH is higher among nonsurgically treated survivors, with annual rates ranging from 2.2% to 3.5%, but rates are lower than expected for surgically treated patients (Winn et al. 1977).

Predictors of late mortality continue to be assessed. Definite predictors include age and cardiac disease, with diabetes and congestive heart failure being other possible factors (Sacco et al. 1994). Stroke worsening is related to outcome. Unfortunately, stroke evolution or worsening is difficult to assess because of the unstable hospital course, differences in stroke subtype, and poor documentation in medical records. Analysts of the Stroke Data Bank suggest that 75% of the cases classified as having an unstable hospital course had worsening of the incident stroke (Sacco et al. 1989b). Among ICH cases, rebleeding may occur, contributing to deterioration; worsening among patients alert on admission was most dependent on hematoma size measured on initial CT (Kassel and Torner 1983;

Olafsson et al. 1997). Recurrence after ICH is thought to be low, but this has not been well documented (Olafsson et al. 1997).

It is more difficult to identify risk factors for recurrent disease. The lower frequency of specific outcomes, greater prevalence of the exposure at onset, and competing effects of mortality make detection of such factors statistically more onerous. Stroke recurrence, particularly after ischemic stroke, varies between 1% and 4% in the first month. Recurrence at 1 year is about 5%–25%, and at 5 years it may be as great as 20% to 40% (Sacco et al. 1994). Recurrence rates vary by subtype and comorbid condition. Early recurrence is tightly associated with stroke subtype. It has been estimated that 8%–9% of strokes that involve large vessels will have early recurrence (Rundek et al. 2000). Likewise, patients with both intracranial and extracranial disease have a greater risk of recurrent stroke (Rundek et al. 2000). Other predictors of early stroke recurrence include elevated blood glucose and hypertension (Sacco et al. 1994).

Late stroke recurrence is more strongly linked to conventional risk factors than to stroke subtype, although atherosclerotic strokes do have a greater risk of late recurrence. Lacunar stroke subtype is associated with the lowest risk of recurrence (O'Donnell et al. 2000). Other risk factors associated with late recurrence include age, hypertension, TIAs, cardiac risk factors, and heavy alcohol consumption. Low albumin/globulin ratio, anticardiolipin antibodies, and aortic arch atheroma are possible risk factors for late recurrence.

Stroke recurrence for primary ICH has rarely been elucidated. Recurrence is uniformly associated with worse disability and greater mortality. Apolipoprotein E (e4 and e2 alleles) may be predictors of recurrent lobar hemorrhage (O'Donnell et al. 2000). The recurrence risk was 28% in 2 years for carriers of the e2 or e4 alleles, compared to 10% for those with the normal variant of e3, with a relative risk of 3.8. Prior symptomatic brain hemorrhage was a strong predictor of recurrence, with a risk of 61% at 2 years and a relative risk of 6.8. This implies that there may be other risk factors—genetic or environmental—which remain to be identified.

Another increasingly important outcome measure is functional status. Measures of the functional status of the stroke survivor are obtained through use of instruments such as the Barthel Index (BI) or modified Rankin Scale.

Future Directions and Conclusions

The Prevention of First Stroke Guidelines outlines evidence that can be used by clinicians for the prevention of first stroke (Gorelick et al. 1999). These guidelines state that "preventing persons from having first stroke will require a comprehensive multidisciplinary strategy to identify and manage major risk factors and to promote adherence to preventive protocols." In addition to standard risk factor studies, the identification of genetic and preclinical markers of disease continues to enhance our knowledge of stroke epidemiology. Genetic markers are of growing importance in the evolving field of molecular epidemiology. Finally, based on the estimated prevalence of risk factors and their attributable risk for stroke in the United States, it is estimated that a significant proportion of strokes could be prevented through the control of modifiable stroke risk factors such as smoking, alcohol, physical activity, and diet. Despite the wealth of data on the importance of stroke risk factors, these conditions are still inadequately controlled because of poor patient compliance and poor adherence to behavior modifications, as well as decreased detection and treatment by health-care providers. The process requires changes in national health policy directed at public health practices to promote healthy lifestyles, recognition of who is at increased risk of stroke, and modification of this risk whenever possible to prevent stroke.

References

Abbott RD, Curb JD, Rodriguez BL, et al. Effect of dietary calcium and milk consumption on risk of thromboembolic stroke in older middle-aged men. The Honolulu Heart Program. *Stroke* 1996;27:813–818.

Abbott RD, Rodriguez BL, Burchfiel CM, Curb JD. Physical activity in older middle-aged men and reduced risk of stroke the Honolulu Heart Program. *Am J Epidemiol* 1994;139: 881–893.

Abbott RD, Yin Y, Reed DM, Yano K. Risk of stroke in male cigarette smokers. *N Engl J Med* 1986;315:717–720.

Adachi H, Hirai Y, Tsuruta M, et al. Is insulin resistance or diabetes mellitus associated with stroke? An 18-year follow-up study. *Diabetes Res Clin Pract* 2001;51:215–223.

Adams HP Jr, Bendixen BH, Kappelle LJ, et al. Classification of subtype of acute ischemic stroke. Definitions for use in a multicenter clinical trial. TOAST. Trial of Org 10172 in Acute Stroke Treatment. *Stroke* 1993;24: 35–41.

Adamson J, Humphries SE, Ostergaard JR, et al. Are cerebral aneurysms atherosclerotic? *Stroke* 1994;25:963–966.

Albers GW, Easton JD, Sacco RL, Teal P. Antithrombotic and thrombolytic therapy for ischemic stroke. *Chest* 1998;114(Suppl): 683S–698S.

Albers GW, Sherman DG, Gress DR, et al. Stroke prevention in nonvalvular atrial fibrillation: a review of prospective randomized trials. *Ann Neurol* 1991;30:511–518.

Amarenco P, Cohen A, Baudrimont M, Bousser MG. Transesophageal echocardiographic detection of aortic arch disease in patients with cerebral infarction. *Stroke* 1992;23: 1005–1009.

American Diabetes Association. Clinical practice recommendations 1998. *Diabetes Care* 1998;21(Suppl 1):S1–S89.

American Heart Association. 1999 Heart and Stroke Statistical Update. Dallas: American Heart Association, 1999.

American Medical Association. International Classification of Diseases, 9th Revision ICD-9. Chicago: Medicode, 1998.

Ansell BJ. Cholesterol, stroke risk, and stroke prevention. *Curr Atheroscler Rep* 2000;2: 92–96.

Balkau B, Shipley M, Jarrett RJ, Pyorala K, et al. High blood glucose concentration is a risk factor for mortality in middle-aged nondiabetic men. 20-year follow-up in the Whitehall Study, the Paris Prospective Study, and the Helsinki Policemen Study. *Diabetes Care* 1998;21:360–367.

Barnett HJ, Taylor DW, Eliasziw M, et al. Benefit of carotid endarterectomy in patients with symptomatic moderate or severe stenosis. North American Symptomatic Carotid Endarterectomy Trial Collaborators. *N Engl J Med* 1998;339:1415–1425.

Barrett-Connor E, Khaw KT. Diabetes mellitus: an independent risk factor for stroke? *Am J Epidemiol* 1988;128:116–123.

Beghi E, Boglium G, Cosso P, et al. Stroke and alcohol intake in a hospital population. A case–control study. *Stroke* 1995;26:1691–1696.

Benfante R, Yano K, Hwang LJ, et al. Elevated serum cholesterol is a risk factor for both coronary heart disease and thromboembolic stroke in Hawaiian Japanese men. Implications of shared risk. *Stroke* 1994;25:814–820.

Benjamin EJ, Plehn JF, D'Agostino RB, et al. Mitral annular calcification and the risk of stroke in an elderly cohort. *N Engl J Med* 1992;327:374–379.

Benjamin EJ, D'Agostino RB, Belanger AJ, et al. Left atrial size and the risk of *Stroke* and death. The Framingham Heart Study. *Circulation* 1995;92:835–841.

Ben-Shlomo Y, Markowe H, Shipley M, Marmot MG. Stroke risk from alcohol consumption using different control groups. *Stroke* 1992;23:1093–1098.

Biller J, Adams HP Jr, Johnson MR, et al. Paradoxical cerebral embolism: eight cases. *Neurology* 1986;36:1356–1360.

Blankenhorn DH, Selzer RH, Crawford DW, et al. Beneficial effects of colestipol-niacin therapy on the common carotid artery. Two- and four-year reduction of intima-media thickness measured by ultrasound. *Circulation* 1993;88:20–28.

Blauw GJ, Lagaay AM, Smelt AH, Westendorp RG. Stroke, statins, and cholesterol. A meta-analysis of randomized, placebo-controlled, double-blind trials with HMG-CoA reductase inhibitors. *Stroke* 1997;28:946–950.

Boden-Albala B, Sacco RL. Lifestyle factors and stroke risk: exercise, alcohol, diet, obesity, smoking, drug use, and stress. *Curr Atheroscler Rep* 2000;2:160–166.

Bonita R. Cigarette smoking, hypertension and the risk of subarachnoid hemorrhage: a population-based case–control study. *Stroke* 1986;17:831–835.

Bonita R, Thompson S. Subarachnoid hemorrhage: epidemiology, diagnosis, management and outcome. *Stroke* 1985;16:591–594.

Bornebroek M, Haan J, Maat-Schieman ML, et al. Hereditary cerebral hemorrhage with amyloidosis-Dutch type (HCHWA-D): I—a review of clinical, radiologic and genetic aspects. *Brain Pathol* 1996;6:111–114.

Boushey CJ, Beresford SA, Omenn GS, Motulsky AG. A quantitative assessment of plasma homocysteine as a risk factor for vascular disease. Probable benefits of increasing folic acid intakes. *JAMA* 1995;274:1049–1057.

Brass LM, Isaacsohn JL, Merikangas KR, Robinette CD. A study of twins and stroke. *Stroke* 1992;23:221–223.

Broderick JP, Brott TG, Duldner JE, et al. Initial and recurrent bleeding are the major causes of death following subarachnoid hemorrhage. *Stroke* 1994;25:1342–1347.

Broderick J, Brott T, Kothari R, et al. The Greater Cincinnati/Northern Kentucky Stroke Study: preliminary first-ever and total incidence rates of stroke among blacks. *Stroke* 1998;29:415–421.

Broderick JP, Brott T, Tomsick T, et al. The risk of subarachnoid and intracerebral hemorrhages in blacks as compared with whites. *N Engl J Med* 1992;326:733–736.

Broderick JP, Brott TG, Tomsick T, et al. Intracerebral hemorrhage more than twice as common as subarachnoid hemorrhage. *J Neurosurg* 1995;45:A365.

Broderick JP, Phillips SJ, Whisnant JP, et al. Incidence rates of stroke in the eighties: the end of the decline in stroke? *Stroke* 1989;20:577–582.

Brott T, Thalinger K, Hertzberg V. Hypertension as a risk factor for spontaneous intracerebral hemorrhage. *Stroke* 1986;17:1078–1083.

Brown RD, Whisnant JP, Sicks JD, et al. Stroke incidence, prevalence, and survival: secular trends in Rochester, Minnesota, through 1989. *Stroke* 1996;27:373–380.

Bruno A, Carter S, Qualls C, Nolte KB. Incidence of spontaneous intracerebral hemorrhage among Hispanics and non-Hispanic whites in New Mexico. *Neurology* 1996;47:405–408.

Bruno A, Carter S, Qualls C, Nolte KB. Incidence of spontaneous subarachnoid hemorrhage among Hispanics and non-Hispanic whites in New Mexico. *Ethn Dis* 1997;7:27–33.

Burchfiel CM, Curb JD, Rodriguez BL, et al. Glucose intolerance and 22-year stroke incidence. The Honolulu Heart Program. *Stroke* 1994;25:951–957.

Burke GL, Evans GW, Riley WA, et al. Arterial wall thickness is associated with prevalent cardiovascular disease in middle-aged adults. The Atherosclerosis Risk in Communities (ARIC) Study. *Stroke* 1995;26:386–391.

Camargo CA Jr. Moderate alcohol consumption and stroke. The epidemiologic evidence. *Stroke* 1989;20:1611–1626.

Camargo CA Jr. Case-control and cohort studies of moderate alcohol consumption and stroke. *Clin Chim Acta* 1996;246:107–119.

Canhao P, Pinto AN, Ferro H, Ferro JM. Smoking and aneurysmal subarachnoid haemorrhage: a case–control study. *J Cardiovasc Risk* 1994;1:155–158.

Caplan LR, Gorelick PB, Hier DB. Race, sex and occlusive cerebrovascular disease: a review. *Stroke* 1986;17:648–655.

Colditz GA, Bonita R, Stampfer MJ, et al. Cigarette smoking and risk of stroke in middle-aged women. *N Engl J Med* 1988;318:937–941.

Collins R, Peto R, MacMahon S, et al. Blood pressure, stroke, and coronary heart disease. Part 2. Short-term reductions in blood pressure: overview of randomised drug trials in their epidemiological context. *Lancet* 1990;335:827–838.

Cooper R, Sempos C, Hsieh SC, Kovar MG. Slowdown in the decline of stroke mortality in the United States, 1978–1986. *Stroke* 1990;21:1274–1279.

Crouse JR III, Byington RP, Bond MG, et al. Pravastatin, lipids, and atherosclerosis in the carotid arteries (PLAC-II). *Am J Cardiol* 1995;76:455–459.

Dahlof B, Lindholm LH, Hansson L, et al. Morbidity and mortality in the Swedish Trial in Old Patients with Hypertension (STOP-Hypertension). *Lancet* 1991;338:1281–1285.

Davila-Roman VG, Barzilai B, Wareing TH, et al. Atherosclerosis of the ascending aorta. Prevalence and role as an independent predictor of cerebrovascular events in cardiac patients. *Stroke* 1994;25:2010–2016.

Davis PH, Dambrosia JM, Schoenberg BS, et al. Risk factors for ischemic stroke: a prospective study in Rochester, Minnesota. *Ann Neurol* 1987;22:319–327.

Denson KW. Passive smoking and an increased risk of acute stroke. *Tob Control* 2000;9:112.

(The) Diabetes Control and Complications Trial Research Group. The effect of intensive treatmen t of diabetes on the development and progression of long-term complications in insulin-dependent diabetes mellitus. *N Engl J Med* 1993;329:977–986.

Diaz MN, Frei B, Vita JA, Keaney JF Jr. Antioxidants and atherosclerotic heart disease. *N Engl J Med* 1997;337:408–416.

Di Tullio M, Sacco RL, Gopal A, et al. Patent foramen ovale as a risk factor for cryptogenic stroke. *Ann Intern Med* 1992;117:461–465.

Di Tullio MR, Sacco RL, Savoia MT, et al. Gender differences in the risk of ischemic stroke associated with aortic atheromas. *Stroke* 2000;31:2623–2627.

Di Tullio MR, Sacco RL, Sciacca RR, et al. Increased left atrial size is an independent risk factor for ischemic stroke. *Stroke* 1998:29;277

Dohlof B Lindholm LH, Hansson L, et al. Morbidity and mortality in the Swedish Trial in Old Patients with Hypertension (STOP-Hypertension). *Lancet* 1991;338:1281–1285.

Donahue RP, Abbott RD, Reed DM, Yano K. Alcohol and hemorrhagic stroke. The Honolulu Heart Program. *JAMA* 1986;255:2311–2314.

Drury I, Whisnant JP, Garraway WM. Primary intracerebral hemorrhage: impact of CT on incidence. *Neurology* 1984;34:653–657.

Elkind MS, Lin IF, Grayston JT, Sacco RL. *Chlamydia pneumoniae* and the risk of first ischemic stroke: the Northern Manhattan Stroke Study. *Stroke* 2000;31:1521–1525.

Executive Committee for the Asymptomatic Carotid Atherosclerosis Study. Endarterectomy for asymptomatic carotid artery stenosis. *JAMA* 1995;273:1421–1428.

Expert Panel on Detection, Evaluation, and Treatment of High Blood Cholesterol in Adults (Adult Treatment Panel II). Summary of the second report of the National Cholesterol Education Program (NCEP) *JAMA* 1993;269:3015–3023.

Feigin VL, Wiebers DO, Nikitin YP, et al. Stroke epidemiology in Novosibirsk, Russia: a population-based study. *Mayo Clin Proc* 1995a;70:847–852.

Feigin VL, Wiebers DO, Whisnant JP, O'Fallon WM. Stroke incidence and 30-day case-fatality rates in Novosibirsk, Russia, 1982 through 1992. *Stroke* 1995b;26:924–929.

Fine-Edelstein JS, Wolf PA, O'Leary DH, et al. Precursors of extracranial carotid atherosclerosis in the Framingham Study. *Neurology* 1994;44:1046–1050.

Foulkes MA, Wolf PA, Price TR, et al. The Stroke Data Bank: design, methods, and baseline characteristics. *Stroke* 1988;19:547–554.

Friday G, Lai SM, Alter M, et al. Stroke in the Lehigh Valley: racial/ethnic differences. *Neurology* 1989;39:1165–1168.

Furberg CD, Adams HP Jr, Applegate WB, et al. Effect of lovastatin on early carotid atherosclerosis and cardiovascular events. Asymptomatic Carotid Artery Progression Study (ACAPS) Research Group. *Circulation* 1994;90:1679–1687.

Furlan AJ, Whisnant JP, Elveback LR. The decreasing incidence of primary intracerebral hemorrhage: a population study. *Ann Neurol* 1979;5:367–373.

Gey KF, Stahelin HB, Eichholzer M. Poor plasma status of carotene and vitamin C is associated with higher mortality from ischemic heart disease and stroke: Basel Prospective Study. *Clin Investig* 1993;71:3–6.

Giles WH, Croft JB, Greenlund KJ, et al. Total homocyst(e)ine concentration and the likelihood of nonfatal stroke: results from the Third National Health and Nutrition Examination Survey, 1988–1994. *Stroke* 1998;29:2473–2477.

Gillman MW, Cupples LA, Gagnon D, et al. Protective effect of fruits and vegetables on development of stroke in men. *JAMA* 1995;273:1113–1117.

Gillman MW, Cupples LA, Millen BE, et al. Inverse association of dietary fat with development of ischemic stroke in men. *JAMA* 1997;278:2145–2150.

Gillum RF. Stroke in blacks. *Stroke* 1988;19:1–9.

Gillum RF, Mussolino ME, Ingram DD. Physical activity and stroke incidence in women and men. The NHANES I Epidemiologic Follow-up Study. *Am J Epidemiol* 1996;143:860–869.

Giroud M, Milan C, Beuriat P, et al. Incidence and survival rates during a two-year period of intracerebral and subarachnoid haemorrhages, cortical infarcts, lacunes and transient ischaemic attacks. The Stroke Registry of Dijon: 1985–1989. *Int J Epidemiol* 1991;20:892–899.

Goldstein LB. Novel risk factors for stroke: homocysteine, inflammation, and infection. *Curr Atheroscler Rep* 2000;2:110–114.

Gorelick PB. Stroke prevention: windows of opportunity and failed expectations? A discussion of modifiable cardiovascular risk factors and a prevention proposal. *Neuroepidemiology* 1997;16:163–173.

Gorelick PB, Rodin MB, Langenberg P, et al. Weekly alcohol consumption, cigarette smoking, and the risk of ischemic stroke: results of a case–control study at three urban medical centers in Chicago, Illinois. *Neurology* 1989;39:339–343.

Gorelick PB, Sacco RL, Smith DB, et al. Prevention of a first stroke: a review of guidelines and a multidisciplinary consensus statement from the National Stroke Association. *JAMA* 1999;281(12):1112–1120.

Greenberg SM, Rebeck GW, Vonsattel JP, et al. Apolipoprotein E epsilon 4 and cerebral hemorrhage associated with amyloid angiopathy. *Ann Neurol* 1995;38:254–259.

Greenberg SM, Vonsattel JP, Segal AZ, et al. Association of apolipoprotein E ε2 and vasculopathy in cerebral amyloid angiopathy. *Neurology* 1998;50:961–965.

Haheim LL, Holme I, Hjermann I, Leren P. Risk factors of stroke incidence and mortality. A 12-year follow-up of the Oslo Study. Stroke 1993;24:1484–1489.

Hankey GJ, Slattery JM, Warlow CP. The prognosis of hospital-referred transient ischaemic attacks. J Neurol Neurosurg Psychiatry 1991;54:793–802.

Hartmann A, Rundek T, Mast H, et al. Mortality and causes of death after first ischemic stroke: the Northern Manhattan Stroke Study. Neurology 2001;57:2000–2005.

Hebert PR, Gaziano JM, Chan KS, Hennekens CH. Cholesterol lowering with statin drugs, risk of stroke, and total mortality. An overview of randomized trials. JAMA 1997;278:313–321.

Hebert PR, Moser M, Mayer J, et al. Recent evidence on drug therapy of mild to moderate hypertension and decreased risk of coronary heart disease. Arch Intern Med 1993;153:578–581.

Hebert R, Lindsay J, Verreault R, et al. Vascular dementia: incidence and risk factors in the Canadian study of health and aging. Stroke 2000;31:1487–1493.

Heiss G, Sharrett AR, Barnes R, et al. Carotid atherosclerosis measured by B-mode ultrasound in populations: associations with cardiovascular risk factors in the ARIC study. Am J Epidemiol 1991;134:250–256.

Higa M, Davanipour Z. Smoking and stroke. Neuroepidemiology 1991;10:211–222.

Hodis HN, Mack WJ, LaBree L, et al. Reduction in carotid arterial wall thickness using lovastatin and dietary therapy: a randomized controlled clinical trial. Ann Intern Med 1996;124:548–556.

Hornig CR, Dorndorf W, Agnoli AL. Hemorrhagic cerebral infarction—a prospective study. Stroke 1986;17:179–185.

Howard G, Wagenknecht LE, Burke GL, et al. Cigarette smoking and progression of atherosclerosis: the Atherosclerosis Risk in Communities (ARIC) Study. JAMA 1998;279:119–124.

Hu FB, Stampfer MJ, Colditz GA, et al. Physical activity and risk of stroke in women. JAMA 2000;283:2961–2967.

Hu HH, Sheng WY, Chu FL, et al. Incidence of stroke in Taiwan. Stroke 1992;23:1237–1241.

Hust MH, Staiger M, Braun B. Migration of paradoxic embolus through a patent foramen ovale diagnosed by echocardiography: successful thrombolysis. Am Heart J 1995;129:620–622.

Hypertension Detection and Follow-up Program Cooperative Group. Five-year findings of the hypertension detection and follow-up program. III. Reduction in stroke incidence among persons with high blood pressure. JAMA 1982;247:633–638.

Inagawa T, Tokuda Y, Ohbayashi N, et al. Study of aneurysmal subarachnoid hemorrhage in Izumo City, Japan. Stroke 1995;26:761–766.

Ingall T, Asplund K, Mahonen M, Bonita R. A multinational comparison of subarachnoid hemorrhage epidemiology in the WHO MONICA stroke study. Stroke 2000;31:1054–1061.

Iribarren C, Jacobs DR, Sadler M, et al. Low total serum cholesterol and intracerebral hemorrhagic stroke: is the association confined to elderly men? The Kaiser Permanente Medical Care Program. Stroke 1996;27:1993–1998.

Iso H, Jacobs DR Jr, Wentworth D, et al. Serum cholesterol levels and six-year mortality from stroke in 350,977 men screened for the multiple risk factor intervention trial. N Engl J Med 1989;320:904–910.

Jerntorp P, Berglund G. Stroke registry in Malmo, Sweden. Stroke 1992;23:357–361.

Juvela S. Alcohol consumption as a risk factor for poor outcome after aneurysmal subarachnoid haemorrhage. BMJ 1992;304:1663–1667.

Juvela S, Hillbom M, Numminen H, Koskinen P. Cigarette smoking and alcohol consumption as risk factors for aneurysmal subarachnoid hemorrhage. Stroke 1993;24:639–646.

Kagan A, Popper JS, Rhoads GG, Yano K. Dietary and other risk factors for stroke in Hawaiian Japanese men. Stroke 1985;16:390–396.

Kamachi I, Colditz GA, Stampfer MJ, et al. Smoking cessation and decreased risk of stroke in women. JAMA 1993;269:232–236.

Kassell NF, Torner JC. Aneurysmal rebleeding: a preliminary report from the Cooperative Aneurysm Study. Neurosurgery 1983;13:479–481.

Kattapong VJ, Becker TM. Ethnic differences in mortality from cerebrovascular disease among New Mexico's Hispanics, Native Americans, and non-Hispanic whites, 1958 through 1987. Ethn Dis 1993;3:75–82.

Khaw KT, Barrett-Connor E. Dietary potassium and stroke-associated mortality. A 12-year prospective population study. N Engl J Med 1987;316:235–240.

Kiely DK, Wolf PA, Cupples LA, et al. Familial aggregation of stroke. The Framingham Study. Stroke 1993;24:1366–1371.

Kiely DK, Wolf PA, Cupples LA, et al. Physical activity and stroke risk: the Framingham Study. Am J Epidemiol.1994;140:608–620.

Kittner SJ, White LR, Losonczy KG, et al.

Black–white differences in stroke incidence in a national sample. The contribution of hypertension and diabetes mellitus. *JAMA* 1990;264:1267–1270.

Kiyohara Y, Kato I, Iwamoto H, et al. The impact of alcohol and hypertension on stroke incidence in a general Japanese population. The Hisayama Study. *Stroke* 1995;26:368–372.

Klatsky AL, Armstrong MA, Friedman GD, Sidney S. Alcohol drinking and risk of hospitalization for ischemic stroke. *Am J Cardiol* 2001;88:703–706.

Knekt P, Reunanen A, Aho K, et al. Risk factors for subarachnoid hemorrhage in a longitudinal population study. *J Clin Epidemiol* 1991;44:933–939.

Kurl S, Laukkanen JA, Rauramaa R, et al. Systolic blood pressure response to exercise stress test and risk of stroke. *Stroke* 2001;32:2036–2041.

Labovitz AJ, Camp A, Castello R, et al. Usefulness of transesophageal echocardiography in unexplained cerebral ischemia. *Am J Cardiol* 1993;72:1448–1452.

Laupacis A, Albers G, Dalen J, et al. Anti-thrombotic therapy in atrial fibrillation. *Chest* 1998;114(Suppl):579S–589S.

Lechat P, Mas JL, Lascault G, et al. Prevalence of patent foramen ovale in patients with stroke. *N Engl J Med* 1988;318:1148–1152.

Lee IM, Hennekens CH, Berger K, et al. Exercise and risk of stroke in male physicians. *Stroke* 1999;30:1–6.

Leppala JM, Virtamo J, Fogelholm R, et al. Vitamin E and beta carotene supplementation in high risk for stroke: a subgroup analysis of the Alpha-Tocopherol, Beta-Carotene Cancer Prevention Study. *Arch Neurol* 2000;57:1503–1509.

Lindegard B, Hillbom M. Associations between brain infarction, diabetes and alcoholism: observations from the Gothenburg population cohort study. *Acta Neurol Scand* 1987;75:195–200.

Lindegard B, Hillbom M, Brody S. High-dose estrogen-progestagen oral contraceptives: a risk factor for aneurysmal subarachnoid hemorrhage? *Acta Neurol Scand* 1987;76:37–45.

(The) LIPID (Long-Term Intervention with Pravastatin in Ischemic Disease) Study Group. Prevention of cardiovascular events and death with pravastatin in patients with coronary heart disease and a broad range of initial cholesterol levels. *N Engl J Med* 1998;339:1349–1357.

Lippmann H, Rafferty T. Patent foramen ovale and paradoxical embolization: a historical perspective. *Yale J Biol Med* 1993;66:11–17.

Longstreth WT Jr. Predicting outcomes after intracerebral hemorrhage. *Stroke* 1991;22:955–956.

Longstreth WT Jr, Manolio TA, Arnold A, et al. Clinical correlates of white matter findings on cranial magnetic resonance imaging of 3301 elderly people. The Cardiovascular Health Study. *Stroke* 1996;27:1274–1282.

Longstreth WT Jr, Nelson LM, Koepsell TD, van Belle G. Cigarette smoking, alcohol use, and subarachnoid hemorrhage. *Stroke* 1992;23:1242–1249.

Longstreth WT Jr, Nelson LM, Koepsell TD, van Belle G. Clinical course of spontaneous subarachnoid hemorrhage: a population-based study in King County, Washington. *Neurology* 1993;43:712–718.

Longstreth WT Jr, Swanson PD. Oral contraceptives and stroke. *Stroke* 1984;15:747–750.

Lucas C, Goullard L, Marchau M Jr, et al. Higher prevalence of atrial septal aneurysms in patients with ischemic stroke of unknown cause. *Acta Neurol Scand* 1994;89:210–213.

MacMahon S, Rodgers A. Blood pressure, antihypertensive treatment and stroke risk. *J Hypertens Suppl* 1994;12:S5–14.

Malarcher AM, Giles WH, Croft JB, et al. Alcohol intake, type of beverage, and the risk of cerebral infarction in young women. *Stroke* 2001;32:77–83.

Manolio TA, Kronmal RA, Burke GL, et al. Magnetic resonance abnormalities and cardiovascular disease in older adults. The Cardiovascular Health Study. *Stroke* 1994;25:318–327.

Mast H, Thompson JL, Lin IF, et al. Cigarette smoking as a determinant of high-grade carotid artery stenosis in Hispanic, black, and white patients with stroke or transient ischemic attack. *Stroke* 1998;29:908–912.

Mayer SA, Sacco RL, Shi T, Mohr JP. Neurologic deterioration in noncomatose patients with supratentorial intracerebral hemorrhage. *Neurology* 1994;44:1379–1384.

Mayeux R, Saunders AM, Shea S, et al. Utility of the apolipoprotein E genotype in the diagnosis of Alzheimer's disease. Alzheimer's Disease Centers Consortium on Apolipoprotein E and Alzheimer's Disease. *N Engl J Med* 1998;338:506–511.

McCarron MO, Nicoll JA, Ironside JW, et al. Cerebral amyloid angiopathy-related hemorrhage. Interaction of APOE ϵ2 with putative clinical risk factors. *Stroke* 1999;30:1643–1646.

McGovern PG, Pankow JS, Burke GL, et al. Trends in survival of hospitalized stroke patients between 1970 and 1985. The Minnesota Heart Survey. *Stroke* 1993;24:1640–1648.

Menghini VV, Brown RD Jr, Sicks JD, et al. Incidence and prevalence of intracranial aneurysms and hemorrhage in Olmsted County, Minnesota, 1965 to 1995. *Neurology* 1998;51:405–411.

Menotti A, Jacobs DR Jr, Blackburn H, et al. Twenty-five-year prediction of stroke deaths in the seven countries study: the role of blood pressure and its changes. *Stroke* 1996;27: 381–387.

Mohr JP, Thompson JL, Lazar RM et al. A comparison of warfarin and aspirin for the prevention of recurrent ischemic stroke. *N Engl J Med* 2001;345:1444–1451.

Morgenstern LB, Spears WD. A triethnic comparison of intracerebral hemorrhage mortality in Texas. *Ann Neurol* 1997;42:919–923.

Morris MC, Manson JE, Rosner B, et al. Fish consumption and cardiovascular disease in the physicians' health study: a prospective study. *Am J Epidemiol* 1995;142:166–175.

MRC Working Party. Medical Research Council trial of treatment of hypertension in older adults: principle results. *BMJ* 1992;304: 405–412.

Murray CJ, Lopez AD. Alternative projections of mortality and disability by cause 1990–2020: Global Burden of Disease Study. *Lancet* 1997;349:1498–1504.

Nelson HD, Humphrey LL, Nygren P, et al. Postmenopausal hormone replacement therapy. Scientific review. *JAMA* 2002;872–881.

Norris JW, Zhu CZ, Bornstein NM, Chambers BR. Vascular risks of asymptomatic carotid stenosis. *Stroke* 1991;22:1485–1490.

North American Symptomatic Carotid Endarterectomy Trial Collaborators. Beneficial effect of carotid endarterectomy in symptomatic patients with high-grade carotid stenosis. *N Engl J Med* 1991;325:445–453.

Nygard O, Vollset SE, Refsum H, et al. Total plasma homocysteine and cardiovascular risk profile. The Hordaland Homocysteine Study. *JAMA* 1995;274:1526–1533.

O'Donnell HC, Rosand J, Knudsen KA, et al. Apolipoprotein E genotype and the risk of recurrent lobar intracerebral hemorrhage. *N Engl J Med* 2000;342:240–245.

Okada H, Horibe H, Ohno Y, Hayakawa N, Aoki N. A prospective study of cerebrovascular disease in Japanese communities, Akabane and Asahi. Part I: evaluation of risk factors in the occurrence of cerebral hemorrhage and thrombosis. *Stroke* 1976;7:599–607.

Olafsson E, Hauser WA, Gudmundsson G, et al. A population-based study of prognosis of ruptured cerebral aneurysm: mortality and recurrence of subarachnoid hemorrhage. *Neurology* 1997;48:1191–1195.

O'Leary DH, Polak JF, Kronmal RA, et al. Distribution and correlates of sonographically detected carotid artery disease in the Cardiovascular Health Study. The CHS Collaborative Research Group. *Stroke* 1992;23: 1752–1760.

O'Leary DH, Polak JF, Kronmal RA, et al. Carotid-artery intima and media thickness as a risk factor for myocardial infarction and stroke in older adults. Cardiovascular Health Study Collaborative Research Group. *N Engl J Med* 1999;340:14–22.

Orencia AJ, Daviglus ML, Dyer AR, et al. Fish consumption and stroke in men. 30-year findings of the Chicago Western Electric Study. *Stroke* 1996;27:204–209.

Phillips LH, Whisnant JP, O'Fallon WM, Sundt TM Jr. The unchanging pattern of subarachnoid hemorrhage in a community. *Neurology* 1980;30:1034–1040.

Pignoli P, Tremoli E, Poli A, et al. Intimal plus medial thickness of the arterial wall: a direct measurement with ultrasound imaging. *Circulation* 1986;74:1399–1406.

Prospective Studies Collaboration. Cholesterol, diastolic blood pressure, and stroke: 13,000 strokes in 450,000 people in 45 prospective cohorts. *Lancet* 1995;346:1647–1653.

Pujia A, Rubba P, Spencer MP. Prevalence of extracranial carotid artery disease detectable by echo-Doppler in an elderly population. *Stroke* 1992;23:818–822.

Qizilbash N, Jones L, Warlow C, Mann J. Fibrinogen and lipid concentrations as risk factors for transient ischaemic attacks and minor ischaemic strokes. *BMJ* 1991;303:605–609.

Qureshi AI, Giles WH, Croft JB. Racial differences in the incidence of intracerebral hemorrhage: effects of blood pressure and education. *Neurology* 1999;52:1617–1621.

Ricci S, Celani MG, La Rosa F, et al. SEPIVAC: a community-based study of stroke incidence in Umbria, Italy. *J Neurol Neurosurg Psychiatry* 1991;54:695–698.

Rosenow F, Hojer C, Meyer-Lohmann C, et al. Spontaneous intracerebral hemorrhage. Prognostic factors in 896 cases. *Acta Neurol Scand* 1997;96:174–182.

Rubattu S, Giliberti R, Volpe M. Etiology and pathophysiology of stroke as a complex trait. *Am J Hypertens* 2000;13:1139–1148.

Ruiz-Sandoval JL, Cantu C, Barinagarrementeria F. Intracerebral hemorrhage in young people: analysis of risk factors, location, causes, and prognosis. *Stroke* 1999;30:537–541.

Rundek T, Mast H, Hartmann A, et al. Predictors of resource use after acute hospitalization: the Northern Manhattan Stroke Study. *Neurology* 2000;55:1180–1187.

Sacco RL. Risk factors, outcomes, and stroke subtypes for ischemic stroke. *Neurology* 1997;49(Suppl 4):S39–S44.

Sacco RL, Benjamin EJ, Broderick JP, et al. American Heart Association Prevention Conference. IV. Prevention and Rehabilitation of stroke. Risk factors. *Stroke* 1997a;28: 1507–1517.

Sacco RL, Benson RT, Kargman DE, et al. High-density lipoprotein cholesterol and ischemic stroke in the elderly: the Northern Manhattan Stroke Study. *JAMA* 2001b;285:2729–2735.

Sacco RL, Boden-Albala B, Abel G, et al. Race-ethnic disparities in the impact of stroke risk factors: the Northern Manhattan Stroke Study. *Stroke* 2001a;32:1725–1731.

Sacco RL, Boden-Albala B, Gan R, et al. Stroke incidence among white, black, and Hispanic residents of an urban community: the Northern Manhattan Stroke Study. *Am J Epidemiol* 1998a;147:259–268.

Sacco RL, Elkind M, Boden-Albala B, et al. The protective effect of moderate alcohol consumption on ischemic stroke. *JAMA* 1999; 281:53–60.

Sacco RL, Ellenberg JH, Mohr JP, et al. Infarcts of undetermined cause: the NINCDS Stroke Data Bank. *Ann Neurol* 1989a;25:382–390.

Sacco RL, Foulkes MA, Mohr JP, et al. Determinants of early recurrence of cerebral infarction. The Stroke Data Bank. *Stroke* 1989b;20:983–989.

Sacco RL, Gan R, Boden-Albala B, et al. Leisure-time physical activity and ischemic stroke risk: the Northern Manhattan Stroke Study. *Stroke* 1998b;29:380–387.

Sacco RL, Homma S, Di Tullio MR. Patent foramen ovale: a new risk factor for ischemic stroke. *Heart Dis Stroke* 1993;2:235–241.

Sacco RL, Roberts JK, Boden-Albala B, et al. Race-ethnicity and determinants of carotid atherosclerosis in a multiethnic population. The Northern Manhattan Stroke Study. *Stroke* 1997b;28:929–935.

Sacco RL, Shi T, Zamanillo MC, Kargman D. Predictors of mortality and recurrence after hospitalized cerebral infarction in an urban community: the Northern Manhattan Stroke Study. *Neurology* 1994;44:626–634

Sacco SE, Whisnant JP, Broderick JP, et al. Epidemiological characteristics of lacunar infarcts in a population. *Stroke* 1991;22:1236–1241.

Sacco RL, Wolf PA, Bharucha NE, et al. Subarachnoid and intracerebral hemorrhage: natural history, prognosis, and precursive factors in the Framingham Study. *Neurology* 1984;34:847–854.

Sacks FM, Pfeffer MA, Moye LA, et al. The effect of pravastatin on coronary events after myocardial infarction in patients with average cholesterol levels. Cholesterol and Recurrent Events Trial investigators. *N Engl J Med* 1996;335:1001–1009.

Salonen R, Nyyssonen K, Porkkala E, et al. Kuopio Atherosclerosis Prevention Study (KAPS). A population-based primary preventive trial of the effect of LDL lowering on atherosclerotic progression in carotid and femoral arteries. *Circulation* 1995;92:1758–1764.

Scandinavian Simvastatin Survival Study Group. Randomised trial of cholesterol lowering in 4444 patients with coronary heart disease: the Scandinavian Simvastatin Survival Study (4S). *Lancet* 1994;344:1383–1389.

Schoenberg BS, Anderson DW, Haerer AF. Racial differentials in the prevalence of stroke in Copiah County, Mississippi. *Arch Neurol* 1986;43:565–568.

Schwartz SM, Petitti DB, Siscovick DS, et al. Stroke and use of low-dose oral contraceptives in young women: a pooled analysis of two US studies. *Stroke* 1998;29:2277–2284.

Segal AZ, Chiu RI, Eggleston-Sexton PM, et al. Low cholesterol as a risk factor for primary intracerebral hemorrhage: a case–control study. *Neuroepidemiology* 1999;18:185–193.

Selhub J, Jacques PF, Bostom AG, et al. Association between plasma homocysteine concentrations and extracranial carotid–artery stenosis. *N Engl J Med* 1995;332: 286–291.

SHEP Cooperative Research Group. Prevention of stroke by antihypertensive drug treatment in older persons with isolated systolic hypertension. Final results of the Systolic Hypertension in the Elderly Program (SHEP). *JAMA* 1991;265:3255–3264.

Shinton R, Beevers G. Meta-analysis of relation between cigarette smoking and stroke. *BMJ* 1989;298:789–794.

Simon JA, Hsia J, Cauley JA, et al. Postmenopausal hormone therapy and risk of stroke: the Heart and Estrogen-progestin Replacement Study (HERS). *Circulation* 2001;103:638–642.

(The) Sixth Report of the Joint National Committee on Prevention, Detection, Evaluation, and Treatment of High Blood Pressure. *Arch Intern Med* 1997;157:2413–2446.

Spence JD, Howard VJ, Chambless LE, et al. Vitamin Intervention for Stroke Prevention (VISP) trial: rationale and design. *Neuroepidemiology* 2001;20:16–25.

Staessen JA, Fagard R, Thijs L, et al. Randomised double-blind comparison of placebo and active treatment for older patients with isolated systolic hypertension. The Systolic Hypertension in Europe (Syst-Eur) Trial Investigators. *Lancet* 1997;350:757–764.

Stampfer MJ, Colditz GA, Willett WC, et al. A prospective study of moderate alcohol consumption and the risk of coronary disease and stroke in women. *N Engl J Med* 1988; 319:267–273.

Staub L, Morgenstern LB. Stroke in Hispanic Americans. *Neurol Clin* 2000;18:291–307.

Stroke Prevention in Atrial Fibrillation Study. Final results. *Circulation* 1991;84:527–539.

Stroke Prevention in Atrial Fibrillation III. Randomised clinical trial. Adjusted-dose warfarin versus low-intensity, fixed-dose warfarin plus aspirin for high-risk patients with atrial fibrillation. *Lancet* 1996;348:633–638.

Tanaka A, Ueno Y, Nakayama Y, et al. Small chronic hemorrhages and ischemic lesions in association with spontaneous intracerebral hematomas. *Stroke* 1999;30:1637–1642.

Terayama Y, Tanahashi N, Fukuuchi Y, Gotoh F. Prognostic value of admission blood pressure in patients with intracerebral hemorrhage. Keio Cooperative Stroke Study. *Stroke* 1997;28:1185–1188.

Teunissen LL, Rinkel GJ, Algra A, van Gijn J. Risk factors for subarachnoid hemorrhage: a systematic review. *Stroke* 1996;27:544–549.

Thrift AG, Donnan GA, McNeil JJ. Heavy drinking, but not moderate or intermediate drinking, increases the risk of intracerebral hemorrhage. *Epidemiology* 1999;10:307–312.

Thorvaldsen P, Asplund K, Kuulasmaa K, et al. Stroke incidence, case fatality, and mortality in the WHO MONICA project. World Health Organization Monitoring Trends and Determinants in Cardiovascular Disease. *Stroke* 1995;26:361–367.

Timsit SG, Sacco RL, Mohr JP, et al. Early clinical differentiation of cerebral infarction from severe atherosclerotic stenosis and cardioembolism. *Stroke* 1992;23:486–491.

Truelsen T, Gronbaek M, Schnohr P, Boysen G. Intake of beer, wine, and spirits and risk of stroke: the Copenhagen city heart study. *Stroke* 1998;29:2467–2472.

Tunick PA, Rosenzweig BP, Katz ES, et al. High risk for vascular events in patients with protruding aortic atheromas: a prospective study. *J Am Coll Cardiol* 1994;23:1085–1090.

U.K. Prospective Diabetes Study Group. Tight blood pressure control and risk of macrovascular and microvascular complications in type 2 diabetes: UKPDS 38. *BMJ* 1998;317:703–713.

U.S. Department of Health and Human Services. Physical Activity and Health: A Report of the Surgeon General. Atlanta, GA: U.S. Department of Health and Human Services, Centers for Disease Control and Prevention, National Center Chronic Disease Prevention and Health Promotion, 1996.

U.S. Department of Health and Human Services. Healthy People 2000: National Health Promotion and Disease Prevention Objectives. Washington, DC, 2000.

Vinters HV. Cerebral amyloid angiopathy. In: Barnett HJM, Mohr JP, Stein BM, Yatsu FM, eds. Stroke—Pathophysiology, Diagnosis, and Management, Third Edition. New York: Churchill Livingstone, 1998.

Watkins PJ, Thomas PK. Diabetes mellitus and the nervous system. *J Neurol Neurosurg Psychiatry* 1998;65:620–632.

Weir CJ, McCarron MO, Muir KW, et al. Apolipoprotein E genotype, coagulation, and survival following acute stroke. *Neurology* 2001;57:1097–1100.

Winn HR, Richardson AE, Jane JA. The long-term prognosis in untreated cerebral aneurysms. 1. The incidence of late hemorrhage in cerebral aneurysm: a 10-year evaluation of 364 patients. *Ann Neurol* 1977; 1:358–70.

Wolf PA, Abbott RD, Kannel WB. Atrial fibrillation as an independent risk factor for stroke: the Framingham Study. *Stroke* 1991; 22:983–988.

Wolf PA, D'Agostino RB, Kannel WB, et al. Cigarette smoking as a risk factor for stroke. The Framingham Study. *JAMA* 1988;259:1025–1029.

Wolf PA, D'Agostino RB, O'Neal MA, et al. Secular trends in stroke incidence and mortality. The Framingham Study. *Stroke* 1992; 23:1551–1555.

Wong KS. Risk factors for early death in acute ischemic stroke and intracerebral hemorrhage: a prospective hospital-based study in Asia. Asian Acute Stroke Advisory Panel. *Stroke* 1999;30:2326–2330.

World Health Organization (WHO). The World Health Report 1997. Conquering Suffering, Enriching Humanity. Geneva: WHO, 1997, pp 1–162.

Writing Group for the Women's Health Initiative Investigators. Risk and benefits of estrogen plus progestin in healthy postmenopausal women. Principal results from the Women's Health Initiative Randomized Clinical Trial. *JAMA* 2002;288:321–333.

10

Brain and Spinal Cord Injury

JESS F. KRAUS AND DAVID L. MCARTHUR

Injuries to the brain and spinal cord are among the most devastating and expensive of all injuries. In the past few years, however, significant advances have been made toward the prevention, medical management, and rehabilitation of brain injuries. This chapter examines particular methodologic issues in the epidemiology of traumatic brain and spinal cord injury and highlights their public health significance.

Brain Injury

Up to 50% of all trauma deaths in the United States involve significant injury to the brain (Sosin et al. 1995). The most common diagnostic rubrics include the *International Classification of Diseases* (ICD), 9th Revision (ICD-9.CM) (1992) and the Abbreviated Injury Scale (Association for the Advancement of Automotive Medicine 1990) for intracranial traumatic injury classification. Though some sectors of the world use the 10th Revision of the ICD (World Health Organization 1992), the 10th Revision gives less specific and descriptive criteria for brain injury compared with the 9th Revision of the ICD and hence is not presented here.

In most of the published literature on neurotrauma, diagnostic subclassifications are lumped together. Studies that have attempted to examine subtypes based on the location of hemorrhage (epidural, subdural, or interparenchymal) have been fraught with problems of cross-classification and cross-aggregation.

Methodological Problems in Published Studies of Brain Injury

Many research papers fail to make a clear distinction between head injuries (which may include non-intracranial, or skull, injuries) and brain injuries (which are only intracranial). In some published reports, for example, the authors' intent was to report on persons with intracranial injury, but the definitions or methods of case finding may have led to the unintentional inclusion of head injuries that were not intracranial.

Example 10–1 One epidemiological report (Annegers et al. 1980) defined head injury as "evidence of presumed brain involvement, i.e., concussion with loss of consciousness, post-traumatic amnesia, or neurologic signs of brain injury. Skull fractures were included, even without altered consciousness." Although the researchers may have intended the mix of brain and non–brain injured patients, the findings from this research are weakened because of possible intracranial injury misclassification of patients included in the study group. Skull facture doesn't necessarily mean brain involvement. Similarly, Macpherson et al. (1990) included all patients with skull fracture in the study group and found that more than one-quarter had no intracranial damage.

Study group inconsistencies permeate the early literature on brain injuries. For example, some papers have restricted the study group to persons with severe brain trauma (Bruce et al. 1978; Auer et al. 1980), persons with mild brain injury (Gronwall and Wrightson 1974; Plaut and Gifford 1976), or persons who were admitted to a hospital alive (Jennett et al. 1979a; Rimel 1981). Other studies (Phonprasert et al. 1980; Klauber et al. 1981a) have excluded persons with penetrating brain injuries, whereas still others included them (Raimondi and Samuelson 1970; Lillard 1978). Certain published reports have focused on brain injuries from specific external causes, such as motor vehicle crashes (Selecki et al. 1968), while other studies failed to describe the external causes of the brain damage. Reports on persons with specific types of injuries (i.e., cerebral hemorrhage) appear frequently in the literature (e.g., Phonprasert et al. 1980), but many studies include a mix of brain trauma diagnoses.

One case ascertainment problem in traumatic brain injury (TBI) studies is the use of functional or clinical criteria to identify patients for study. In the absence of objective evidence, some brain injury diagnoses are determined by clinical judgment. Whether or not concussion is diagnosed, for example, may depend on the patient's presenting symptoms and/or functional status at discharge. Acute brain trauma is often the cause of paralysis or amnesia but other psychological states, such as diminished cognitive ability or behavior deviation, have less certain etiologies. Diagnosing acute brain trauma solely on the basis of neuropsychological symptoms might lead to case misclassification and distort the findings.

Other Problems Affecting Brain Injury Incidence, Severity, and Outcome Measures

Although most of the studies reviewed in this chapter attempted to describe the nature of the study group or population, some left unclear how the cases were found or from what sources they were selected (Cambria et al. 1979; Phonprasert et al. 1980). This failure is not crucial to a case series study, which doesn't report injury rates, but it is a major problem in incidence studies, which do report rates. The problem emerges in two ways. The first is the failure to achieve complete case ascertainment (Kalsbeek et al. 1980; Klauber et al. 1981a); the second is the assumption that the incidence of brain injury in a hospital's catchment area is the same as in a defined population (Jagger et al. 1984b). Complete case ascertainment in a defined population is a hallmark of distinguished epidemiological research; incidence can then be accurately calculated since all cases within an entire population at risk are identified. Only a small proportion of TBI studies can make such a claim, however. In many communities around the world, there are multiple hospitals and ambiguous catchment districts, leaving uncertainty as to whether every case stemming from the study population has been enumerated, and whether every person at risk has been identified.

The failure of these studies to make clear their case-selection procedures has serious implications for subsequent calculation of case fatality rates (CFRs, e.g., the number

of fatalities among the total number of patients admitted with brain injury over a defined period of time).

> *Example 10–2*   In one region, all TBI pa-
> tients admitted to hospitals with medically
> verified brain injury are the basis (de-
> nominator) for determining death before
> hospital discharge. In another region only
> those admitted to neurosurgical units are
> included as the patient group. The CFRs
> derived under these two situations neces-
> sarily have different interpretations, yet
> the death rates derived are often com-
> pared. The comparison almost invariably
> suggests that the latter group was more
> severely injured, in more need of aggres-
> sive treatment, and/or more disabled upon
> discharge if the patients survive, com-
> pared to the former group. Whether the
> latter group would also be more or less
> likely to die might depend, however, on
> unrelated factors such as the policies for
> admitting a patient from the emergency
> department to the neurosurgical unit.

Another methodological problem is the
manner in which severity of TBI is determined or classified. For decades, different
systems were used to classify severity, ren-
dering findings nonreproducible. One of
the criteria most consistently used in the
past to evaluate severity of TBI was duration of unconsciousness (Jagger et al.
1984a). However, focal injury can cause focal neurological dysfunction without loss of
consciousness (Jennett and Teasdale 1981).
More than 25 years ago, Teasdale and Jennett (1974) introduced the Glasgow Coma
Scale (GCS) to assess the degree of impaired
consciousness (see Table 10–1). A variety
of extensions to improve the utility of the
GCS have been proposed. For example, the
World Health Organization Advisory
Group on the Prevention and Treatment of
Neurotrauma has supported recent work to
extend the mild end of the GCS by additional scoring of the patient's amnesia immediately after the injury event (Nell et al.
2000).

Several problems are inherent in the
GCS. The advisory panel recommends ap-

plying the Scale between 4 and 8 hours
post-injury, and many recommend repeating the measurement. But the time between
the occurrence of the injury and the application of baseline GCS can vary widely, especially if alcohol is involved (Jagger et al.
1984a). The component parts of the GCS
are subject to a variety of phenomena that
may vary substantially in minutes or hours,
such as the blossoming of a secondary injury or the use of intubation. Thus, it is
common to see disagreement between the
GCS scores gathered by emergency medical
technicians on the scene of the injury event,
the scores gathered by the emergency department staff, and the scores observed in
the neurosurgical unit, even when these
were obtained within a short time of one
another. Alcohol's depressive effects on the
nervous system can be (but are not necessarily) a major contributor to reduced
scores in each of the three components of
the GCS.

The GCS has other limitations. For example, eye opening may be restricted due
to facial swelling, verbal response may be
precluded by an endotracheal tube, and the
use of drugs to reduce intracranial pressure
can profoundly affect the patient's verbal
and motor responses. The use of the GCS
is questionable in infants and very young
children, those who do not understand English, and those having chronic conditions
that affect motor, verbal, or eye response.

Assessing the consequences of brain injury is problematic as well. Many studies
have evaluated brain injury outcomes with
the Glasgow Outcome Scale (GOS) (Jennett
and Bond 1975), which is a crude measure
of medical (neurological) complications or
residual effects in the patient on discharge
from the primary treatment facility or during follow-up contacts (see Table 10–1).
The categories of the GOS include death,
persistent vegetative state (no cerebral cortical function as judged behaviorally), severe disability (disabled and wholly or partially dependent on assistance), moderate
disability (disabled but independent), and
good recovery (intact function or mild im-

Table 10–1 The Glasgow Coma Scale and the Glasgow Outcome Scale

GLASGOW COMA SCALE*		GLASGOW COMA SCALE EXTENDED†	
Ability assessed	Points	Memory assessed	Points
Eye Opening		**Amnesia**	
Not open	1	>3 months	0
To pain	2	31 to 90 days	1
To speech	3	8 to 30 days	2
Spontaneous	4	1 to 7 days	3
		3 to 24 hours	4
Verbal Response		$^{1}/_{2}$ to 3 hours	5
Silence	1	<30 minutes	6
Sounds	2	No amnesia	7
Nonsense	3		
Confused	4		
Conversation	5		
Motor Response			
To pain: no response	1		
Arm extension	2		
Arm flexion	3		
Withdrawal	4		
Localizing	5		
To command	6		
Total score = eye opening + verbal response + motor response			

GLASGOW OUTCOME SCALE*		GLASGOW OUTCOME SCALE EXTENDED‡	
Condition assessed	Points	Condition assessed	Points
Dead	1	Dead	1
Vegetative	2	Vegetative state	2
Severely disabled	3	Lower severe disability	3
		Upper severe disability	4
Moderately disabled	4	Lower moderate disability	5
		Upper moderate disability	6
Good recovery	5	Lower good recovery	7
		Upper good recovery	8

*Source: Jennett and Teasdale (1981).
†Source: Nell et al. (2000).
‡Source: Wilson et al. (1998).

pairment with persistent sequelae that do not rule out a normal social life). The GOS includes some measures that are subjective, and some of the complications or sequelae identified may not be a result of the brain injury or related injuries.

The GOS has also been criticized as being insensitive to "subtle changes in functional status" (see Wilson et al. 1998 for expanded discussion of limitations of the GOS). To counter this problem, an 8-point version of the GOS has been proposed and tested (Table 10–1). This new version, the Glasgow Outcome Scale Extended (GOSE), purportedly clarifies and simplifies the criteria at each of the disability levels (Wilson et al. 1998).

The GOS is the most widely used single indicator of general outcome after TBI. Less crude measures have been introduced, however, such as the Functional Independence Measure (FIM) (Granger et al. 1995), an 18-item scale that includes assessments of motor and cognitive impairments and the average minutes of assistance required from another person each day. In persons with

TBI, the FIM's motor score is closely associated with the need for direct aid, and the FIM's cognitive score is closely associated with the need for supervisory assistance (Corrigan et al. 1997). Another instrument for measuring TBI outcome is the 29-item Neurobehavioral Rating Scale (Levin et al. 1987), which measures difficulties in higher cerebral functioning, such as confusion, memory loss, and depression.

Brain-injured persons may have a wide variety of sequelae that are not captured by the GOS. More refined instruments for assessing outcomes after TBI are needed. In the United States, The National Institute on Disability and Rehabilitation Research (NIDRR) has long funded the Traumatic Brain Injury Model Systems, which in turn have recently developed The Center for Outcome Measurement in Brain Injury (COMBI) as a collaborative project (see http://www.tbims.org/combi/). This collaboration aims to develop, test, and disseminate new measures that are appropriate to TBI patients, readily applicable in the clinical context, and psychometrically validated for the needs of TBI researchers.

Measures of Occurrences, Persons at Risk and External Causes of Brain Injury

Prevalence Estimates for Brain Injury

Prevalence is a measure of all persons at a specific point (or period) of time having the condition of interest and includes those newly diagnosed and those with residual disability or impairment. There are few published prevalence estimates for brain-injured persons. The most recent estimates, based on data obtained in 1996 as part of the Colorado Traumatic Brain Injury Registry and Follow-up System (Brooks et al. 1997), are that overall prevalence in the United States is 2%, or 5.3 million persons living with a TBI-related disability (Guerrero et al., unpublished).

Estimates of Incidence

Fatal Brain Injury. About 1 in 12 deaths in the United States results from injury and

more than 146,400 injury-related deaths (6.3% of the total of 2,314,245) were recorded for 1997 (Hoyert et al. 1999). The exact proportion of those deaths that resulted from brain injury is unknown, but if death rate estimates from Olmsted County, Minnesota (Annegers et al. 1980), San Diego County, California (Kraus et al. 1984), and data from 13 states in the United States (Thurman and Guerrero 1999) are averaged, the annual death rate from brain injuries is about 23 per 100,000 per year or roughly 42% of the overall crude injury death rate of 55 per 100,000 per year for 1997. The most recent estimates from the National Center for Health Statistics suggest that, mostly due to a 38% decrease in deaths related to transportation since 1980, the TBI-associated death rate for 1994, as identified only from ICD-9 codes, was 19.8 per 100,000 (Thurman et al. 1999).

Several studies have reported fatality rates from brain injury (Klauber et al. 1981a, 1981b; Cooper et al. 1983; Jagger et al. 1984b; Kraus et al. 1984; Whitman et al. 1984; MacKenzie et al. 1989; Sosin et al. 1989; Schuster 1994; Thurman et al. 1999). Sosin et al. (1989) reported a brain injury death rate in the United States of about 17 per 100,000 per year. Excluding the Massachusetts study (Schuster 1994) and the study from the north-central Virginia area (Jagger et al. 1984b), reported rates range from 17 to 30 per 100,000 per year with an average brain injury death rate of 22 per 100,000 per year. Thus one can extrapolate that about 59,400 of the 146,400 injury deaths in 1997 involve damage to the brain, or about 41% of the total. This estimate could reasonably vary by as much as 6000 persons, however, due to the paucity of up-to-date population-based TBI studies.

Sosin et al. (1989) estimated the percentage of head injury–related deaths in the United States to be 28% of all injury deaths. The investigators acknowledged that the case finding process may have underestimated head injury–associated deaths by as much as 44%. Nevertheless, head (brain) injury is associated with more trauma deaths than injury to any other body region. There are no accurate data on the annual incidence of all fatal and non-fatal brain injuries combined for the United States. An estimate for 1991 reported by the U.S. Centers for Disease Control and Prevention (CDC) (Centers for Disease Control and Prevention 1998) gives a total of 1.54 million U.S. civilians reporting non-fatal concussions, skull fractures, brain hemorrhages, contusions, lacerations, and other intracranial injuries needing profes-sional medical care but not institutional-ized. This estimate includes patients with head trauma but without brain injury.

Total (Fatal and Nonfatal) Brain Injury. The only national data available on the number of brain injuries in the United States come from the U.S. Hospital Dis-charge Survey (Graves 1995), which in-cludes information from a large sample of non-military and non-veterans hospitals. In 1993, there were 396,000 patients dis-charged with a diagnosis of brain injury for a rate of about 154 per 100,000 per year. Unfortunately, this estimate may include multiple admissions and discharges of the same person from the same or different hos-pitals, as well as patients with a date of original injury in a prior year. Some pa-tients with head injury but without neuro-logical injuries may be included, while per-sons dying at the scene of the injury or dead on arrival may be excluded. Therefore the estimate may be skewed by the degree to which the number of persons in the first three categories is larger or smaller than the number of persons who die before reach-ing a hospital.

Data from all available resources can be used to estimate the total number of per-sons sustaining a medically treated and di-agnosed brain injury each year. Each year in the United States, for each individual who dies from a brain injury, 6 persons are admitted to a hospital and 24 persons seek medical treatment for TBI (Kraus and

McArthur 2000). Incidence data for 23 re-ports are summarized in Tables 10–2 and 10–3. Rates (and methods of case defini-tion and ascertainment) vary significantly. Guerrero et al. (2000) reported the highest incidence rate of 392 per 100,000 per year, excluding persons who were hospitalized or died before reaching a hospital. This rate was estimated from data obtained in the National Hospital Ambulatory Medical Care Survey, in which cases with qualify-ing ICD codes were identified in a multi-stage probability sampling design of almost 400 emergency departments across the United States. The 1981 San Diego findings (Klauber et al. 1981a) also show a high rate (294 per 100,000 per year); however, they reflect an unknown percent of non-neuro-logical cases and non-residents. It is note-worthy that the incidence rates reported af-ter 1990 are generally lower than those published in the 1970s and 1980s.

The variations in definitions of brain in-juries, case ascertainment, methods of de-lineation of the populations at risk, geo-graphic study area, and time of study could account for some of the variation in re-ported rates. Increasing wide-scale avail-ability of injury-reducing technologies such as airbags in vehicles may contribute as well. Lack of adjustment in rates for age, gender, or race in some studies further ac-counts for some of the differences. But at present it must be acknowledged that the underlying reasons for such a broad range of rates are not yet fully understood. The overall incidence estimate based on the U.S. studies, after eliminating the highest and lowest values, is in the range of 150 per 100,000 per year. This rate applied to the 1998 U.S. population of 270 million results in about 405,000 cases of brain injury. This rate includes those admitted to a hospital for treatment as well as those who die be-fore reaching a hospital.

Earlier reports from Europe and Aus-tralia indicated rates from 200 to 377 per 100,000 per year but newer data from In-dia, Taiwan, and New South Wales show rates that are considerably less, in the range

Table 10–2 Brain Injury Incidence Data for the United States: Selected Reports

Report	Year of study	Place	No. of cases	Population (×1000)	Rate per 10⁵ per year	Comments
Annegers et al. 1980	1965–1974	Olmsted County, MN	3587	NS	193	Age-adjusted to 1970 U.S. population
Kalsbeek et al. 1980	1974	U.S.	422,000	210,725	200	Based on sample of about 9000 cases
Jagger et al. 1984b	1978	North-central Virginia	735	354	208	Rate includes residents and nonresidents; no prehospital deaths
Klauber et al. 1981a	1978	San Diego County, CA	5055	NS	294	Includes some nonresidents; excludes some external causes
Whitman et al. 1984	1979–1980	Inner-city Chicago and Evanston, IL	782	213	367	Composite rate from data in original paper
Cooper et al. 1983	1980–1981	Bronx, NY	1209	NS	249	Estimate based on sample, age-adjusted
Kraus et al. 1984	1981	San Diego County, CA	3358	1862	180	Population-based, non–age-adjusted
Schuster 1994	1990	Massachusetts	27,816	6016	10	Fatal
					86	Hospitalized
					366	Emergency department treatment only
Thurman et. al. 1996	1990–1992	Utah	5782	NS	106	Age-adjusted
					20	Fatal
Gabella et. al. 1997b	1991–1992	Colorado	7056	NS	101	Age-adjusted
Gabella et. al. 1997a	1990–1993	Colorado, Missouri, Oklahoma, Utah	13,978	13,687	103	Age-adjusted
					23	Fatal
Thurman et al. 1999	1994–1995	U.S.	NS	NS	98	Hospitalized cases only
Schootman et al. 2000	1993	Iowa	2559	NS	90.9	Crude severe injury rate based on capture–recapture method
Guerrero et al. 2000	1995–1996	U.S.	449	NS	392	Emergency department visits with TBI diagnoses, without subsequent hospitalization

NS, not stated.

Table 10–3 Brain Injury Incidence Data for Europe and Asia: Selected Reports

Report	Year of study	Place	No. of cases	Population (×1000)	Rate per 10^5 per year	Comments
Jennett and MacMillan 1981	1974	England, Wales, Scotland	NS	NS	270* 313†	Rates not age-adjusted
Selecki et al. 1982	1977	New South Wales, Australia	NS	4960	377	Includes non-neurological cases; pre-hospital deaths excluded
Edna and Cappelen 1984	1979–1980	Trondelag, Norway	1124	NS	200	Includes unknown percent non-neurological head injuries; excludes pre-hospital deaths
Wang et al. 1986	1983	Six cities in People's Republic of China	35	63	56	Rate based on samples of defined communities located within the cities
Tiret et al. 1990	1986	Aquitaine, France	30,310	2700	281	Rate based on sample of hospitals and weeks of observation in 1986
Hillier et al. 1997	1987	South Australia	4486	1392	322	Excludes pre-hospital deaths
Gururaj et al. 1993	1991–1992	Bangalore, India	2897	NS	122	Excludes pre-hospital deaths
Wang et al., 1995	1993	Central Taiwan	7050	5970	118	Includes non-neurological cases
Tate et al. 1998	1988	New South Wales	413	343,140	100	Hospital admitted cases only
Engberg and Teasdale 2001	1979–1996	Denmark	166,443	5120	265‡ 224** 157***	Hospital admitted cases only
Masson et al. 2001	1996	Aquitaine, France	479	2.8 million	17.3	Severe TBI only

NS, not stated.

*England and Wales (includes emergency room visits).

†Scotland (all primary surgical ward admissions).

‡1979–81.

**1985–87.

***1991–93.

of 100 to 122 per 100,000 per year (Table 10–4). Findings from South Australia for 1987 (Hillier et al. 1997) are more consistent with some of the earlier reports showing rates in excess of 300 per 100,000 per year. In Denmark in 1979–1981, the incidence rate of hospitalized TBI was 265 per 100,000, but this declined 41% by 1991–1993, due in large measure to large decreases in concussions and cranial fractures (Engberg and Teasdale 2001). The reasons for these dramatic differences in reported rates are not clear but could reflect differences in case definitions, case finding, and/or hospitalization practices for patients with the less severe form of injury. There may also be important large-scale changes in safety practices especially regarding motor vehicles and traffic, as well as regional and cultural influences (for example, the mixing of vehicles and pedestrians in urban India defies most Western precepts about injury prevention), but these have yet to be investigated in detail.

Inconsistencies in studying persons at risk for TBI make it difficult to compare findings. Age intervals used by investigators vary, for example. In one incidence study (Jagger et al. 1984b), persons aged 10 to 20 are grouped together, combining two very different life-cycle periods of exposure to injury. Teenagers, who are often beginning drivers, face risk exposures that are different from those faced by their pre-teen siblings.

Age. Brain injury incidence peaks in the young and the elderly. The U.S. population-based reports that have age-specific data show a peak incidence of 250 or more per 100,000 in young adults aged 15–24. Persons over age 70 have a peak incidence of about 200 per 100,000, nearly twice that of persons in their 50s. In many studies, two additional peaks in incidence include infants and young children (Cooper et al. 1983; Whitman et al. 1984; Fife 1987; MacKenzie et al. 1989) and those over age 64 (Annegers et al. 1980; Cooper et al. 1983; Fife et al. 1986). This pattern gener-

ally remains consistent in reports published in the 1990s with the exception of findings in rural Colorado for 1991–92 (Gabella et al. 1997b), where the TBI rate was lower by a factor of at least 5 among infants and children less than 5 years of age. Reasons for this variation were not evident; further study is required.

The distribution of incident cases by age depends on the external causes most common in the population. For example, in most studies, motor vehicle accidents account for the major proportion of brain injuries and involve a disproportionately large number of young persons. In the Bronx, New York, however (Cooper et al. 1983), the major cause of injury was interpersonal violence and involved older adults.

Gender. Almost all U.S. reports show a male-to-female incidence rate ratio of 2.0 or more. Males predominate in high-risk work settings, high-risk sports, and high-risk driving; consequently, males, regardless of age, are more frequently exposed to risk than females. One exception is the U.S. National Head and Spinal Cord Injury (NHSCI) Survey (Kalsbeek et al. 1980), which showed a male-to-female rate ratio of 1:1. One possible explanation for this finding is that a large number of head injuries without neurological injury in females were included in the data set.

External Cause

The percentage distribution of brain injuries by major external cause categories from brain injury incidence studies is given in Table 10–4. Major differences are found in the classification scheme used in all reports with respect to the description of the external cause. For purposes of Table 10–4, brain injuries have been classified by event (e.g., crash), place (e.g., domicile), or activity (e.g., sports), hence only the broadest external cause categories could be used (as finer gradations cannot be reliably constructed). Eight of 10 U.S. incidence reports show transport-related events as the single largest cause of new cases of brain injury

Table 10-4 Percentage Distribution of Brain Injuries by External Cause—Selected Case Series Reports from U.S. and non-U.S. Studies

Study location, year (reference)	Transport (%)	Falls (%)	Firearms or assaults (%)	Sports (%)	Other (%)	Comments
Indiana, 1965–69 (Schulhof et al. 1972)	36	36	19	NS	10	Cases from one general hospital
Washington, D.C. 1966–1972 (Barber et al. 1974)	14	33	37	NS	16	Cases from one general hospital
Norway, 1974 (Nestvold et al. 1988)	58	NS	NS	4	38	Other includes at work and home
Taiwan, 1977–1987 (Lee et al. 1990)	90	5	NS	NS	5	Other includes at work; falls include suicides
Aquitaine, France, 1986 (Tiret et al. 1990)	60	32	1	NS	7	Other includes 6.1% "struck by object"
South Africa, 1986–1987 (Nell and Brown 1991)	41	3	43	NS	13	Other includes explosion, suicide, legal intervention
Pakistan, 1986–1991 (Raja 1993)	58	16	22	1	3	
Taiwan, 1987–1988 (Lee et al. 1990)	68	22	5	NS	5	
Central Taiwan, 1991–1993 (Wang et al. 1995)	76	17	5	1	1	Other includes struck by fallen object
Malawi, 1995 (Adeloye et al. 1997)	45	9	40	NS	6	Other includes occupational injuries

NS, not stated.

and falls routinely are the second leading cause. The remaining two studies represent high-density urban areas, where assaults and firearms were the single largest cause. It is important to note characteristics of both the population and the environment when considering these studies because, once again, exposure to risk is often markedly different.

Motor vehicle crash–related brain injuries involve a number of different exposures. Although there are few data on crash-related factors, there are some reports available that give major subcategories by external cause of injury. Among the U.S. incidence studies, five reports show motor vehicle–related brain injuries by status— i.e., occupant of a motor vehicle (mostly passenger cars), motorcyclist (including scooter/moped), pedestrian, or bicyclist. Four of these five reports show that 75%–81% of the injured were occupants of cars or trucks and 8% to 15% were pedestrians. These studies reflect conventional Western settings and may not readily translate to regions of the world where passenger cars are rare and two- or three-wheeled vehicles predominate.

Thurman et al. (1998) recently assessed the epidemiology of sports-related TBI. Two different systematically collected U.S. data sources estimate that 20% of all brain injuries occur during sports and recreation, with one-third occurring in competitive sports and two-thirds in recreational activities. Among organized sports, brain injuries occurred most frequently in basketball, baseball, and football, with each accounting for 20% of the total brain injuries from competitive sports. In recreational settings, playground activities predominated, causing more than one-third of all such injuries.

Powell and Barber-Foss (1999) studied reports collected from athletic trainers at 235 U.S. high schools and found that, in 63% of the cases in which mild TBI was suspected, the individual was playing football. Noting that, between 1931 and 1986, over 800 deaths were directly attributable to playing American football, Cantu (1996) stated that changes in rules, equipment, conditioning, and on-scene medical services have precipitated a dramatic decrease in the most serious sports-related head injuries in the last two decades. Significant problems remain, however. The "second impact syndrome," in which an athlete sustains a second blow to the head before symptoms of the first injury have cleared, remains a topic of controversy. Cantu (1996) has reported that this second impact syndrome is more common than previously thought. Collins et al. (1999) have shown that both learning disability and concussion history are significant factors in reduced neuropsychological performance among university football players. (Readers interested in the topic of head and spine injuries to the athlete are referred to Cantu 2000).

Alcohol. Alcohol consumption can be a critical factor in brain injury in at least three ways. First, alcohol intoxication greatly increases the risk of all types of injury (especially motor vehicle crashes, falls, assaults, and self-inflicted injuries) by impairing gross and fine motor skills, reaction times, and judgment (e.g., Waller et al. 1986; Kraus et al. 1989; Miller and Pentland 1989; Modell and Mountz 1990). Second, alcohol intoxication can complicate diagnosis in the emergency department by lowering the level of consciousness independent of brain injury severity (Galbraith et al. 1976; Jagger et al. 1984a). Finally, both pathophysiological and cognitive consequences of acute and chronic alcohol consumption may affect outcomes after brain injury (e.g., Ward et al. 1982; Zink et al. 1993).

Reports from San Diego (Klauber et al. 1981b), Seattle (Gale et al. 1983), and north-central Virginia (Rimel 1981) have documented the association of alcohol with brain injuries to be 9%, 49%, and 72%, respectively. The problem is not unique to the United States, as seen in the report from Norway (Edna 1982), in which 32% of brain-injured patients were intoxicated.

Nearly half of the patients older than 15 years in the study reported by Kraus et al. (1989) showed blood alcohol concentrations (BAC) >80 mg%. Evidence of intoxication was most frequent among the 25–44 age group and among those with a mild brain injury. The reasons for the extreme diversity in proportions are not well documented but could represent important variation in alcohol drinking practices.

Of concern is the impact of alcohol on the accuracy of diagnosis, selection and implementation of therapy, and outcome after brain injury. Galbraith et al. (1976), Brismar et al. (1983), and Jagger et al. (1984a) found that alcoholic intoxication at the time of diagnosis interferes with the assessment of brain injury severity because of depression of the GCS score. Tate et al. (1999) reported that after controlling for pre-injury history of alcohol abuse, blood alcohol levels in TBI patients upon hospital admission were directly related to delays in verbal memory, decrements in verbal memory over time, and reductions in visuospatial functioning during recovery. However, information on the effect of alcohol on therapeutic efficacy or eventual outcome after brain injury is equivocal. A few reports indicate that alcohol is positively correlated with fatal and nonfatal neurological outcomes, while other studies show opposite results. A carefully organized study of this question is needed, with standardization of both alcohol measure and alcohol history.

Example 10–3 Kraus et al. (1989, 1994) found that among residents who died from or required hospitalization for a brain injury, injury severity and hospital mortality were inversely related to admission blood alcohol level. Upon initial assessment, a protective effect appeared to be provided by acute alcohol intoxication. The authors concluded, however, that this relationship was likely due to differential rates of blood alcohol level testing. In survivors with more severe injuries, intoxication with BAC >100 mg% was associated with a higher prevalence of physician-diagnosed neurological impairment at discharge compared with sober individuals. Gurney et al. (1992) found that brain-injured adults who were intoxicated at the time of injury were more likely to develop respiratory distress and/or pneumonia secondary to decreased immune function from ethanol exposure than brain-injured adults who were not intoxicated at the time of injury.

Blood alcohol level determination in TBI. Because of alcohol's purported effect on the outcome of brain injury, we recommend estimating BAC at the time of injury, based on analyses by Wagner et al. (1990). A "standard drink" (e.g., 360 ml of beer, 150 ml of wine, 44 ml of distilled liquor) contains about 15 grams of alcohol. Using an estimated blood alcohol level at time of injury provides a more accurate measure of degree of intoxication than relying on admission BAC, which does not account for elimination of alcohol that has occurred since injury. After ingestion, peak blood concentrations are achieved in 30 to 90 minutes, with longer periods required when alcohol is taken on a full stomach. One drink will result in a BAC ranging from 20 mg% to 40 mg%, depending on the rates of ingestion and absorption. Alcohol is eliminated from the body on average at the rate of 7 grams per hour, i.e., 2 hours for complete elimination of one drink as defined above. Most importantly, the rate of elimination of alcohol is considered constant once equilibrium has been established: expressed as mg% per hour, it ranges from 9.75 to 37.34, with an average of 20 mg% per hour. The rate is generally higher in chronic drinkers without liver disease and lower in occasional drinkers. The BAC at time of injury can be estimated by using the BAC on admission and the time elapsed from injury to when the blood was drawn for alcohol level determination adjusted for elimination. Extrication and transport time after injury can be over an hour and occasionally is considerably longer. This time can generally be determined from paramedic records and/or witness accounts. For patients who have a BAC of zero upon admission to the emergency department, they or their relatives ought to be questioned as to whether any alcohol use occurred within 12 hours of the injury; if there was none, such patients can be declared as having a BAC of zero.

There have been relatively few studies concerning other drugs as a factor in TBI, acting separately from alcohol. For example, Drubach et al. (1993) reported that TBI patients with either drug or drug and alcohol abuse appear more likely than others to sustain violent injuries such as gunshot wounds. Corrigan (1995) reported, however, that the current literature on this topic is sparse.

Severity

Some U.S. studies report the severity distribution of hospitalized patients with brain injury. A study in the Chicago area (Whitman et al. 1984) used a clinical definition for classifying brain injury severity, whereas studies in San Diego (Klauber et al. 1981a; Kraus et al. 1984) and north-central Virginia (Rimel 1981) used the GCS and a Maryland study used the ICD (MacKenzie et al. 1989). In north-central Virginia, 49% of the hospital-admitted cases were mild head injuries (Rimel 1981), compared with 86% for the Chicago area study (Whitman et al. 1984). Overall, about 80% of persons with brain injury have mild trauma. On average, less than 10% of persons admitted to the hospital for brain injury have severe, life-threatening injuries.

The severity distribution of TBI in the United States appears to be shifting from 80% mild, 10% moderate, and 10% severe to 60% mild, 20% moderate, and 20% severe. These shifting proportions are a reflection of increased stringency in hospital admission criteria, which bar mildly injured persons from being seen at a hospital (Thurman and Guerrero 1999), rather than of true increases in moderate and severe injuries. Patients with only a mild brain injury, however, may still have serious health problems (Murshid 1998), including in-

tracranial hematomas (Dacey et al. 1986) and seizures (Lee and Liu 1992).

Brain Injury Case Fatality Rates

In-hospital case fatality rates (CFRs) from eight U.S. incidence studies (Klauber et al. 1981a, 1981b; Jagger et al. 1984b; Kraus et al 1984; MacKenzie et al. 1989; Thurman et al. 1996; Gabella et al. 1997b; Tate et al. 1998; Masson et al. 2001) range from 3% to 20%. Variable admissions standards for mildly brain-injured persons could explain the inconsistent rates. The CFR has also been used to evaluate and compare outcomes and quality of care among institutions. The CFR results should be interpreted with caution, however, because of possible differences in hospital admission practices, selection of patients for follow-up, level of care available, time to admission after injury, follow-up durations, or some combination of these factors.

Disability after Brain Injury

There are no published data at the national level that accurately estimate the number of persons in the United States who sustain disability, impairment, or functional limitation from acute brain trauma. Although estimates for some types of physical limitations are reported periodically from the National Health Interview Survey (Collins 1985), epidemiological findings on physical limitations specific to acute brain injury are not available. Studies conducted at the regional level have indicated incidence rates for disability following brain injury that vary from as low as 3.3 per 100,000 (Johnson and Gleave 1987) to as high as 40 per 100,000 (Bryden 1989).

Several analyses have been conducted of a stratified sample of 71,900 disabled persons living in Canada, who were the target of a health and activity limitation survey administered in 1986 by Statistics Canada, the national statistical agency (Moscato et al. 1994; Dawson and Chipman 1995; Lubinski et al. 1997). Using a methodology standardized on the *International Classification of Impairment, Disability, and*

Handicap (ICIDH) (World Health Organization 1980), 60% of the respondents with a history of TBI had a physical-independence handicap. Speech and hearing disabilities persisted for more than 10 years for 43.2% and 45% of respondents, respectively. Males reported speaking and hearing disabilities more frequently than females (61.1% vs. 38.9% and 70.6% vs. 29.3%, respectively). Ninety-five percent of those with TBI had a working handicap (although 25% indicated they were employed). Ninety percent had one or more difficulties in social integration. Motor disorders were identified in 76% of the TBI respondents, and communication difficulties in 61%. Factors with significant influence on physical independence among TBI respondents included gender (females were more disadvantaged overall than males), education (those with only a primary school education were more disadvantaged), living with greater numbers of people in the household, presence of physical barriers in the environment, and disabilities in features of personal care. The level of handicap experienced by TBI respondents in relation to work was especially notable, and was more prevalent among older persons and those with environmental barriers or motor disabilities.

Measures of disability are neither definitive nor interchangeable (McPherson and Pentland 1997). The Barthel Index (Mahoney and Barthel 1965), which scores level of dependence in 10 activities of daily living, has been extensively used, but has a relatively restricted focus and is relatively insensitive to change. The Disability Scale of the British Office of Population, Censuses and Surveys (Martin et al. 1988) assesses 13 areas of mobility, dexterity, self-care, communication, intellectual functioning, behavior, and related topics. The Functional Independence Measure (Granger et al. 1986) determines function at four levels of dependence in a variety of skills, and for brain-injured individuals is often accompanied by the Functional Assessment Measure (Hall 1992) to expand the range of cognitive and psychosocial topics assessed. The European Brain Injury Questionnaire (Deloche et al. 2000), focusing almost exclusively on subjective features of cognition, emotion, and social life as reported by both TBI patients and their families, represents another distinctive approach to the challenge of assessing disability following TBI. However, Gordon et al.'s (2000) recent demonstration of complex variations in self-reported symptoms between mild and moderate/severe TBI groups a year or more after injury suggests caution in interpreting subjective reporting. In part because there continue to be huge differences in defining disability, breaking the term into discrete components and measuring them, the task of executing simple cost-effective epidemiological studies of disability after brain injury has not been easily accomplished.

Prognosis after Brain Injury

Although there is extensive literature on prognosis after severe head injury (Jennett et al. 1979b), there were no published follow-up studies of a representative TBI cohort until recently. Investigators (Thornhill et al. 2000) in Glasgow, Scotland followed a large cohort of TBI hospital-discharged patients for 1 year to determine frequency of disability. Disability was 47% (measured using the GOS), and exceeded 54% if patients who had died or were in a vegetative state were not included in the analysis. Findings from this new report contradict the conventionally held belief that the prevalence of disability increases with increased initial TBI severity. The proportions disabled were 47%, 45%, and 48% for mildly, moderately, and severely brain injured persons, respectively, 1 year postinjury.

Though longitudinal follow-up studies have been conducted for as many as 25 years on some small samples, extreme loss during the follow-up period has prohibited generalizations from these studies. Even the recent Scottish study (Thornhill et al. 2000) had a 30% non-response rate.

Spinal Cord Injury

The epidemiological study of spinal cord injury (SCI) is less encumbered by definitional and diagnostic uncertainty than is TBI, because the two leading SCI classification systems are widely accepted and applicable. The scale provided by Frankel et al. (1969) details the degree of lesion completeness within each of five discrete gradations of preservation of neurological functioning. The scale provided by the American Spinal Injury Association (Ditunno et al. 1994) is an internationally accepted series of definitions, procedures for neurological examination in SCI, sensory and motor scoring considerations, and scales for case assessment. Prior to the acceptance of these scales, work on SCI was limited by the lack of agreement on case definition and diagnostic codes, making comparisons among studies difficult, and uncertainties about the extent to which debilitating weaknesses or transient impairments were to be included or excluded (Kraus et al. 1996). Work continues in refining these scales and their use (Capaul et al. 1994; Cohen et al. 1998).

Although it is important to know which factors, if any, are associated with SCI occurrence and are predictive of specific outcomes, few reports have examined the role of pre-injury factors with immediate and longer-term consequences. Researchers from Alabama (Novack et al. 2001) identified a significant relationship between the pre-injury factors of age, education, employment status, alcohol and drug use, and social history (e.g., history of arrests, suicide attempts) and injury severity and functional and cognitive outcomes measured at 1 year post-injury. Information on pre-injury factors was obtained from family members. The importance of these findings are diminished somewhat because of a 37% loss to follow-up in the original cohort, as well as a significant difference in age between those followed to 1 year (mean age 34) and those not followed (mean age 41).

Incidence of Spinal Cord Injury

The first well-documented effort to determine SCI incidence rates in the United States was a detailed population-based study of 18 counties in northern California conducted in the early 1970s (Kraus et al. 1975). Since that time there have been several studies in the United States and elsewhere to estimate national or regional incidence; these vary substantially in methods but results are similar. The generally accepted rate of about 30 hospitalized cases per million per year stems from several statewide registries and hospital surveys conducted in the United States (Go et al. 1995); the figure for other countries is, on average, about one-third lower (see Table 10–5).

A recently published article from Australia reports a nationwide rate of 14.5 per million population for 1998–1999 (O'Connor 2002). The basis for case finding was the countrywide SCI registry, which uses the case definition from the U.S. CDC, namely, "an acute, traumatic lesion of neural elements in the spinal canal (spinal cord and corda equina) resulting in temporary or permanent sensory deficit, motor deficit, or bladder/bowel dysfunction" (Thurman et al. 1995). It is noteworthy that while all adult cases are referred to specialist treatment units, and subsequently the national register, the reporting of pediatric cases is likely to be incomplete. In addition, possible cases referred to the coroner may be missed in the national registry.

Prevalence of Spinal Cord Injury

A recent review found international prevalence rates of SCI ranging from 11 to 112 per 100,000, based on a variety of sources covering the United States and eight other countries published between 1975 and 1992 (Blumer and Quine 1995). The average of new and existing cases reported in the U.S. studies is about 700 per million population, yielding a total of about 165,000 nationwide in 2000. From the

Table 10–5 Selected Studies of Spinal Cord Injury Incidence, by Year(s) Studied

Country	Reference	Year(s) studied	Source of case identification	Population at risk	Incidence rate per 10^6
U.S.	Kraus et al. 1975	1970–1971	Records from all hospitals, coroners, and state agencies for 18 California counties	1970 U.S. county-level census data	53.4, 33.1[†]
U.S.	Bracken et al. 1981	1970–1977	National Hospital Discharge Survey	1979 U.S. Census estimates	40.1[†]
U.S.	Fine et al. 1979	1973–1978 (latter date assumed)	Case series from one model SCI center	Not stated	29.4[†]
The Netherlands	Schönherr et al. 1996	1982–1993	Case series from the only SCI rehabilitation unit in region	Not stated	16[†]
Fiji	Maharaj 1996	1985–1994	All cases drawn from the only SCI rehabilitation unit in country	Ministry of Health, 1991	10.0[‡]
U.S.	Thurman et al. 1995	1989–1991	State injury reporting system	1980 U.S. Census	47[*]
Japan	Shingu et al. 1995	1990–1992	Nationwide survey of medical institutions	1990–92 Japanese census estimates (assumed)	40.2[‡]
U.S.	Warren et al. 1995	1991–1993	State trauma registry	Alaska Department of Labor statistics	83[†]
Taiwan	Chen et al. 1997	1992–1996	Nationwide survey of SCI facilities	1994 Taiwan census (assumed)	18.8[‡]
Australia	O'Connor 2002	1998–1999	Nationwide SCI register	Entire Australian population	14.5[†]

[*] All persons including deaths before hospitalization.

[†] All persons reaching hospital alive.

[‡] All persons registered in hospital.

most recent U.S. studies, a prevalence estimate of 232,000 individuals can be calculated. This is more than 40% higher than
the previous figure and 16% above the figure of 200,000 in 1998 quoted without ci-
tation by Zigler and Capen (1998). Controlling for both incidence and prevalence
within specific age cohorts by year, Lasfargues et al. (1995) have projected an increase
of 20% in SCI prevalence in the United
States from 1994 through 2010.

Causes of Spinal Cord Injury

According to the collaborative program
called the Model Spinal Cord Injury Systems and its National Spinal Cord Injury
Database (Richards et al. 1995), the predominant causes of SCI in the United States
during 1970 through 1990 were motor vehicle crashes (44.5%), falls (18.1%), violence (16.6%), and sports (12.7%) (Go et
al. 1995). Automobiles constitute 80.5% of
motor vehicle–related causes, while motor-
cycles account for 13.7% of such injuries.
Eighty-eight percent of violent SCI injuries
were due to gunshot wounds. Sixty-seven
percent of all SCIs related to sports were
caused by diving incidents. There has been
a decrease in motor vehicle–related causes
of SCI and a concomitant increase in violence as a cause. While in the 1970s motor
vehicle crash–related SCI constituted 43.1%
of the etiology of all SCI, during the period
1994–1998 it declined to 37.7%, but increases were seen in new SCI cases caused
by falls (16.9% to 21.3%) and by violence
(12.9% to 20.1%) (Nobunaga et al. 1999).
This latter increase was also reported by
Farmer et al. (1998), who found gunshot
wounds as a cause of SCI to have risen from
9.4% of all hospital admissions in 1984 to
become the leading cause in 1993 (28.6%)
in a single regional institution in Delaware.

Motor vehicle crashes are the predominant cause of SCI in other countries. A notable exception is the very low rate of SCI
injuries from motor vehicle accidents in Silberstein and Rabinovich's (1995) study
conducted in Novosibirsk, Russia; motor
vehicle usage is much rarer there than in

most other nations, and, correspondingly,
they reported elevated rates for falls
(40.4%) and sports-related SCI (32.9%).

In countries outside of the United States,
falls are a more common cause of SCI and
violent causes are much lower (see Table
10–6). In the survey by Ramsey and Hilson
(1995) in Australia, for instance, SCIs due
to all violent events were less than half the
usual proportions found in U.S. studies
(6.8%), and firearms as a cause of SCI
made up less than 1% of all SCIs in Australia. It appears that interpersonal violence, as a root cause of SCI, is essentially
an American phenomenon. Gunshot injuries of the spine are sustained in an ap-
preciable proportion in Jordan (Otom et al.
1997), but these injuries appear to be due
to a long-standing national tradition involving discharging guns in celebration.

In a recent study of SCI by McKinley et
al. (1999), 39% of SCI patients discharged
from one regional program were found to
have acquired their disability through nontraumatic illnesses, including spinal stenosis, tumor, ischemia, transverse myelitis,
and infection. The average age of those
with nontraumatic SCI was significantly
higher than that of persons with traumatic
causes (61.2 vs. 38.6 years), and the
male/female ratio for nontraumatic SCI was
1:1 while traumatic SCI occurred predominantly in males (5:1). Tetraplegics with
nontraumatic causes of injury had significantly briefer stays in rehabilitation relative
to those with traumatic causes; paraplegics
with nontraumatic causes had better motor
scores on discharge.

Mortality after Spinal Cord Injury

Mortality rates, including immediate deaths
and deaths occurring in the hospital, continue to be elevated compared with those
of the general population of the same age,
but overall mortality has declined significantly (DeVivo and Stover 1995), even
among persons with high-level injuries and
dependency on automated ventilators (De-
Vivo and Ivie 1995). Improvement in survival after spinal cord injury can be linked

Table 10–6 Selected U.S. and International Studies of SCI: Age and Proportion by Gender and Selected Causes

Country	Reference	Year(s) studied	Age group with highest incidence	Male (%)	Motor vehicle (%)	Falls (%)	Sports (%)	Violence (%)
U.S.	Kraus et al. 1975	1970–1971	20–29	74	56	19	7	12
France	Minaire et al. 1979	1970–1975	20–25	79	30	25	9	1
U.S.	Fine et al. 1979	1973–1978	15–29	60	40	27	7	21
U.S.	Nobunaga et al. 1999	1973–1998	16–30	82	43	19	11	19
Nigeria	Igun et al. 1999	1984–1997	1–30	93	57	22	0	3
Fiji	Maharaj 1996	1985–1994	16–30	80	29	39	3[a]	3[a]
U.S.	Velmahos et al. 1995	1988–1992	15–30	78	30	9[b]	9[b]	61
Jordan	Otom et al. 1997	1988–1993	21–30	85	44	21	3	28
Portugal	Martins et al. 1998	1989–1992	15–24, 55–74	77	57	37	5[a]	5[a]
Russia	Silberstein and Rabinovich 1995	1989–1993	20–29	78	25	40	33	2
Japan	Shingu et al. 1995	1990–1992	~20, 50–70	80	44	42	3[a]	3[a]
Turkey	Karamehmetoglu et al. 1995	1992	20–29	76	41	43	NS	5
New South Wales	Ramsey and Hilson 1995	1992	15–24	NS	54	8	3	7
U.S.	Warren et al. 1995	1991–1993	15–24	83	32	49	NS	6
Taiwan	Chen et al. 1997	1992–1996	24–34, 65+	75	46	44	1	2
Thailand	Pajareya 1996	1994	NS	89	51	31	<1	9
The Netherlands	van Asbeck et al. 2000	1994	21–30	77	31	49	9	NS
Australia	O'Connor 2002	1998–1999	15–24	76	43	23	5	5

NS, not stated.

[a]Combines sports and violence.

[b]Combines falls and sports.

to improvements in emergency medical services, medicines, development of dedicated medical units for SCI, improved professional training, and dramatic changes in control and prevention of secondary complications—especially infection—and use of regular follow-up. Recent data from a small-scale Canadian study of skiing and snowboarding spinal injuries indicated survival prior to reaching a hospital to be over 98% (Tarazi et al. 1999), but the average figure from older studies is about 94%. Data on survival during acute hospitalization are readily available from a number of studies and range from to 73.5% in a Nigerian study (Igun et al. 1999) to over 97% in a South African study (Velmahos et al. 1995). If we ignore the highest and lowest values, the mean proportion that survive acute hospitalization is about 93.0% (Bracken et al. 1981; Warren et al. 1995; Pajareya 1996; Chen et al. 1997; Martins et al. 1998).

Example 10–4 In a detailed study of SCI over 50 years in Great Britain, Frankel et al. (1998) computed standardized mortality ratios for four groupings of injury by gender and age. Their data indicate that mortality in persons with C1–C4 injuries was up to 7.8 times greater than that in the general population, with C5–C8 level injuries being up to 8.4 times greater, and thoracic and lumbar injuries up to 3.7 times greater. Analyses showed that males were at significantly elevated risk of death compared with females (risk ratio [RR] = 1.23, 95% confidence interval [CI] = 1.03–1.47), that tetraplegics and paraplegics were significantly elevated compared to those with full recovery of muscles below their injury (RR = 2.22, 95% CI 1.85–2.66, and RR = 1.46, 95% CI 1.23–1.73, respectively), and that each year of age at which the injury occurs added incrementally to the risk of death (RR = 1.07, 95% CI 1.07–1.08). Additionally, their data show a marked decline in mortality over time: persons injured between 1943 and 1952, for example, were up to 9 times more likely to die than persons injured between 1982 and 1990. The current

odds of dying in the first year after injury, according to evidence from the U.S. National SCI Database Project, are only one-third those recorded 20 years ago (DeVivo et al. 1999). The same researchers have found, however, that overall long-term mortality after the fifth year following injury has not changed appreciably, and an upswing in deaths in the period of 2 to 5 years post-injury has also been identified. Hartkopp et al. (1997) studied long-term survival after SCI in Denmark and found that standardized mortality ratios were reduced 18% for males and 53% for females in the period 1972–1990 as compared to the period 1953–1971. Confidence limits, however, were too large to interpret these findings as statistically significant.

Data from the National SCI Database show that pneumonia and influenza are the most common cause of death among SCI patients, accounting for 16.3% of all deaths, followed by nonischemic heart disease (12.2%) and septicemia (8.7%) (DeVivo and Stover 1995). The comparable figures for the general U.S. population are substantially lower for pneumonia and influenza (3.7%) and for septicemia (0.3%), but are about the same for nonischemic heart disease (14.6%) (Hoyert et al. 1999).

Recent data from Sydney, Australia (Soden et al. 2000) show cause-specific standardized mortality ratios (SMRs) among SCI patients to be significantly elevated for septicemia, pneumonia and influenza, diseases of the urinary system, suicide, and cardiovascular disease. The researchers also report that while mortality following SCI from septicemia and pneumonia have declined in recent decades, those from suicide have increased.

Future Directions and Conclusions

Much research on SCI focuses on prevention, treatment, and rehabilitation. While no cures for SCI are imminent, numerous advances have arisen from the marriage of basic and clinical neuroscience (Marwick 1999). Laboratory studies have shown that spinal cord function can be restored in animals through nerve regeneration, and researchers are eager to mimic this effect in humans. The routes to regeneration are complex, involving neurotrophic factors, anti-scarring and anti-neuroinhibitory agents, embryonic and other specialized cell transplants, and collateral nerve sprouting (Ramer et al., 2000). However, one widely regarded pharmacological therapy—the use of the corticosteroid methylprenisolone in high dosages during the acute phase of injury—has recently been shown by a systematic meta-analysis to be noneffective (Short et al. 2000), despite its success in other neurologic diseases (e.g., multiple sclerosis, see Miller et al. 2000). Epidemiological studies examining injury surveillance, risk and prognostic factors, and long-term outcome through carefully controlled trials have yet to be conducted. The finding of SCI in more than 5% of TBI patients in a recent study (Holly et al. 2002) is also an important topic for further exploration.

Epidemiologic methods can be used to determine the proportion of SCI cases that could have been prevented. Tyroch et al. (1997) showed that 71% of 150 motor vehicle–related SCI cases from one level I trauma center could have been prevented had the individuals used restraint devices or not been impaired from intoxication. They also showed that 54% of the SCIs due to gunshot wounds were related to illegal possession or accidental discharge of a firearm and could have been prevented. More work in this area, using large representative databases and sound epidemiological methods, is clearly indicated.

ACKNOWLEDGMENTS

Work on this chapter was supported by the Southern California Injury Prevention Research Center, CDC Grant No. R49/CCR903622, and the UCLA Brain Injury Research Center, National Institute of Neurological Diseases and Stroke Grant No. FDP-NIH NS30308.

References

Adeloye A, Ssembatya-Lule GC. Aetiological and epidemiological aspects of acute head injury in Malawi. *East Afr Med* 1997;74: 822–828.

Annegers JF, Grabow HD, Kurland LT, Laws ER Jr. The incidence, causes, and secular trends of head trauma in Olmsted County, Minnesota, 1935–1974. *Neurology* 1980; 30:912–919.

Association for the Advancement of Automotive Medicine. The Abbreviated Injury Scale, 1990 revision. Des Plaines, IL: Association for the Advancement of Auotomotive Medicine, 1990.

Auer L, Gell G, Richling B, et al. Predicting lethal outcome after severe head injury—a computer-assisted analysis of neurological symptoms and laboratory values. *Acta Neurochir* 1980;52:225–238.

Barber JB, Webster JC. Head injuries, review of 150 cases. *J Natl Med Assoc* 1974;66:201–204.

Blumer CE, Quine, S. Prevalence of spinal cord injury: an international comparison. *Neuroepidemiology* 1995;14:258–268.

Bracken MB, Freeman DH, Hellenbrand K. Incidence of acute traumatic hospitalized spinal cord injury in the United States, 1970–1977. *Am J Epidemiol* 1981;113:615–622.

Brismar B, Engstrom A, Rydberg U. Head injury and intoxication: a diagnostic and therapeutic dilemma. *Acta Chir Scand* 1983;149: 11–14.

Brooks CA, Gabella B, Hoffman R, et al. Traumatic brain injury: designing and implementing a population-based follow-up system. *Arch Phys Med Rehabil* 1997;78:S26–S30.

Bruce DA, Schut L, Bruno L, et al. Outcome following severe head injuries in children. *J Neurosurg* 1978;48:679–688.

Bryden J. How many head-injured. The epidemiology of post head injury disability. In: Wood R, Eames P, eds. Models of Brain Injury Rehabilitation. London: Chapman & Hall, 1989, pp 17–27.

Cambria S, Cardia E, Tomasello F, Moraci A. Considerations on the operative results in a group of elderly neurosurgical patients. *J Neurosurg Sci* 1979;23:121–123.

Cantu RC. Head injuries in sport. *Br J Sports Med* 1996;30:289–296.

Cantu RC. Cervical spine injuries in the athlete. *Semin Neurol* 2000;20:173–178.

Capaul M, Zollinger H, Satz N, et al. Analyses of 94 consecutive spinal cord injury patients using ASIA definition and modified Frankel score classification. *Paraplegia* 1994;32: 583–587.

Centers for Disease Control and Prevention. Traumatic Brain Injury in the United States: An Interim Report to Congress. Atlanta, GA:

Centers for Disease Control and Prevention, 1998.

Chen H, Chiu W, Chen S, et al. A nationwide epidemiological study of spinal cord injuries in Taiwan from July 1992 to June 1996. *Neurol Res* 1997;19:617–622.

Cohen ME, Ditunno JF Jr, Donovan WH, Maynard FM Jr. A test of the 1992 International Standards for Neurological and Functional Classification of Spinal Cord Injury. *Spinal Cord* 1998;36:554–560.

Collins JG. Persons Injured and Disability Days due to Injuries, United States, 1980–81. Vital and Health Statistics, Series 10, No. 149. DHHS Pub No (PHS) 85-1577. Washington, D.C., U.S. Government Printing Office, March 1985.

Collins MW, Grindel SH, Lovell MR, et al. Relationship between concussion and neuropsychological performance in college football players. *JAMA* 1999;282:964–970.

Cooper JD, Tabaddor K, Hauser WA. The epidemiology of head injury in the Bronx. *Neuroepidemiology* 1983;2:70–88.

Corrigan, JD. Substance abuse as a mediating factor in outcome from traumatic brain injury. *Arch Phys Med Rehabil* 1995;76:302–309.

Corrigan JD, Smith-Knapp K, Granger CV. Validity of the Functional Independence Measure for persons with traumatic brain injury. *Arch Phys Med Rehabil* 1997;78:828–834.

Dacey RG Jr, Alves WM, Rimel RW, et al. Neurosurgical complications after apparently minor head injury. Assessment of risk in a series of 610 patients. *J Neurosurg* 1986;65:203–210.

Dawson DR, Chipman M. The disablement experienced by traumatically brain-injured adults living in the community. *Brain Inj* 1995;9:339–353.

Deloche G, Dellatolas G, Christensen A-L. The European Brain Injury Questionnaire: patient's and family's subjective evaluation of brain-injured patients' current and prior injury difficulties. In: Christensen A-L, Uzzell BP, eds. International Handbook of Neuropsychological Rehabilitation. New York: Kluwer Academic/Plenum, 2000, pp 81–92.

DeVivo MJ, Ivie CS 3rd. Life expectancy of ventilator-dependent persons with spinal cord injuries. *Chest* 1995;108:226–232.

DeVivo M, Krause JS, Lammertse D. Recent trends in mortality and causes of death among persons with spinal cord injury. *Arch Phys Med Rehabil* 1999;80:1411–1419.

DeVivo MJ, Stover SL. Long-term survival and causes of death. In: Stover SL, DeLisa JA, Whiteneck GG, eds. Spinal Cord Injury: Clinical Outcomes from the Model Systems.

Gaithersburg, MD: Aspen Publishers, 1995, pp 289–316.

Ditunno JF Jr, Young W, Donovan WH, Creasy G. The international standards booklet for neurological and functional classification of spinal cord injury. *Paraplegia* 1994;32:70–80.

Drubach DA, Kelly MP, Winslow MM, Flynn JP. Substance abuse as a factor in the causality, severity, and recurrence rate of traumatic brain injury. *Md Med J* 1993;42:989–993.

Edna T-H. Alcohol influence and head injury. *Acta Chir Scand* 1982;148:209–212.

Edna TH, Cappelen J. Hospital admitted head injury. A prospective study in Trondelag, Norway, 1979–80. *Scand J Soc Med* 1984;12:7–14.

Engberg AW, Teasdale TW. Traumatic brain injury in Denmark. A national 15-year study. *Eur J Epidemiol* 2001;17:437–442.

Farmer JC, Vaccaro AR, Balderston RA, et al. The changing nature of admissions to a spinal cord injury center: violence on the rise. *J Spinal Disord* 1998;11:400–403.

Fife D. Head injury with and without hospital admission: comparisons of incidence and short-terms disability. *Am J Public Health* 1987;7:810–812.

Fife D, Faich G, Hollenshead W, Boynton W. Incidence and outcome of hospital-treated head injury in Rhode Island. *Am J Public Health* 1986;76:773–778.

Fine PR, Kuhlemeir KV, DeVivo MJ, Stover SL. Spinal cord injury: an epidemiologic perspective. *Paraplegia* 1979;17:237–250.

Frankel HL, Coll JR, Charlifue SW, et al. Long-term survival in spinal cord injury: a fifty-year investigation. *Spinal Cord* 1998;36:266–274.

Frankel JL, Hancock DO, Hyslop G, et al. The value of postural reduction in the initial management of closed injuries of the spine with paraplegia and tetraplegia: Part I. *Paraplegia* 1969;7:179–192.

Gabella B, Hoffman R, Land G, et al. Traumatic brain injury—Colorado, Missouri, Oklahoma, and Utah, 1990–1993. *MMWR Morb Mortal Wkly Rep* 1997a;46:8–11.

Gabella B, Hoffman RE, Marine WW, Stallones L. Urban and rural traumatic brain injuries in Colorado. *Ann Epidemiol* 1997b;7:207–212.

Galbraith S, Murray WR, Patel AR, et al. The relationship between alcohol and its effect on the conscious level. *Br J Surg* 1976;63:128–130.

Gale JL, Dikmen S, Wyler A, et al. Head injury in the Pacific Northwest. *Neurosurgery* 1983;12:487–491.

Go BK, DeVivo MJ, Richards JS. The epidemiology of spinal cord injury. In: Stover SL, DeLisa JA, Whiteneck GG, eds. Spinal Cord Injury: Clinical Outcomes from the Model Systems, Gaithersburg, MD: Aspen Publishers, 1995, pp 21–55.

Gordon WA, Haddad L, Brown M, et al. The sensitivity and specificity of self-reported symptoms in individuals with traumatic brain injury. *Brain Inj* 2000;14:21–33.

Granger CV, Divan N, Fiedler RC. Functional assessment scales: a study of persons after traumatic brain injury. *Arch Phys Med Rehabil* 1995;74:107–113.

Granger CV, Hamilton BB, Keith RA. Advances in functional assessment for medical rehabilitation. *Top Geriatr Rehabil* 1986;1:59–74.

Graves E. Detailed diagnoses and procedures, National Hospital Discharge Survey, 1993. Vital Health Statistics. No. 122, 1995.

Gronwall SL, Wrightson P. Delayed recovery of intellectual function after minor head injury. *Lancet* 1974;2:605–609.

Guerrero JL, Leadbetter S, Thurman DJ, et al. A method for estimating the prevalence of disability from traumatic brain injury. Atlanta: Centers for Disease Control and Prevention, National Center for Injury Prevention and Control, unpublished manuscript.

Guerrero JL, Thurman DJ, Sniezek JE. Emergency department visits associated with traumatic brain injury. *Brain Inj* 2000;14:181–186.

Gurney JG, Rivara FP, Mueller BH, et al. The effects of alcohol intoxication on the initial treatment and hospital course of patients with acute brain injury. *J Trauma* 1992;33:709–713.

Gururaj G, Das BS, Channabasavanna SM, Kaliaperumal VG. A descriptive epidemiological study of head injuries in Bangalore. In: Chiu W-T, Choi K, Hung C-C, Shih C-J, LaPorte RE, eds. Epidemiology of Head and Spinal Cord Injury in Developing and Developed Countries. Proceedings of The First International Symposium of The Epidemiology of Head and Spinal Cord Injury. Yuan, Republic of China: Department of Health Executive, 1993, pp 121–128.

Hall KM. Overview of functional assessment scales in brain injury rehabilitation. *Neurorehabilitation* 1992;2:97–112.

Hartkopp A, Br*nnum-Hansen H, et al. Survival and cause of death after traumatic spinal cord injury, a long-term epidemiological survey from Denmark. *Spinal Cord* 1997;35:76–85.

Hillier SL, Hillier JE, Metzer J. Epidemiology of traumatic brain injury in South Australia. *Brain Inj* 1997;11:649–659.

Holly LT, Kelly DF, Counelis GJ, et al. Cervical spine trauma associated with moderate and severe head injury: incidence, risk factors, and injury characteristics. *J Neurosurg* 2002;96:285–291.

Hoyert DL, Kochanek KD, Murphy SL. Deaths: final data for 1997. Hyattsville, MD: National Center for Health Statistics, 1999. (National Vital Statistics Reports, v. 47, no. 19) (DHHS publication no. (PHS) 99-1120).

Igun GO, Obekpa OP, Ugwu BT, Nwadiaro HC. Spinal injuries in the Plateau State, Nigeria. *East Afr Med J* 1999;76:75–79.

International Classification of Diseases, 9th revision, 4th edition. Clinical Modification. Karaffa MC, ed. Los Angeles: Practice Management Information Corp., 1992.

Jagger J, Fife D, Vernberg K, Jane JJ. Effect of alcohol intoxication on the diagnosis and apparent severity of brain injury. *Neurosurgery* 1984a;15:303–306.

Jagger J, Levine J, Jane J, Rimel RW. Epidemiologic features of head injury in a predominantly rural population. *J Trauma* 1984b;24:40–44.

Jennett B, Bond M. Assessment of outcome after severe brain damage. *Lancet* 1975;1:480–484.

Jennett B, MacMillan R. Epidemiology of head injury. *BMJ* 1981;282:101–104.

Jennett B, Murray A, Carlin J, et al. Head injuries in three Scottish neurosurgical units. *BMJ* 1979a;2:955–958.

Jennett B, Teasdale G. Management of Head Injuries. Philadelphia, FA Davis Co., 1981, pp 77–93.

Jennett B, Teasdale G, Braakman R, et al. Prognosis in series of patients with severe head injury. *Neurosurgery* 1979b;4:283–289.

Johnson R, Gleave J. Counting the people disabled by head injury. *Injury* 1987;18:7-9.

Kalsbeek WD, McLaurin RL, Harris BS 3d, Miller JD. The National Head and Spinal Cord Injury Survey: major findings. *J Neurosurg* 1980;Suppl:S19-S31.

Karamehmetoglu SS, Unal S, Karacan I, et al. Traumatic spinal cord injuries in Istanbul, Turkey. An epidemiological study. *Paraplegia* 1995;33:469–471.

Klauber MR, Barrett-Connor E, Marshall LF, Bowers SA. The epidemiology of head injury. A prospective study of an entire community: San Diego County, California, 1978. *Am J Epidemiol* 1981a;113:500–511.

Klauber MR, Marshall LF, Barrett-Connor E. Prospective study of patients hospitalized with head injury in San Diego County, 1978. *Neurosurgery* 1981b;9:236–241.

Kraus JF, Black MA, Hessol N, et al. The incidence of acute brain injury and serious impairment in a defined population. *Am J Epidemiol* 1984;119:186–201.

Kraus JF, Franti CE, Riggins RS, et al. Incidence of traumatic spinal cord lesions. *J Chron Dis* 1975;28:471–492.

Kraus JF, McArthur DL. Epidemiology of brain injury, 4th edition. In: Cooper PR, Golfinos JG, eds. Head Injury. New York: McGraw-Hill, 2000, pp 1–27.

Kraus JF, McArthur DL, Silberman TA. Epidemiology of mild head injury. *Semin Neurol* 1994;14:1–7.

Kraus JF, Morgenstern H, Fife D, et al. Blood alcohol tests, prevalence of involvement, and outcomes following brain injury. *Am J Public Health* 1989;79:294–299.

Kraus JF, Silberman TA, McArthur DL. Epidemiology of spinal cord injury. In: Menezes AH, Sontagg VKH, eds. Principles of Spinal Surgery. New York: McGraw-Hill, 1996, pp 41–58.

Lasfargues JE, Custis D, Morrone F, et al. A model for estimating spinal cord injury prevalence in the United States. *Paraplegia* 1995;33:62–68.

Lee ST, Lui TN. Early seizures after mild closed head injury. *J Neurosurg* 1992;76:435–439.

Lee S, Liu T, Chang C, et al. Features of head injury in a developing country—Taiwan (1977–1987). *J Trauma* 1990;30:194–199.

Levin HS, High WM, Goethe KE, et al. The Neurobehavioral Rating Scale: assessment of the behavioral sequelae of head injury by the clinician. *J Neurol Neurosurg Psychiatry* 1987;50:183–193.

Lillard PL. Five years experience with penetrating craniocerebral gunshot wounds. *Surg Neurol* 1978;9:79–83.

Lubinski R, Moscato BS, Willer BS. Prevalence of speaking and hearing disabilities among adults with traumatic brain injury from a national household survey. *Brain Inj* 1997;11:103-114.

MacKenzie EJ, Edelstein SL, Flynn JP. Hospitalized head-injured patients in Maryland: incidence and severity of injuries. *Md Med J* 1989;38:725–732.

Macpherson BC, Macpherson P, Jennett B. CT evidence of intracranial contusion and haematoma in relation to the presence, site and type of skull fracture. *Clin Radiol* 1990;42:321–326.

Maharaj JC. Epidemiology of spinal cord paralysis in Fiji: 1985–1994. *Spinal Cord* 1996;34:549–559.

Mahoney FI, Barthel DW. Functional evaluation: the Barthel Index. *Md State Med J* 1965;14:61–68.

Martin J, Meltzer H, Elliot D. The Prevalence of Disability Among Adults. London: Her Majesty's Stationary Office, 1988.

Martins F, Freitas F, Martins L, et al. Spinal cord injuries—epidemiology in Portugal's central region. *Spinal Cord* 1998;36:574–578.

Marwick C. Spinal cord injury research shows promise. *JAMA* 1999;282:2108–2110.

Masson F, Thicoipe M, Aye P, Mokni T, Senjean P, Schmitt V, Dessalles PH, Cazaugade M, Labadens P. Epidemiology of severe brain injuries: a prospective population-based study. *J Trauma* 2001;51:481–489.

McKinley WO, Seel RT, Hardman JT. Nontraumatic spinal cord injury: incidence, epidemiology, and functional outcome. *Arch Phys Med Rehabil* 1999;80:619–623.

McPherson KM, Pentland B. Disability in patients following traumatic brain injury—which measure? *Int J Rehabil Res* 1997;20:1–10.

Miller DM, Weinstock-Guttman B, Béthoux F, et al. A meta-analysis of methylprednisolone in recovery from multiple sclerosis exacerbations. *Mult Scler* 2000;6:267–273.

Miller JD, Pentland B. The factors of age, alcohol, and multiple injury in patients with mild and moderate head injury. In: Hoff J, Anderson T, Cole T, eds. Mild to Moderate Head Injury. Boston: Blackwell Scientific, 1989, pp 125–133.

Minaire P, Castanier M, Girard R, Berard E, Didier C, Bourret J. Epidemiology of spinal cord injury in the Rhone-Alpes Region, France, 1970–1975. *Paraplegia* 1979;16:76–87.

Modell JG, Mountz JM. Drinking and flying—the problem of alcohol use by pilots. *N Engl J Med* 1990;323:455–461.

Moscato BS, Trevisian M, Willer B. The prevalence of traumatic brain injury and co-occurring disabilities in a national household survey of adults. *J Neuropsychiatry Clin Neurosci* 1994;6:134–142.

Murshid WR. Management of minor head injuries: admission criteria, radiological evaluation and treatment of complications. *Acta Neurochir (Wien)* 1998;140:56–64.

Nell V, Brown DSO. Epidemiology of traumatic brain injury in Johannesburg—II. Morbidity, mortality and etiology. *Soc Sci Med* 1991;33:289–296.

Nell V, Yates DW, Kruger J. An extended Glasgow Coma Scale (GCS-E) with enhanced sensitivity to mild brain injury. *Arch Phys Med Rehabil* 2000;81:614–617.

Nestvold K, Lundar T, Blikra G, Lonnum A. Head injuries during one year in a central hospital in Norway. A prospective study:

epidemiologic features. *Neuroepidemiology* 1988;7:134–144.

Nobunaga AI, Go BK, Karunas RB. Recent demographic and injury trends in people served by the Model Spinal Cord Injury Care Systems. *Arch Phys Med Rehabil* 1999;80: 1372–1382.

Noguchi T. A survey of spinal cord injuries resulting from sport. *Paraplegia* 1994;32:170–173.

Novack TA, Bush BA, Meythaler JM, Canupp K. Outcome after traumatic brain injury: pathway analysis of contributions from premorbid, injury severity, and recovery variables. *Arch Phys Med Rehabil* 2001;82:300–305.

O'Connor P. Incidence and patterns of spinal cord injury in Australia. *Accid Anal Prev* 2002; 34:405–415.

Otom AS, Doughan AM, Kawar JS, Hattar EZ. Traumatic spinal cord injuries in Jordan—an epidemiological study. *Spinal Cord* 1997; 35:253–255.

Pajareya K. Traumatic spinal cord injuries in Thailand: an epidemiologic study in Siriraj Hospital, 1989–1994. *Spinal Cord* 1996;34: 608–610.

Phonprasert C, Suwanwela C, Hongsaprabhas C, et al. Extradural hematoma: analysis of 138 cases. *J Trauma* 1980;20:679–683.

Plaut MR, Gifford RR. Trivial head trauma and its consequences in a perspective of regional health care. *Mil Med* 1976;141:244–247.

Powell JW, Barber-Foss KD. Traumatic brain injury in high school athletes. *JAMA* 1999; 282:958–963.

Raimondi AD, Samuelson GH. Craniocerebral gunshot wounds in civilian practice. *J Neurosurg* 1970;32:647–683.

Raja IA. Epidemiology of head injury in Pakistan. In: Chiu W-T, Choi K, Hung C-C, Shih C-J, LaPorte RE, eds. Epidemiology of Head and Spinal Cord Injury in Developing and Developed Countries. Proceedings of The First International Symposium of The Epidemiology of Head and Spinal Cord Injury. Yuan, Republic of China: Department of Health Executive, 1993, pp 37–58.

Ramer MS, Harper GP, Bradbury EJ. Progress in spinal cord research, a refined strategy for the International Spinal Research Trust. *Spinal Cord* 2000;38:449–472.

Ramsey M, Hilson F. Community integration—redefining life after brain injury. Parramatta NSW, Michael Ramsey and Associates Pty Ltd, 1995, cited in Brain Injury Association of New South Wales, Brain Injury—The Statistics. Parramatta NSW, Disability Information & Resource Centre Inc., 2000 (www.dircsa.org.au/pub/docs/factsht9.htm).

Richards JS, Go BK, Rutt RD, Lazarus PB. The National Spinal Cord Injury Collaborative Database. In: Stover SL, DeLisa JA, Whiteneck GG, eds. Spinal Cord Injury: Clinical Outcomes from the Model Systems. Gaithersburg, MD: Aspen Publishers, 1995, pp 10–20.

Rimel RW. A prospective study of patients with central nervous system trauma. *J Neurosurg Nurs* 1981;13:132–141.

Schönherr MC, Groothoff JW, Mulder GA, Eisma WH. Rehabilitation of patients with spinal cord lesions in The Netherlands: an epidemiological study. *Spinal Cord* 1996;34: 679–683.

Schootman M, Harlan M, Fuortes L. Use of capture–recapture method to estimate severe traumatic brain injury rates. *J Trauma* 2000; 48:70–75.

Schulhof LA, Rivet R, Maroon JC. Severe head injuries: a retrospective review of 100 consecutive cases. Marian County General Hospital. *J Indiana State Med Assoc* 1972;65: 739–746.

Schuster M. Traumatic Brain Injury in Massachusetts. Boston, MA: Injury Prevention and Control Program, Massachusetts Department of Public Health, 1994.

Selecki BR, Hoy RJ, Ness P. Neurotraumatic admissions to a teaching hospital: a retrospective survey. Part 4. Neurotrauma after road accidents. *Med J Aust* 1968;2:490–493.

Selecki BR, Ring IT, Simpson DA, et al. Trauma to the central and peripheral nervous system: Part I: an overview of mortality, morbidity and cost; New South Wales, 1977. *Aust N Z J Surg* 1982;52:93–102.

Shingu H, Ohama M, Ikata T, et al. A nationwide epidemiological survey of spinal cord injuries in Japan from January 1990 to December 1992. *Paraplegia* 1995;33:183–188.

Short DJ, El Masry WS, Jones PW. High does methylprednisolone in the management of acute spinal cord injury—a systematic review from a clinical perspective. *Spinal Cord* 2000;38:273–286.

Silberstein B, Rabinovich. Epidemiology of spinal cord injuries in Novosibirsk, Russia. *Paraplegia* 1995;33:322–325.

Soden RJ, Walsh J, Middleton JW, et al. Causes of death after spinal cord injury. *Spinal Cord* 2000;38:604–610.

Sosin DM, Sacks JJ, Smith SM. Head injury–associated deaths in the United States from 1979 to 1986. *JAMA* 1989;262: 2251–2255.

Sosin DM, Sniezek JE, Waxweiler RJ. Trends in death associated with traumatic brain injury, 1979 through 1992: success and failure. *JAMA* 1995;273:1778–1780.

Tarazi F, Dvorak FS, Wing, PC. Spinal injuries in skiers and snowboarders. *Am J Sports Med* 1999;27:177–180.

Tate PS, Freed DM, Bombardier CH, Harter SL, Brinkman S. Traumatic brain injury: influence of blood alcohol level on post-acute cognitive function. *Brain Inj* 1999;13:767–784.

Tate R, McDonald S, Lulham J. Incidence of hospital-treated traumatic brain injury in an Australian community. *Aust N Z J Public Health* 1998;22:419–423.

Teasdale G, Jennett B. Assessment of coma and impaired consciousness: a practical scale. *Lancet* 1974;2:81–84.

Thornhill S, Teasdale GM, Murray GD, et al. Disability in young people and adults one year after head injury: prospective cohort study. *BMJ* 2000;320:1631–1635.

Thurman DJ, Alverson CA, Dunn KA, et al. Traumatic brain injury in the United States: a public health perspective. *J Head Trauma Rehabil* 1999;14:602–615.

Thurman D, Guerrero J. Trends in hospitalization associated with traumatic brain injury. *JAMA* 1999;282:954–957.

Thurman DJ, Jeppson L, Burnett CL, et al. Surveillance of traumatic brain injuries in Utah. *West J Med* 1996;135:192–196.

Thurman DJ, Sniezek JE, Johnson D, et al. Guidelines for surveillance of central nervous system injury. Atlanta, GA: U.S. Department of Health and Human Services, Centers for Disease Control and Prevention, 1995.

Tiret L, Hausherr E, Thicoipe M, et al. The epidemiology of head trauma in Aquitaine (France), 1986: A community-based study of hospital admissions and deaths. *Int J Epidemiol* 1990;19:133–140.

Tyroch AH, Davis JW, Kaups KL, Lorenzo M. Spinal cord injury, a preventable public health burden. *Arch Surg* 1997;1323:778–781.

van Asbeck FWA, Post MWM, Pangalila RF. An epidemiological description of spinal cord injuries in The Netherlands in 1994. *Spinal Cord* 2000;38:420–424.

Velmahos GC, Degiannis E, Hart K, et al. Changing profiles in spinal cord injuries and risk factors influencing recovery after penetrating injuries. *J Trauma* 1995;38:334–337.

Wagner JG, Wilkinson PK, Ganes DA. Estimation of the amount of alcohol ingested from a single blood alcohol concentration. *Alcohol Alcohol* 1990;25:379–384.

Waller PF, Stewart JR, Hansen AR, et al. The potentiating effects of alcohol on driver injury. *JAMA* 1986;256:1461–1466.

Wang C-C, Schoenberg BS, Li S-C, Yang Y-C, Cheng X-M, Bolis L. Brain injury due to head trauma. Epidemiology in urban areas of the People's Republic of China. *Arch Neurol* 1986;43:570–572.

Wang YC, P'eng FK, Yang DY, et al. Epidemiological study of head injuries in Central Taiwan. *Chin Med J* 1995;55:50–57.

Ward RE, Flynn TC, Miller PW, Blaisdell WF. Effects of ethanol ingestion on the severity and outcome of trauma. *Am J Surg* 1982;144:153–157.

Warren S, Moore M, Johnson MS. Traumatic head and spinal cord injuries in Alaska (1991–1993). *Alaska Med* 1995;37:11–19.

Whitman S, Coonley-Hoganson R, Desai BT. Comparative head trauma experiences in two socioeconomically different Chicago-area communities. A population study. *Am J Epidemiol* 1984;119:570–580.

Wilson JT, Pettigrew LE, Teasdale GM. Structured interviews for the Glasgow Outcome Scale and the Extended Glasgow Outcome Scale: guidelines for their use. *J Neurotrauma* 1998;15:573–585.

World Health Organization. International Classification of Impairments, Disabilities, and Handicaps: A Manual of Classification Relating to the Consequences of Disease. Geneva: World Health Organization, 1980.

World Health Organization. International Statistical Classification of Diseases and Related Health Problems, Tenth Revision. Geneva: World Health Organization, 1992.

Zigler JE, Capen DA. Epidemiology of spinal cord injury: a perspective on the problem. In: Levine AM, Eismont FJ, Garfin SR, Zigler JE, eds. Spine Trauma. Philadelphia: WB Saunders, 1998, pp 2–8.

Zink BJ, Walsh RF, Feustel PJ. Effects of ethanol in traumatic brain injury. *J Neurotrauma* 1993;10:275–286.

11

Peripheral Neuropathy

GARY M. FRANKLIN

Peripheral neuropathy can be defined as any disorder of the nervous system distal to the brain stem (cranial nerves) or spinal cord (dorsal and ventral nerve roots, sensory ganglia, and peripheral nerves). Peripheral neuropathies can be classified by the anatomic region involved (e.g., radiculopathy is a compression of a nerve root by an extruded disc), the type of nerve involved (e.g., sensory, motor, or autonomic), or by cause (e.g., entrapment, metabolic) (Dyck 1982). A few neuropathies are very common. Carpal tunnel syndrome is the most common entrapment neuropathy; diabetic neuropathy is the most common metabolic neuropathy; and Guillain-Barré syndrome is the most common inflammatory neuropathy.

A number of large-scale studies to determine the population burden of neurologic disease have been reported from various nations (Osuntokun et al. 1987; Rajput et al. 1988; Cruz Gutierrez-del-Olmo et al. 1989; Tekle-Haimanot et al. 1990; Munoz et al. 1995). Despite dramatic differences in methods and international venue, these studies have consistently reported neuropathy as the third or fourth leading type of neurologic disorder even among the elderly (Munoz et al. 1995). Because the underlying etiology or precipitating events of peripheral neuropathy are identifiable in most affected individuals, epidemiologic research on neuropathies has largely focused on descriptive studies of disease frequency, or on identifying potential risk factors for neuropathy occurrence.

Classification of Peripheral Neuropathies

The approach to the classification of peripheral neuropathies has been based on anatomic localization, pathology, natural history, or underlying cause (Dyck 1982; Dyck et al. 1993). The taxonomic approach taken here relates to both the frequency and underlying cause of the neuropathy (Table 11–1). Within each underlying cause category, only those disorders for which incidence/prevalence data are available, which

279

Table 11–1 Taxonomy of Peripheral Neuropathy

Neuropathies Associated with Systemic (Metabolic) Disorders

Diabetic neuropathy
Uremic neuropathy
Hypothyroid neuropathy

Infectious Neuropathies

Leprosy—*Mycobacterium leprae* (Tekle-Haimanot et al. 1990)
HIV-1 (Parry et al. 1997)
Hepatitis C
Herpes zoster—shingles
Lyme disease—*Borrelia burgdorferi*

Traumatic or Compressive Neuropathies

Carpal tunnel syndrome—median nerve entrapment
Cervical radiculopathy (Radhakrishnan et al. 1994)
Lumbar radiculopathy (sciatica)
Perioperative neuropathies (Warner et al. 1994)

Toxin- and Drug-induced Neuropathies

Alcohol
Chemotherapy agents—cisplatin (van der Hoop et al. 1990), etc.
Antiretroviral agents—dideoxycytidine
Heavy metals—arsenic, lead, mercury
Acrylamide
Short-chain hexacarbons—*n*-hexane, methyl-*n*-butyl ketone
Pyridoxine-associated neuropathy
Carbon disulfide
Organophosphates—triorthocresyl phosphate (Morgan 1982)

Immune-mediated or Inflammatory Neuropathies

Guillain-Barré syndrome
Brachial neuritis (neuralgic amyotrophy) (Beghi et al. 1985)

Nutritional Deficiency Neuropathies

Vitamin B_{12}
Epidemic optic neuropathy—Cuba (Cuba Neuropathy Field Investigation Team 1995), Tanzania (Bourne et al. 1998)
Thiamine—beriberi

Hereditary Neuropathies

Hereditary motor and sensory neuropathy (Charcot-Marie-Tooth) (Holmberg 1993)

Idiopathic Neuropathies

Bell's palsy (Hauser et al. 1971)
Trigeminal neuralgia—tic douloureux (Yoshimasu et al. 1972)

Neuropathies Associated with Aging

Distal sensory neuropathy (Italian Longitudinal Study 1997)
Optic neuropathy (Johnson and Arnold 1994)

are emerging as common disorders of potential public health importance, or which are of epidemiologic interest for other reasons are included in Table 11–1.

Of the more than 130 neuropathies recently enumerated in *A Guide to the Peripheral Neuropathies* (Neuropathy Association 1999), incidence/prevalence rates have been reported for fewer than 20. The main reason for this paucity of epidemiologic research is that we have insufficient data on ambulatory conditions, including most peripheral neuropathies. The best available population-based rates are derived from (1) the records linkage system of the Mayo Clinic (Hauser et al. 1971; Yoshimasu et al. 1972; Beghi et al. 1985; Stevens et al. 1988), (2) community studies based on intensive case finding of the underlying condition with secondary retrospective or prospective ascertainment of peripheral neuropathy (Maser et al. 1989; Franklin et al. 1990), (3) door-to-door (Savettieri et al. 1993) or mail (Atroshi et al. 1999) surveys with a two-stage screening/validation procedure, (4) large insurance databases (Franklin et al. 1991), and (5) intensive case finding related to endemic (Schonberger et al. 1979) or epidemic (Cuba Neuropathy Field Investigation Team 1995) neuropathy.

Three of the leading neuropathies in the United States and worldwide will be covered here in detail: diabetic neuropathy, carpal tunnel syndrome, and Guillain-Barré syndrome. Earlier epidemiologic reviews have summarized the available data on all neuropathies (Haerer et al. 1991; Martyn and Hughes 1997), as well as on the neuropathies reviewed here (Franklin 1994). The methods underlying the epidemiologic study of these three neuropathies are the subject of this chapter and are generally applicable to the study of all neuropathies.

Diabetic Neuropathy

Disease Description

Four principal clinical types of neuropathy have been described in association with diabetes (Thomas and Tomlinson 1993), but only two of these, distal symmetrical sensory neuropathy (DSN) and autonomic neuropathy (AN), are common enough to have been addressed in population-based studies. These conditions tend to develop with later, more severe cases of diabetes and often co-occur with two other important late complications of diabetes, nephropathy and retinopathy. Complications relate to both the metabolic disorder and microvascular anatomic changes seen

most commonly in the endothelial basement membrane (Dyck 1992). The relative contribution of these two pathogenetic mechanisms to neuropathy is unknown.

Distal symmetrical sensory neuropathy typically presents as numbness, tingling, or aberrant pain (dysesthesias) in the distalmost part of the feet and slowly progresses proximally, in a "stocking and glove" fashion. The patient will lose ankle reflexes early in the course of DSN; as the condition progresses, the patient may experience motor weakness in the legs and sensory symptoms in the distal upper extremities. This pattern of progression with the longest nerves (lower extremities) involved first is termed "dying back" neuropathy and is the most common presentation of neuropathy due to toxic/metabolic disorders. Distal symmetrical sensory neuropathy appears to involve greater axonal destruction than demyelination (Partanen et al. 1995), a worse portent for potential recovery of nerve function. Abnormal findings on electrodiagnostic studies may be present even before symptoms of DSN are noticed and may worsen with clinical progression (Thomas and Tomlinson 1993; Partanen et al. 1995).

Autonomic neuropathy, in contrast to DSN, is rarely prominent clinically until very late in the disease course of diabetes when impotence, gastroparesis, orthostatic hypotension, or other clinical concomitants of dysautonomia may occur. Special tests specific to the measurement of autonomic dysfunction are required to assess more accurately the presence or absence of AN (Mackay et al. 1980). The most commonly used test in field-based studies is computerized assessment of (cardiac) R-R interval variability after deep breathing (Ewing et al. 1981).

Because neither DSN nor AN exhibit a pattern of neuropathy unique to diabetes, case definitions depend on both (1) a set of common clinical or test criteria defining DSN or AN and (2) validated criteria for the presence of diabetes, such as those developed by the World Health Organization (1985).

Descriptive Studies of Diabetic Neuropathy

Incidence rates for diabetic neuropathy have rarely been reported in population-based studies because of resource and methodologic constraints. A well-designed study of diabetic neuropathy incidence would require following a large population of non-neuropathic diabetics for a period sufficient for the development of neuropathy, or 5 to 20 years in most cases.

> *Example 11–1* One such study, the San Luis Valley Diabetes Study, tracked 231 people free of DSN at baseline for a mean of 4.7 years (Sands et al. 1997). Only 14/239 (6%) developed consistently present neuropathy. Overall reported incidence of DSN was 6.1 per 100 person-years (95% confidence interval [CI] 4.7–7.8), based on 66 cases who met clinical criteria on at least one follow-up visit.

The Diabetes Control and Complication Trial (DCCT) followed 1441 patients with insulin-dependent diabetes mellitus (IDDM) for the development of complications (DCCT Research Group 1993). At 5 years, the incidence rate of DSN among those free of neuropathy at baseline ranged from 3.1 per 100 person-years to 16.1 per 100 person-years in four treatment subgroups. The case definition of DSN in this study required presence of DSN on physical examination by a neurologist and either abnormal nerve conduction in two separate nerves or unequivocally abnormal autonomic function test results. More recently, the Epidemiology of Diabetes Complications study reported DSN incidence among a cohort of 463 IDDM patients followed with biennial neurologic examinations. After a mean follow-up of 5.3 years, DSN incidence was reported to be 2.8 per 100 person-years (Forrest et al. 1997).

Numerous cross-sectional studies of DSN prevalence have been reported with prevalence ratios ranging between 4% and 80% (Haerer et al. 1991). The higher prevalence ratios are from hospital and clinic-based studies or from using overly sensitive criteria for the detection of neuropathy. Studies with more conservative criteria have reported rates of DSN in the range of 10% (Fry et al. 1962; Pirart 1978).

Table 11–2 outlines criteria useful in epidemiologic studies of diabetic DSN. For the purposes of population-based studies of prevalence, a national consensus of experts in diabetic neuropathy recommended that diagnosis be based on a screening examination consisting of at least a validated report of symptoms and at least one objective test (reflexes, sensory loss, electrodiagnostic studies) (Proceedings of a Consensus Development Conference 1992). When specificity rather than sensitivity is desirable, such as in clinical trials and studies of diagnostic test accuracy, more objective study is desirable, such as requiring a positive history of neuropathy symptoms and abnormal physical exam findings (e.g., decreased reflexes and abnormal electrodiagnostic tests) (Dyck et al. 1991; DCCT Research Group 1993; Feldman et al. 1994). Dyck et al. (1991) carried out an intensive examination of 380 out of 870 diabetics in Rochester, Minnesota on January 1, 1986. Symptomatic DSN was found in 13%–15% of diabetics and was twice as common as AN (7%). A less technically demanding and resource-intensive screening examination

Table 11–2 Criteria for Case Definition of Distal Symmetric Neuropathy

Criterion	Method
Self-reported symptoms of DSN	Validated questionnaire
Reduced or absent ankle reflexes	Assessment by trained examiner
Sensory loss in the distal lower extremities	Assessment by trained examiner or by quantitative sensory tests
Reduced sensory nerve action potential	Electrodiagnostic studies

for DSN has been applied in most other recent prevalence studies of DSN (Table 11–3). The first population-based study of diabetic neuropathy, based on a retrospective chart review of 1028 diabetics aged >30 years at diagnosis, in Rochester, Minnesota, reported that 4% within 5 years and 15% within 20 years of disease onset had neuropathy (Palumbo et al. 1978). The vast majority (72%) with neuropathy had DSN, while only 3% had clinical AN. Other neuropathies were more common than AN (carpal tunnel syndrome, 12%; isolated mononeuropathy, 6%).

A large registry-based study of younger persons with IDDM in Allegheny County, Pennsylvania used a case definition requiring any two of three screening criteria (Table 11–3) (Maser et al. 1989). Overall DSN prevalence was 34%, 18% in 18- to 29-year-olds and 58% in those ≥30 years old. In a subsequent substudy, the authors demonstrated strong correlations of this case definition of DSN with both quantitative sensory testing and electrodiagnostic testing.

Another geographically based study in south-central Colorado that used a similar case definition reported an age-adjusted prevalence of DSN of 4% in controls, 11% in those with impaired glucose tolerance, and 26% in those with non–insulin-dependent diabetes mellitus (NIDDM) (Franklin et al. 1990). The screening neuropathy criteria were strongly correlated with quantitative sensory tests and had 90% agreement (kappa 0.79) with a neurologist's examination.

A somewhat lower prevalence for DSN (3% of controls, 16% of diabetics) was identified in a community-based study in England that combined NIDDM and IDDM patients (Walters et al. 1991). Twenty-four percent of the defined neuropathy cases were asymptomatic, so an explanation for the lower prevalence is not entirely clear.

A door-to-door survey was used to screen for all neurological disorders in two Sicilian communities. A two-stage method to ascertain cases of neuropathy consisted of both a screening questionnaire and a follow-up standardized examination by a neurologist. Only 39/810 (5%) of adults who screened positive for neuropathy were classified with diabetic neuropathy. The population prevalence was estimated to be 268 per 100,000 (Savettieri et al. 1993).

Harris et al. (1993) accessed a representative sample of the U.S. population through the National Health Interview Survey. Persons with self-reported diabetes who could be interviewed (2405 subjects) responded to structured questions regarding sensory symptoms in their feet during the past 3 months. Reported prevalence of DSN was 30% in persons with IDDM, 37% in those with NIDDM, and 10%–12% in nondiabetic persons.

Several other large clinic- or hospital-based studies of DSN outside of the United States have reported prevalence rates ranging from 21% to 29%: Italy, 21% (Veglio and Sivieri 1993); Spain, 23% (Cabezas-Cerrato 1998); Europe, 28% (Tesfaye et al. 1996); and United Kingdom, 29% (Young et al. 1993).

Studies of the prevalence of AN in diabetics have been limited by the relatively low frequency of reported symptoms of AN and the need to add additional tests for its detection. Only 2%–3% of diabetics have been reported to have symptomatic AN in population-based studies (Palumbo et al. 1978; Neil et al. 1989). The only geographically based prevalence estimate of AN was provided by the Oxford (England) Community Diabetes Study (Neil et al. 1989). After excluding patients with underlying cardiovascular disease or those who were taking antihypertensives, 14% had at least one abnormal heart rate variation test.

Analytical Studies of Diabetic Neuropathy

Analytic studies of potential risk factors for diabetic neuropathy are limited primarily to clinic-based observational studies and population-based studies of prevalent cases. Duration of diabetes and poor glycemic control have been consistently

Table 11–3 Population-Based Prevalence Studies of Diabetic Neuropathy

Reference	Population	Type of diabetic neuropathy	Case definition	Prevalence	Comments
Palumbo et al. 1978	1028 patients with NIDDM in Rochester, MN	DSN	Symmetrical sensory symptoms and/or decreased vibratory sense with or without reflex change	4% within 5 years 15% after 20 years	Prevalence of other types of neuropathy less common (CTS 1.3%); autonomic neuropathy 0.3%)
Maser et al. 1989	400 registry patients with IDDM in Allegheny County, PA	DSN	Two of three criteria: 1. Sensory symptoms in legs or feet 2. Sensory or motor signs 3. Absent or decreased tendon reflexes	34% overall 18%, age 18–29 years 58%, age >30 yrs	Case criteria validated in subsequent substudy (Maser et al. 1992) by psychophysical and NCV measures
Neil et al. 1989	245/412 diabetics ≥20 years of age in Oxford, U.K.	AN	Heart rate variability <2.5 percentile for age-related norms	14%	
Franklin et al. 1990	279 cases with NIDDM, 577 controls, in San Luis Valley, CO	DSN	Two of three criteria: 1. Sensory symptoms in legs or feet 2. Decreased or absent ankle reflexes 3. Decreased or absent thermal sensation in feet	4% in controls 11% in those with impaired glucose tolerance 26% in diabetics	Field case definition had 90% agreement with standard neurological examination
Walters et al. 1991	1077 diabetics (NIDDM and IDDM) and 480 controls in an English community	DSN	At least two of the following: 1. Neuropathic symptoms in both feet 2. Decreased light touch in the feet 3. Impaired pain perception in the feet 4. Absent ankle reflexes 5. Elevated vibration threshold	3% in controls 17% in diabetics	76% of defined neuropathy cases were symptomatic
Savettieri et al. 1993	796 subjects who screened positive for neuropathy, door-to-door survey in two Sicilian municipalities	All diabetic neuropathies	Two-phase study: 1. Screen (+) for neuropathy 2. Neurologist exam by protocol	No % available; prevalence ratio 268/100,000	Patient self-report of diabetes status
Harris et al., 1993	2405 persons with self-reported diabetes identified through National Health Interview Survey	DSN	Structured interview for at least one of the following: 1. Numbness in hands or feet 2. Pain or tingling in hands or feet 3. Decreased hot or cold perception in hands or feet	30% in IDDM 37% in NIDDM 10%–12% in controls	

AN, autonomic neuropathy; CTS, carpal tunnel syndrome; DSN, distal symmetric neuropathy; IDDM, insulin dependent diabetes; NCV, nerve conduction velocity; NIDDM, non–insulin-dependent diabetes demonstrated to be related to prevalent DSN. In a large case series, Pirart (1978) was the first to report a strong association between longer duration and higher prevalence of DSN. This strong association has been confirmed for both IDDM (Maser et al. 1989) and NIDDM (Franklin et al. 1994) in population-based studies of prevalent neuropathy and in one incidence study in an IDDM cohort (Forrest et al. 1997). In the younger IDDM population, Maser et al. (1989) found a 15% increased risk of DSN for each 10-year increase in duration. In an older NIDDM population, Franklin et al. (1994) reported a 30% increase in risk for each 5-year increase of diabetes duration. Older age has also been positively and independently associated with DSN prevalence (Nathan et al. 1986; Franklin et al. 1994) but less consistently associated than duration of diabetes. The strong correlation between age and duration has led some investigators to use duration, not age, in multivariate modeling of DSN risk (Forrest et al. 1997).

The strongest and most important risk factor for DSN is poor glycemic control, usually measured as % HbA1c (glycosylated hemoglobin), a cumulative marker of recent glycemia (within 60–90 days). Even after adjustment for duration of diabetes, the risk of prevalent DSN is increased 35%–50% for each 1%–2% increase in HbA1c in both IDDM (Maser et al. 1989) and NIDDM (Franklin et al. 1994). The relative risk (RR) of incident DSN related to HbA1c in an IDDM cohort was reported to be 2.6 (95% CI 1.6–4.3) after adjustment for duration or diabetes (Forrest et al. 1997). The most forceful demonstration that glycemic control is one key to the etiology of DSN lies in the results of the Diabetes Control and Complications Trial, a randomized controlled clinical trial of an intervention aimed at strictly controlling blood glucose in IDDM patients (DCCT Research Group 1993)— incident clinical DSN was reduced by 60% (95% CI 38%–74%).

While many other risk factors for DSN have been investigated, studies have been inconsistent. This is partly due to differences in the two types of diabetes studied. For example, hypertension (Maser et al. 1989; Forrest et al. 1997), smoking (Maser et al. 1989; Mitchell et al. 1990; Forrest et al. 1997; Misra et al. 1999), and lipid status (Maser et al. 1989) have been associated with DSN in IDDM but not in NIDDM (Franklin et al. 1994). Hypertension was a particularly strong risk for incident DSN in a cohort with IDDM (RR 3.9, 95% CI 2.2–6.9) (Forrest et al. 1997). Hypertension may thus be an important preventable factor, other than hyperglycemia, that is worth pursuing, particularly in studies of younger IDDM patients.

Height is of some theoretical interest as a risk factor for DSN, since longer axons might be at greater risk in "dying-back" neuropathies. While a positive association between height and DSN has been suggested in case series (Sosenko et al. 1988; Robinson et al. 1992) and in one study of incident DSN (Forrest et al. 1997), it has not been corroborated in population-based studies (Maser et al. 1989).

Genetic susceptibility to neuropathy has not been clearly demonstrated. Although diabetes per se and its cardiovascular complications are noted to be more frequent among minority populations (Carter et al. 1996), this is likely related to nongenetic factors. More specific investigation through population-based studies has found no association between neuropathy and ethnicity (Franklin et al. 1990; Harris et al. 1993). Recent investigations of various genetic markers, including acetylation phenotypes (Misra et al. 1999), a Na-K-ATPase gene polymorphism (Vague et al. 1997), an aldose reductase gene polymorphism (Heesom et al. 1998), and an HLA-DR3/4 phenotype for AN (Barzilay et al. 1992), are very much exploratory. The genetic relevance of regulation of nerve growth factors and the relationship of neural growth factors to the development of DSN remain largely speculative (Brewster et al. 1994).

The principal prognostic issues relevant to diabetic neuropathy are (1) chronic, painful sensory disturbances in the feet that may affect quality of life, (2) the association of DSN with diabetic foot ulcer and amputation, and (3) the association of AN with excess mortality.

Melton and Dyck (1987) estimated that disabling (painful) neuropathy affects more than a half million diabetics in the United States. Neuropathy and peripheral vascular disease contribute significantly to the estimated 50,000 lower extremity amputations per year in diabetic populations (Bild et al. 1989).

Example 11-2 In a recent prospective study of 776 U.S. veterans followed for a median of 3.3 years, both peripheral vascular disease (RR 3.0, 95% CI 1.3–7.1) and DSN, measured as insensitivity to monofilament testing (RR 2.9, 95% CI 1.1–7.8), independently predicted amputation among diabetics (Adler et al. 1999). Prior foot ulcers were also a significant risk for amputation (Adler et al. 1999), and DSN independently predicted foot ulceration (RR 2.2, 95% CI 1.5–3.1) (Boyko et al. 1999). While reduced morbidity via prevention of foot ulcer and amputation is a high priority for diabetes education strategies (Bild et al. 1989), few randomized trials have demonstrated the cost-effectiveness of this approach (McCabe et al. 1998).

While most excess mortality among diabetics relates to cardiovascular disease and nephropathy (Moss et al. 1991), AN may be associated with excess mortality as well (Page and Watkins 1978; Ewing et al. 1980; Boyko et al. 1999). In a prospective clinic-based study of 484 IDDM patients, O'Brien et al. (1991) found significantly reduced 5-year survival in diabetics with AN compared to those without AN at baseline; however, competing comorbidities such as renal failure and hypertension were also significantly associated with premature death. QT prolongation may relate AN to excess mortality, but QT prolongation may be present even in the absence of AN (Veglio et al. 1999). While heart rate variability correctly identifies AN, such variability in combination with other cardiac risk factors probably more clearly predicts a high risk of mortality (Stein and Kleiger 1999).

Directions for Future Research of Diabetic Neuropathy

Various criteria for neuropathy, in differing combinations, have led to substantial variation in reported prevalence. Standard epidemiologic case definitions for detecting DSN and AN in population-based studies would be useful for future studies. Such a case definition for DSN, as in the epidemiologic case definition for carpal tunnel syndrome (Rempel et al. 1998), would include both validated clinical measures (e.g., structured questionnaire, sensory loss diagram) and objective measures of peripheral nerve dysfunction (electrodiagnostic studies). While quantitative sensory testing, such as vibrometry, thermal threshold, or monofilament perception, are in widespread use, their accuracy for detecting individuals with DSN is only modest. These tests, however, are useful in validating the presence or absence of DSN in populations of diabetics and controls because group mean threshold measures may differentiate groups with neuropathy from groups without neuropathy. In addition, threshold distributions are often skewed and analyses may require the use of log-normal values (Franklin et al. 1990). The use of electrodiagnostic studies in field studies would have to be weighed against their cost and problems with patient acceptance of discomfort.

Etiologic studies of diabetic neuropathy should focus on incident cases. Population-based, prospective studies of newly diagnosed diabetics, with baseline and follow-up collection of data, should be conducted in both IDDM and NIDDM populations. Prospective studies of incident cases are needed to identify preventable risk factors other than glycemic control and duration.

On the basis of results from the Diabetes Control and Complications Trial (DCCT Research Group 1993), many states in the

United States have passed laws mandating health benefits to improve glycemic control among diabetics. It is not clear, however, that the dramatic results of the DCCT can be duplicated in general practice. Community-based clinical trials are necessary to demonstrate that less intensive resources, such as education, could accomplish equivalent glycemic control and prevention of complications. For the purpose of early intervention, formal screening programs for early detection of diabetes in the general population may be justified (U.K. Prospective Diabetes Study Group 1998). More recently, persons with impaired glucose tolerance, a prediabetic state, have become the focus of prospective intervention studies (Adler and Turner 1999).

Carpal Tunnel Syndrome

Disease Description

Carpal tunnel syndrome (CTS), the most common entrapment neuropathy, is characterized by numbness, tingling, or, most commonly, painful dysesthesias such as burning sensations that occur in the distribution of the median nerve in one or both hands (Rosenbaum and Ochoa 1993). Patients with CTS are frequently awakened by nocturnal paresthesias (Stevens et al. 1988). Mild but painful symptoms appear to persist for months or years. In later stages, definitive loss of sensation (digits I–III) and weakness (abductor pollucis brevis, opponens pollucis) in the median nerve distribution in the hand may be detected by neurologic examination and corroborated by electrodiagnostic studies. Despite accurate knowledge of symptoms, the natural history of CTS has not been well described.

The median nerve becomes entrapped in the wrist beneath the transverse carpal ligament as the nerve courses through the tight "tunnel" with all of the flexor tendons of the digits. Median nerve dysfunction at the point of entrapment in the wrist slows nerve conduction at that point and is the basis for specific electrodiagnostic study testing parameters (American Academy of Neurology 1993; American Association of Electrodiagnostic Medicine Quality Assurance Committee 1993). The ulnar nerve, on the median side of the wrist, courses outside the tunnel and is spared by entrapment. The pathogenesis of median nerve dysfunction likely relates to both increased pressure and ischemia, although the relative contribution of each factor is unknown (Sunderland 1976; Gelberman et al. 1988; Szabo and Chidgey 1989).

Descriptive Studies of Carpal Tunnel Syndrome

Similar to diabetic neuropathy, an ideal case definition for CTS would include symptoms *and* signs *and* objective tests (such as nerve conduction studies). An early surveillance case definition of work-related CTS, dependent on provocative test findings (Tinel's, Phelan's), was found to incorrectly classify 38% of workers with CTS (Cummings et al. 1989; Katz et al. 1991). Thus, in the absence of the late and relatively rare signs of axonal degeneration, such as loss of sensation and weakness, a case definition representative of typical CTS must accurately reflect symptoms alone in the median nerve distribution. Katz et al. (1990) developed a structured, self-administered hand symptom diagram that classifies cases by median nerve symptom distribution and is reasonably accurate compared to electrodiagnostic studies.

Example 11–3 Consensus criteria for the classification of CTS in epidemiologic studies were recently developed by combining the hand symptom diagram (classic/probable versus possible versus unlikely symptoms) with electrodiagnostic studies for the most accurate classification of CTS (Rempel et al. 1998) (Table 11–4). Mildly abnormal electrodiagnostic studies alone, in the absence of likely symptoms, are commonly found in working populations and do not predict presence or future development of symptomatic CTS (Werner et al. 1997). Epidemiologic studies based either on symptoms alone or electrodiagnostic studies alone are there-

Table 11–4 Estimated Likelihood of Carpal Tunnel Syndrome (CTS) for Case Definitions that Include Electrodiagnosis Studies

Symptoms of CTS*	Electrodiagnostic study	Ordinal likelihood of CTS
Classic/probable	Positive	+++
Possible	Positive	++
Classic/probable	Negative	+/−†
Possible	Negative	−
Unlikely	Positive	−
Unlikely	Negative	−

*The criteria require symptom classification according to a hand symptom diagram (classic/probable versus possible versus unlikely symptoms) (Rempel et al. 1998).

†No consensus achieved on whether likelihood should be − or +.

Adapted with permission from Rempel D, Evanoff B, Amadio PC, et al. Consensus criteria for the calssification of carpal tunnel syndrome in epidemiologic studies. *Am J Public Health* 1998;88:1447–1451.

fore likely to significantly overestimate true prevalence of CTS. In a study of Japanese furniture workers, for example, Nathan et al. (1994) used a very sensitive electrodiagnostic test and found that 18% had abnormal nerve conduction velocity while only 2% had clinically definite CTS.

Incidence of CTS has been reported in four population-based studies (Stevens et al. 1988; Franklin et al. 1991; Nordstrom et al. 1998; Silverstein et al. 1998). The first such study, using the records linkage system of the Mayo Clinic, identified 1016 patients, all but 3 of whom had at least two appropriate symptoms or signs, or abnormal electrodiagnostic studies. The crude average annual incidence, 99 per 100,000 person-years, reflected a 42% increase in age-adjusted rates between 1961 and 1980. The mean age at diagnosis was 51 years and the female-to-male ratio was 3:1 (149/100,000 compared to 52/100,000).

Two population-based studies from Washington State reported CTS incidence for the years 1984–1988 (Franklin et al. 1991) and 1987–1995 (Silverstein et al. 1998) based on workers' compensation administrative data. The annualized incidence rates for these time periods revealed a dramatic increase in incidence, from 174 per 100,000 person-years (Franklin et al. 1991) to 273 per 100,000 person-years (Silverstein et al. 1998), but the increase stabilized during 1992–1995. The mean age of CTS

cases (37 years) (Franklin et al. 1991) and the female-to-male ratio of 1.2:1 (Franklin et al. 1991; Silverstein et al. 1998) were substantially different from those of the general population (Stevens et al. 1988), reflecting the demographics of the injured worker population. Validation studies comparing the administrative classification of CTS to medical record substantiation showed that the two sources were concordant for the diagnosis of CTS in 80% of cases (Franklin et al. 1991). Nordstrom et al. (1998), using an administrative clinic database for the Marshfield, Wisconsin area, identified all new CTS diagnoses made during 1991–1993. Using the strictest case definition, based on physician diagnosis and at least one clinical finding documented in the medical record, 309 cases were identified, for an annualized incidence rate of 346 per 100,000 person-years. The rate rose with age, as the rate among persons over 64 years was 1.65-fold that of persons aged 18–29 years. The female-to-male ratio (1.1:1) was much lower than that reported for Rochester, Minnesota (Stevens et al. 1988).

Four population-based prevalence studies of CTS have been reported since 1992. Using an age- and sex-stratified random sample of one district in The Netherlands, deKrom et al. (1992) identified 6% of women and 0.6% of men as having CTS according to reported symptoms and electrodiagnostic studies. A low response rate led the investigators to regard these as minimal rates. In a U.S. national health survey, Tanaka et al. (1995) used questions from an occupational health supplement to ascertain cases of medically diagnosed CTS among persons with self-reported prolonged hand discomfort. The overall prevalence of CTS was estimated to be 0.53% among recent workers and was somewhat higher among females (0.67%) than males (0.42%). A three- to fourfold increased prevalence of CTS was observed among females in older (≥55 years) age groups.

Ferry et al. (1998) used a two-stage procedure to estimate the prevalence of CTS in a suburban population of Manchester, U.K., served by a family practice. A baseline mail survey was sent to a random sample of 100 18- to 75-year-olds, requesting that a hand symptom diagram (Katz et al. 1990) be completed. Seventy-nine percent responded to the mailed questionnaire, and of these, a weighted sample based on symptoms received electrodiagnostic studies (155/250 invitees). Depending on the electrodiagnostic study cut point used and adjusting for bias due to non-participation, a prevalence of 7%–16% was estimated on the sole basis of electrodiagnostic findings. The prevalence of electrodiagnostic study abnormalities was reported to be higher in older age groups (>54 years) but no different by gender. This study is limited in that only 20% of persons with abnormal electrodiagnostic studies had classic or probable hand pain diagrams, so that the true prevalence of clinical CTS would only have been about 3%–4%.

Example 11–4 Atroshi and colleagues (1999) conducted a rigorous population-based study on CTS prevalence in southern Sweden. An age- and gender-stratified random sample of 3000 subjects (25–74 years) was sent a mail survey regarding symptoms of pain, numbness, and tingling occurring in any part of the body. Eighty-three percent responded, and 81% of these agreed to a clinical examination and electrodiagnostic studies. While 14% reported symptoms in the median nerve

distribution, only 3% overall had both clinical and electrodiagnostic study confirmation of CTS. Electrodiagnostic study abnormality in asymptomatic persons was common (18%) and its prevalence increased with age.

Analytic Studies of Carpal Tunnel Syndrome

Carpal tunnel syndrome has classically been described in clinical case series to occur in association with a number of underlying disorders (wrist fracture, crush injury, diabetes, hypothyroidism), and it is clear that these disorders may cause structural damage to the median nerve (Stewart and Aguayo 1984). For example, diabetic nerves appear to be more susceptible to compression (Ozaki et al. 1988). In a population-based study in which medical record verification was used to identify associated disorders, Stevens et al. (1992) found elevated standardized morbidity ratios (SMRs) for rheumatoid arthritis (SMR 3.6), diabetes (SMR 2.3), and pregnancy (SMR 2.5) among individuals with CTS. Other conditions frequently noted but without elevated SMRs were Colle's fracture, oophorectomy, and excessive occupational use of the hands. Very high prevalence of CTS (2%–7%) has been reported in hospital-based series of pregnant women, especially among third-trimester primiparas (Ekman-Ordeberg et al. 1987; McLennan et al. 1987). Carpal tunnel syndrome is also common in persons undergoing long-term hemodialysis (Kessler et al. 1992). Most strikingly, though, Stevens et al. (1992) could find no documented CTS-associated condition in the medical record for nearly 50% of the Mayo Clinic cases.

Aside from fracture, pregnancy, diabetes, and the rarer conditions mentioned above, it is likely that most CTS in working-age populations is related to exposures at work. While this has been a relatively contentious area of investigation (Silverstein et al. 1996), only one nonoccupational personal factor, obesity, has been clearly demonstrated to be significantly associated with

CTS. In a case–referent study, Wieslander et al. (1989) found that the risk of CTS related to work factors *and* obesity (odds ratio [OR] 7.1) was almost threefold greater than the risk related to obesity alone (OR 2.6). In a population-based incident case–control study, Nordstrom et al. (1997) found that obesity, after controlling for work factors, was significantly associated with CTS risk (OR 1.08 per each unit increase in body mass index [BMI], $p <$ 0.02). In a population-based prevalent case–control study, Tanaka et al. (1997) found that a BMI ≥ 25 increased risk for CTS twofold (OR 2.0, 95% CI 1.3–3.0).

Other nonoccupational factors are likely to be less important than obesity. While smaller carpal canal size has been suggested as a risk factor in a case–control study (Bleecker 1987), this has not been corroborated in more recent investigations (Winn and Habes 1990; Pierre-Jerome et al. 1997). An association of CTS with exposure to smoking was not found in a population-based incident case–control study (Nordstrom et al. 1997); however, Tanaka et al. (1997) reported an increased risk (OR 1.6) associated with smoking for self-reported prevalent CTS, and, using standardized first referral rates, Vessey et al. (1990) found a threefold risk for CTS referral related to smoking. In a large cross-sectional study of workers, Nathan et al. (1996) reported that exposure to tobacco and other drugs (caffeine) would explain at most only 5% of the risk for CTS, and only in women. Increased risk of CTS related to oophorectomy and/or hysterectomy (Bjorkquist et al. 1977; Cannon et al. 1981; deKrom et al. 1990; Pascual et al. 1991; Giersiepen et al. 2000) or oral contraceptive use (Vessey et al. 1990; Ferry et al. 2000) has also been reported in case–control studies. In a nested case–control study of 1214 women with CTS and 1214 age-matched control women without CTS, Ferry et al. (2000) found that a prior history of another musculoskeletal complaint was also associated with CTS (OR 2.0).

The relationship of work to the develop-ment of CTS has been the subject of numerous recent reviews (Stock 1991; Hagberg et al. 1992; Cumulative Trauma Disorders in the Workplace 1995). Rossignol et al. (1997) estimated the proportion of all persons receiving CTS surgery on the island of Montreal whose condition was likely related to work. In 53% of cases, CTS was possibly work related, 12% was associated with diabetes, 9% with thyroid disease, 8% with a history of wrist fracture, and 5% with pregnancy. This population may over-represent the work-related fraction, since most pregnant women with CTS do not require CTS surgery.

In general, population-based studies have assessed work-related risk factors for CTS using brief self-reported questionnaires. More detailed assessment of risk from direct observation at work has only been reported from industry-based cross-sectional studies, which tend to have a relatively small number of subjects and are often underpowered.

In a national survey, Tanaka et al. (1997) reported an increased risk of self-reported CTS in relation to bending or twisting the hands and wrists many times an hour (OR 5.5, 95% CI 3.2–9.4) and to working with handheld vibrating tools (OR 1.9, 95% CI 1.2–2.8). In a questionnaire given to community-based incident CTS cases and controls, Nordstrom et al. (1997) were able to explore the relationship to work in greater detail. Significant positive associations were seen for bending and twisting the hands at least 3.5 hours per day, but not for the mean workday use of power tools. This study also found a significant association with a job organization factor, less job control.

Smaller cross-sectional case–control studies have conducted exposure assessment with greater specificity. In the first substantial study, Armstrong and Chaffin (1979) reported a significant association between CTS and repetitive, forceful exertions of the hand, measured by electromyogram (EMG) and cinematography. Silverstein et al. (1987) categorized exposure in 39 jobs ($n = 652$ workers) based on the predominance of high force, high repetition, both, or neither, with the latter serving as the reference group. High repetition was more significantly associated with CTS than high force, but the combination yielded a 15-fold increased risk for CTS.

In a case–control study of male workers (34 received CTS surgery, 143 controls matched by age), Wieslander et al. (1989) reported an increased risk for both hand-held vibrating tools (OR 2.9) and repetitive movements of the wrist (OR 2.1). Recently, in detailed blind assessment of physical exposure risks based on benchmarked criteria, Latko et al. (1999) found a nonsignificant association of repetition with a strict case definition of CTS (Rempel et al. 1998). Only 19/352 study subjects met the CTS criteria, however, so that despite sophisticated exposure assessment, the study was likely underpowered.

Industry-specific CTS incidence rates estimated from large administrative databases also support the association between physical factors at work and CTS (Franklin et al. 1991; Silverstein et al. 1998). Industries such as food processing and meatpacking have extremely high rates of CTS (10- to 15-fold higher than the industry-wide rate). The moderate to high rates found in certain industries likely reflect a combination of physical factors that have been studied both epidemiologically and experimentally in relation to CTS (Viikari-Juntura and Silverstein 1999). One case–control study reported a dramatic increase in CTS risk with increasing numbers of occupational risk factors (Roquelaure et al. 1997). Blanc et al. (1996) estimated a national prevalence of 240,578 persons with CTS-related work disability in 1988.

Giersiepen et al. (2000) conducted a population-based case–control study of CTS in Bremen, Germany among 808 persons (50% women <65 years old) who received surgery for CTS, matched by age and gender to population registry controls. Both repetitive movement of the hands (OR 2.9 for men, OR 2.2 for women) and forceful grip (OR 2.7 for men, OR 2.3 for women) were significant risk factors, even after controlling for BMI. These authors estimated that the proportion of the CTS population (<65 years of age) in which CTS was attributable to work was 33% for men and 15% for women.

Genetic factors in CTS have not been well studied. One recent study among female twin pairs suggested that up to one-half of the disability of CTS in women may be genetically determined (Hakim et al. 2002). The case definition for CTS in this study was weak, however, since only a pain diagram, but no electrodiagnostic studies, was used to define cases.

In terms of both the number of cases and days of work lost among workers, CTS and hearing loss account for greater morbidity than any other illness (Leigh and Miller 1998). Prognosis in CTS is likely mostly dependent on whether appropriate treatment, such as surgery to decompress the tight canal, is done early (Cseuz et al. 1966; Hybbinette and Mannerfelt 1975; Gelberman et al. 1980; Kaplan et al. 1990; Kruger et al. 1991; Adams et al. 1994) and whether the case is related to workers' compensation. In a 10-year follow-up study of cases in the general population, 22% of persons who did not receive surgery had symptoms for at least 8 years (DeStefano et al. 1997). Persons not receiving surgery or undergoing surgery 3 or more years following CTS diagnosis were less likely to have resolution of symptoms. Katz et al. (1998) developed predictive models of long-term work disability due to CTS: worse functional status at baseline and a contested workers' compensation claim were the strongest predictors of work absence.

Directions for Future Research of Carpal Tunnel Syndrome

While a large number of descriptive and analytic studies on CTS have been conducted, the vast majority were based in working populations. There are few data on CTS incidence or prevalence in persons older than 60 years, among ethnic minorities, or from developing countries. The increased risk among females may be greater in the aged than in working populations.

Precise estimates of the relative contribution of work versus non-work factors to CTS causation in the general population have not been well studied. Large prospective studies of at-risk populations are necessary to more clearly determine a more comprehensive risk model. In addition, familial and genetic studies may help to determine whether gene–environment interactions play a role in CTS.

Primary, secondary, and tertiary intervention trials should be conducted to reduce the incidence and disability burden of CTS. Randomized trials of work modification (Tittiranonda et al. 1999) and clinical interventions (Cook et al. 1995) are warranted. In injured worker populations with CTS, comprehensive risk reduction models should be developed and tested, with a focus on modifiable factors such as reduced exposure, improved health-care delivery, and reorganization of work.

Guillain-Barré Syndrome

Disease Description

Guillain-Barré syndrome (GBS), previously termed *acute inflammatory polyradiculoneuritis,* is the most common cause of acute neuromuscular paralysis in children and adults (Arnason and Soliven 1993). The most common form, a demyelinating neuropathy, affects 85% of persons with GBS. The presentation is typically with a progressive motor deficit, with minimal sensory findings, over days to weeks. Distinctive clinical and laboratory (spinal fluid, electrodiagnostic) findings contribute to a consensus case definition (Asbury et al. 1978). More recently, variants of GBS have been more clearly described and comprise 10%–15% of cases (Emilia-Romagna Study Group on Clinical and Epidemiological Problems in Neurology 1998; Hahn 1998). The various subtypes exhibit distinctive neuropathologic changes in the pe-

ripheral nervous system (Griffin et al. 1995).

Descriptive Studies of Guillain-Barré Syndrome

With a clear case definition (Asbury et al. 1978) and generally easy access to hospital-based records for an acute disorder that usually requires hospitalization, numerous incidence studies have been published worldwide (Alter 1990; Franklin 1994). Table 11–5 summarizes the reported incidence rates in more recent studies. Both crude and age- and gender-adjusted incidence rates are quite narrow worldwide, generally ranging between 1 and 2 per 100,000, with a slight male preponderance. Most studies demonstrate increasing incidence rates with age, or a bimodal age distribution, with peaks in the 20- to 30-year and greater than 50-year age groups. There is little evidence of a temporal change in rates over time.

The use of hospital discharge data is the predominant case-finding method used in incidence studies of GBS. Studies that supplement these methods with medical record validation report a false-positive rate of 20%–25% (McLean et al. 1994). Studies based on voluntary surveillance have estimated underreporting by as much as 25% (Rees et al. 1998). Some recent studies, particularly in children, are primarily surveillance efforts aimed at identifying polio; as polio has declined, GBS has become the predominant cause of acute flaccid paralysis (Olive et al. 1997). Prevalence ratios for GBS have not been reported, primarily because most of cases recover fully.

Analytic Studies of Guillain-Barré Syndrome

The likeliest etiology of most cases of GBS is antecedent viral or bacterial exposures that induce an immunological cross-reaction with peripheral nerve tissue (Hahn 1998). Such molecular mimicry likely occurs because the cellular and humoral immune responses induced by the infecting exposure also react against epitopes on the myelin sheath or axonal membranes.

Table 11-5 Incidence of Guillain-Barré Syndrome Worldwide

Region (reference)	Incident years	Methods	No.	Incidence rate (cases per 100,000 persons per year)	Comments
Southwest Stockholm, Sweden (Jiang et al. 1995)	1973–1991	Hospital discharge records and ambulatory medical record review	103	(1.5–1.9)	Bimodal age distribution (peaks at 20–30 years, 50–70 years) M/F ratio = 1.1:1
Cantabria, northern Spain (Sedano et al. 1994)	1975–1988	One regional hospital	69	0.95	57% with antecedent "events," no seasonal pattern M/F ratio = 1:1
Sweden (Jiang et al. 1997)	1978–1993	Population-based hospital discharge data	2257	1.77	Increased incidence with age and bimodal distribution (peaks at 20–24 years, 70–74 years) M/F ratio = 1:1
Finland (Kinnunen et al. 1998)	1981–1986	Hospital discharge registry	247	0.82	
Ferrara, northern Italy (Paolina et al. 1991)	1981–1987	Intensive hospital and clinic-based case finding, medical record review	16	1.3 (0.7–2.0)	38% with antecedent infection, no seasonal pattern M/F ratio = 1.7:1
Ontario and Quebec, Canada (McLean et al. 1994)	1983–1989	Records linkage of all hospitals, sample record review	2333	1.5 Ontario 1.8 Quebec	Adjustment for false-positive rates, no seasonal pattern, peak incidence over age 60
United States (Prevots and Sutter 1997)	1985–1991	National hospital discharge database, national death certificate data	10,453	3.0	Increased incidence with 3770 GBS-related deaths
Latin America, 7 countries (Olive et al. 1997)	1989–1991	Acute flaccid paralysis registry	1527	0.9 among children (<15 years old)	
Paraguay (Hart et al. 1994)	1990–1991	National surveillance program for polio	37	1.1 among children (<15 years old)	Only 57% hospitalized, 78% with onset January–April
The Netherlands (Oostvogel et al. 1998)	1992–1994	Dutch Pediatric surveillance system for acute flaccid paralysis	52	0.7 among children (<15 years old)	Modest seasonal peak in younger age groups
Southeast England (Rees et al. 1998)	1993–1994	British Neurological Surveillance Unit, voluntary reporting, multiple sources	79	1.5	Adjusted for undetected cases by capture-recapture technique
Lombardy, Italy (Beghi et al. 1996)	1994–1995	Hospital-based registry	109	0.9	

The case–control design is the most appropriate method for exploring risk associations between antecedent infections and a relatively rare disorder such as GBS. A multicenter case–control study of GBS in Italy (Guillain-Barré Syndrome Study Group 2000) reported a positive association between GBS and having had an antecedent flu-like syndrome (OR 7.1, 95% CI 3.3–15.5) or gastroenteritis (OR 3.6, 95% CI 1.3–9.7). The most common antecedent event appears to be enteric infection with *Campylobacter jejuni*, a common bacterial cause of diarrheal illness worldwide. In a prospective case–control study of GBS and variants, Rees et al. (1995a) identified 26% of cases with bacteriologic and serologic evidence of recent *Campylobacter* infection. In comparison, only 2% of household controls and 1% of age-matched hospital controls had evidence of such antecedent exposure. In addition, the majority (70%) of GBS patients with laboratory-supported antecedent *Campylobacter* infection had reported diarrheal illness in the 12 weeks preceding onset of GBS. In another large case–control study using serologic determination of antecedent infection, Jacobs et al. (1998) reported that 32% of 154 GBS patients had antecedent *Campylobacter* compared to 12% of 154 age- and gender-matched neurological disease controls (OR 3.1, 95% CI 1.7–5.9) and 8% of 50 healthy subjects (OR 5.4, 95% CI 1.9–15.1). The estimated attributable risk related to *Campylobacter* was 0.22 (i.e., 22% of GBS cases in the population were attributable to infection with *C. jejuni*). Other antecedent infections significant in multivariate models (with their attributable risks) were cytomegalovirus (0.12), Epstein-Barr virus (0.09), and *Mycoplasma pneumoniae* (0.04). Earlier studies had also reported increased risk related to both cytomegalovirus (Kaplan et al. 1983) and Epstein-Barr virus (Horwitz et al. 1983). McCarthy and Giesecke (2001) conducted a retrospective cohort study of 29,563 cases of *C. jejuni* infection in the Swedish national laboratory reporting system and

found 9 cases of GBS in the cohort—a rate of 30.4 per 100,000 (95% CI 13.9–57.8). The expected incidence of GBS in a 2-month period in the general population was 0.3 per 100,000 population, indicating that the risk of developing GBS within a 2-month period following a *C. jejuni* infection was approximately 100 times higher than the rate of GBS in the general population. This study was based on diagnosed cases of *C. jejuni* infection and it is not known whether asymptomatic infection with *C. jejuni* is followed by a similarly enhanced risk of developing GBS.

The demonstration of molecular mimicry as the link between antecedent infection and GBS has been extensively investigated only for *C. jejuni*. Oomes et al. (1995) showed that specific *Campylobacter* serotype isolates could inhibit antibody (anti GM1-IgG) for epitopes of peripheral nerve. Prendergast et al. (1998) demonstrated that the structural oligosaccharide core of *Campylobacter* serotype 0:41 was structurally similar to GM1 ganglioside. Nachamkin et al. (1999) reported that 26% of a population-based sample of *Campylobacter* enteritis isolates contained the GM1-like epitopes and concluded that host factors must also play a role in determining whether GBS develops in persons exposed to the common potentially offending strains. Rees et al. (1995b) showed that one such host factor, a specific HLA-class II allele (HLA DBQ1*03), was significantly more frequent in persons with *Campylobacter*-positive GBS (25/30, 83%) than in those with *Campylobacter*-negative GBS (33/67, 49%, $p = 0.05$). This association was not confirmed, however, in a study of Japanese GBS patients (Ma et al. 1998).

Endemics of GBS have also been reported, the most striking of which occurred in late 1976 in the United States following a nationwide vaccination program for A1 New Jersey swine influenza. Schoenberger et al. (1979) reported an increased risk of GBS (OR 7.6) within a 6-week window of receipt of vaccination. The excess was estimated to be one additional GBS case per

100,000 vaccines during October 1976 to January 1977. Later reanalysis of a subset of the original data with blind validation of cases by medical chart review confirmed the original estimate of risk (Safranek et al. 1991). Subsequent investigations have revealed no increased risk of GBS related to other influenza vaccination programs (Hurwitz et al. 1981; Kaplan et al. 1982; Roscelli et al. 1991; Lasky et al. 1998).

An association of GBS with diphtheria, tetanus toxoid, and oral poliovirus vaccines has been suggested (Stratton et al. 1994) but unconfirmed in more recent investigations (Tuttle et al. 1997; Ismail et al. 1998; Kinnunen et al. 1998). Exposure to various drugs, including gangliosides (used to *treat* peripheral neuropathy in Europe), has also been reported as positively associated with GBS in case–control studies (Stricker et al. 1994; Raschetti et al. 1995). Finally, similar to other immune-mediated disorders such as multiple sclerosis, GBS risk decreases during pregnancy but is significantly elevated during the immediate post-partum period (Jiang et al. 1996; Cheng et al. 1998).

Prognosis in GBS is generally excellent despite substantial weakness often requiring intensive care, including ventilatory assistance. While most patients recover fully, 3% die (Loffel et al. 1977) and up to 20% have significant impairment (Smith and Hughes 1992; Sedano et al. 1994). Deaths in the United States estimated from a national surveillance program average 628 per year (Prevots and Sutter 1997). Worse outcome has been associated with older age (Rees et al. 1998) and prognosis is better in children (Olive et al. 1997). Recovery does not appear to differ by GBS subtype (Ho et al. 1997).

Directions for Future Research of Guillain-Barré Syndrome

The increasing availability of hospital discharge data in electronic form should allow population-based surveillance of GBS at little cost in future studies. Such surveillance would allow recognition and action in the event of a large increase in incidence in GBS like that which occurred in the United States in 1976 with the swine flu vaccine. Substantial morbidity and mortality could have been avoided had the pandemic been recognized earlier. Similar surveillance methods have been used in conjunction with surveillance for polio in developing countries.

Hospital-based registries would allow more detailed access to records and the self-report and laboratory collection of willing patients. Careful matching of such patients to both other hospital neurological cases and to normal controls are important in designing case–control studies. In addition, the assessment of comorbid conditions in the neurological disease groups is critical.

Future investigations should pursue the exciting development of the putative etiologic role of *Campylobacter jejuni* infection and the molecular mimicry hypothesis of disease causation, as well as similar evidence of mimicry for other putative antecedent infections (e.g., cytomegalovirus, Epstein-Barr virus). Studies designed to further explore gene–*Campylobacter* interactions and the impact of other host factors on the development of GBS in persons exposed to *Campylobacter* serotypes that commonly cross-react with nerve epitopes are warranted. The development of animal models may enhance the study of molecular mimicry in the development of forms of GBS, as demonstrated by a recent study that sensitized rabbits with GM1 ganglioside and produced an axonal neuropathy similar to axonal GBS with acute onset of flaccid limb weakness, a monophasic course, and predominant Wallerian-like degeneration of the peripheral nerves (Yuki et al. 2001). Finally, the question of risk related to pharmacologic use of gangliosides should be further investigated given the widespread use of these agents in Europe.

References

Adams ML, Franklin GM, Barnhart S. Outcome of carpal tunnel surgery in Washington State workers' compensation. *Am J Ind Med* 1994;25:527–536.

Adler AI, Boyko EJ, Ahroni JH, Smith DG. Lower-extremity amputation in diabetes. The independent effects of peripheral vascular disease, sensory neuropathy, and foot ulcers. *Diabetes Care* 1999;22:1029–1035.

Adler AI, Turner RC. The diabetes prevention program. *Diabetes Care* 1999;22:543–545.

Alter M. The epidemiology of Guillain-Barré syndrome. *Ann Neurol* 1990;27(Suppl): S7–S12.

American Academy of Neurology, American Association of Electrodiagnostic Medicine, American Academy of Physical Medicine and Rehabilitation. Practice parameter for electrodiagnostic studies in carpal tunnel syndrome. *Neurology* 1993;43:2404–2405.

American Association of Electrodiagnostic Medicine Quality Assurance Committee. Literature review of the usefulness of nerve conduction studies and electromyography for the evaluation of patients with carpal tunnel syndrome. *Muscle Nerve* 1993;16:1392–1414.

Armstrong TJ, Chaffin DB. Carpal tunnel syndrome and selected personal attributes. *J Occup Med* 1979;21:481–486.

Arnason BGW, Soliven B. Acute inflammatory demyelinating polyradiculoneuropathy. In: Dyck PJ, Thomas PK, Griffin JW, Low PA, Poduslo JF, eds. Peripheral Neuropathy. Philadelphia: WB Saunders, 1993, pp 1437–1497.

Asbury AK, Arnason BGW, Karp HR, McFarlin DE. Criteria for diagnosis of Guillain-Barré syndrome. *Ann Neurol* 1978;3:565–566.

Atroshi I, Gummesson L, Johnsson R, et al. Prevalence of carpal tunnel syndrome in a general population. *JAMA* 1999;282:153–158.

Barzilay J, Warram JH, Rand LI, et al. Risk for cardiovascular autonomic neuropathy is association with the HLA-DR 3/4 phenotype in type I diabetes mellitus. *Ann Intern Med* 1992;116:544–549.

Beghi E, Bogliun G. The Guillan-Barré syndrome (GBS). Implementation of a register of the disease on a nationwide basis. Italian GBS Study Group. *Ital J Neurol Sci* 1996; 17:355–361.

Beghi E, Kurland LT, Mulder DW, Nicolosi A. Brachial plexus neuropathy in the population of Rochester, Minnesota, 1970–1981. *Ann Neurol* 1985;38:134–138.

Bild DE, Selby JV, Sinnock P, et al. Lower extremity amputation in people with diabetes. Epidemiology and prevention. *Diabetes Care* 1989;12:24–31.

Bjorkqvist SE, Lang AH, Punnonen R, Rauramo L. Carpal tunnel syndrome in ovariectomized women. *Acta Obstet Gynecol Scand* 1977; 56:127–130.

Blanc PD, Faucett J, Kennedy JJ, et al. Self-reported carpal tunnel syndrome: predictors of work disability from the National Health Interview Survey Occupational Health Supplement. *Am J Ind Med* 1996;30:362–368.

Bleecker ML. Medical surveillance for carpal tunnel syndrome in workers. *J Hand Surg* 1987;12:845–848.

Bourne RR, Dolin PJ, Mtanda AT, Plant GT, Mohamed AA. Epidemic optic neuropathy in primary school children in Dar es Salaam, Tanzania. *Br J Opthalmol* 1998;82:232–234.

Boyko EJ, Ahroni JH, Stensel V, et al. A prospective study of risk factors for diabetic foot ulcer. The Seattle Diabetic Foot Study. *Diabetes Care* 1999;22:1036–1042.

Brewster WJ, Fernyhough P, Diemel LT, et al. Diabetic neuropathy, nerve growth factor and other neurotrophic factors. *Trends Neurosci* 1994;17:321–325.

Cabezas-Cerrato J. The prevalence of clinical diabetic polyneuropathy in Spain: a study in primary care and hospital clinic groups. Neuropathy Spanish Study Group of the Spanish Diabetes Society (SDS). *Diabetologia* 1998;41:1263–1269.

Cannon L, Bernacki EJ, Walter SD. Personal and occupational factors associated with carpal tunnel syndrome. *J Occup Med* 1981;23: 255–258.

Carter JS, Pugh JA, Monterrosa A. Non-insulin dependent diabetes mellitus in minorities in the United States. *Ann Intern Med* 1996; 125:221–232.

Cheng Q, Jiang GX, Fredrikson S, et al. Increased incidence of Guillain-Barré syndrome postpartum. *Epidemiology* 1998;9: 601–604.

Cook AC, Szabo RM, Birkhole SW, King EF. Early mobilization following carpal tunnel release. A prospective randomized study. *J Hand Surg* 1995;20:228–230.

Cruz Gutierrez-del-Olmo M, Schoenberg BS, Portera-Sanchez A. Prevalence of neurological diseases in Madrid, Spain. *Neuroepidemiology* 1989;8:43–47.

Cseuz KA, Thomas JE, Lambert EH, et al. Long-term results of operation for carpal tunnel syndrome. *Mayo Clin Proc* 1966;41:232–241.

Cuba Neuropathy Field Investigation Team. Epidemic optic neuropathy in Cuba—clinical characterization and risk factors. *N Engl J Med* 1995;333:1176–1182.

Cummings K, Maizlish N, Rudolph L, et al. Occupational disease surveillance: carpal tunnel syndrome. *MMWR Morb Mortal Wkly Rep* 1989;38:485–489.

Cumulative Trauma Disorders in the Workplace Bibliography. Department of Health and Human Services (Publication No. 95-119). Cincinnati, OH: National Institute for Occupational Safety and Health 1995.

DCCT Research Group. The effect of intensive treatment of diabetes on the development and progression of long-term complications in insulin-dependent diabetes mellitus. *N Engl J Med* 1993;329:977–986.

de Krom MC, Kester AD, Knipschild PG, Spaans F. Risk factors for carpal tunnel syndrome. *Am J Epidemiol* 1990;132:1102–1110.

de Krom MC, Knipschild PG, Kester AD, et al. Carpal tunnel syndrome: prevalence in the general population. *J Clin Epidemiol* 1992; 45:373–376.

DeStefano F, Nordstrom DL, Vierbant RA. Long-term symptom outcomes of carpal tunnel syndrome and its treatment. *J Hand Surg* 1997;22:200–210.

Dyck PJ. The causes, classification, and treatment of peripheral neuropathy. *N Engl J Med* 1982;307:283–286.

Dyck PJ. New understanding and treatment of diabetic neuropathy. *N Engl J Med* 1992; 326:1287–1288.

Dyck PJ, Kratz KM, Lehman KA, et al. The Rochester Diabetic Neuropathy Study: design criteria for types of neuropathy, selection bias, and reproducibility of neuropathic tests. *Neurology* 1991;41:799–807.

Dyck PJ, Thomas PK, Lambert EH, Bunge R, eds. Peripheral Neuropathy, 3rd edition. Philadelphia: WB Saunders, 1993.

Ekman-Ordeberg G, Salgeback S, Ordeberg G. Carpal tunnel syndrome in pregnancy. A prospective study. *Acta Obstet Gynecol Scand* 1987;66:233–235.

Emilia-Romagna Study Group on Clinical and Epidemiological Problems in Neurology. Guillain-Barré syndrome variants in Emilia-Romagna, Italy, 1992–3: incidence, clinical features, and prognosis. *J Neurol Neurosurg Psychiatry* 1998;65:218–224.

Ewing DJ, Borsey DQ, Bellavere F, Clarke BF. Cardiac autonomic neuropathy in diabetes: comparison of measures of R-R interval variation. *Diabetologia* 1981;21:18–24.

Ewing DJ, Campbell IW, Clarke BF. The natural history of diabetic autonomic neuropathy. *Q J Med* 1980;49:95–108.

Feldman EL, Stevens MD, Thomas PK, et al. A practical two-step quantitative clinical and electrophysiological assessment for the diagnosis and staging of diabetic neuropathy. *Diabetes Care* 1994;17:1281–1289.

Ferry S, Hannaford P, Warskyj M, et al. Carpal tunnel syndrome: a nested case–control study of risk factors in women. *Am J Epidemiol* 2000;151:566–574.

Ferry S, Pritchard T, Kennana J, Croft P, Silman AJ. Estimating the prevalence of delayed median nerve conduction in the general population. *Br J Rheumatol* 1998;37:630–635.

Forrest KY, Maser RE, Pombianco G, et al. Hypertension as a risk factor for diabetic neuropathy: a prospective study. *Diabetes* 1997;46:665–670.

Franklin GM. Peripheral neuropathy. In: Gorelick P, Alter M, eds. Handbook of Neuroepidemiology. New York: Marcel Dekker, 1994, pp 381–403.

Franklin GM, Haug JA, Heyer N, et al. Occupational carpal tunnel syndrome in Washington State, 1984–1988. *Am J Public Health* 1991;81:741–746.

Franklin GM, Kahn L, Baxter J, et al. Sensory neuropathy in non–insulin-dependent diabetes mellitus. The San Luis Valley Diabetes Study. *Am J Epidemiol* 1990;131:633–643.

Franklin GM, Shetterly SM, Cohen JA, et al. Risk factors for distal symmetric neuropathy in NIDDM. The San Luis Valley Diabetes Study. *Diabetes Care* 1994;17:1172–1177.

French Cooperative Group on Plasma Exchange in Guillain-Barré syndrome. Efficiency of plasma exchange in Guillain-Barré syndrome: role of replacement fluids. *Ann Neurol* 1987;22:753–761.

Fry IK, Harwick C, Scott GW. Diabetic neuropathy: a survey and follow-up of 66 cases. *Guy's Hosp Rep* 1962;3:113–129.

Gelberman RH, Aronson D, Weisman MH. Carpal tunnel syndrome: results of a prospective trial of steroid injection and splinting. *J Bone Joint Surg* 1980;62A:1181–1184.

Gelberman RH, Rydevik BL, Pess GM, et al. Carpal tunnel syndrome: a scientific basis for clinical care. *Orthop Clin North Am* 1988; 19:115–124.

Giersiepen K, Eberle A, Pohlabeln H. Gender differences in carpal tunnel syndrome? Occupational and non-occupational risk factors in a population-based case–control study. *Ann Epidemiol* 2000;10:481.

Griffin JW, Li CY, Ho TW, et al. Guillain-Barré syndrome in northern China. The spectrum of neuropathological changes in clinically defined cases. *Brain* 1995;118:577–595.

Guillain-Barré Syndrome Study Group. Guillain-Barre syndrome: an Italian multicenter case–control study. *Neurol Sci* 2000;21: 229–234.

Haerer AF, Conwell DE, Subramony SH. Epidemiology of peripheral neuropathies. In: Anderson DW, Schoenberg DG, eds. Neuroepidemiology: A Tribute to Bruce Schoenberg. Boston: CRC Press, 1991, pp 146–166.

Hagberg M, Morgenstern H, Kelsh M. Impact of occupations and job tasks on the prevalence of carpal tunnel syndrome. *Scand J Work Environ Health* 1992;18:337–345.

Hahn AF. Guillan-Barré syndrome. *Lancet* 1998;352:635–641.

Hakim AJ, Cherkas L, El Zayet S, et al. The genetic contribution to carpal tunnel syndrome in women: a twin study. *Arthritis Rheum* 2002;47:275–279.

Harris M, Eastman R, Corvic C. Symptoms of sensory neuropathy in adults with NIDDM in the U.S. population. *Diabetes Care* 1993; 16:1446–1452.

Hart DE, Rojas LA, Rosario JA, et al. Childhood Guillain-Barré syndrome in Paraguay, 1990 to 1991. *Ann Neurol* 1994;36:859–863.

Hauser WA, Karnes WE, Arnnis J, Kurland LT. Incidence and prognosis of Bell's palsy in the population of Rochester, Minnesota. *Mayo Clin Proc* 1971;46:258–264.

Heesom AE, Millward A, Demaine AG. Susceptibility to diabetic neuropathy in patients with insulin dependent diabetes mellitus is associated with a polymorphism at the 5' end of the aldose reductose gene. *J Neurol Neurosurg Psychiatry* 1998;64:213–216.

Ho TW, Li CY, Cornblath DR, et al. Patterns of recovery in the Guillain-Barré syndromes. *Neurology* 1997;48:695–700.

Holmberg BH. Charcot-Marie-Tooth disease in northern Sweden: an epidemiological and clinical study. *Acta Neurol Scand* 1993;87:416–422.

Horwitz CA, Henle W, Henle G, et al. Infectious mononucelosis in patients aged 40 to 72 years: report of 27 cases, including 3 without heterophile-antibody responses. *Medicine* 1983;62:256–262.

Hurwitz ES, Schonberger LB, Nelson DB, Holman RC. Guillain-Barré syndrome and the 1978–1979 influenza vaccine. *N Engl J Med* 1981;304:1557–1561.

Hybbinette CH, Mannerfelt L. The carpal tunnel syndrome. A retrospective study of 400 operated patients. *Acta Orthop Scand* 1975;46:610–620.

Ismail EA, Shabani IS, Badawi M, et al. An epidemiologic, clinical, and therapeutic study of childhood Guillian-Barré syndrome in Kuwait: is it related to the oral polio vaccine? *J Child Neurol* 1998;13:488–492.

Italian Longitudinal Study Group. Prevalence of chronic diseases in older Italians: comparing self-reported and clinical diagnoses. The Italian Longitudinal Study on Aging Working Group. *Int J Epidemiol* 1997;26:995–1002.

Jacobs BC, Rothbarth PH, van der Meche FG, et al. The spectrum of antecedent infections in Guillain-Barré syndrome: a case–control study. *Neurology* 1998;51:1110–1115.

Jiang GX, Cheng Q, Link H, dePedro-Cuesta J. Epidemiological features of Guillain-Barré syndrome in Sweden, 1978–93. *J Neurol Neurosurg Psychiatry* 1997;62:447–453.

Jiang GX, dePedro-Cuesta J, Fredrikson S. Guillan-Barré syndrome in south-west Stockholm, 1973–1991. 1. Quality of registered hospital diagnoses and incidence. *Acta Neurol Scand* 1995;91:109–117.

Jiang GX, dePedro-Cuesta J, Strigard K, et al. Pregnancy and Guillian-Barré syndrome: a nationwide register cohort study. *Neuroepidemiology* 1996;15:192–200.

Johnson LN, Arnold AC. Incidence of nonarteritic and arteritic anterior ischemic optic neuropathy. Population-based study in the state of Missouri and Los Angeles County, California. *J Neurophthalmol* 1994;14:38–44.

Kaplan JE, Greenspan JR, Bomgaars M, et al. Simultaneous outbreaks of Guillain-Barré syndrome and Bell's palsy in Hawaii in 1981. *JAMA* 1983;250:2635–2640.

Kaplan JE, Katona P, Hurwitz ES, Schonberger LB. Guillain-Barré syndrome in the United States, 1979–1980 and 1980–1981. Lack of an association with influenza vaccination. *JAMA* 1982;248:698–700.

Kaplan SJ, Glickel SZ, Eaton RG. Predictive factors in the non-surgical treatment of carpal tunnel syndrome. *J Hand Surg (Br)* 1990;15:106–108.

Katz JN, Larson MG, Fossel AH, Liang MH. Validation of a surveillance case definition of carpal tunnel syndrome. *Am J Public Health* 1991;81:189–193.

Katz JN, Lew RA, Bessette L, et al. Prevalence and predictors of long-term work disability due to carpal tunnel syndrome. *Am J Ind Med* 1998;33:543–550.

Katz JN, Stirrat CR, Larson MG, et al. A self-administered hand symptom diagram for the diagnosis and epidemiologic study of carpal tunnel syndrome. *J Rheumatol* 1990;17:1495–1498.

Kessler M, Netter B, Azoulay E, et al. Dialysis associated arthropathy: a multicentre survey of 171 patients receiving hemodialysis for over 10 years. The Cooperative Group on Dialysis-associated Arthropathy. *Br J Rheumatol* 1992;31:157–162.

Kinnunen F, Junttila O, Haukka J, Hovi T. Nationwide oral poliovirus vaccination campaign and the incidence of Guillain-Barré syndrome. *Am J Epidemiol* 1998;147:69–73.

Kruger VL, Kraft GH, Deitz JC, et al. Carpal tunnel syndrome: objective measures and splint use. *Arch Phys Med Rehabil* 1991;72: 517–520.

Lasky T, Terracciano GJ, Magder L, et al. The Guillain-Barré syndrome and the 1992–1993 and 1993–1994 influenza vaccines. *N Engl J Med* 1998;339:1797–1802.

Latko WA, Armstrong TJ, Franzblau A, et al. Cross-sectional study of the relationship between repetitive work and the prevalence of upper limb musculoskeletal disorders. *Am J Ind Med* 1999;36:248–259.

Leigh JP, Miller TR. Occupational illnesses within two national data sets. *Int J Occup Environ Health* 1998;4:99–113.

Loffel NB, Rossi LN, Mumentaler, Lutsch GJ, Ludin HP. The Landry-Guillain-Barré syndrome: complications, prognosis and natural history in 123 cases. *J Neurol Sci* 1977; 33:71–79.

Ma JJ, Nishimura M, Mine H, et al. HLA and T-cell receptor gene polymorphisms in Guillain-Barré syndrome. *Neurology* 1998;51: 379–384.

Mackay JD, Page MM, Cambridge J, Watkins PJ. Diabetic autonomic neuropathy: the diagnostic value of heart rate monitoring. *Diabetologia* 1980;18:471–478.

Martyn CN, Hughes RAC. Epidemiology of peripheral neuropathy. *J Neurol Neurosurg Psychiatry* 1997;62:310–312.

Maser RE, Steenkiste AR, Dorman JS, et al. Epidemiological correlates of diabetic neuropathy: report from Pittsburgh Epidemiology of Diabetes Complications Study. *Diabetes* 1989;38:1456–1461.

McCabe CJ, Stevenson RC, Dolan AM. Evaluation of a diabetic foot screening and protection programme. *Diabet Med* 1998;15: 80–84.

McCarthy N, Giesecke J. Incidence of Guillain-Barré syndrome following infection with *Campylobacter jejuni*. *Am J Epidemiol* 2001; 153:610–614.

McLean M, Duclos P, Jacob P, Humphreys P. Incidence of Guillain-Barré syndrome in Ontario and Quebec, 1983–1989, using hospital service databases. *Epidemiology* 1994;5: 443–448.

McLennan HG, Oats JN, Walstab JE. Survey of hand symptoms in pregnancy. *Med J Aust* 1987;147:542–544.

Melton LJ, Dyck PJ. Epidemiology. In: Dyck PJ, Thomas PK, Asbury AK, Winegard AI, Porte D, eds. Diabetic Neuropathy. Philadelphia: WB Saunders, 1987, pp 27–35.

Misra A, Mittal V, Jain S, Bajaj JS. Correlation of acetylator phenotype with peripheral, autonomic and central neuropathy in Northern Indian non–insulin-dependent diabetes mellitus patients. *Eur J Clin Pharmacol* 1999;55: 419–424.

Mitchell BD, Hawthorne VM, Vinik AI. Cigarette smoking and neuropathy in diabetic mellitus. *Diabetes Care* 1990;13:434–437.

Morgan JP. The Jamaica ginger paralysis. *JAMA* 1982;242:1864–1867.

Moss SE, Klein R, Klein BE. Cause-specific mortality in a population-based study of diabetes. *Am J Public Health* 1991;81:1158–1162.

Munoz M, Boutros-Toni F, Preux PM, et al. Prevalence of neurological disorders in Haute-Vienne department (Limousin region–France). *Neuroepidemiology* 1995;14:193–198.

Nachamkin I, Ung H, Moran AP, et al. Ganglioside GM1 mimicry in *Campylobacter* strains from sporadic infections in the United States. *J Infect Dis* 1999;179:1183–1189.

Nathan DM, Singer DE, Godine JE, Perlmuter LC. Non–insulin dependent diabetes in older patients. *Am J Med* 1986;81:837–842.

Nathan PA, Kenison RC, Lockwood RS, Meadows KD. Tobacco, caffeine, alcohol, and carpal tunnel syndrome in American industry. A cross-sectional study of 1464 workers. *J Occup Environ Med* 1996;38:280–298.

Nathan PA, Takigawa K, Keniston RC, et al. Slowing of sensory conduction of the median nerve and carpal tunnel syndrome in Japanese and American industrial workers. *J Hand Surg* 1994;19:30–34.

Neil HA, Thompson AV, John S, et al. Diabetic autonomic neuropathy: the prevalence of impaired heart rate variability in a geographically defined population. *Diabet Med* 1989; 6:20–24.

Neuropathy Association. A Guide to the Peripheral Neuropathies. New York: The Neuropathy Association, 1999, pp 1–24 (www.neuropathy.org).

Nordstrom DL, DeStefano F, Vierkant RA, Layde PM. Incidence of diagnosed carpal tunnel syndrome in a general population. *Epidemiology* 1998;9:342–345.

Nordstrom DL, Vierkant RA, DeStefano F, Layde PM. Risk factors for carpal tunnel syndrome in a general population. *Occup Environ Med* 1997;54:734–740.

O'Brien IA, McFadden JP, Corrall RJ. The influence of autonomic neuropathy on mortality in insulin-dependent diabetes. *Q J Med* 1991;79:495–502.

Olive JM, Castillo C, Castro RG, deQuadros CA. Epidemiologic study of Guillain-Barré syndrome in children <15 years of age in Latin America. *J Infect Dis* 1997;175(Suppl): S110–S164.

Oomes PG, Jacobs BC, Hazenberg MP, et al. Anti-GM1 IgG antibodies and *Campylobacter* bacteria in Guillain-Barré syndrome: evidence of molecular mimcry. *Ann Neurol* 1995;38:170–175.

Oostvogel PM, Spaendonck MA, Hirasing RA, van Loon AM. Surveillance of acute flaccid paralysis in The Netherlands, 1992–94. *Bull World Health Organ* 1998;76:55–62.

Osuntokun BO, Adeuja AO, Schoenberg BS, et al. Neurological disorders in Nigerian Africans: a community-based study. *Acta Neurol Scand* 1987;75:13–21.

Ozaki I, Baba M, Matsunaga M, Takebe K. Deleterious effect of the carpal tunnel on nerve conduction in diabetic polyneuropathy. *Electromyogr Clin Neurophysiol* 1988;28:301–306.

Page MM, Watkins PJ. Cardiorespiratory arrest and diabetic autonomic neuropathy. *Lancet* 1978;1:14–16.

Palumbo PJ, Elvehack LR, Whisnant JP. Neurologic complications of diabetes mellitus: transient ischemic attack, stroke and peripheral neuropathy. In: Schoenberg BS. Neurological Epidemiology: Principals and Clinical Applications. New York: Raven Press, 1978, pp 593–601.

Paolino E, Govoni V, Tola MR, et al. Incidence of the Guillain-Barré syndrome in Ferrara, northern Italy, 1981–1987. *Neuroepidemiology* 1991;10:105–111.

Parry O, Mielke J, Latif AS, et al. Peripheral neuropathy in individuals with HIV infection in Zimbabwe. *Acta Neurol Scand* 1997;96:218–222.

Partanen J, Niskanen L, Lehtinen J, et al. Natural history of peripheral neuropathy in patients with non–insulin-dependent diabetes mellitus. *N Engl J Med* 1995;333:89–94.

Pascual E, Giner V, Arostegui A, et al. Higher incidence of carpal tunnel syndrome in oophorectomized women. *Br J Rheumatol* 1991;30:60–62.

Pierre-Jerome C, Bekkelund SI, Mellgren SI, Nordstrom R. Quantitative MRI and electrophysiology of preoperative carpal tunnel syndrome in a female population. *Ergonomics* 1997;40:642–649.

Pirart J. Diabetes mellitus and its degenerative complications: a prospective study of 4,400 patients observed between 1947 and 1973. *Diabetes Care* 1978;1:168–188.

Prendergast MM, Lastovica AJ, Moran AP. Lipopolysaccharides from *Campylobacter jejuni* 0:41 strains association with Guillain-Barré syndrome exhibit mimicry of GM1 ganglioside. *Infect Immunol* 1998;66:3649–3655.

Prevots DR, Sutter RW. Assessment of Guillain-Barré syndrome mortality and morbidity in the United States: implications for acute flaccid paralysis surveilance. *J Infect Dis* 1997; 175(Suppl):S151–S155.

Proceedings of a Consensus Development Conference on standardized measures in diabetic neuropathy. *Neurology* 1992;42:1823–1839.

Radhakrishnan K, Litchy WJ, O'Fallon WM, Kurland LT. Epidemiology of cervical radiculopathy: a population-based study from Rochester, Minnesota. *Brain* 1994; 117:325–335.

Rajput AH, Uitti RJ, Rajput AH. Neurological disorders and services in Saskatchewan—a report based on provincial health care records. *Neuroepidemiology* 1988;7:145–151.

Raschetti R, Maggini M, Popoli P, et al. Gangliosides and Gullain-Barré syndrome. *J Clin Epidemiol* 1995;48:1399–1405.

Rees JH, Soudain SE, Gregson NA, Hughes RA. *Campylobacter jejuni* infection and Guillain-Barré syndrome. *N Engl J Med* 1995a;333: 1374–1379.

Rees JH, Thompson RD, Smeeton NC, Hughes RA. Epidemiological study of Guillan-Barré syndrome in southeast England. *J Neurol Neurosurg Psychiatry* 1998;64:74–77.

Rees JH, Vaughan RW, Kondeatis E, Hughes RAC. HLA-class II alleles in Guillain-Barré syndrome and Miller Fisher syndrome and their association with preceding *Campylobacter jejuni* infection. *J Neuroimmunol* 1995b;62:53–57.

Rempel D, Evanoff B, Amadio PC, et al. Consensus criteria for the classification of carpal tunnel syndrome in epidemiologic studies. *Am J Public Health* 1998;88:1447–1451.

Robinson LR, Stolov WC, Rubner DE, et al. Height is an independent risk factor for neuropathy in diabetic men. *Diabetes Res Clin Pract* 1992;16:97–102.

Roquelaure Y, Mechali S, Dano C, et al. Occupational and personal risk factors for carpal tunnel syndrome in industrial workers. *Scand J Work Environ Health* 1997;23:364–369.

Roscelli JD, Bass JW, Pang L. Guillain-Barré syndrome and influenza vaccination in the US Army, 1980–1988. *Am J Epidemiol* 1991; 133:952–955.

Rosenbaum RB, Ochoa J. Carpal Tunnel and Other Disorders of the Median Nerve. Boston: Butterworth-Heineman, 1993.

Rossignol M, Stock S, Patry L, Armstrong B. Carpal tunnel syndrome: what is attributable to work? The Montreal Study. *Occup Environ Med* 1997;54:519–523.

Safranek TJ, Lawrence DN, Kurland LT, et al. Reassessment of the association between Guillain-Barré syndrome and receipt of swine influenza vaccine in 1976–1977: results of a two-state study. Expert Neurology Group. *Am J Epidemiol* 1991;133:940–951.

Sands ML, Shetterly SM, Franklin GM, Hamman RF. Incidence of distal symmetric (sensory) neuropathy in NIDDM. The San Luis Valley Diabetes Study. *Diabetes Care* 1997;20:322–329.

Savettieri G, Rocca WA, Salemi G, et al. Prevalence of diabetic neuropathy with somatic symptoms: a door-to-door survey in two Sicilian municipalities. *Neurology* 1993;43:1115–1120.

Schonberger LB, Bregman DJ, Sullivan-Bolyai JZ, et al. Guillain-Barré syndrome following vaccination in the National Influenza Immunization Program. United States, 1976–1977. *Am J Epidemiol* 1979;110:105–123.

Sedano MJ, Calleja J, Canga E, Berciano J. Guillain Barré syndrome in Cantabria, Spain. An epidemiological and clinical study. *Acta Neurol Scand* 1994;89:287–292.

Silverstein B, Welp E, Nelson N, Kalat J. Claims incidence of work-related disorders of the upper extremities: Washington State, 1987 through 1995. *Am J Public Health* 1998;88:1827–1833.

Silverstein BA, Fine LJ, Armstrong TJ. Occupational factors and carpal tunnel syndrome. *Am J Ind Med* 1987;11:343–358.

Silverstein MA, Silverstein BA, Franklin GM. Evidence for work-related musculoskeletal disorders: a scientific counter-argument. *J Occup Environ Med* 1996;38:477–484.

Smith GD, Hughes RA. Plasma exchange treatment and prognosis of Guillain-Barré syndrome. *QJ Med* 1992;85:751–760.

Sosenko JM, Boulton AJ, Gadia MT, et al. The association between symptomatic sensory neuropathy and body stature in diabetic patients. *Diabetes Res Clin Pract* 1988;16:97–102.

Stein PK, Kleiger RE. Insights from the study of heart rate variability. *Annu Rev Med* 1999;50:249–261.

Stevens J, Beard CM, O'Failon WM, Kurland LT. Conditions associated with carpal tunnel syndrome. *Mayo Clin Proc* 1992;67:541–548.

Stevens JC, Sun S, Beard CM, et al. Carpal tunnel syndrome in Rochester, Minnesota, 1961–1980. *Neurology* 1988;38:134–138.

Stewart JD, Aguayo AJ. Peripheral Neuropathy. Philadelphia: WB Saunders, 1984.

Stock SR. Workplace ergonomic factors and the development of musculoskeletal disorders of the neck and upper limbs: a meta-analysis. *Am J Ind Med* 1991;19:87–107.

Stratton KR, Howe CJ, Johnson RB. Adverse events associated with childhood vaccines other than pertussis and rubella. Summary of a report from the Institute of Medicine. *JAMA* 1994;271:1602–1605.

Stricker BH, van der Klauw MM, Ottervanger JP, van der Meche FG. A case–control study of drugs and other determinants as potential causes of Guillain-Barré syndrome. *J Clin Epidemiol* 1994;47:1203–1210.

Sunderland S. The nerve lesion in the carpal tunnel syndrome. *J Neurol Neurosurg Psychiatry* 1976;39:615–626.

Szabo RM, Chidgey LK. Stress carpal tunnel pressures in patients with carpal tunnel syndrome and normal patients. *J Hand Surg* 1989;14A:624–627.

Tanaka S, Wild DK, Cameron LL, Freund E. Association of occupational and non-occupational risk factors with the prevalence of self-reported carpal tunnel syndrome in a national survey of the working population. *Am J Ind Med* 1997;32:550–556.

Tanaka S, Wild DK, Seligman PJ, et al. Prevalence and work-relatedness of self-reported carpal tunnel syndrome among US workers: analysis of the Occupational Health Supplement Data of 1988 National Health Interview Survey. *Am J Ind Med* 1995;27:451–470.

Tekle-Haimanot R, Abebe M, Gebre-Mariam A, et al. Community-based study of neurological disorders in rural central Ethiopia. *Neuroepidemiology* 1990;9:263–277.

Tesfaye S, Stevens LK, Stephenson JM, et al. Prevalence of diabetic peripheral neuropathy and its relation to glycaemic control and potential risk factors: the EURODIAB IDDM Complications Study. *Diabetologia* 1996;39:1377–1384.

Thomas PK, Tomlinson DR. Diabetic and hypoglycemic neuropathy. In: Dyck PJ, Thomas PK, Griffin J, Low PA, Poduslo JF, eds. Peripheral Neuropathy. Philadelphia: WB Saunders, 1993, pp 1219–1250.

Tittiranonda P, Rempel D, Armstrong T, Borastero S. Effect of four computer keyboards in computer users with upper extremity musculoskeletal disorders. *Am J Ind Med* 1999;35:647–661.

Tuttle J, Chen RT, Rautala H, et al. The risk of Guillain-Barré syndrome after tetanus-toxoid–containing vaccines in adults and children in the United States. *Am J Publ Health* 1997;87:2045–2048.

U.K. Prospective Diabetes Study (UKPDS) Group. Intensive blood-glucose control with sulphonylureas or insulin compared with conventional treatment and risk of complications in patients with type 2 diabetes. *Lancet* 1998;352:837–853.

Vague P, Dufayet D, Coste T, et al. Association of diabetic neuropathy with Na/K ATPase gene polymorphism. *Diabetologia* 1997;40: 6–11.

van der Hoop RG, van der Burg ME, ten Bokkel Huinink WW, et al. Incidence of neuropathy in 395 patients with ovarian cancer treated with or without cisplatin. *Cancer* 1990;66: 1697–1702.

Veglio M, Borra M, Stevens LK, et al. The relation between QTc interval prolongation and diabetic complications. The EURODIAB IDDM Complication Study Group. *Diabetologia* 1999;42:68–75.

Veglio M, Sivieri R. Prevalence of neuropathy in IDDM patients in Piemonte, Italy. The Neuropathy Study Group of the Italian Society for the Study of Diabetes, Piemonte Affiliate. *Diabetes Care* 1993;16:456–461.

Vessey MP, Villard-Mackintosh L, Yeates D. Epidemiology of carpal tunnel syndrome in women of childbearing age. Findings in a large cohort study. *Int J Epidemiol* 1990;19: 655–659.

Viikari-Juntura E, Silverstein B. Role of physical load factors in carpal tunnel syndrome. *Scand J Work Environ Health* 1999;25:163–185.

Walters DP, Gatling E, Mullee MA, Hill RD. The prevalence of diabetic distal sensory neuropathy in an English community. *Diabet Med* 1991;9:349–353.

Warner MA, Warner ME, Martin JT. Ulnar neuropathy. Incidence, outcome, and risk factors in sedated or anesthetized patients. *Anesthesiology* 1994;81:1332–1340.

Werner RA, Franzblau A, Albers JW, et al. Use of screening nerve conduction studies for predicting future carpal tunnel syndrome. *Occup Environ Med* 1997;54:96–100.

Wieslander G, Norback D, Gothe C-J, Juhlin L. Carpal tunnel syndrome (CTS) and exposure to vibration, repetitive wrist movements, and heavy manual work: a case–referent study. *Br J Ind Med* 1989;46:43–47.

Winn FJJ, Habes DJ. Carpal tunnel area as a risk factor for carpal tunnel syndrome. *Muscle Nerve* 1990;13:254–258.

World Health Organization (WHO). Diabetes Mellitus, Report of a WHO Study Group. Geneva: World Health Organization, 1985.

Yoshimasu F, Kurland LT, Elveback LR. Tic douloureux in Rochester, Minnesota, 1945–1969. *Neurology* 1972;22:952–956.

Young MJ, MacLeon AF, Williams DR, Sonksen PH. A multicentre study of the prevalence of diabetic peripheral neuropathy in the United Kingdom hospital clinic population. *Diabetologia* 1993;36:150–154.

Yuki NM, Yamada M, Koga K, et al. Animal model of axonal Gullain-Barré syndrome induced by sensitization with a GM1 ganglioside. *Ann Neurol* 2001;49:712–720.

12

Epilepsy

J. FRED ANNEGERS

In this chapter, *seizure* or *seizure disorder* will refer to the broad category of disorders in which excessive neural discharges lead to altered consciousness. Epilepsy is a disorder marked by recurrent, unprovoked seizures. Although some investigators have required more than two seizures to diagnose epilepsy (Beran et al. 1982; Sillanpaa et al. 1995) in most studies two seizures at different times are considered both necessary and sufficient for this diagnosis (Hauser et al. 1998).

Seizures are usually described by either clinical manifestation or etiology. Generalized seizures are those that involve the entire brain, whereas in partial or focal seizures or epilepsy, the abnormal discharge is limited to a part of the brain. A partial seizure can develop into a generalized seizure if it spreads to the entire brain. The latter would be termed a secondary generalized seizure. Other terms used to describe seizures include petit mal or absence seizures (few general motor symptoms with short-term lack of conscious activity), myo-clonic (single or repetitive jerking), tonic (stiffening), clonic (jerking), or grand mal or tonic–clonic (involves entire body with rigidity, violent rhythmic jerking, and loss of consciousness) seizures. These latter terms are typically used to categorize generalized seizures.

A second axis of classification is clinical seizure type—sometimes including information from electroencephalograms (EEGs)—as proposed by the International League Against Epilepsy (1989). The international classification of epilepsy is designed mainly to assist clinicians in identifying specific syndromes that will aid in treatment decisions and prognosis. Implementation in population-based epidemiologic studies is problematic, however, because the extensive clinical monitoring and EEG information will not be consistently available; and even with such information, many cases cannot be specifically classified (Manford et al. 1992; Oka et al. 1995; Zarrelli et al. 1999).

On evaluation, many patients who appear to have had a seizure are found instead to have had syncope, pseudoseizures, breath-holding spells, or loss of consciousness (LOC) from other causes (Fig. 12–1). If a seizure has occurred, the next step is to establish whether a concurrent central nervous system (CNS) insult is responsible. "Acute symptomatic seizures" have specific structural (e.g., head trauma) or metabolic (e.g., ethanol withdrawal) causes. Febrile seizures in children differ from other acute symptomatic seizures by virtue of their ubiquitous cause, recurrent nature, and strong familial aggregation. Afebrile seizures without an acute cause are considered unprovoked, and when they recur, epilepsy. If unprovoked seizures are attributable to a prior neurologic insult, the disorder is considered secondary to that insult, representing remote symptomatic seizures. When there is no probable predisposing factor, the seizure disorder is idiopathic or cryptogenic. Seizure disorders with radiologic evidence of a possible cause but no known antecedent insult are classified as cryptogenic; those with neither are called idiopathic.

Disease Description

Clinical Features that Affect Epidemiologic Studies

In contrast to static cognitive or motor deficits, the episodic nature of seizure disorders makes ascertainment and classification in epidemiologic studies more difficult than with most neurologic diseases. A clinical history of the event is required to establish the occurrence of prior seizures as well as their proper classification by seizure type and etiology. The vast majority of seizure disorders—all acute symptomatic seizures by definition, single unprovoked seizures, and even most (perhaps 70%) epilepsy cases—are self-limiting and cannot be captured by patient monitoring. The proper syndrome classification is usually limited to intractable seizures that can be observed by video and EEG monitoring. Patients with only a remote seizure history are difficult to classify.

Example 12–1 Hauser and colleagues (1991) defined prevalent cases of seizures as those individuals with a history of a seizure within the last 5 years or those taking antiepileptic drugs (for seizure) in that same period. There is no perfect answer to this issue of what constitutes a prevalent case. Individuals with only a history long ago probably represent a condition that has little clinical or public health significance. Thus, most population studies have restricted prevalence cases to individuals with seizures or use of antiepileptic medication within 5 years (Hauser et al. 1991), since those that have successfully discontinued antiepileptic medication for 5 years or longer are considered to be in remission.

Methods of Ascertaining and Verifying Cases

Epidemiologic studies of epilepsy and seizure disorders must deal with the inadequacy of the *International Statistical Classification of Disease*, Ninth Revision (ICD-9) classification system to ascertain seizures and epilepsy (World Health Organization 1977). The designated epilepsy code 345 includes not only epilepsy but other seizure diagnoses, including acute symptomatic seizures. The ICD-9 code 780.1 was intended for febrile convulsions, but in practice many epilepsy cases are signed out as convulsive disorder and coded as 780.1 or convulsions. In population-based studies, ascertaining all cases of seizure and epilepsy

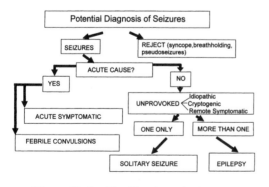

Figure 12–1 Classification of seizures.

requires reviewing further broad rubrics of ICD-9 categories that include syncope, LOC, and breath-holding spells.

> *Example 12–2* To accurately find all cases of epilepsy can be labor intensive. Only 10% of cases of syncope, LOC, and recorded breath-holding spells will ultimately be determined to be seizure and less than half of seizure will be epilepsy (Hauser et al. 1991; Annegers et al. 1999). Nonetheless, if one's goal is to accurately find all cases within a population, it is necessary to search to the extent possible in all relevant categories where cases may be misdiagnosed.

The EEG is diagnostic of certain types of epilepsy, notably absence, infantile spasms, photo-sensitive seizures, and rolandic epilepsy, but the interictal EEG is of limited value in the diagnosis of most seizure disorders. The prevalence of EEG abnormalities varies with age so that the diagnostic value of this instrument is further limited in population-based studies of the prevalence of seizure disorders.

Types of Populations Studied

There are many prevalence surveys available for communities throughout the world (see Table 12–1). The United States National Health Interview Surveys include questions on epilepsy and seizure (Adams and Marano 1995) and provide a national estimate of the prevalence of epilepsy, though this estimate is probably low be-cause of underreporting. There have also been prevalence surveys of children in the United States (Rose et al. 1973; Baumann et al. 1977; Murphy et al. 1995) and special populations such as military recruits (Love and Davenport 1920). Incidence studies of epilepsy are less common because epilepsy is not reported and cannot be easily determined from hospital or outpatient ICD codes. Incidence studies are available from relatively small, defined populations such as Rochester, Minnesota (Hauser et al. 1991); Umea, Sweden (Sidenvall et al. 1993; Forsgren et al. 1996); Aarhus, Denmark (Juul-Jensen and Ipsen 1975); and Martinique (Jallon 1999). The National General Practice Study of Epilepsy cohort provides a national sample for incidence studies of seizures in the United Kingdom (Sander et al. 1990; Manford et al. 1992). Managed care organizations provide defined populations for incidence studies, but this is a selected subset of the general population (Annegers et al. 1999) as many members belong as a condition of employment and epileptics represent a smaller portion of the workforce than in the general population.

Descriptive Studies

Prevalence Studies

The prevalence of epilepsy has been assessed in numerous populations (Table 12–1). Most studies in the United States, Europe, and Asia have reported overall

Table 12–1 Prevalence Studies of Epilepsy (Prevalence per 1000)

Country	Reference	Year	Crude	Age-adjusted*
			PREVALENCE	
Denmark	Juul-Jensen et al. 1975	1972	6.90	—
Poland	Zielinski 1974	1974	7.80	7.69
Mississippi	Haerer et al. 1986	1978	6.78	6.96
Rochester, MN	Haerer et al. 1986	1980	6.66	6.48
Nigeria	Osuntokun et al. 1987	1982	5.30	5.40
China	Li et al. 1985	1983	4.57	4.36
Bombay, India	Bharucha et al. 1988	1985	3.70	—
Pakistan	Aziz et al. 1994	1987	9.99	9.75

*Age-adjusted to U.S. 1970 population.

prevalences of 5 to 9 per 1000, although these studies were not strictly comparable in terms of case definitions, case ascertainment, and population structure. Some studies in tropical countries noted foci of exceptionally high prevalences, e.g., 57 per 1000 in an Amerindian community in Panama (Gracia et al. 1990).

If the 1980 prevalence in Rochester, Minnesota of 6.66 per 1000 (Hauser et al. 1991) was extrapolated to the total population, in 2000 about 1,800,000 persons in the United States would have epilepsy. The age-specific prevalences for Rochester, Minnesota are given in Figure 12–2 (Hauser et al. 1996). In this and most other studies, prevalence rises sharply from birth to adolescence, reaching between 5 and 10 per 1000. Prevalence remains fairly constant to age 65 despite the continued occurrence of new incidence cases, because their addition after adolescence is compensated by remission and, to a lesser extent, by increased mortality rates among people with epilepsy. The prevalence of epilepsy increases rapidly after age 65, as the incidence rises sharply in the elderly.

In the United States, limited data support ethnic differences in the occurrence of epilepsy. Studies of New Haven, Connecticut and of a rural Mississippi county reported a higher prevalence of epilepsy in African Americans than in whites (Shamansky and Glaser 1979; Haerer et al. 1986).

Incidence Studies

The age-specific incidence rates of afebrile unprovoked seizures is high in childhood, declining between ages 20 and 50, and increases after age 50 (Hauser et al. 1991; Sidenvall et al. 1993; Forsgren et al. 1996; Annegers et al. 1999; Jallon 1999). The rates in populations from Sweden; Martinique; Rochester, Minnesota; and Houston, Texas are remarkably similar despite ethnic and geographical diversity. In each of these studies about 75% of the cases were epilepsy and about 25% were single unprovoked seizures. These studies were comparable in case definition and ascertainment. The managed care cohort (Annegers et al. 1999) has a progressively lower rate with advancing age, probably due to the population being selected to

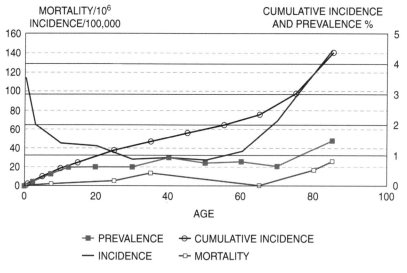

Figure 12–2 Measures of epilepsy (Rochester Minnesota, 1935–1984): age-specific incidence per 100,000 person-years; cumulative incidence (percent); age-specific prevalence (percent); and age-specific mortality per 100,000 person-years.

(Reprinted with permission from Hauser WA, Annegers JF, Rocca WA. Descriptive epidemiology of epilepsy: contributions of population-based studies from Rochester, Minnesota. *Mayo Clin Proc* 1996;71:576–586.)

increasingly include healthy working members.

Epilepsy begins at all ages, but it will appear to be largely a disease of childhood in populations with a young age structure and of the elderly populations with an older one. In Rochester, Minnesota, the proportion of incident cases of epilepsy in persons aged 65 or older has increased from 14% between 1935 and 1944 to 34% between 1985 and 1994 (Hauser et al 1996)—a trend expected to continue as the U.S. population ages.

Incidence by Seizure Type. Epilepsy can be classified into five broad categories of clinical seizure types—partial (focal), generalized tonic-clonic, myoclonic, absence, and others—that can be applied to population studies (Hauser et al. 1991). Although more detailed classifications are sometimes desirable, small numbers in most categories and the lack of necessary documentation for all members of a defined population limit subclassification. The age-specific incidence rates of epilepsy by seizure type are shown in Figure 12–3. Myoclonic seizures, most common during the first year of life, diminish in incidence rapidly thereafter. The inci-

dence of generalized tonic-clonic epilepsy is 15 per 100,000 in children younger than age 1 year and gradually declines to 10 per 100,000 for children aged 10 to 14 years, remaining at that level until the rates increase in persons older than 65. The incidence of partial seizures, with or without secondary generalization, remains remarkably consistent at 20 per 100,000 from infancy through age 65, but then increases sharply. The proportion of new cases of partial epilepsy progressively rises with age. The incidence of absence epilepsy with or without generalized tonic-clonic seizures is 11 per 100,000 from ages 1 through 10 years, whereas its onset is uncommon after age 14.

The incidence rates of epilepsy are about 15% higher in men than in women at all ages and for most seizure types. In contrast to other major seizure types, absence epilepsy has an incidence twice as high in girls than in boys.

Cumulative Risk. Cumulative incidence expresses risk and is a useful summary of occurrence. Figure 12–2 presents cumulative incidence of epilepsy over the life span on the basis of the Rochester data. The risk

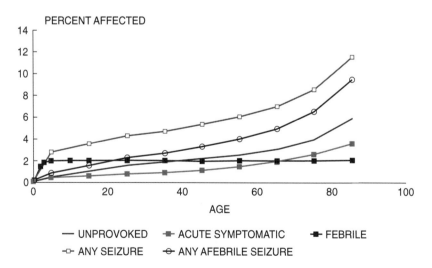

Figure 12–3 Percent of population affected by epilepsy by age and seizure type. (Reprinted with permission from Hauser WA, Annegers JF, Rocca WA. Descriptive epidemiology of epilepsy: contributions of population-based studies from Rochester, Minnesota. *Mayo Clin Proc* 1996; 71:576–586.)

of epilepsy starts at 1% from birth through age 20 and reaches 3% by age 75. Thus, about 3% of the population can be expected to have epilepsy at some time during their lives. Unlike prevalence, cumulative incidence progressively increases with age because epilepsy may begin at any age. Cumulative incidence provides the total epilepsy risk following specific etiologic events and exposures. For example, the 5-year risk of epilepsy after severe head trauma is about 15% (Annegers et al. 1980).

Analytic Studies

Methodologic Issues

Historical cohort studies have contributed more to our understanding of neurologic insults as risk factors for epilepsy than have case–control studies. Case–control studies are problematic because the neurologic insults that might cause epilepsy are rare and their severity and type are difficult to gauge by interviews conducted years after the fact. Historical cohort studies, in contrast, can follow individuals with a specific insult over time to observe and characterize the incidence of epilepsy. Historical cohort studies have also been used to evaluate prognosis and familial aggregation (see below).

Case–Control Studies

Case–control studies have been used largely in two areas: (1) perinatal risk factors for epilepsy and (2) risk factors for idiopathic epilepsy.

Case–Control Studies of Etiologic Factors. Only prior events with epidemiologic evidence of causality (an established relative risk [RR] of 2 or more) are considered etiologies of epilepsy; potential risk factors with an inconclusive causal association, such as perinatal insults and trivial head trauma, are not. Case–control studies of childhood epilepsy have inconsistently identified perinatal insults—long presumed to be a major cause of childhood-onset

epilepsy, especially of partial complex seizures (Lilienfeld and Pasamanick 1954; Nelson and Ellenberg 1986; Rocca et al. 1987). The second major application of the case–control design to the etiology of epilepsy has been to evaluate possible risk factors for adult-onset idiopathic epilepsy. These studies have suggested some new risk factors, especially hypertension and/or its treatment (Hesdorffer et al. 1996).

Cohort Studies of Etiologic Factors

Over the past 20 years, a number of cohort studies have determined the magnitude of the relative risk of epilepsy associated with brain trauma and with the duration of unconsciousness following brain trauma.

Example 12–3 Annegers and colleagues (1998) followed up 4541 children and adults who had suffered brain trauma defined by a loss of consciousness, post-traumatic amnesia, or skull fracture. They reported that, when compared to population rates, the overall standardized incidence ratio (SIR) was 3.1 (95% confidence interval [CI] 2.5–3.8). The SIR increased as the seriousness of the injury increased. These investigators used a retrospective cohort approach to follow up a large cohort with considerable detail about the injury. Similar detail would mostly likely not be available in a case–control approach, where the injury might have occurred many years or decades in the past.

Prognostic Studies

At one time, most of the information available on the prognosis of epilepsy and seizure disorders was derived from clinical series of patients referred to tertiary centers. Epidemiologic studies have made major contributions to our understanding of the prognosis of epilepsy, specifically, through population-based cohort studies of incidence cases in which life-table and, more recently, Cox proportional hazards methods were used. These contributions have been reviewed by Berg and Shinnar (1994).

Risks Predictors of Epilepsy after Febrile Convulsions

Cohort studies of patient with febrile convulsions have shown the risk of developing epilepsy to be about 4% to age 7 and 7% to age 25 (Nelson and Ellenberg 1986; Annegers et al. 1987). These studies have shown the risks to be much higher for children with complex febrile convulsions and quite modest for those with simple febrile convulsions.

Prospects and Predictors for Remission in Epilepsy

Although it has long been known that many children outgrow their epilepsy, the prognosis of epilepsy for intractable cases referred to tertiary centers is bleak. Cohort studies have now established that most epilepsy, about 70% of new-onset epilepsy, is self-limiting while about 15% of cases have persistent but rare seizures, and another 15% develop intractable epilepsy (Annegers et al. 1979; Sander et al. 1990). These studies have been less successful, however, in identifying predictors for prognosis, with a known etiology being the only strong and consistent predictor of prognosis (unfavorable).

First Seizure Prognosis

The nature of some types of epilepsy, such as absence and infantile spasms, are not recognized until recurrent seizures are established. However, about half of new-onset unprovoked seizures are recognized from the initial seizure—usually a primary or secondary generalized tonic-clonic seizure. A number of cohort studies have been conducted to evaluate the risk of recurrence after first seizure, which is on the order of 50% over the first 5 years of follow-up (Annegers et al. 1987; Hart et al. 1990; Hauser et al. 1990; Cockerell et al. 1995; Shinnar et al. 1996). Another application has been to assess the prospects of seizure recurrence after discontinuation of antiepileptic medications (Emerson et al. 1981; Shinnar et al. 1985; Calligan et al. 1988).

Mortality and Causes of Death in Epilepsy

Epilepsy is rarely listed as the underlying cause of death, although patients with epilepsy are known to have standardized mortality ratios (SMRs) on the order of 2.5 (Zielinski 1974; Hauser et al. 1980; Cockerell et al. 1994). The SMRs are highest at younger ages, for acquired epilepsy, and for childhood-onset epilepsy with the presence of other neurologic deficits, such as cerebral palsy and/or mental retardation (Hauser et al. 1980; Cockerell et al. 1994). There are several reasons for the increased mortality in people with epilepsy. First, the causes of epilepsy, especially brain tumors and cerebral vascular disease, are related to excess mortality. Second, seizures themselves can cause death through accident, especially drowning, and rarely fatal status epilepticus. Recently, a phenomenon of unexpected, unexplained death in epilepsy has been established in various cohort studies of patients with intractable epilepsy (Lip and Brodie 1992; Klenerman et al. 1993; Timmings 1993; Nashef et al. 1995a, 1995b; Derby et al. 1996), surgical patients (Dasheiff 1991; Hennessy et al. 1999), and cohorts receiving new antiepileptic drugs (AEDs) or vagus nerve stimulation (Dreifuss 1989; Kaufman et al. 1997; Annegers et al. 1999). These deaths typically occur in bed or during other normal activity, presumably proceeded by a brief seizure, and are not explained by other causes such as asphyxiation or coronary heart disease (Leestma et al. 1997). Adult patients with severe epilepsy have an incidence of sudden unexplained death in epilepsy (SUDEP) of 2 to 10 per 1000 person-years, which is many times that of individuals without known seizure disorders (Ficker et al. 1998).

Nongenetic Risk Factors

Although many definitive causes of epilepsy are known, only about one-third of all incidence cases of epilepsy (see Fig. 12–4) have a definite antecedent neurologic insult

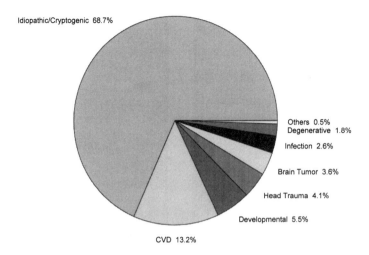

Figure 12–4 Etiology of epilepsy in 888 cases. Incidence in Rochester, Minnesota, 1935–1984. CVD, cardiovascular disease. (Reprinted with permission from Annegers JF, Rocca WA, Hauser WA. Causes of epilepsy: contributions of the Rochester epidemiology project. *Mayo Clin Proc* 1996;71:570–575.)

that is believed to be causal. The remaining two-thirds are idiopathic/cryptogenic. At this time, there is no standardized definition that differentiates cryptogenic from idiopathic for use in epidemiologic studies; work on this issue is greatly needed to improve the research in this area.

Example 12–4 In a detailed examination of 2952 men and women with epilepsy, Ng et al. (2001) found that 59.9% were cryptogenic, 35.1% were symptomatic, and 3.9% were idiopathic. Zarelli et al. (1999) found that among localization-related epilepsies, cryptogenic and symptomatic forms were similar in occurrence and about 86 times more common than idiopathic epilepsy. They also reported that among generalized epileptics, the three categories occurred with about the same frequency. While these may be real differences due to population differences, each group used a different definition and had different levels of medical testing (e.g., EEGs, imaging) that may also account for the contrast. Having a standardized definition would help avoid the difficulties in interpreting results from various sites.

Traumatic Brain Injury

The incidence of epilepsy after traumatic brain injury (TBI) has been extensively studied in military cohorts since World War I (Salazar et al. 1985). These studies show a high risk of epilepsy after penetrating head injuries, increasing from about 30% in World War I to 50% during the Vietnam War. The increased risks in recent conflicts presumably reflect more successful treatment and survival of more serious wounds. Studies of closed head injuries in civilian populations report lower risks of post-traumatic epilepsy. Series of neurosurgical patients indicate average risks of 3% to 7% (Jennett 1975).

One historical cohort study that followed cases of TBI for 53,222 person-years found that trauma with LOC, amnesia, or a skull fracture is somewhat common (Annegers et al. 1998). For all patients with mild TBI, the SIR was 3.1 in the first year after the injury and 2.1 for the next 4 years, but there was no increase thereafter. The SIR during the first 5 years after injury was slightly higher, 2.5 (95% CI 1.2–4.4), among the patients with mild traumatic brain injuries with LOC, as compared with 2.1 (95% CI 0.7–4.9) among those with only post-traumatic amnesia (PTA). Among those with severe TBI, the risk of seizures was elevated during the first year of follow-up (standardized incidence ratio 96.9) and remained significantly elevated throughout follow-up. In those patients with moderate TBI, an increased incidence was apparent for the first 10 years after injury, but not after that time.

Brain contusion or subdural hematoma remained the strongest risk factor for post-traumatic seizures. Loss of consciousness or PTA of 1 day or more, linear skull fracture in ages 5 years and older, depressed skull fracture, age of 65 years or older, and early seizure were strong factors. The presence of early seizures in 117 patients was also a strong univariate risk factor (RR 5.5), but the relative risk for early seizures was 1.4 when adjusted for the other factors.

Only 4% of all epilepsy cases are post-traumatic, however, as relatively few people survive severe head trauma. Brain injury accounts for 13% of epilepsy of presumed cause and occurs at all ages (Fig. 12–5). Trauma is the most important cause of remote symptomatic epilepsy in persons aged 15 to 24 years and is an important contributing factor in epilepsy in children and young adults.

Central Nervous System Infections

Prior CNS infections are presumed to cause 1% to 5% of epilepsy cases (Hauser et al. 1986). The incidence is highest in children, with a second peak noted among the elderly (Nicolosi et al. 1986). These infections are a major contributor of acquired epilepsy through age 35 (see Fig. 12–5), even though the illness responsible usually occurs in early childhood. Survivors of CNS infections have a threefold increase overall in risk for epilepsy (Annegers et al. 1988), independent of age at infection, but the risk varies greatly by type of infection and presence of early seizures.

No discernible increase in risk for epilepsy follows aseptic meningitis; bacterial meningitis, however, increases risk by approximately fivefold, with most of this risk occurring in the first 2 years after the infection. As with moderate head injury, the increase in risk may be limited to the first 5 years after the infection. Viral encephalitis increases the risk tenfold, and this increased risk persists at least 15 years after the infection. For patients with encephalitis and early seizures, the risk of epilepsy is 10% by 5 years and 22% by 20 years after the infection. The 20-year risk of unprovoked seizures is 10% in encephalitis patients without early seizures. Bacterial meningitis involves a 20-year risk of 13% and 2% for cases with and without early seizures, respectively (Annegers et al. 1988).

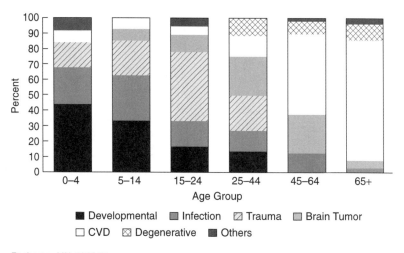

Rochester, MN, 1935-84

Figure 12–5 Remote symptomatic epilepsy. Proportions by age and etiology in Rochester, Minnesota, 1935–1984. CVD, cardiovascular disease. (Reprinted with permission from Hauser WA, Annegers JF, Kurland LT. Incidence of epilepsy and unprovoked seizures in Rochester, Minnesota; 1935–1984. *Epilepsia* 1993;34:453–468.)

Cerebrovascular Disease

Cerebrovascular disease is the major cause of seizures and epilepsy in the elderly (Lesser et al. 1985; Hauser et al. 1991). In Rochester, Minnesota, 55% of all newly diagnosed seizures in persons older than 65 were attributed to the acute or late effects of cerebrovascular disease (Hauser et al. 1991). Cerebrovascular disease is the major cause of acquired epilepsy in people aged 45 to 64.

The incidence of cerebrovascular disease increases with age. Beyond age 75, more than 1% of the population previously unaffected will suffer a cerebrovascular insult annually (Broderick et al. 1989); this is the major reason for the sharp rise in epilepsy incidence rates after age 65. Although many reports note the relationship between epilepsy and stroke, few give an accurate picture of the magnitude, duration, and prognostic factors. Most reports also fail to distinguish between acute symptomatic seizures at the time of stroke and subsequent unprovoked seizures. The reported proportion of stroke patients experiencing late seizures is 3% to 8% (Richardson and Dodge 1954; Fentz 1971; Olsen et al. 1987). Viitanen et al. (1988) observed a population-based cohort of stroke patients admitted to a university hospital in Sweden. Patients with transient ischemic attacks (13%), intracerebral hemorrhage (11%), and brain infarctions (76%) were included. The cumulative risk of epilepsy was 3% to 1 year and 5% to 5 years after stroke.

Cortical lesions detected on computed tomography (CT) or postmortem examination are predictive of late seizures (Olsen et al. 1987; Burri et al. 1989). In 1987, Olsen et al. reported a 2-year incidence of poststroke seizures of 9%. Of 23 patients with cortical lesions, 6 experienced epilepsy, whereas only 1 of 42 patients with subcortical lesions and none of 12 with no lesions had late seizures.

Brain Tumors

Brain tumors account for 3.6% of all cases of epilepsy (see Fig. 12–4) and 12% of acquired epilepsy. Epilepsy from brain tumors occurs at all ages but is proportionately greatest in ages 25 to 64 (see Fig. 12–5). In addition, brain tumors are responsible for a substantial proportion of epilepsy in the elderly (Luhdorf et al. 1986), although in many of these cases the seizures may be more appropriately considered provoked. A newly identified seizure disorder, particularly in adults, invariably raises concern about a brain tumor. In fact, about 30% of patients with brain tumors have acute symptomatic seizures either as an initial symptom or postoperatively (Foy et al. 1981; Franceschetti et al. 1988). A much smaller proportion of brain tumor patients have subsequent unprovoked seizures. More difficult to categorize are cases of long-standing epilepsy in individuals with cerebral neoplasms. Prior to the availability of CT or magnetic resonance imaging (MRI), case series of patients undergoing epilepsy surgery reported unsuspected neoplasms in 15% to 45% (Mathieson 1975; Blume et al. 1982; Spencer et al. 1984).

Degenerative Central Nervous System Diseases

Epilepsy associated with a degenerative process accounts for only about 2% of all cases of epilepsy and 6% of epilepsy with a presumed cause. The incidence of degenerative neurologic disease increases with age, and at least some of these illnesses are associated with an increased incidence of epilepsy. Each year, Alzheimer's disease affects 0.5% of the population aged 70 to 79 and 2% of those older than 80 (Kokmen et al. 1988). This disease is associated with a 10-fold increase in risk of epilepsy, and an estimated 10% of long-term Alzheimer's survivors eventually develop epilepsy (Hauser et al. 1986; Romanelli et al. 1990).

Even though epilepsy is generally considered to involve neurons, individuals with demyelinating disease appear to be at increased risk. In clinical series, up to 5% of patients with multiple sclerosis had seizures or epilepsy—at least a 10-fold increase over the expected proportion. In fact, multiple sclerosis is the major contributor to epilepsy from a degenerative disorder in patients of ages 25 through 64. Two studies have quantified the risk (Kinnunen and Wikstrom 1986; Olaffsson et al 1999); epilepsy occurred at the time of or soon after the diagnosis of multiple sclerosis in 1.8% of patients, or 3.4 times the expected rate.

Developmental Deficits

Developmental disorders are associated with about 5.5% of all new cases of epilepsy and account for 18% of all epilepsy with a presumed cause. They are the most important secondary cause in children but are relevant in young adults as well (see Fig. 12–5). Approximately 3 to 6 children per 1000 live births are affected with cerebral palsy or moderate or severe mental retardation, or both, and one-third of them will have epilepsy (Nelson and Ellenberg 1986). Cerebral palsy and mental retardation, therefore, should be considered markers for underlying brain abnormalities responsible for both the neurologic handicap and the epilepsy. Most cases of both conditions have no readily identifiable etiology, and there is little insight into either the basic mechanisms or preventive strategies for epilepsy in these groups. Individuals with mental retardation or cerebral palsy retain an increased incidence of epilepsy into adulthood. Down's syndrome in adults, which could also be regarded as a degenerative etiology, is an important contributor to the older-onset cases in this category. The prevalence of epilepsy in Down's syndrome patients increases progressively from about 5% at ages 18 to 29 to about 50% at ages 50 to 60 (McVicker et al. 1994). A recent study found that spontaneous abortions were associated with a four- to five-fold increase in risk of epilepsy among the offspring of epileptic mothers (Schupf and Ottman 2001).

Familial Aggregation and the Genetics of Seizures

Like other chronic diseases, seizure disorders have been shown to aggregate in families, but only rare syndromes show a Mendelian pattern of inheritance. The familial aggregation is strongest for febrile convulsions, with about a fourfold relative risk or 10% absolute risk for first-degree relatives of affected individuals (Hauser et al. 1985). Idiopathic epilepsy, and especially generalized onset seizures starting in childhood, has an overall level of familial aggregation in first-degree relatives of about threefold, or a 5% risk, to about age 20 (Annegers et al. 1982). The levels of familial aggregation decrease and presumably approach relative risks of close to 1.0 for older or partial-onset epilepsies (Ottman et al. 1996). Twin studies in a variety of epilepsy classifications have suggested that the concordance rate between monozygotic twins is greater than for dizygotic twins, thus there may be genetic contributions to the onset of epilepsy (Kaneko et al. 2002). Knowledge of the genetics of the familial forms has greatly increased since 1995 (Leppert et al. 1989; Hirose et al. 2002). The genetics of partial epilepsy is probably the best described at this point. Rare polymorphic genes on 20q, 1q, and 15q have been associated with nocturnal frontal lobe epilepsy (Phillips et al. 1995, 1998; Hirose et al. 2002; Ottman 2001). Mutations in genes for the gamma amniobutyric acid (GABA) receptor and the calcium channels appear to contribute to childhood-absence epilepsy (Robinson et al. 2002). While there have been other successes (see Ottman 2001; Hirose et al. 2002; Kalachikov et al. 2002; Kaneko et al. 2002), these genetic influences are likely to contribute to only a small portion of idiopathic or cryptogenic causes of epilepsy. Nonetheless, these types of studies greatly enhance insight into treatment and pathophysiology in idiopathic and cryptogenic epilepsy. Furthermore, the facts that epilepsy phenotypes vary in families and generalized-onset epilepsy co-aggregates strongly with febrile convulsions suggest the existence of several different seizure-predisposing alleles (Annegers et al. 1982; Berkovic and Scheffer 1998). The relationship between genetic and environmental causes of epilepsy has been explored but may be difficult to detect, as the combined effects of genetic predisposition and environmental insults appear to result in additive relative risks (Ottman et al. 1996). The discovery and confirmation of genes that play a role in a large number of idiopathic and cryptogenic epilepsy cases will require the use of modern genetic epidemiologic techniques, including assessment of the prevalence of newly discovered genes in large unselected populations and functional genetic studies (Berkovic and Ottman 2000). The former studies often require large sample sizes and are expensive to conduct.

Knowledge of the genetics of epilepsy will greatly expand with increasing rigor in the phenotype definitions and their use in genetic studies. For example, describing autosomal dominant partial epilepsy as having auditory features resulted in identification of susceptibility genes on 10q (Ottman et al. 1995; Kalachikov et al. 2002). There is likely to be more success in identifying genetic factors when rigorous case definitions or phenotypes are used.

Future Directions and Conclusions

Methodologies to Improve Epidemiologic Studies

Standardized Definitions. A system of classification of major seizure disorder types in epidemiologic studies has been developed and applied. Additional classification areas that need to be developed are (1) definitions of presumed etiologies, (2) radiologic evidence for cryptogenic features, and (3) syndrome classification that can be applied to populations.

For presumed etiology, epidemiologists must consider the following questions: What must the relative risk be to conclude causality? For example, is a relative risk of 2.0 sufficient? And how long do risks remain elevated after certain types of neurologic insults such as moderate traumatic brain injury?

Seizure disorders with radiologic evidence of a lesion but no known antecedent neurologic insult are considered cryptogenic seizures. However, the nature of the lesions that can be considered causal is not established. Perhaps a case–control study with MRI findings of risk factors would help remedy the problem.

There are difficulties in applying the syndrome classification to population-based studies, such as the following: the necessary information may not be available; syndromes are classified in part by prognosis and are therefore not applicable to incidence cases; and a large proportion of population-based cases may not fit the classification system. A system incorporating the syndrome classification as reasonably as possible into population-based studies is needed.

Understudied Populations. A recent Centers For Disease Control Consensus Conference on Epilepsy identified two major populations in the United States that are understudied for the epidemiology of seizure disorders: minority groups and the elderly. Given the age-specific pattern of incidence and the demographic changes in the United States and elsewhere, epilepsy is becoming more a disease of the elderly. In fact, about one-third of the 120,000 incidence cases of epilepsy occurring each year in the United States are in individuals over age 65, and this proportion is expected to increase. The few studies with comparable definitions of epilepsy indicate that the incidence of epilepsy, and especially of unprovoked seizure disorders, does not vary by ethnicity (Hauser et al. 1993; Sidenvall et al. 1993; Forsgren et al. 1996; Annegers et al. 1999; Jallon et al. 1999). However, data are limited.

Areas for Additional Etiologic Investigations

To evaluate the prognosis and treatment alternatives for people with seizures, it is important to develop and design studies that will permit better prediction of intractable seizures. Such studies are complicated, however, by the lack of consensus of a working definition for "intractable" (Berg and Shinnar 1994).

The appropriateness of prophylactic AEDs for traumatic brain injury has been studied in far greater depth than other causes of epilepsy (Temkin et al. 1990), such as stroke, brain tumors, and CNS infections. Although practices vary widely, studies are needed to evaluate the benefits and risks of prophylactic AEDs.

Through post-marketing surveillance of AEDs, important adverse effects have been identified, including aplastic anemia with felbamate (Kaufman et al. 1997), liver toxicity with sodium valproate (Dreifuss 1989), and visual field defects with vigabatrin (Stefan et al. 1999). A national registry of pregnancies (North American Registry for Epilepsy and Pregnancy 1998) is being compiled and a large prospective cohort study (NEAD 2003) of women exposed to AEDs in utero is currently underway to evaluate the teratogenicity of old and new AEDs. The recent introduction of many new drugs for epilepsy and the broader use of these drugs for indications other than epilepsy necessitate continued post-marketing surveillance for adverse effects. A survey of nursing homes across the United States showed a high prevalence of AEDs for any indication (Garrard et al. 2000).

For significant progress to be made in our knowledge of the etiology of epilepsy, large population-based studies will be needed that marry the modern techniques of genetics with rigorous ascertainment of environmental exposures. While our understanding of the causes and progression of epilepsy has greatly advanced over the last several decades, additional improvements in the methodological aspects of the research are needed to move the field forward.

References

Adams PF, Marano MA. Current estimates from the National Health Interview Survey, 1994. National Center for Health Statistics. *Vital Health Stat* 1995;10.

Annegers JF, Dubinsky S, Coan SP, et al. The incidence of epilepsy and unprovoked seizures in multiethnic, urban health maintenance organizations. *Epilepsia* 1999;40: 502–506.

Annegers JF, Grabow JD, Groover RV, et al. The incidence, causes, and secular trends of head trauma in Olmsted County, Minnesota, 1935–1974. *Neurology* 1980;30:912–919.

Annegers JF, Hauser WA, Anderson VE. The risks of seizure disorders among relatives of patients with childhood onset epilepsy. *Neurology* 1982;32:174–179.

Annegers JF, Hauser WA, Beghi E, et al. The risk of unprovoked seizures after encephalitis and meningitis. *Neurology* 1988;38: 1407–1410.

Annegers JF, Hauser WA, Coan SP, Rocca WA. A population-based study of seizures after traumatic brain injuries. *N Engl J Med* 1998;338:20–24.

Annegers JF, Hauser WA, Elveback LR. Remission of seizures and relapse in patients with epilepsy. *Epilepsia* 1979;20:729–737.

Annegers JF, Hauser WA, Shirts SB, Kurland LT. Factors prognostic of unprovoked seizures after febrile convulsions. *N Engl J Med* 1987;316:493–498.

Annegers JF, Rocca WA, Hauser WA. Causes of epilepsy: contributions of the Rochester epidemiology project. *Mayo Clin Proc* 1996; 71:570–575.

Aziz H, Ali SM, Frances P, et al. Epilepsy in Pakistan: a population-based epidemiologic study. *Epilepsia* 1994;35:950–958.

Baumann RJ, Marx BM, Leonidakis MG. An estimate of the prevalence of epilepsy in a rural Appalachian population. *Am J Epidemiol* 1977;106:42–52.

Begley CE, Famulari M, Annegers JF, et al. The cost of epilepsy in the United States: an estimate from population-based clinical and survey data. *Epilepsia* 2000;41:342–351.

Beran RG, Hall L, Pesch A, et al. Population prevalence of epilepsy in Sydney, Australia. *Neuroepidemiology* 1982;1:201–208.

Berg AT, Shinnar S. The contributions of epidemiology to the understanding of childhood seizures and epilepsy. *J Child Neurol* 1994; 9(Suppl 2):19–26.

Berkovic SF, Ottman R. Molecular genetics of the idiopathic epilepsies: the next steps. *Epileptic Disord* 2000;2:179–181.

Berkovic SF, Scheffer IE. Febrile seizures: genetics and relationship to other epilepsy syndromes. *Curr Opin Neurol* 1998;11:129–134.

Bharucha NE, Bharucha AE, Bharucha EP. Prevalence of epilepsy in the Parsi community of Bombay. *Epilepsia* 1988;29:111–115.

Blume WT, Girvin JP, Kaufmann JCE. Childhood brain tumors presenting as chronic uncontrolled focal seizure disorders. *Ann Neurol* 1982;12:538–541.

Broderick JP, Phillips SJ, Whisnant JP, et al. Incidence rates of stroke in the eighties: the end of the decline in stroke? *Stroke* 1989;20:577–582.

Burri H, Schaffler L, Karbowski K. Epileptic seizures in patients with a cerebrovascular infarction [in German]. *Schweiz Med Wochenschr* 1989;119:500–507.

Callaghan N, Garrett A, Goggin T. Withdrawal of anticonvulsant drugs in patients free of seizures for two years. A prospective study. *N Engl J Med* 1988;318:942–946.

Cockerell OC, Johnson AL, Sander JW, et al. Mortality from epilepsy: results from a prospective population-based study. *Lancet* 1994;344:918–921.

Cockerell OC, Johnson AL, Sander JW, et al. Remission of epilepsy: results from the National General Practice Study of Epilepsy. *Lancet* 1995;346:140–144.

Dasheiff RM. Sudden unexpected death in epilepsy: a series from an epilepsy surgery program and speculation on the relationship to sudden cardiac death. *J Clin Neurophysiol* 1991;8:216–222.

Derby LE, Tennis P, Jick H. Sudden unexplained death among subjects with refractory epilepsy. *Epilepsia* 1996;37:931–935.

Dreifuss FE. Valproic acid hepatic fatalities: revised table [letter]. *Neurology* 1989;39:1558.

Emerson R, D'Souza BJ, Vining EP, et al. Stopping medication in children with epilepsy: predictors of outcome. *N Engl J Med* 1981;304:1125–1129.

Fentz V. Epileptic seizures in patients with cerebrovascular disease. *Abstr Nord Med* 1971;86:1023–1025.

Ficker DM, So EL, Shen WK, et al. Population-based study of the incidence of sudden unexplained death in epilepsy. *Neurology* 1998;51:1270–1274.

Forsgren L, Bucht G, Eriksson S, Bergmark L. Incidence and clinical characterization of unprovoked seizures in adults: a prospective population-based study. *Epilepsia* 1996;37:224–229.

Foy PM, Copeland GP, Shaw MDM. The incidence of postoperative seizures. *Acta Neurochir* 1981;55:252–264.

Franceschetti S, Battagha G, Lodrini S, Avanzini G. Relationship between tumors and epilepsy. In: Broggi G, ed. The Rational Basis of the Surgical Treatment of Epilepsies. London: John Libbey Eurotext, 1988, pp 97–102.

Garrard J, Cloyd J, Gross C, et al. Factors associated with antiepileptic drug use among elderly nursing home residents. *J Gerontol A Biol Sci Med Sci* 2000;55:M384–M392.

Gracia F, Loode Lao S, Castillo L, et al. Epidemiology of epilepsy in Guaymi Indians from Bocas del Toro Province, Republic of Panama. *Epilepsia* 1990;31:718–723.

Haerer AF, Anderson DW, Schoenber BS. Prevalence and clinical features of epilepsy in a biracial United States population. *Epilepsia* 1986;27:66–75.

Hart YM, Sander JW, Johnson AL, Shorvon SD. National General Practice Study of Epilepsy: recurrence after a first seizure. *Lancet* 1990;336:1271–1274.

Hauser WA, Annegers JF, Anderson VE, Kurland LT. The risk of seizure disorders among relatives of children with febrile convulsions. *Neurology* 1985;35:1268–1273.

Hauser WA, Annegers JF, Elveback LR. Mortality in patients with epilepsy. *Epilepsia* 1980;21:399–412.

Hauser WA, Annegers JF, Kurland LT. The prevalence of epilepsy in Rochester, Minnesota, 1940–1980. *Epilepsia* 1991;32:429–445.

Hauser WA, Annegers JF, Kurland LT. Incidence of epilepsy and unprovoked seizures in Rochester, Minnesota: 1935–1984. *Epilepsia* 1993;34:453–468.

Hauser WA, Annegers JF, Rocca WA. Descriptive epidemiology of epilepsy: contributions of population-based studies from Rochester, Minnesota. *Mayo Clin Proc* 1996;71:576–586.

Hauser WA, Morris ML, Heston LL, Anderson VE. Seizures and myoclonus in patients with Alzheimer's disease. *Neurology* 1986;36:1226–1230.

Hauser WA, Rich SS, Annegers JF, Anderson VE. Seizure recurrence after a 1st unprovoked seizure: an extended follow-up. *Neurology* 1990;40:1163–1170.

Hauser WA, Rich SS, Lee JR, et al. Risk of recurrent seizures after two unprovoked seizures. *N Engl J Med* 1998;338:429–434.

Hennessy MJ, Langan Y, Elwes RDC, et al. A study of mortality after temporal lobe epilepsy surgery. *Neurology* 1999;53:1276–1283.

Hesdorffer DC, Hauser WA, Annegers JF, Rocca WA. Severe, uncontrolled hypertension and adult-onset seizures: a case–control study in Rochester, Minnesota. *Epilepsia* 1996;37:736–741.

Hirose S, Okada M, Yamakawa K, et al. Genetic abnormalities underlying familial epilepsy syndromes. *Brain Dev* 2002;24:211–222.

International League Against Epilepsy. Proposal for revised classification of epilepsies and epileptic syndromes. Commission on Classification and Terminology of the International League Against Epilepsy. *Epilepsia* 1989;30:389–399.

Jallon P, Smadja D, Cabre P, et al. EPIMART: prospective incidence study of epileptic seizures in newly referred patients in a French Carribean island (Martinique). *Epilepsia* 1999;40:1103–1109.

Jennett WB. Epilepsy After Non-missile Head Injuries, 2nd ed. London: Heinemann Medical Books, 1975.

Juul-Jensen P, Ipsen J. Prevalence and incidence of epilepsy in greater Aarhus. *Ugeskr Laeg* 1975;137:2380–2388.

Kalachikov S, Evgrafov O, Ross B, et al. Mutations in *LGI1* cause autosomal-dominant partial epilepsy with auditory features. *Nat Genet* 2002;30:335–341.

Kaneko S, Okada M, Iwasa H, et al. Genetics of epilepsy: current status and perspectives. *Neurosci Res* 2002;44:11–30.

Kaufman DW, Kelly JP, Anderson T, et al. Evaluation of case reports of aplastic anemia among patients treated with felbamate. *Epilepsia* 1997;38:1265–1269.

Kinnunen E, Wikstrom J. Prevalence and prognosis of epilepsy in patients with multiple sclerosis. *Epilepsia* 1986;27:729–733.

Klenerman P, Sander JW, Shorvon SD. Mortality in patients with epilepsy: a study of patients in long-term residential care. *J Neurol Neurosurg Psychiatry* 1993;56:149–152.

Kokmen E, Chandra V, Schoenberg BS. Trends in incidence of dementing illness in Rochester, Minnesota, in three quinquennial periods, 1960–1974. *Neurology* 1988;38:975–980.

Leestma JE, Annegers JF, Brodie MJ, et al. Sudden unexplained death in epilepsy: observations from a large clinical development program. *Epilepsia* 1997;38:47–55.

Leppert M, Anderson VE, Quattlebaum T, et al. Benign familial neonatal convulsions linked to genetic markers on chromosome 20. *Nature* 1989;337:647–648.

Lesser RP, Lüders H, Dinner DS, Morris HH. Epileptic seizures due to thrombotic and embolic cerebrovascular disease in older patients. *Epilepsia* 1985;26:622–630.

Li S, Schoenberg BS, Wang C, et al. Epidemiology of epilepsy in urban areas of the People's Republic of China. *Epilepsia* 1985;26:391–394.

Lilienfeld AM, Pasamanick B. Association of maternal and fetal factors with the development of epilepsy. *JAMA* 1954;155:719–724.

Lip GY, Brodie MJ. Sudden death in epilepsy: an avoidable outcome? *J R Soc Med* 1992;85:609–611.

Love AG, Davenport CB. Defects found in drafted men. Statistical information compiled from the draft records showing the physical condition of the men registered and examined in pursuance of the requirements of the Selective Service Act. Washington, DC: Surgeon-General's Office, United States Printing Office, 1920.

Luhdorf K, Jensen LK, Plesner AM. Etiology of seizures in the elderly. *Epilepsia* 1986;27:458–463.

Manford M, Hart YM, Sander JW, Shorvon SD. The National General Practice Study of Epilepsy. The syndromic classification of the International League Against Epilepsy applied to epilepsy in a general population. *Arch Neurol* 1992;49:801–808.

Mathieson G. Pathologic aspects of epilepsy to the surgical pathology of focal cerebral seizures. *Adv Neurol* 1975;8:107–138.

McVicker RW, Shanks OEP, McClelland RJ. Prevalence and associated features of epilepsy in adults with Down's syndrome. *Br J Psychiatry* 1994;164:528–532.

Murphy CC, Trevathan E, Yeargin-Allsopp M. Prevalence of epilepsy and epileptic seizures in 10-year-old children: results from the Metropolitan Atlanta Developmental Disabilities Study. *Epilepsia* 1995;36:866–872.

Nashef L, Fish DR, Garner S, et al. Sudden death in epilepsy: a study of incidence in a young cohort with epilepsy and learning difficulty. *Epilepsia* 1995a;36:1187–1194.

Nashef L, Fish DR, Sander JW, Shorvon SD. Incidence of sudden unexpected death in an adult outpatient cohort with epilepsy at a tertiary referral centre. *J Neurol Neurosurg Psychiatry* 1995b;58:462–464.

NEAD. Neurodevelopmental Effects of Antiepileptic Drug Study (NEAD Study), Georgetown University, 2003 (http://www.neadstudy.com/epilepsy/index.html).

Nelson KB, Ellenberg JH. Antecedents of seizure disorders in early childhood. *Am Dis Child* 1986;40:1053–1061.

Ng KK, Ng PW, Tsang KL, for Hong Kong Epilepsy Study Group. Clinical characteristics of adult epilepsy patients in the 1997 Hong Kong epilepsy registry. *Chin Med J* 2001;114:84–87.

Nicolosi A, Hauser WA, Beghi E, Kurland LT. The epidemiology of central nervous system infections in Olmsted County, Minnesota, 1950–1981. *J Infect Dis* 1986;154:399–408.

North American Registry for Epilepsy and Pregnancy, a unique public/private partnership of health surveillance. *Epilepsia* 1998;39:793–798.

Oka E, Ishida S, Ohtsuka Y, Ohtahara S. Neuroepidemiological study of childhood epilepsy by application of international classification of epilepsies and epileptic syndromes (ILAE, 1989). *Epilepsia* 1995;36:658–661.

Olafsson E, Benedikz J, Hauser WA. Risk of epilepsy in patients with multiple sclerosis: a population-based study in Iceland. *Epilepsia* 1999;40:745–747.

Olsen TS, Hagenhaven H, Thage O. Epilepsy after stroke. *Neurology* 1987;37:1209–1211.

Osuntokun BO, Adeuja AOG, Nottidge VA, et al. Prevalence of the epilepsies in Nigerian Africans: a community-based study. *Epilepsia* 1987;28:272–279.

Ottman R. Progress in the genetics of the partial epilepsies. *Epilepsia* 2001;42 (Suppl 5):24–30.

Ottman R, Annegers JF, Risch N, et al. Relations of genetic and environmental factors in the etiology of epilepsy. *Ann Neurol* 1996; 39:442–449.

Ottman R, Risch N, Hauser WA, et al. Localization of a gene for partial epilepsy to chromosome 10q. *Nat Genet* 1995;10:56–60.

Phillips HA, Scheffer IE, Berkovic SF, et al. Localization of a gene for autosomal dominant nocturnal frontal lobe epilepsy to chromosome 20q 13.2. *Nat Genet* 1995;10:117–118.

Phillips HA, Scheffer IE, Crossland KM, et al. Autosomal dominant nocturnal frontal-lobe epilepsy: genetic heterogeneity and evidence for a second locus at 15q24. *Am J Hum Genet* 1998;63:1108–1116.

Richardson EP, Dodge PR. Epilepsy in cerebrovascular disease. *Epilepsia* 1954;3: 49–74.

Robinson R, Taske N, Sander T, et al. Linkage analysis between childhood absence epilepsy and genes encoding GABA$_A$ and GABA$_B$ receptors, voltage-dependent calcium channels, and the *ECA1* region on chromosome 8q. *Epilepsy Res* 2002;48:169–179.

Rocca WA, Sharbrough FW, Hauser WA, et al. Risk factors for complex partial seizures: a population-based case–control study. *Ann Neurol* 1987;21:22–31.

Romanelli MF, Morris JC, Ashkin K, Coben LA. Advanced Alzheimer's disease is a risk factor for late onset seizures. *Arch Neurol* 1990;47:847–850.

Rose SW, Penry JK, Markush RE, et al. Prevalence of epilepsy in children. *Epilepsia* 1973;14:133–152.

Salazar AM, Jabbari B, Vance SC, et al. Epilepsy after penetrating head injury, I: clinical correlates. *Neurology* 1985;35:1406–1414.

Sander JW, Hart YM, Johnson AL, Shorvon SD. National General Practice Study of Epilepsy: newly diagnosed epileptic seizures in a general population. *Lancet* 1990;336:1267–1271.

Schupf N, Ottman R. Risk of epilepsy in offspring of affected women: association with maternal spontaneous abortion. *Neurology* 2001;57:1642–1649.

Shamansky SL, Glaser GH. Socioeconomic characteristics of childhood seizure disorders in the New Haven area: an epidemiologic study. *Epilepsia* 1979;20:457–474.

Shinnar S, Berg AT, Moshe SL, et al. The risk of seizure recurrence after a first unprovoked afebrile seizure in childhood: an extended follow-up. *Pediatrics* 1996;98:216–225.

Shinnar S, Vining EP, Mellits ED, et al. Discontinuing antiepileptic medication in children with epilepsy after two years without seizures. A prospective study. *N Engl J Med* 1985;313:976–980.

Sidenvall R, Forsgren L, Blomquist HK, Heijbel J. A community-based prospective incidence study of epileptic seizures in children. *Acta Paediatr* 1993;82:605.

Sillanpaa M, Camfield P, Camfield C. Predicting long-term outcome of childhood epilepsy in Nova Scotia, Canada, and Turku, Finland. Validation of a simple scoring system. *Arch Neurol* 1995;52:589–592.

Spencer DD, Spencer SS, Mattson RH, Williamson PD. Intracerebral masses in patients with intractable partial epilepsy. *Neurology (Cleve)* 1984;34:432–436.

Stefan H, Bernatik J, Knorr J. Visual field defects due to antiepileptic drugs [in German]. *Nervenarzt* 1999;70:552–555.

Temkin NR, Dikmen SS, Wilensky AJ, et al. A randomized, double-blind study of phenytoin for the prevention of post-traumatic seizures. *N Engl J Med* 1990;323:497–502.

Timmings PL. Sudden unexpected death in epilepsy: a local audit. *Seizure* 1993;2:287–290.

Viitanen M, Eriksson S, Asplund K. Risk of recurrent stroke, myocardial infarction and epilepsy during long-term follow-up after stroke. *Eur Neurol* 1988;28:227–231.

World Health Organization. International Statistical Classification of Diseases, Ninth Revision (ICD-9). Geneva: World Health Organization, 1977.

Zarrelli MM, Beghi E, Rocca WA, Hauser WA. Incidence of epileptic syndromes in Rochester, Minnesota: 1980–1984. *Epilepsia* 1999;40:1708–1714.

Zielinski JJ. Epidemiology and medical-social problems of epilepsy in Warsaw. Warsaw, Psychoneurological Institute, 1974.

13

Migraine and Tension-Type Headache

RICHARD B. LIPTON, SANDRA W. HAMELSKY,
AND WALTER F. STEWART

Headache is a pain symptom that virtually everyone experiences at one time or another. In 1988, the International Headache Society (IHS) (Olesen 1988) categorized the many causes of headaches, and two broad groups of headache disorders were distinguished: primary headache disorders and secondary headache disorders. In primary headache disorders, the headache disorder is the fundamental problem; it is not symptomatic of another cause. The two most common types of primary headache disorders are episodic tension-type headache (ETTH) and migraine. Secondary headache disorders are a consequence of an underlying condition, such as a brain tumor, a systemic infection, or a head injury. The underlying causes of secondary headaches determine their epidemiology; therefore, most neuroepidemiologic research has focused on the epidemiology of primary headache.

Approximately 36% of men and 42% of women aged 18 to 65 suffer from ETTH (Schwartz et al. 1998), while 18% of women and 6% of men aged 12 to 80 suffer from migraine (Stewart et al. 1992; Lipton and Stewart 1993). Tension-type headache has a modest impact on the individual; because the disorder is so prevalent, however, the aggregate impact of ETTH on society is high. Tension-type headaches (TTH) may also be chronic (CTTH) instead of episodic. Migraine headache is less common than tension-type headaches, but attacks are considerably more painful and disabling, often resulting in lost work time. Because the societal impact of both tension-type headache and migraine is significant, this chapter will focus on the epidemiology of these two disorders.

Migraine

Case Definition

Migraine is a chronic disorder with episodic manifestations; it is characterized by attacks of head pain and various combinations of neurological, gastrointestinal, and autonomic changes. Although the IHS defines seven subtypes of migraine, by far, the two most important are migraine without aura and migraine with aura (see Table 13–1). Migraine is both a diagnosis of inclusion and exclusion. It is a diagnosis of inclusion because specific diagnostic features are required. It is a diagnosis of exclusion since secondary headache disorders have to be eliminated on the basis of the history, physical examination, or laboratory studies.

The gold standard for diagnosing migraine is assigned by a headache expert applying IHS criteria. In studies using videotaped patient encounters, the reliability of headache diagnosis is good to excellent (mean kappa = 0.74) but far from perfect (Granella et al. 1994). In epidemiology studies, a diagnosis of migraine is often assigned on the basis of a telephone interview or self-administered questionnaire. Using a clinical assessment as the gold standard, telephone interviews have sensitivities of approximately 85% and specificities of approximately 93% for migraine (Stewart et al. 1996a).

The migraine attack is often divided into four phases: the premonitory phase, the

Table 13–1 International Headache Society Diagnostic Criteria for Migraine with and without Aura

a. Migraine without aura	b. Migraine with aura
Description	Description
Idiopathic, recurring disorder manifesting with attacks of neurological symptoms unequivocally localizable to cerebral cortex or brain stem, usually gradually developed over 5–20 minutes and usually lasting less than 60 minutes. Headache, nausea, and/or photophobia usually follow neurological aura symptoms directly or after a free interval of less than an hour. The headache usually lasts 4–72 hours, but may be completely absent.	Idiopathic, recurring disorder manifesting with attacks of neurological symptoms unequivocally localizable to cerebral cortex or brain stem, usually gradually developed over 5–20 minutes and usually lasting less than 60 minutes. Headache, nausea, and/or photophobia usually follow neurological aura symptoms directly or after a free interval of less than an hour. The headache usually lasts 4–72 hours, but may be completely absent.
Diagnostic Criteria	Diagnostic Criteria

A. At least five attacks fulfilling B–D
B. Headache attacks lasting 4–72 hours (untreated or unsuccessfully treated)
C. Headache has at least two of the following characteristics:
  1. Unilateral location
  2. Pulsating quality
  3. Moderate or severe intensity inhibits or prohibits daily activities
  4. Aggravation by walking stairs or similar routine physical activity
D. During headache at least one of the following:
  1. Nausea and/or vomiting
  2. Photophobia and phonophobia
E. At least one of the following:
  1. History and physical and neurological examinations do not suggest symptomatic headache.
  2. History and/or physical and/or neurological examinations do suggest such disorder, but it is ruled out by appropriate investigations.
  3. Such disorder is present, but migraine attacks do not occur for the first time in close temporal relation to one another.
	A. At least two attacks fulfilling B
	B. At least three of the following four characteristics:
	  1. One or more fully reversible aura symptoms indicating focal cerebral cortical and/or brain stem dysfunction
	  2. At least one aura symptom develops gradually over more than four minutes or 2 or more symptoms occur in succession.
	  3. No aura symptom lasts more than 60 minutes. If more than one aura symptom is present, accepted duration is proportionally increased.
	  4. Headache follows aura with a free interval of less than 60 minutes. (It may also begin before or simultaneously with aura.)
	C. At least one of the following:
	  1. History and physical and neurological examinations do not suggest symptomatic headache.
	  2. History and/or physical and/or neurological examinations do suggest such disorder, but it is ruled out by appropriate investigations.
	  3. Such disorder is present, but migraine attacks do not occur for the first time in close temporal relation to the disorder.

aura, the headache phase, and the resolution phase. None of these phases is obligatory for diagnosis and most people with migraine do not have all four phases. The premonitory phase (prodrome) usually begins hours to days before headache onset. Symptoms are variable but may include changes in mood, hyperactivity, yawning, food cravings, and thirst (Silberstein et al. 1998). Premonitory features occur in about 60% of migraine sufferers.

In migraine with aura, focal neurological symptoms precede or accompany the attack. The aura develops over a period of 5–20 minutes and typically lasts less than 1 hour. Auras are usually visual and may include a mix of positive features (spots of light, zig-zag lines) and negative features (regions of visual loss). Auras may also involve other features, including motor, language, or brain stem disturbances. The aura is usually, but not always, followed by a headache. Approximately 20%–25% of migraine sufferers have migraine with aura. Most individuals who have migraine with aura also have attacks of migraine without aura (Johannes et al. 1995).

The third phase of the migraine attack is the headache phase. The headache of migraine is typically one-sided, throbbing, moderate to severe in intensity, and aggravated by routine physical activity. The headache phase may be accompanied by photophobia (sensitivity to light), phonophobia (sensitivity to sound), nausea, and vomiting, in variable combinations.

During the final phase, the resolution phase, the pain and accompanying symptoms subside. Many migraine sufferers report mood changes (euphoria, lethargy, fatigue) and scalp tenderness, even after spontaneous pain has subsided.

Incidence

Estimating the incidence of a chronic disorder with episodic manifestations is challenging. Since diagnostic criteria for migraine without aura require at least five lifetime attacks, should incidence be esti-

mated using the time of the first or fifth attack? Further, the disease affects individuals of all ages and the incidence rate varies substantially by age. To accurately describe incidence requires a large cohort study of individuals across the life span. There have been few studies of migraine incidence and no studies that systematically ascertain new migraine cases across a broad range of ages. The ideal study design for estimating the incidence of migraine would be prospective in design, ascertaining prevalent migraine cases at baseline and newly incident migraine cases as the study proceeded. As yet, no study has achieved this ideal in an inception cohort across a broad age span, but one study of migraine incidence was conducted in an inception cohort of young adults.

Example 13–1 Breslau et al. (1996) conducted a prospective study in 1007 members of a health maintenance organization. The inception cohort ranged in age from 21 to 30 years. Most of the sample (972/1007) completed follow-up interviews 3.5 and 5.5 years after enrollment. The at-risk population was composed of 848 participants who did not meet the criteria for migraine at baseline. The 5.5-year cumulative incidence was 8.4% (71/848; 60 female cases; 11 male cases), for a rate of 17.0 per 1000 person-years (24.0/10^2 female, 6.0/10^2 male). Of interest is that the female/male ratio of incidence rates was 4:1 in this study of young adults.

Two other population-based studies estimated the incidence of migraine using the reported age of migraine onset and reconstructed cohort methods. Using this method, a prevalence sample of migraine sufferers is identified and age of onset is determined, often by self-report. Self-reported age of onset is used to estimate age-specific incidence as described below.

Example 13–2 In Washington County, Maryland, telephone interviews were conducted among 10,169 residents between the ages of 12 and 29 to identify 392 males and 1018 females with migraine (Stewart et al. 1991). In both males and females, the incidence rate of migraine with aura peaked 3 to 5 years earlier than migraine without aura (Fig. 13–1). In addition, the incidence of migraine in females peaked at a later age than in males. The phenomenon of telescoping, or the tendency to report the occurrence of events in the past at times closer to the present (Brown et al. 1985), complicates incidence estimates de-

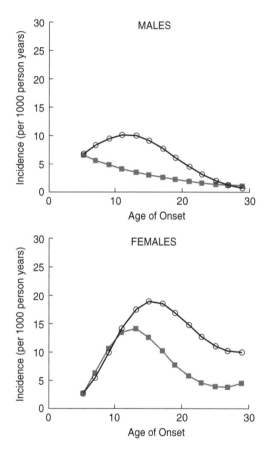

Figure 13–1 Age- and gender-specific incidence of migraine headache with and without aura among 10,131 survey respondents 12–29 years of age, Washington County, Maryland, 1987. Upper curve (O), migraine without aura; lower curve (■), migraine with aura. (Reprinted with permission from Stewart WF, Linet M, Celentano D, et al. Age- and sex-specific incidence rates of migraine with and without aura. *Am J Epidemiol* 1991;134:1111–1120.)

rived using reconstructed cohort methods. Studies that estimate the age-specific incidence of migraine based on recall would likely be biased toward older ages of headache onset (Brown et al. 1985; Cummings et al. 1990). In the Washington County study, age-specific incidence rates were adjusted for the time lag between the reported age of onset and the age at interview. This study is still limited by the narrow age range of the participants.

Another population-based study, conducted by Rasmussen (1995), reported that the age-adjusted annual incidence of migraine was 3.7 per 1000 person-years (females $5.8/10^2$; males $1.6/10^2$). Neither age-specific incidence nor incidence by migraine subtypes was reported.

A third approach to estimating migraine incidence used medical records to ascertain cases. In the linked medical records system in Olmstead County, Minnesota, a review of 6400 patient records yielded 629 individuals who fulfilled criteria for migraine (Stang et al. 1992). The age-adjusted incidence rates were 1.37 per 1000 person-years for males and 2.94 per 1000 person-years for females. Only individuals who consulted a health-care provider for headache were included in this study, which may explain why these incidence rates are lower than in the previously discussed studies.

Prevalence

Although incidence studies of migraine have been few, many studies have estimated the prevalence of migraine. *Prevalence* is defined as the proportion of a given population that has migraine over a defined period of time. Studies have focused on lifetime and 1-year period prevalence.

Prevalence estimates for migraine have varied widely, largely because of differences in case definitions and demographic features of study populations. Since migraine prevalence varies by age, gender, race, geography, and socioeconomic status, prevalence differences among studies may be influenced by these factors (Stewart et al. 1995; Scher et al. 1999). The variations in migraine prevalence across studies could be due to many factors, including differences in case definition and study population features (i.e., age and gender distribution, geographic location).

Example 13–3 We conducted two meta-analyses of published population-based studies to examine the variation in prevalence among studies (Stewart et al. 1995; Scher et al. 1999). Our 1995 meta-analysis included 24 studies published prior to 1994, only 5 of which used the IHS di-

agnostic criteria. Figure 13–2 presents the age-specific migraine prevalence estimates among males (Fig. 13–2a) and females (Fig. 13–2b) from these population-based studies of migraine prevalence (Stewart et al. 1995). Clearly the prevalence estimates vary considerably among studies, making it difficult to draw conclusions about the true prevalence of migraine in the population. We used linear regression to estimate the proportion of variance in the age- and gender-specific prevalence ratios according to factors such as age, gender,

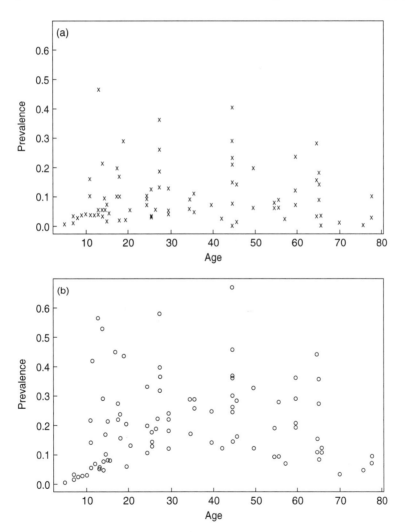

Figure 13–2 a: Age-specific estimates of migraine prevalence among males from 24 population-based studies of migraine. **b.** Age-specific estimates of migraine prevalence among females from 24 population-based studies of migraine.

(Reprinted with permission from Stewart W, Simon D, Schechter A, Lipton R. Population variation in migraine prevalence: a meta analysis. *J Clin Epidemiol* 1995;48:269–280.)

case definition criteria, method of selecting the sample, source of sample, response method, response rate, time period for estimating prevalence, and whether the case was clinically confirmed. Interestingly, we found that over 65% of the variation in migraine prevalence among studies can be explained by remarkably few factors. The single most important factor, case definition, accounted for the largest portion of variation in prevalence (36%) among studies. Other important factors included gender (15%) and age (age 3%; age^2 14%). Migraine was more prevalent among females than males, peaking between 35 and 55 years of age in both genders. Methodologic factors, such as the source of the population, the response rate, and whether diagnoses were confirmed by a clinical examination, did not have significant explanatory power.

In a second meta-analysis conducted in 1998, we included 18 population-based studies, all based on the IHS criteria (Scher et al. 1999). In this meta-analysis, case definition was held relatively constant and separate meta-analyses were conducted for males and females. Thus, the two most important explanatory factors in the first meta-analysis (case definition and gender) were eliminated. In this second meta-analysis, among both females and males, prevalence peaked during the third and fourth decades of life. For females, age and geographic location of the study population accounted for 74% of the variation in migraine prevalence. For males, these two variables accounted for 58% of the variation in migraine prevalence. Assessment of geographic location revealed that migraine prevalence was highest in North America, South America, and Western Europe, intermediate in Africa, and lowest in Asia, as discussed below. Once again, variation in migraine prevalence was not explained by methodological factors such as sampling method, response method, response rate, and recall period. Socioeconomic status, cultural differences in symptom reporting, or other unmeasured factors may help account for the residual variation in migraine prevalence (Stewart et al. 1995; Scher et al. 1999).

Prevalence by Age and Gender. Migraine prevalence varies by age and gender. At post-pubertal ages, migraine prevalence is consistently higher in females than males (Scher et al. 1999). The prevalence of migraine varies with age, peaking between the ages of 35 to 45 years. Overall, prevalence is highest from 25 to 55, the peak years for economic productivity. This age distribution may account for the enormous economic impact of migraine due to absenteeism and reduced productivity at work.

Prevalence by Race and Geographic Region. Race and geographic region contribute to variation in migraine prevalence. A population-based study in the United States compared the prevalence of migraine among Caucasians, African Americans, and Asian Americans living in Baltimore County, Maryland. Both before and after adjusting for sociodemographic covariates, prevalence of migraine was lowest in Asian Americans (female 9.2%, male 4.8%), intermediate in African Americans (female 16.2%, male 7.2%), and highest among Caucasians (female 20.4%, male 8.6%). These results mirror the meta-analytic finding that prevalence is lowest in Asia and Africa, with considerably higher prevalence in Europe, Central/South America, and North America (Scher et al. 1999).

What accounts for the international variation in migraine prevalence? Sociocultural factors, such as diet, stress, or other environmental factors, may account for the variation. Alternatively, differences in genetic susceptibility may play a role. The relative contributions of genetic and environmental risk factors or their interactions to the observed patterns of migraine prevalence remain to be determined.

Prevalence by Education and Income. Population-based studies conducted in North America indicate that migraine prevalence is inversely related to household income or education (Stewart et al. 1992, 1996a; Lipton and Stewart 1993; Kryst and Scherl 1994). That is, as income or education increases, migraine prevalence declines. This population finding contradicts prior beliefs regarding a direct relationship between income and migraine prevalence. This discrepancy may be explained by patterns of health-care utilization. Migraine may appear to be a disease of high income in the doctor's office, because medical diagnosis of migraine is more common among high-income groups (Lipton et al. 1992). Results of the National Health Interview Survey (NHIS) (Stang and Osterhaus 1993) support the hypothesis that patterns of consultation may shape physicians' perceptions. In the NHIS study, migraine prevalence was lower in the low-income group than in the middle-income group, and was highest in the high-income group. Since this study relies on self-reported medical diagnosis, the higher prevalence among the high-income group may be due to an increased likelihood of diagnosis of migraine as income rises. Studies outside the United States have not generally reported the inverse relationship between migraine prevalence and income (Rasmussen 1992; Abu-Arefeh and Russell 1994; Gobel et al. 1994; O'Brien et al. 1994). Reasons for this international variation are unclear.

Risk Factors for Developing Migraine

Risk factors for migraine should be distinguished from risk factors that trigger the episodic attacks of headache within people who suffer from migraine (Olesen et al. 1993; Rasmussen 1995). Positive family history, female gender, epilepsy, depression, and low socioeconomic status are associated with developing chronic migraine (Rasmussen 1995; Breslau and Rasmussen 2001).

Over the last decade, some progress has been made in defining risk factors for the disease. Numerous studies have examined the socioeconomic profiles, comorbidities, and genetics of migraine (Olesen 1993; Lipton and Stewart 1997; Breslau and Rasmussen 2001). Migraine is emerging as a clinically and biologically heterogenous disorder, however, further advances are still needed to identify and quantify the contributions of factors that cause the development of migraine.

Genetic risk factors may be involved in migraine. Studies have found that various headache types and migraine tend to aggregate within families (Russell and Olesen 1995, 1996; Stewart et al. 1997; Russell et al. 1999). This has raised the question of whether this is due to environmental or genetic origins (or both). While an active search is underway to identify genes that cause migraine, no definitive results have been published.

Triggering Factors among Migraine Sufferers

For an individual who suffers from migraine headaches, certain factors may trigger an attack (see Table 13–2), including endogenous (e.g., menses) and exogenous factors (e.g., diet, fatigue, stress, and seasonal changes) (Lipton 2000; Breslau and Rasmussen 2001). Migraine sufferers are eager to understand what initiates their attack. Identifying the precipitating factors can lead to preventive strategies such as trigger avoidance, stress management, and short-term prophylaxis of menstrual migraine, and can enhance feelings of self-control (Olesen 1993; Lipton and Stewart 1997).

The most common method used to investigate trigger factors is patient surveys (Van den Bergh et al. 1987; Rasmussen 1993) in which migraine sufferers are asked to list their headache triggers and whether specific listed factors trigger their migraine attacks. In some cases, a clinician may conduct an N-of-1 study that helps suggest whether a factor triggers headaches or not. However, these studies are notorious for not providing clear evidence.

Example 13–4 In a study to determine the effect of Chinook weather conditions on the probability of developing a mi-

Table 13–2 Risk Factors and Triggering Factors for Migraine

Risk factor or trigger	Examples
Food	Xanthine-containing foods (wine, chocolate, tea, coffee, colas)
	Tyramine-containing foods (cheese, bean pods)
	Preservatives (sulfites, nitrates)
	Pickled or fermented foods
	Flavor enhancers (aspartame, MSG)
	Alcohol
Environment	Weather
	Exposure to smoke
	Air pollution
	Noise
	Odors
Behaviors	Activity level
	Food consumption patterns (e.g., meal skipping)
Medications	Hormones
	Antihistamines
	Diurectics
	Vasodilators
	Bronchodilators
	Hypoglycemic agents
	Chemotherapy
	Sympathomimetic agents
	Overuse of pain or analgesic agents
Physiological and psychological factors	Stress
	Depression
	Sleep disturbances
	Hormone cycles

graine headache, 88% of the participants reported that the Chinook weather influenced their migraine (Cooke et al. 2000). However, using rigorous diary methods, Chinook weather precipitated migraine in only 29% of the participants. Thus, migraine sufferers may differentially recall only the attacks that support their belief that a particular putative factor triggered their migraine headache.

Randomized clinical trials are often conducted to examine exogenous triggers of migraine (Lipton 2000). Subjects are exposed to a placebo or to a trigger factor, such as aspartame, chocolate, or nitroglycerine (Olesen 1993; Van Den Eeden et al. 1994; Rasmusssen 1995). When only one trigger is tested, inferences about between-group differences in migraine occurrence with and without exposure to the factor may be possible. However, multiple exposures to the trigger factor for each

patient is a better design to support inferences about individual patients. In any case, well-controlled trials that are blinded and adequately controlled are needed to assess these factors. Study designs such as crossover trials, if appropriate, or diary studies that have the participants blinded to the hypothesis can greatly enhance the believability of these putative associations.

Individual Impact-Frequency and Severity of Attacks

Migraine is a disabling disorder with an impact on both the individual and society. The individual impact of migraine is measured by quantifying the symptom profile and the frequency and severity of attacks, as well as through quality of life studies.

The individual impact of migraine has been evaluated in numerous studies (Stewart et al. 1992, 1994, 1996b; Lipton and

Stewart 1993). In a population study of 1748 migraine sufferers identified by telephone interview, approximately 40% of subjects (female 39%; male 46%) reported severe pain, while an additional 40% reported very severe pain (female 43%; male 32%). The remainder of subjects reported pain that ranged from mild to moderate.

Most migraine sufferers reported a range of symptoms other than pain including photophobia (overall 82%; female 84%; male 77%) and phonophobia (overall 78%; female 79%; male 73%). More than half (59%) of migraine sufferers reported nausea that accompanies their migraine headache more than half of the time (female 62%; male 47%), while only a small proportion reported vomiting.

Most subjects reported one to two migraine attacks per month. The duration of an untreated attack varies considerably by gender. Among females, approximately 71% of attacks last longer than 24 hours. In contrast, 48% of males reported attacks that last longer than 24 hours. These results are comparable to the results of previous studies (Stewart et al. 1992, 1994; Lipton and Stewart 1993).

There have been at least three population-based studies of health related quality of life (HRQoL) in migraine cases versus controls (Terwindt et al. 1998; Lipton et al. 1999a; Steiner et al. 1999). In all of these studies, migraine sufferers had substantially lower HRQoL relative to population controls. In addition, HRQoL was inversely related to attack frequency and disability (Terwindt et al. 1998; Lipton et al. 1999a). One clinic-based study (Osterhaus et al. 1994) found that migraine sufferers have HRQoL scores similar to patients with osteoarthritis, hypertension, or diabetes. However, HRQoL measured in clinic-based samples may differ from that of migraine sufferers in the community. In addition, many studies conducted in clinic-based samples lack a contemporaneous control group derived from the same source population or sample (e.g., neurology clinic).

Economic Impact of Migraine Headache

The direct costs of migraine care may include outpatient visits, hospitalization, the use of emergency department services, the cost of prescriptions and diagnostic tests, as well as other treatments. For migraine, most of the direct costs are due to outpatient visits and the cost of prescription medications, rather than hospitalization (Stang and Osterhaus 1993; Clouse and Osterhaus 1994), or are due to the use of emergency department services (Celentano et al. 1992; Edmeads et al. 1993; Clouse and Osterhaus 1994).

Few studies have assessed medical care for migraine in economic terms. In a population sample, Hu et al. (1999) estimated the annual costs of migraine treatment. They found that the annual treatment costs for migraine were over $1 billion, about $100 per migraine sufferer per year. These are likely to be underestimates because the figures were derived from 1994 data, and consultation and medication use have increased substantially over recent years (Lipton et al. 1999b). Clouse and Osterhaus (1994) reported similar, though slightly higher, average claim costs per member per month ($145). Since migraine sufferers are likely to have comorbid conditions, the increased costs may reflect the costs due to the treatment of migraine as well as other medical conditions.

Lost productivity time is the major determinant of the indirect economic impact of migraine. When estimating indirect costs, it is important to account not only for lost workdays due to migraine (absenteeism) but also reduced productivity while at work. Some studies have asked patients to report absenteeism or reduced production over 1 year; however, the accuracy of recall over this period is uncertain (Rasmussen et al. 1992; Stewart et al. 1996b; Schwartz et al. 1997). For some purposes, it is desirable to combine lost workdays (absenteeism) and reduced effectiveness days into an overall measure, often termed lost workday equivalent (LWDE). The

LWDE equals the total days of missed work plus the number of days at work with headache multiplied by the estimated decrease in percent effectiveness for working with headache (Stewart et al. 1996b).

Example 13–5 To circumvent limitations of prior studies, Von Korff et al. (1998) conducted a population-based diary study. Individuals recorded missed time from work and reduced productivity on a daily basis for 3 months. During this 3-month period, migraine sufferers missed an average of 1.1 days per month due to headache. Subjects who worked during a migraine attack reported work effectiveness that was reduced by an average of 41%. The missed workday and LWDE estimates reported by Von Korff et al. (1998) are higher than those reported in other population-based studies (Osterhaus et al. 1992, Stang and Osterhaus 1993; van Roijen et al. 1995, Stewart et al. 1996b). The use of a daily diary may have improved the accuracy of reporting, which is inherently limited by asking people to recall events over the past 3 to 12 months. A relatively small percentage of migraine sufferers account for the majority of lost work time. In this study, the most disabled 20% of the participants accounted for 77% of the missed workdays; 40% of subjects accounted for 75% of the total LWDEs (Von Korff et al. 1998).

Recently, Hu et al. (1999) used the human capital method to estimate the indirect costs of migraine. These studies assume that the economic value of a missed day of work is equivalent to the lost wages for that day. According to the results of this population-based study, Hu et al. estimated that migraine costs American employers $13 billion per year because of absenteeism and reduced effectiveness at work. Approximately 62% of the cost was due to absenteeism. Importantly, the greatest indirect costs were found among middle-age (30–49) individuals. Although this study provided important information, the human capital method values the indirect costs of the disease according to the sufferers' salary. A lost workday is valued by the individuals' wages for that day, therefore the impact of the disease in a laborer or homemaker would be valued lower than that of a business executive with a high salary. A limitation of all studies reported to date is that reduced productivity while at work when suffering from a migraine is based on self-report. No studies to date have actually quantified reductions in productivity.

Tension-type Headache

Case Definition

Tension-type headache (TTH) is diagnosed on the basis of a characteristic symptom profile and the exclusion of secondary headache (Table 13–3). In TTH, there is no prodrome or aura. The headache is usually bilateral, with pressing, tightening, or squeezing pain of mild to moderate intensity. Tension-type headaches are of two major forms, episodic tension-type headache (ETTH) and chronic tension-type headache (CTTH) (see Table 13–3). The major difference between these disorders is the frequency of headache attacks. If headaches occur less than 15 days per month, they are classified as ETTH, while those that occur 15 or more days per month are classified as CTTH. For ETTH, nausea excludes the diagnosis but one of either photophobia or phonophobia is permitted. For CTTH, any one of nausea, photophobia, or phonophobia may occur; if more than one of these features is present, the diagnosis is excluded.

Most subjects with ETTH (90%) report mild to moderate headache pain; attacks typically occur 3 times per month (Rasmussen et al. 1991; Gobel et al. 1994; Lavados and Tenhamm 1998; Schwartz et al. 1998). Chronic tension-type headache, by contrast, is typically associated with higher pain intensity and more frequent attacks. By definition, CTTH headache frequency ranges from 15 to 30 headaches per

Table 13–3 International Headache Society Diagnostic Criteria for Episodic Tension-Type Headache and Chronic Tension-Type Headache

a. Episodic tension-type headache	b. Chronic tension-type headache
Description	Description
Recurrent episodes of headache lasting minutes to days. The pain is typically pressing/tightening in quality, of mild or moderate intensity, and bilateral in location, and it does not worsen with routine physical activity. Nausea is absent, but photophobia or phonophobia may be present.	Headache is present for at least 15 days a month for at least 6 months. The headache is usually pressing/tightening in quality, mild or moderate in severity, and bilateral, and it does not worsen with routine physical activity. Nausea, photophobia, or phonophobia may occur.
Diagnostic Criteria	Diagnostic Criteria

A. At least 10 previous headache episodes fulfilling criteria B–D listed below. Number of days with headache <180 per year (<15 per month)
B. Headache lasting from 30 minutes to 7 days
C. At least two of the following pain characteristics:
  1. Pressing/tightening (non-pulsating) quality
  2. Mild or moderate intensity (may inhibit, but does not prohibit activities)
  3. Bilateral location
  4. No aggravation by walking stairs or similar routine physical activity
D. Both of the following:
  1. No nausea or vomiting (anorexia may occur)
  2. Photophobia and phonophobia are absent, or one but not the other is present
E. At least one of the following:
  1. History and physical and neurological examinations do not suggest symptomatic headache.
  2. History and/or physical and/or neurological examinations do suggest such disorder, but it is ruled out by appropriate investigations.
  3. Such disorder is present, but tension-type headache does not occur for the first time in close temporal relation to the disorder.
	A. Average headache frequency 15 days per month (180 days per year) for 6 months fulfilling criteria B–D listed below
	B. At least two of the following pain characteristics:
	  1. Pressing/tightening quality
	  2. Mild or moderate intensity (may inhibit, but does not prohibit activities)
	  3. Bilateral location
	  4. No aggravation by walking stairs or similar routine physical activity
	C. Both of the following:
	  1. No vomiting
	  2. No more than one of the following: nausea, photophobia, phonophobia
	D. At least one of the following:
	  1. History and physical and neurological examinations do not suggest symptomatic headache.
	  2. History and/or physical and/or neurological examinations do suggest such disorder, but it is ruled out by appropriate investigations.
	  3. Such disorder is present, but tension-type headache does not occur for the first time in close temporal relation to the disorder.

month (Gobel et al. 1994; Schwartz et al. 1998). In one study, 86% of subjects with CTTH reported moderate or severe pain (moderate, 44%; severe, 42%) (Gobel et al. 1994). Using a 10-point scale, Schwartz et al. (1998) found significantly higher pain intensity scores among CTTH subjects than among ETTH subjects (CTTH, 5.55; ETTH, 4.98; $p < 0.001$).

The clinical profile of TTH varies by gender. Bilateral pain occurs in most TTH sufferers, but occurs with even greater frequency among women than among men (Lavados and Tenhamm 1998). Throbbing pain occurs approximately equally in 66%

of men and 57% of women; this feature, often viewed as a hallmark of migraine, poorly discriminates the two disorders. Pressing pain is also frequently reported. Many subjects with TTH report that pain is exacerbated with movement (men, 70%; women, 76%), which is surprising since pain that is exacerbated by movement is normally associated with migraine rather than TTH. Photophobia or phonophobia is common, especially in women. If both features are present simultaneously, the diagnosis of TTH is excluded; however, each feature occurs in isolation with surprising frequency.

Prevalence

Published studies of the epidemiology of TTH have produced estimates for the 1-year period prevalence, which range between 14% (Lavados and Tenhamm 1998) and 93% (Rasmussen et al. 1991) for ETTH and 0% (Tekle-Haimanot et al. 1995; Lavados and Tenhamm 1998) to 8% (Tekle-Haimanot et al. 1995) for CTTH. Variation in prevalence estimates may be due in part to differences in study methodology. Lifetime prevalences are higher than 1-year period prevalences. Demographic factors, such as age of the population, influence prevalence estimates, and case definition, also plays a role. Studies have used various levels of diagnostic specificity; some studies group all TTH (IHS 2.0) subjects together, while other studies distinguish between subjects with ETTH, (IHS 2.1), those with CTTH (IHS 2.2), and those with headache of the tension type fulfilling all criteria except one (IHS 2.3). Data collection methods may also influence prevalence estimates. Methods of data collection (e.g., self-administered questionnaires, telephone interviews, and clinical examinations) as well as the quality of data collection contribute to variation in diagnostic accuracy. Finally, the source of the study population, community based or clinic based, is likely to cause varying prevalence estimates.

There has been one large-scale population survey in the United States describing the epidemiology of IHS-defined ETTH and CTTH (Schwartz et al. 1998). Data from a telephone interview survey of 13,345 residents of the Baltimore County, Maryland area (Stewart et al. 1996a) were used to estimate the 1-year period prevalence of ETTH and CTTH by gender, age, education, and race. The 1-year period prevalence of ETTH in the past year was 38%.

In Santiago, Chile, Lavados and Tenhamm (1998) conducted in-person interviews in a representative sample of 1385 adults (>14 years old). Subjects reported details about the type of headache they suffered most often. The 1-year prevalence of ETTH was 24%. The lower prevalence in this study compared to the U.S. study (Schwartz et al. 1998) may be explained by differences in case definition. In Santiago, only a subject's most common type of headache was eligible to be classified. Classification based on a single headache type in the U.S. study yielded a prevalence estimate of 25% vs. 38% after the second headache type was classified.

In a Danish study, prevalence estimates for ETTH were higher than in most other studies (Rasmussen et al. 1991). Potential participants were identified from the Danish National Central Person Registry and invited to a general health examination, with an emphasis on headache. In this study of 740 subjects, the 1-year period prevalence of ETTH was 74%. Since potential subjects were invited to a health exam with an emphasis on headache, individuals who had headaches may have been more likely to participate.

The prevalence of CTTH is markedly lower than that of ETTH. Across studies, 1-year period prevalence estimates range from 1.7%–2.2% (Rasmussen et al. 1991; Takle-Haimanot et al. 1995; Lavados and Tenhamm 1998; Schwartz et al. 1998; Castillo et al. 1999). Overall, 4% to 5% of the population reports headaches 15 or more days per month (Castillo et al. 1999).

Prevalence by Age and Gender. The prevalence of both ETTH and CTTH varies with gender and age. Tension-type headache is slightly more common among females than among males. For example, in the United States, 42% of females and 36% of males have ETTH, yielding an overall gender prevalence ratio of 1.16 (Schwartz et al. 1998). The female preponderance occurs at all ages and educational levels and in all races. Several other studies also reported a higher prevalence of TTH among women (Rasmussen et al. 1991; Pryse-Phillips et al. 1992; Wong et al. 1995; Barea et al. 1996; Wang et al. 1997; Lavados and Tenhamm 1998), with female-to-male gender ratios ranging from 1.25 (Rasmussen et al. 1991) to 1.9 (Lavados and Tenhamm 1998).

The female preponderance for CTTH is substantially greater than that of ETTH. For example, in the United States, the prevalence of CTTH was reported at 2.8% in women and 1.4% in men, for an overall gender prevalence ratio of 2.0 (Schwartz et al. 1998). Other studies have also reported a female preponderance in CTTH (Tekle-Haimanot et al. 1995; Lavados and Tenhamm 1998; Castillo et al. 1999). The female preponderance in CTTH falls between that of ETTH and migraine.

The prevalence of TTH may vary by age, though results are inconsistent across studies. Several studies showed that TTH prevalence peaks in the 30s and 40s, with a decline thereafter (Pryse-Phillips et al. 1992; Wong et al. 1995; Lavados and Tenhamm 1998; Schwartz et al. 1998). One study suggested that prevalence decreases with age (Rasmussen et al. 1991), and one found no difference in prevalence by age (Gobel et al. 1994). The lack of association with age in the latter study may be due to the use of wider age groupings than that in the other studies (20-year intervals vs. 10-year intervals).

Several authors reported that the prevalence of CTTH increases with age (Tekle-Haimanot 1995; Lavados and Tenhamm 1998; Schwartz et al. 1998). Perhaps individuals develop ETTH, which gradually increases over time until criteria for CTTH are met (Langemark et al. 1988; Rasmussen 1995).

Prevalence by Race and Geographic Region. Geographic and racial differences may account for part of the variation in the prevalence of TTH among studies. According to the results of reported studies, prevalence appears to be highest in the Western Hemisphere (Pryse-Phillips et al. 1992; Lavados and Tenhamm 1998; Schwartz et al. 1998) and Denmark (Rasmussen et al. 1991), and lowest in the Asian countries (Wong et al. 1995).

A U.S. study examined prevalence of TTH by race (Schwartz et al. 1998). The prevalence of ETTH was significantly higher in whites than in African Americans in both men (40% vs. 23%) and women (47 vs. 31%). The prevalence of CTTH by race paralleled the observations for ETTH: prevalence was higher in whites than in African Americans in both men (1.6% vs. 1.0%) and women (3.0% vs. 2.2%).

Prevalence by Education. The relationship between socioeconomic status and the prevalence of ETTH varies among studies. Schwartz et al. (1998) used educational level as a measure of socioeconomic status. Prevalence was directly related to education, peaking in those with a graduate-level education (men 48.5%; women 48.9%). Similarly, Lavados and Tenhamm (1998) found a direct relationship between ETTH prevalence and socioeconomic status. Other studies have not found this direct association (Pryse-Phillips et al. 1992; Gobel et al. 1994). A German study using only two educational categories (i.e., basic and secondary) did not find such a relationship (Gobel et al. 1994), but this approach may have lacked the power to detect an effect. The influence of socioeconomic status may also vary by country.

The socioeconomic pattern for CTTH is different from that of ETTH. Two studies reported that the prevalence of CTTH declined with increasing educational level, especially among women (Lavados and Tenhamm 1998; Schwartz et al. 1998). This pattern is similar to findings in migraine. Schwartz et al. (1998) suggested that the epidemiology of CTTH, with its higher risk in women and strong relationship to socioeconomic status, has an epidemiologic profile intermediate between that of ETTH and migraine and may reflect the progression of both headache types to a chronic form.

Economic Impact of Tension-type Headache

The first population-based study to examine work loss data in ETTH was reported by Rasmussen et al. (1992) in Denmark.

Among employed participants, 12% were absent from work at least once during the previous year because of ETTH. Of those who missed work, the majority (68%) were absent from 1 to 7 days during the previous year. Twenty-five percent (25%) were absent between 8 and 14 days during the year, and only 16% were absent more than 14 days during the previous year.

Schwartz et al. also measured the impact of headache in the workplace in a study conducted in Baltimore County, Maryland (Schwartz et al. 1997, 1998). Reduced ability to function and inability to function (actual missed work) were measured separately. Of the lost work time associated with headache, 19% of the missed workdays and 22% of the reduced-effectiveness days were specifically due to ETTH (Schwartz et al. 1997). Among subjects with ETTH, 8% reported missed workdays (absenteeism), while 44% reported reduced-effectiveness days at work due to headache. Among those with missed workdays, an average of 8.9 missed workdays were reported, while subjects with reduced-effectiveness days reported approximately 5.0 reduced-effectiveness days per person. Lavados and Tenhamm (1998) found higher levels of missed work among their sample of TTH sufferers: 25% of males and 39% of females reported missed work due to their headaches.

The proportions of subjects with CTTH and ETTH who report lost and reduced-effectiveness days were similar: 12% of CTTH sufferers reported lost workdays and 47% reported reduced-effectiveness days. Sufferers of CTTH reported more frequently lost workdays and reduced-effectiveness days in comparison with ETTH sufferers. Subjects with lost workdays reported an average of 27.4 lost workdays per person; subjects with reduced-effectiveness days reported approximately 20.4 reduced-effectiveness days per person.

Future Directions and Conclusions

For individuals with headache, particularly chronic headaches or migraine, the ques-

tion remains: why do most of these individuals suffer while others exposed to the same factors do not develop migraine? The etiology of these conditions is in need of focused studies that use the best epidemiologic study methods, including rigorous case definition. Genetic studies will provide a set of clues that should prove helpful to the prevention and treatment of the disease. These studies will need to be expanded to not only affected families but also broader population-based studies or other innovative designs so that the genetic components can be identified, as well as the environmental features. In the future, descriptive epidemiology needs to give way to analytic epidemiology to identify risk factors, possible susceptibility genes, and factors that trigger episodes among people who suffer from migraine headaches.

Migraine has been studied far more often than tension-type headache. Future research should also seek to expand our understanding of the variation in tension-type headache prevalence among certain subgroups, as well as to heighten our awareness of the impact tension-type headache has on the individual and society.

References

Abu-Arefeh I, Russell G. Prevalence of headache and migraine in schoolchildren. *BMJ* 1994; 309:765–769.

Arregui A, Cabrera J, Leon-Velarde F, et al. High prevalence of migraine in a high-altitude population. *Neurology* 1991;41: 1668–1669.

Barea L, Tannhauser M, Rotta N. An epidemiologic study of headache among children and adolescents of southern Brazil. *Cephalalgia* 1996;16:545–549.

Breslau N, Chilcoat H, Andreski P. Further evidence on the link between migraine and neuroticism. *Neurology* 1996;47:663–667.

Breslau N, Davis G, Andreski P. Migraine, psychiatric disorders, and suicide attempts: an epidemiologic study of young adults. *Psychiatry Res* 1991;37:11–23.

Breslau N, Rasmussen BK. The impact of migraine. Epidemiology, risk factors, and co-morbidities. *Neurology* 2001;56:S4–S12.

Brown N, Rips L, Shevell S. The subjective dates of natural events in very long–term memory. *Cognit Psychol* 1985;17:139–177.

Castillo J, Munoz P, Guitera V, Pascual J. Epidemiology of chronic daily headache in the general population. *Headache* 1999;39:190–196.

Celentano D, Stewart W, Lipton R, Reed M. Medication use and disability among migraineurs: a national probability sample survey. *Headache* 1992;32:223–228.

Clouse J, Osterhaus J. Healthcare resource use and costs associated with migraine in a managed healthcare setting. *Ann Pharmacother* 1994;28:659–664.

Cooke LJ, Rose MS, Becker WJ. Chinook winds and migraine headache. *Neurology* 2000;54:302–307.

Cummings R, Kelsey J, Nevitt M. Methodologic issues in the study of frequent and recurrent health problems. *Ann Epidemiol* 1990;1:49–56.

Edmeads J, Findlay H, Tugwell P, et al. Impact of migraine and tension-type headache on life-style, consulting behavior, and medication use: a Canadian population survey. *Can J Neurol Sci* 1993;20:131–137.

Franceschi M, Colombo B, Rossi P, Canal N. Headache in a population-based elderly cohort: an ancillary study to the Italian Longitudinal Study of Aging (ILSA). *Headache* 1997;37:79–82.

Gobel H, Petersen-Braun M, Soyka D. The epidemiology of headache in Germany: a nationwide survey of a representative sample on the basis of the headache classification of the International Headache Society. *Cephalalgia* 1994;14:97–106.

Hu X, Markson L, Lipton R, et al. Burden of migraine in the United States: disability and economic costs. *Arch Intern Med* 1999;159:813–818.

Johannes C, Linet M, Stewart W, et al. Relationship of headache to phase of the menstrual cycle among young women: a daily diary study. *Neurology* 1995;45:1076–1082.

Kryst S, Scherl E. A population-based survey of the social and personal impact of migraine. *Headache* 1994;34:344–350.

Langemark M, Olesen J, Poulsen D, Bech P. Clinical characterization of patients with chronic tension headache. *Headache* 1988;28:590–596.

Lavados P, Tenhamm E. Epidemiology of tension-type headache in Santiago, Chile: a prevalence study. *Cephalalgia* 1998;18:552–558.

Lipton RB. Fair winds and foul headaches. *Neurology* 2000;54:280–281.

Lipton R, Liberman J, Kolodner K, et al. Migraine headache disability and quality of life: a population-based case–control study. *Headache* 1999a;39:365.

Lipton RB, Stewart WF. Migraine in the United States: a review of epidemiology and health care use. *Neurology* 1993;43(suppl 3):S6–S10.

Lipton R, Stewart W. Epidemiology and comorbidity of migraine. In: Goadsby PJ, Silberstein SD, eds. Headache. London: Butterworth-Heineman, 1997, pp 201–226.

Lipton R, Stewart W, Celentano D, Reed M. Undiagnosed migraine headaches: a comparison of symptom-based and reported physician diagnosis. *Arch Intern Med* 1992;152:1273–1278.

Lipton R, Stewart W, Kolodner K, Liberman J. Epidemiology and patterns of health care use for migraine in the United States. *Headache* 1999b;39:363–364.

Lipton R, Stewart W, Simon D. Medical consultation for migraine: results of the American migraine study. *Headache* 1998;38:87–90.

O'Brien B, Goeree R, Streiner D. Prevalence of migraine headache in Canada: a population-based survey. *Int J Epidemiol* 1994;23:1020–1026.

Olesen J. Classification and diagnostic criteria for headache disorders, cranial neuralgias and facial pain. Classification Committee of the International Headache Society. *Cephalalgia* 1988;8(Suppl 7):1–96.

Olesen J, Tfelt-Hansen P, Welch KMA. The Headache. New York: Raven Press, 1993.

Osterhaus JT, Gutterman DL, Plachetka JR. Healthcare resource and lost labour costs of migraine headache in the US. *PharmacoEconomics* 1992;1:67–76.

Osterhaus J, Townsend R, Gandek B, Ware J. Measuring functional status and well-being of patients with migraine headache. *Headache* 1994;34:337–343.

Pryse-Phillips W, Findlay H, Tugwell P, et al. A Canadian population survey on the clinical, epidemiologic and societal impact of migraine and tension-type headache. *Can J Neurol Sci* 1992;19:333–339.

Rasmussen B. Migraine and tension-type headache in a general population: psychosocial factors. *Int J Epidemiol* 1992;21:1138–1143.

Rasmussen B. Epidemiology of headache. *Cephalalgia* 1995;15:45–68.

Rasmussen B, Jensen R, Olesen J. Impact of headache on sickness absence and utilisation of medical services: a Danish population study. *J Epidemiol Commun Health* 1992;46:443–446.

Rasmussen B, Jensen R, Schroll M, Olesen J. Epidemiology of headache in a general population: a prevalence study. *J Clin Epidemiol* 1991;44:1147–1157.

Russell MB, Olesen J. Increased familial risk and evidence of genetic factor in migraine. *BMJ* 1995;311:541–544

Russell MB, Olesen J. Migrainous disorder and its relation to migraine without aura and migraine with aura. A genetic epidemiological study. *Cephalalgia* 1996;16:431–435.

Russell MB, Ostergaard S, Bendtsen L, Olesen J. Familial occurrence of chronic tension-type headache. *Cephalalgia* 1999;19:207–210

Scher A, Stewart W, Lipton R. Migraine and headache: a meta-analytic approach. In: Crombie I, ed. Epidemiology of Pain. Seattle: IASP Press, 1999, pp 159–170.

Schwartz B, Stewart W, Lipton R. Lost workdays and decreased work effectiveness associated with headache in the workplace. *J Occup Environ Med* 1997;39:320–327.

Schwartz BS, Stewart WF, Simon D, Lipton RB. Epidemiology of tension-type headache. *JAMA* 1998;279:381–383.

Silberstein S, Lipton R, Goadsby P. Headache in Clinical Practice. Oxford: Isis Medical Media Ltd., 1998.

Stang P, Osterhaus J. Impact of migraine in the United States: data from the National Health Interview Survey. *Headache* 1993;33:29–35.

Stang P, Yanagihara T, Swanson J, et al. Incidence of migraine headache: a population-based study in Olmstead County, Minnesota. *Neurology.* 1992;42:1657–1662.

Steiner TJ, Lipton RB, Liberman JN, et al. Work and family impact of migraine: a population-based case–control study. *Neurology* 1999; 52(Suppl 2):A470–A471.

Stewart WF, Linet M, Celentano D, et al. Age- and sex-specific incidence rates of migraine with and without visual aura. *Am J Epidemiol* 1991;134:1111–1120.

Stewart WF, Lipton RB, Celentano DD, Reed ML. Prevalence of migraine headache in the United States: relation to age, income, race, and other sociodemographic factors. *JAMA* 1992;267:64–69.

Stewart WF, Lipton RB, Liberman J. Variation in migraine prevalence by race. *Neurology* 1996a;16:231–238.

Stewart W, Lipton R, Simon D. Work-related disability: results from the American migraine study. *Cephalalgia* 1996b;16:231–238.

Stewart W, Schechter A, Lipton R. Migraine heterogeneity: disability, pain intensity, and attack frequency and duration. *Neurology* 1994;44(Suppl 4):S24–S39.

Stewart W, Simon D, Schechter A, Lipton R. Population variation in migraine prevalence: a meta-analysis. *J Clin Epidemiol* 1995;48: 269–280.

Stewart WF, Staffa J, Lipton RB, Ottman R. Familial risk of migraine: a population-based study. *Ann Neurol* 1997;41:166–172.

Tekle-Haimanot R, Seraw B, Forsgren L, et al. Migraine, chronic tension-type headache, and cluster headache in an Ethiopian rural community. *Cephalalgia* 1995;15:482–488.

Terwindt G, Launer L, Ferrari M. The impact of migraine on quality of life in the general population: the GEM study. *Neurology* 1998;50(Suppl 4):A434.

Van den Bergh V, Amery WK, Waalkens J. Trigger factors in migraine: a study conducted by the Belgian Migraine Society. *Headache* 1987;27:191–196.

Van Den Eeden SK, Koepsell TD, Longstreth WT Jr, et al. Aspartame ingestion and headaches: a randomized crossover trial. *Neurology* 1994;44:1787–1793.

van Roijen L, Essink-Bot M, Koopmanschap M, et al. Societal perspective on the burden of migraine in the Netherlands. *PharmacoEconomics* 1995;7:170–179.

Von Korff M, Stewart WF, Simon DS, Lipton RB. Migraine and reduced work performance: a population-based diary study. *Neurology* 1998;50:1741–1745.

Wang S, Liu H, Fuh J, et al. Prevalence of headaches in a Chinese elderly population in Kinmen: age and gender effect and cross-cultural comparisons. *Neurology* 1997;49: 195–200.

Wong T, Wong K, Yu T, Kay R. Prevalence of migraine and other headaches in Hong Kong. *Neuroepidemiology* 1995;14:82–91.

14

Intracranial Neoplasms

MARGARET WRENSCH, YURIKO MINN, TERRI CHEW,
AND MELISSA BONDY

Primary intracranial tumors account for 95% of all primary nervous system tumors; extracranial nervous system tumors have rarely, if ever, been the subject of separate epidemiologic study. Therefore, this chapter deals mainly with primary brain (not other nervous system) tumors.

Primary brain tumors are benign or malignant tumors that arise in the brain or its meningeal lining. Although primary brain tumors are relatively rare compared to more common cancers, such as lung, breast, prostate, and colorectal, about 36,000 people in the United States are diagnosed annually with primary brain tumors, and nearly 13,000 people die from these tumors (Central Brain Tumor Registry of the United States 2002). One-fourth of all cancer deaths in children are from brain tumors (Grovas et al. 1997).

Much work remains to discover the causes of most human brain tumors. Established environmental and genetic risk factors account for only a small proportion of these diseases. However, increasing in-terest in and knowledge about both neurobiology and cancer, improved tools for molecular classification of tumors, and the recent availability of etiologically relevant polymorphisms may help to determine who gets brain tumors and why.

Taxonomy of Intracranial Neoplasms

Table 14–1 shows the currently accepted taxonomy of primary brain and central nervous system tumors. Most primary brain tumors are gliomas (48%) or meningiomas (24%). Gliomas are tumors of the non-neuronal, or glial, cells of the brain; they are usually malignant. Meningiomas occur in the meningeal lining of the brain; while usually noninvasive, they can cause permanent neurologic damage and can be lethal.

Over the past decade, we and others have reviewed brain tumor epidemiology (Bondy et al. 1994; Berleur and Cordier 1995; Inskip et al. 1995; Preston-Martin and Mack 1996; Wrensch et al. 2000b, 2002).

Table 14–1 Taxonomy of Primary Brain and Central Nervous System Tumors

Histologic group*	Median age at diagnosis (years)	Alternate names used in epidemiologic literature	Review articles
I. Tumors of neuroepithelial tissue		Glioma: I1–I4 and	Wrensch et al. 2002
1. Astrocytoma		some of I6	Wrensch et al. 1993
Glioblastoma	64	Brain cancer or	Inskip et al. 1995
Anaplastic astrocytoma	50	primary malignant	Preston-Martin and
Diffuse astrocytoma	49	brain tumor refers to	Mack 1996
(protoplasmic, fibrillary)		all primary tumors of	Berleur and Cordier 1995
Pilocytic astrocytoma	12	malignant behavior	Bondy et al. 1994
Unique astrocytoma variants	30	regardless of tissue type.	SEER: http://www.
Astrocytoma, NOS	48		seer.ims.nci.nih.gov/
2. Oligodendroglioma			publications/
Anaplastic oligodendroglioma	47		
Oligodendroglioma	39		
3. Ependymoma			
Ependymoma/anaplastic	37		
ependymoma			
Ependymoma variants	36		
4. Mixed glioma	39		
5. Embryonal/primitive/	8.5		
medulloblastoma			
6. Other			
Glioma malignant, NOS	48		
Choroid plexus	7		
Neuroepithelial	41		
Benign and malignant neuronal/	23		
glial, neuronal, and mixed			
Pineal parenchymal	27		
II. Tumors of the meninges		Benign brain tumor,	Bondy et al. 1996
1. Meningioma	65	meningioma	
2. Other mesenchymal, benign	42		
and malignant			
3. Hemangioblastoma	45		
III. Tumors of the sellar region		None	None
1. Pituitary	49		
2. Craniopharyngioma	36		
IV. Tumors of the cranial and spinal nerves		None	None
1. Nerve sheath, benign, and	52		
malignant			
2. Other tumors of cranial and	—		
spinal nerves			
V. Lymphomas and hemopoietic neoplasms		None	None
1. Lymphoma	55		
VI. Other		None	None
1. Germ cell tumors and cysts			
Germ cell tumors, cysts, and	17		
heterotopias			
2. Local extensions from regional			
tumors			
Chordoma/chondrosarcoma	65		
3. Unclassified tumors			
Hemangioma	43		
Neoplasm, unspecified	71		
Other	50		

NOS, not otherwise specified.

*Histologic groupings used are according to the Central Brain Tumor Registry of the United States, and Surawicz et al. (1999).

Preston-Martin and Mack (1996) provide the most comprehensive tables of results of general analytic epidemiologic studies published through 1994, listing risk factor or occupation/industry, study design, group and place studied, and estimated odds ratio(s) or other measures of relative risk. Bondy et al. (1994) provide a detailed overview of familial and inherited syndromes involved in brain tumors, with brief updated information on the potential etiologic role of polymorphisms in carcinogen metabolizing, DNA repair, or other genes. Berleur and Cordier (1995) provide superb overviews of pertinent experimental studies in animals and physiologic aspects of neurocarcinogenesis, including discussion of the blood–brain barrier. In their comprehensive review of adult brain tumors, Inskip et al. (1995) highlight the descriptive epidemiology of different subtypes of brain cancer and provide a particularly good discussion of molecular mechanisms in brain tumor pathogenesis. More recently, Wrensch et al. (2000b, 2002) and Davis and McCarthy (2000) have discussed the promising areas for research in etiology and prognosis and have emphasized the need for tumor markers to reduce heterogeneity of classifications. Bondy and Lignon (1996) has reviewed meningioma epidemiology, and Bunin (2000) has reviewed issues in childhood brain tumor epidemiology. Davis et al. (1999a) have reviewed issues in descriptive epidemiology of brain tumors.

In this chapter, we will not attempt to duplicate the detail presented in these reviews. Our primary aim is to give an overview of the basic epidemiology of brain tumors and to discuss commonly encountered methodologic issues and problems.

Gliomas include astrocytomas, oligodendrogliomas, and ependymomas, each named to reflect the type of glial cell from which they are thought to derive—i.e., astrocytes, oligodendrocytes, and ependymal cells, respectively. Mixed gliomas usually contain features of astrocytoma and oligodendroglioma, and are often referred to as oligoastrocytoma. Other mixed types, such as astrocytoma and ependymoma, have been reported. Clinical presentation varies widely depending on a tumor's location and size, and whether it is malignant or benign.

Astrocytomas account for about 39% of primary brain tumors, 60% of neuroepithelial tumors, and 83% of gliomas (Surawicz et al. 1999). The most commonly accepted grading nomenclature for astrocytomas is that used by the World Health Organization (WHO) (Kleihues and Cavenee 2000) (see Table 14–2). Higher grades predict worse prognosis (that is, shorter recurrence-free interval and survival). The four WHO grades are based on several histologic features, including nuclear features, mitotic activity, cellularity, vascular proliferation, and necrosis. WHO grade I (pilocytic) astrocytomas rarely undergo neoplastic transformation; grade II (low-grade astrocytomas or astrocytomas) tumors are infiltrative; grade III (anaplastic) astrocytomas are highly malignant gliomas and have an increased tendency to progress to glioblastoma; and WHO grade IV (glioblastoma multiforme) tumors are extremely aggressive brain tumors with very poor prognosis, largely because the tumor rapidly spreads to other regions of the brain. The median ages of onset of grade I–IV tumors are 12, 30–49, 50, and 64, respectively.

Oligodendrogliomas (WHO grade II) and anaplastic oligodendrogliomas (WHO grade III) account for about 3%–18% of primary brain tumors (Surawicz et al. 1999; Kleihues and Cavenee 2000) and are composed of cells that resemble oligodendroglia. About 2% of primary brain tumors are ependymomas arising from ependymal cells lining the ventricals of the brain (Kleihues and Cavenee 2000).

The histologic origins and classification of embryonal tumors such as medulloblastoma and other primitive neuroectodermal tumors remain controversial (Kleihues and Cavenee 2000). These tumors account for a large proportion of intracranial tumors in young children.

Meningiomas can be graded according to WHO criteria, and grades I–III are called

Table 14-2 Comparisons of Fibrillary Astrocytoma Grading Systems

Bailey and Cushing (1926)	Kernohan et al. (1949)	Ringertz (1950)	University of California, San Francisco	Modified Ringertz	St. Anne-Mayo (Daumas-Duport et al. 1988)	WHO2* (Kleihues et al. 1993)
Astrocytoma	Astrocytoma grade 1	Astrocytoma	Mildly anaplastic astrocytoma	Astrocytoma	Astrocytoma grade I	Astrocytoma (grade II)
	Astrocytoma grade 2		Moderately anaplastic astrocytoma		Astrocytoma grade II	
Astroblastoma		Intermediate type	Highly anaplastic astrocytoma	Anaplastic astrocytoma	Astrocytoma grade 3	Anaplastic astrocytoma (grade III)
Spongioblastoma multiforme	Astrocytoma grade 3 Astrocytoma grade 4	Glioblastoma multiforme	Glioblastoma multiforme	Glioblastoma multiforme	Astrocytoma grade 4	Glioblastoma multiforme (grade IV)

*(Kleihues, 1993) This is the currently accepted standard.

Reprinted with permission from Fuller (1996). Central nervous system tumors. In: Parham DM, ed. Pediatric Neoplasia: Morphology and Biology. Philadelphia: Lippincott-Raven.

meningioma, atypical meningioma, and anaplastic or malignant meningioma, respectively. Most (90%) of these are benign (grade I) tumors. Autopsy data have shown that a large proportion of meningiomas do not reach clinical detection, although the number that are being diagnosed secondarily to computed tomography (CT) and magnetic resonance imaging (MRI) is increasing (Bondy and Ligon 1996; Kleihues and Cavenee 2000).

Diagnostic Issues

Alternatives to the WHO criteria for grading astrocytomas (Table 14–2) complicate the descriptive epidemiology of gliomas. For example, the Kernohan system names tumors that would be called "glioblastoma" or "astrocytoma, grade 4 or IV" in other systems "astrocytoma, grade 3." Without help from a neuropathologist or other specialist, there is no simple way to determine which grading system a particular pathologist has used.

The use of molecular tumor markers may help to develop more objective, replicable, and consistently applied diagnostic criteria. Molecular subsets might be identified that could be useful in predicting prognosis or preferred treatment regimens.

> *Example 14–1* Patients whose oligodendrogliomas show losses of chromosomes 1p and 19q respond more favorably to chemotherapy than patients without this chromosomal loss (Cairncross et al. 1998). Also, certain etiologic factors might be more likely to lead to particular molecular changes, so subsets of tumors based on molecular changes might be more etiologically homogeneous than subsets based on histologic categories.

Molecular classification is such a rapidly developing field that any list of findings is soon out of date, but some important and durable observations are noteworthy. Glioblastoma multiforme appears to have at least two forms. One form seems to progress from lower-grade astrocytomas, has a longer clinical course measured in years, occurs in younger adult patients, and more likely involves p53 modification or loss of chromosome 17p (Kleihues and Cavenee 2000). Another form appears to arise de novo, has a shorter clinical course, occurs in older patients, and more likely involves amplification of epidermal growth factor receptor (EGFR) and loss of all or parts of chromosome 10 (which is thought to contain several tumor suppressor genes) (Kleihues and Cavenee 2000). There are likely to be other forms of glioblastoma. Phosphatase and tensin homologue deleted on chromosome 10 (PTEN) is commonly altered in glioblastoma but rarely in lower-grade tumors, a finding suggesting that this marker is involved in progression to higher-grade tumors (James et al. 2002). Meningiomas have long been observed to have deletions of chromosome 22. Since about 60% of meningiomas have alterations in the neurofibromatosis-2 (NF2) gene (Kleihues and Cavenee 2000), this is believed to be a major tumor suppressor gene on chromosome 22. Other genes on chromosome 22 and elsewhere are likely to be involved in the development of meningiomas.

Descriptive Studies

Methodologic Issues

Two major methodologic issues for descriptive epidemiology of brain tumors are diagnostic discrepancies and incomplete disease registration or ascertainment. Diagnostic discrepancies, as discussed above, pose a major difficulty in comparing rates of brain tumors among different regions of the United States and the world. Even within a relatively small geographic region, such as the San Francisco Bay Area, diagnostic discrepancies for some types of tumors can be substantial.

> *Example 14–2* A recent report by Aldape et al. (2000) found agreement among 77% of 457 diagnoses made by a review neuropathologist with the original diagnoses given in a population-based series

of adult neuroepithelial tumors. Although 95% of subjects originally diagnosed with glioblastoma were diagnosed with glioblastoma upon review, only 57% and 38% of subjects originally diagnosed with anaplastic astrocytoma or astrocytoma, respectively, received the identical diagnosis upon review. Bruner and colleagues (1997) found some disagreement in review and original diagnosis in 214/500 (43%) of consecutive brain or spinal cord biopsies submitted for neuropathology consultation, indicating that diagnostic discrepancies can be substantial.

Ascertainment biases introduced through geographic and socioeconomic variation in access to medical care, availability of sophisticated imaging equipment, and case registration criteria lead to enormous difficulties in interpreting international comparisons or temporal trends. For example, very high brain tumor rates of 21 per 100,000 (nearly double that found in even high-incidence areas) were recently found in two English Counties, which the authors attributed to exhaustive case-finding efforts (Pobereskin and Sneyd 2000). Given these concerns and the further problem that some countries present data for both benign and malignant brain tumors while others provide data only for malignant tumors, we will not present geographic comparisons here.

Several data sources exist for descriptive information about brain tumors. The Scandinavian tumor registries historically have had the most complete national ascertainment of primary brain tumors (Kreftregisteret 2002). The Connecticut Cancer Registry is the oldest in the United States, dating back to 1935 (Connecticut Department of Public Health 2002). The Surveillance, Epidemiology, and End Results (SEER) program of the National Cancer Institute has registered primary malignant brain tumors in the United States since 1973 (Surveillance, Epidemiology, and End Results 2002a). The Central Brain Tumor Registry of the United States (CBTRUS) database is the largest population-based source for primary brain tumor incidence in the United States and currently includes data from 12 state cancer registries, which collect information for both benign and malignant brain tumors.

The overall annual age-adjusted incidence rate of primary brain tumors in the United States is 11–12 per 100,000 individuals, and for primary malignant brain tumors is 6–7 per 100,000 (Central Brain Tumor Registry of the United States 2002). In addition to geographic variation, descriptive epidemiologic studies show variations in brain tumor incidence and mortality by age, gender, histologic type, time, intracranial site, and ethnicity.

Age and Gender

Overall, the average age of onset of primary brain tumors is 53. As shown in Table 14–1, the median ages of onset for glioblastoma and meningioma are 64 and 65, respectively. The age distributions of primary brain tumors vary considerably by site and histologic types, as shown in Figures 14–1 and 14–2. The peak observed in incidence of all brain tumors around age 65–75, due to peaks in this age group for glioblastoma and astrocytoma, has been attributed to incomplete diagnosis in the elderly, a contention supported by the observation that the peak has shifted to older ages with time. The incidence rate of meningioma does not drop off in the oldest age groups. As with other types of cancer, that incidence of most types of brain tumors increases with age could be due to the duration of exposure required for malignant transformation, the need for many genetic alterations prior to disease onset, or poorer immune surveillance with age. Age distributions for the three most common histologic types of primary childhood brain tumors show decreasing incidence with age, with higher rates in those 0–4 years of age and lowest rates in those 15–19 years of age (Fig. 14–2). Although risks of ependymoma, medulloblastoma, and pilocytic astrocytoma decrease substantially with age, these diseases occasionally occur even in middle age and late adulthood.

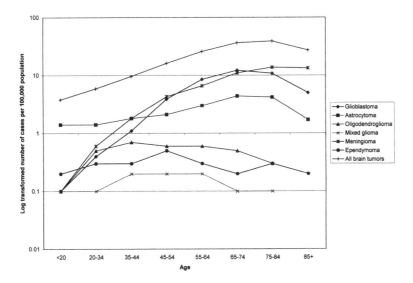

Figure 14–1 Primary brain tumor incidence rates by age for all and the most common histologic types, according to the Central Brain Tumor Registry of the United States, 1990–1994 (Central Brain Tumor Registry of the United States, 2000).

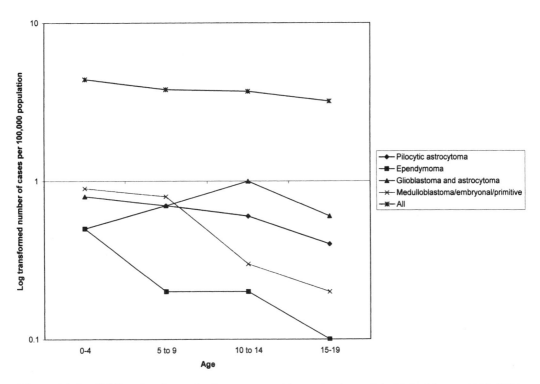

Figure 14–2 Childhood primary brain tumor incidence by age for all and the most common histologic types, according to the Central Brain Tumor Registry of the United States, 1990-1994 (Central Brain Tumor Registry of the United States, 2000).

341

Higher rates of glioma among males (Fig. 14–3) and of meningioma among females (Central Brain Tumor Registry of the United States 2002) are perhaps the most consistent epidemiologic findings for primary brain tumors. These gender differences are consistent across almost all ages and populations studied and should be accounted for in any comprehensive theory of the causes of brain tumors. McKinley et al. (2000) showed that the gender differential in glioblastoma begins around the age of menarche, is greatest around the age of menopause, and decreases thereafter, suggesting a protective effect of female hormones.

Time Trends and Ethnic Differences

The dramatic rise in malignant brain tumor rates between 1973 through the mid-1980s (Fig. 14–3) was apparent in most industrialized countries. Several recent articles have characterized, in depth, the increase in primary brain tumor rates in the United States (Smith et al. 1998; Legler et al. 1999; Gurney and Kadan-Lottick 2001). Much of the increase has been attributed to diagnostic improvements with computerized axial tomography (CAT) scanning and MRI, increased availability of neurosurgeons, and changing attitudes towards diagnosis in the elderly (Wrensch et al. 1993; Inskip et al. 1995; Preston-Martin and Mack 1996). However, many researchers also suggest that some of the increase (especially in childhood) may be due to changes in causal factors. Because inherited genes do not change in a single generation, environmental factors are suspect, but major candidates have yet to be identified.

Problems in exploring and understanding future temporal trends in brain tumor incidence can be minimized through rigorous registration to accurately track without bias changes in occurrence and survival of both benign and malignant brain tumors

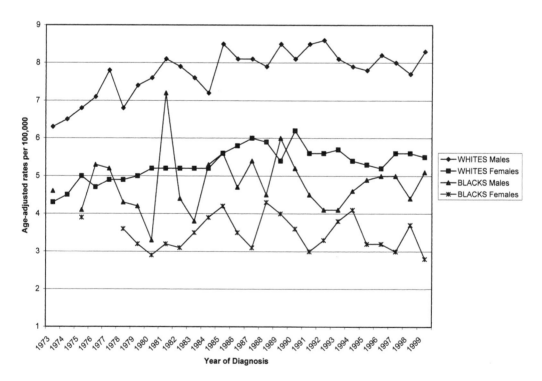

Figure 14–3 Age-adjusted incidence rates of primary malignant brain tumors by year and gender among blacks and whites (Surveillance, Epidemiology, and End Results, 2002b).

(Davis et al. 1996, 1997; Smith et al. 1998; Legler et al. 1999; Gurney and Kadan-Lottick 2001).

Malignant brain tumor rates are higher among whites than African Americans in the United States, and this is true for both men and women (Fig. 14–3). In contrast, meningioma rates are approximately equivalent among African Americans and whites in the United States (Central Brain Tumor Registry of the United States 2002).

Survival

For primary malignant brain tumors, improved survival is associated with lower histologic grade and younger age within each histologic grade. The location of a tumor and the extent of tumor resection are also factors predicting overall or progression-free survival (Curran et al. 1993; Davis et al. 1999b; Horn et al. 1999; Lopez-Gonzalez and Sotelo 2000; Nakamura et al. 2000). Although some progress has been made in treatment of lower-grade astrocytomas, oligodendrogliomas, and medulloblastoma, there has been essentially no improvement in survival for the most lethal and common type of brain tumor, glioblastoma multiforme, in the past 20 years (Davis et al. 1998). Overall 5-year survival for primary malignant brain tumors is about 27%, but remains a very dismal 4%–5% for people diagnosed at age 65 or older. Although there is much current research focusing on discovery of prognostic markers (Cairncross et al. 1998; Hagel et al. 1999; Mizumatsu et al. 1999; Strojnik et al. 1999; Huncharek and Kupelnick 2000; Grotzer et al. 2001; Simmons et al. 2001), age and grade remain the strongest predictors of survival.

Analytic Studies

Methodologic Issues in Identifying Brain Tumor Risk Factors

A PubMed search of key words ("brain neoplasms", "brain tumor", "glioblastoma", or "meningioma" and "epidemiology" or "risk factors") resulted in 3723 articles since 1990, 1154 in the 1980s, and 935 articles between 1966 and 1980. Despite the enormous increase in the numbers of studies, few risk factors for brain tumors have been consistently identified (Table 14–3). Furthermore, convincingly linked factors probably explain a relatively small proportion of the disease.

Part of the problem in identifying risk factors lies in methodologic difficulties arising from the nature of brain tumors. Brain tumors are relatively rare, thus the use of cohort studies is generally prohibited. Exceptions are cohort studies conducted in countries with population registration and socialized medicine that permit linking of population and patient data (e.g., Inskip et al. 1998) and some occupational and industrial cohort studies. Even these studies may have too few affected individuals to analyze interesting exposure subgroups. Therefore, most investigations have relied on case–control methodology, with concomitant problems involving misclassification of prior exposures and differential selection of cases and controls.

Malignant brain tumors are often rapidly fatal, and population-based studies must rely on proxy respondents for information on a substantial proportion of cases, leading to further inaccuracies in prior exposures or characteristics. Some studies have avoided this problem by conducting studies of cases seen at particular hospitals. Hospital-based studies eliminate the need for proxy respondents and facilitate the collection of blood specimens for genetic or serologic studies. However, the case group may not be representative of all cases (e.g., academic specialty centers tend to see patients who are on average younger and for whom a smaller proportion have glioblastoma than in the community as a whole [Aldape et al. 2000]), and selecting an appropriate control group may be problematic. Concerns with either population-based or hospital-based studies are further compounded by heterogeneity of primary brain tumors and the paucity of large-scale studies of homogeneous subtypes. In addition

Table 14–3 Factors Studied in Relations to Risk of Primary Brain Tumors of Neuroepithelial Tissue or Meninges

• Hereditary syndromes*: tuberous sclerosis, neurofibromatosis types 1 and 2, nevoid basal cell carcinoma syndrome, and adenomatous polyposis syndromes, Li-Fraumeni cancer family syndrome (inherited *p53* mutations)	• Epilepsy, seizures, or convulsions
	• Drugs and medications
• Family history of brain tumors	• Diet and vitamins: nitrosamine, nitrosamide, nitrate, or nitrite consumption, calcium, food frequency, cured foods
• Constitutive polymorphisms in glutathione transferases, cytochrome p450 2D6 and 1A1, n-acetyltransferase, ERCC1 and ERCC2, other carcinogen metabolizing, DNA repair, and immune function genes	• Tobacco smoke exposures
	• Alcohol
	• Hair dyes and sprays
	• Traffic-related air pollution
• Lymphocyte mutagen sensitivity to gamma radiation	• Occupations and industries: synthetic rubber manufacturing, vinyl chloride, petroleum refining/production work, licensed pesticide applicators, agricultural work, parental workplace exposures
• Prior cancers	
• Infectious agents or immunologic response: viruses (common colds, influenza, varicella zoster virus, BK, JC, others), *Toxoplasma gondii*	• Ionizing radiation Therapeutic*
• Allergies	Diagnostic and Other Sources
• Head trauma	• Cellular telephones
	• Other radio frequency exposures
	• Power frequency electromagnetic field

*These are the only factors that have been proven to cause primary brain tumors of neuroepithelial tissue or meninges. See text for evidence for or against associations of other factors.

Reproduced with permission from Wrensch M, Minny Y, Chew TC, et al. Epidemiology of brain tumors: current concepts and review of the literature. *Neurooncology* 2002;4:278–299.

to histologic and site heterogeneity, molecular studies suggest that there may be substantial etiologic heterogeneity even within a single category such as glioblastoma. If this is true, future studies may require more rigorous phenotypic classifications and may require very large source populations to ensure adequate numbers in each subgroup.

Another major impediment in retrospective exposure assessment is that the pertinent latency periods for most types of primary brain tumors remain undefined. As noted above, some glioblastomas progress from lower-grade tumors with a relatively long clinical course and presumably have long latency, whereas others seem to develop in a very short time frame.

Despite these obstacles, brain tumors are easier to study than many neurologic diseases because malignant types have been registered in SEER program regions in the United States since 1973. Furthermore, several of these registries have rapid case ascertainment programs enabling population-based studies. Knowledge garnered from the study of more common cancers may also help to elucidate causes of brain tumors.

Current models of carcinogenesis assert that cancers develop through accumulation of genetic errors or epigenetic misregulation that allows cells to grow out of control of normal regulatory mechanisms and/or escape destruction by the immune system. Candidate carcinogens include chemical, physical, and biologic agents that damage DNA, and inherited changes in cell-cycle control genes, such as *p53*. Developments in molecular biology, genetics, immunology, and virology will help elucidate molecular causes of brain tumors. Continuing epidemiologic work will clarify the relative roles of different mechanisms for the full scope of human brain tumors.

A few rare genes with high penetrance for causing cancer (Table 14–3) and exposures to therapeutic ionizing radiation (Table 14–3) are the only undisputed causes of primary brain tumors. They are undisputed because most studies of these factors show a positive association and there is biologic plausibility based on currently accepted conceptual models of carcinogenesis.

Although viruses are known to induce brain tumors in experimental animals, their role in human brain tumors has received little consideration, perhaps because the right concepts and tools have not been available to permit such study.

With regard to chemical carcinogens, Preston-Martin proposed study of N-nitroso compounds because these compounds are potent neurocarcinogens in experimental animals (reviewed in Preston-Martin and Mack 1996). Despite biologic plausibility for this class of chemical carcinogens, little progress has been made in determining its specific role in human brain tumors, partly because there are so many different sources of exposure to N-nitroso compounds that determining any individual's lifetime exposure is at best problematic and may be impossible. For other classes of chemical carcinogens, the primary exposures often come from occupational sources. However, because occupational or industrial cohorts usually have many relevant exposures, identifying which chemicals or processes are responsible for observed increased risks is complex. Although tobacco smoke is a known carcinogen for lung and other tissues, it has not consistently been shown to increase risk of brain tumors.

Even more equivocal than the risks associated with suspected chemical carcinogens are the risks from factors for which there is limited established biologic plausibility, such as extremely low-frequency electromagnetic fields (EMF) associated with the distribution and use of electricity.

Other seemingly relevant factors exhibit additional methodologic problems. Head injury and seizures, for example, are two possible, but not established, risk factors for brain tumors. Complexities in teasing apart the roles of these two factors involve bias, confounding, and order in the causal chain: head trauma might be subject to differential recall by those with and without a brain tumor, head trauma can cause seizures, and seizures may be an early symptom of brain tumors. Other factors that may be important, such as the role of the immune system in protecting against tumors, have received little attention until recently.

Given these problems, we present only a brief summary of genetic and environmental risk factors that have been studied in association with brain tumors (Table 14–3).

Genetic and Familial Factors

Genetic Predisposition. We refer to *genetically predisposed* individuals as those who have a rare gene or chromosomal abnormality that greatly increases their chances of developing a disease compared with the general population. As summarized in Table 14–3, hereditary syndromes such as tuberous sclerosis, neurofibromatosis types 1 and 2, nevoid basal cell carcinoma syndrome, and syndromes involving adenomatous polyps confer predisposition to brain or central nervous system tumors (Bondy et al. 1994). In addition, gross congenital malformations have been associated with brain tumors in case reports. For example, gastrointestinal and genitourinary system abnormalities have co-occurred with medulloblastoma. Also, some individuals with Down's syndrome, a disorder involving chromosome 21, have been reported to have central nervous system tumors.

Cancer family syndromes are heritable syndromes in which individuals in affected families have a greatly increased risk of developing certain types of cancers. One example is Li-Fraumeni syndrome (LFS), which predisposes individuals to brain tumors, sarcomas, breast cancer, and cancer of the adrenal gland. A copy of a defective gene (which in some families is the gene for *p53*, a protein involved in various aspects of cell-cycle control and programmed cell death) in LFS individuals may be passed from parent to child. Germline *p53* mutations also appear to be more common in patients with multifocal glioma, glioma and another primary tumor, or glioma plus a family history of cancer (Kyritsis et al. 1994). Furthermore, adult glioma patients with *p53* mutation-positive tumors may be more likely than those whose tumors were *p53* mutation negative to have had a first-degree relative affected with cancer and to have personal history of a previous cancer (Li et al. 1998). Inherited predisposition, though well documented as a causal etiologic factor, probably accounts for only a small percentage (5%–10%) of brain tumors (Narod et al. 1991; Wrensch et al. 1997a).

Familial Aggregation. Epidemiologic studies that compare family medical histories of brain tumor cases with those of controls provide further evidence of familial etiology. Relative risks for any cancer in families of brain tumor cases compared with control families have ranged from 1.0 to 1.8 and the relative risks of brain tumors in these families have ranged from nearly 1 to 10 (Bondy et al. 1994; Wrensch et al. 1997a; Malmer et al. 1999; Hemminki et al. 2000; Paunu et al. 2002).

The statistical genetics approach of segregation analysis has not yielded evidence for an effect of a single major gene in either childhood (Bondy et al. 1994) or adult brain tumors (de Andrade et al. 2001). This result, combined with the limited role of strong genetic predisposition, suggests that common familial exposures to environmental agents (Grossman et al. 1999), multifactorial genetic inheritance, and/or gene–environment interactions contribute to a majority of brain tumors.

Genetic Susceptibility. We use the term *genetic susceptibility* to refer to increased cancer risk arising from common genetic alterations that influence oxidative metabolism, carcinogen detoxification, DNA stability and repair, and immune function. We distinguish genetic predisposition from genetic susceptibility by the extent of in-

creased risk that arises from the inherited genetic alterations, referring to very high individual risk as predisposition and to lower-risk as susceptibility.

The role of genetic polymorphisms (alternate variants of genes that occur in >1% of the population) in modulating susceptibility to carcinogenic exposures has been of increasing interest. Due to rapid developments in genetic technology, genes involved in carcinogen detoxification, oxidative metabolism, DNA repair genes, and immune response are among an increasing number of potentially relevant polymorphisms available for epidemiologic evaluation. To date, the role of genetic polymorphisms has been the subject of some tobacco-related tumor studies, but has been less prominent in brain tumor research.

Example 14–3 Certain polymorphisms of the genes cytochrome p450 2D6, glutathione transferases θ and μ, rapid *n*-acetyltransferase acetylation, and excision repair cross-complementing (*ERCC1* and *ERCC2*) have been associated with brain tumors in some studies but not in others. Studies of other polymorphisms have found no association with glioma (Elexpuru-Camiruaga et al. 1995; Wiencke et al. 1997; Caggana et al. 2001; Peters et al. 2001). In population-based case–control studies it has been difficult to distinguish associations related to survival from those related to etiology because patients with poorest survival often do not live long enough for investigators to obtain blood or buccal specimens. This is an example of incidence-prevalence bias that may be particularly problematic with disorders such as brain tumors when survival is very short.

People inherit differences in their ability to repair DNA damaged by gamma-radiation. This mutagen sensitivity appears to be one of the few genetic susceptibilities for brain tumors that has been replicated in independent populations (Bondy et al. 1996, 2001). Other types of mutagen sensitivity might also be relevant to brain tumors (Shadan and Koziol 2000).

Several authors are currently investigating these and other potentially relevant markers. For example, El-Zein et al. (1999) found that glioma patients had much higher rates of chromosome instability in lymphocytes than controls. Future studies examining panels of relevant markers integrated with epidemiologic data on a large number of study subjects might help to clarify the role of genetic susceptibility and brain tumor risk.

Personal Medical History

Infections. The etiologic role of viruses in human neuro-oncogenesis has not been adequately evaluated (Wrensch et al. 1993; Berleur and Cordier 1995), but interest in this area is increasing. Although retroviruses, papovaviruses, and adenoviruses have been shown to cause brain tumors in experimental animals, the topic has received little attention in epidemiologic studies. Possible reasons for this include difficulties of designing meaningful studies, a scarcity of appropriately trained investigators, and emphases on other etiologic hypotheses. SV40 has been linked to brain tumors in epidemiologic studies, but determining whether SV40 precedes or follows tumor development has posed a major challenge. The polyomavirus BK and JC (a virus similar to SV40), and herpes virus 6 have also been investigated in relation to brain tumors (Huang et al. 1999; Krynska et al. 1999; Zhen et al. 1999; Cuomo et al. 2001; Del Valle et al. 2001; Wrensch et al. 2002), with no consensus on a causal connection.

Varicella zoster virus, which causes chicken pox and shingles, is another agent that has been considered in relation to brain tumors (reviewed in Wrensch et al. 2002). One study found that adults with glioma in the San Francisco Bay Area were significantly less likely to report having had either chicken pox or shingles than controls and also were less likely to have immunoglobulin G antibody to varicella zoster virus (Wrensch et al. 2001). Although several noncausal explanations are possible, these results, combined with studies showing that people with brain cancer are less likely than controls to report allergies (see below) and common infections, suggest that further study of the role of common infections and allergies in preventing brain tumors is justified.

Space–time clustering of childhood astrocytoma and ependymoma in England suggests the possibility of an infectious culprit (McNally et al. 2002). Colds and influenza have been studied in relation to brain tumors with mixed results (Linos et al. 1998; Fisher et al. 2000)

Antibodies to *Toxoplasma gondii*, an infectious agent that may cause gliomas in experimentally exposed animals, were linked to astrocytoma in one study (reviewed in Wrensch et al. 1993). However, a more recent study found an association with meningioma, but not with adult glioma (Ryan et al. 1993).

Allergies. An inverse association of history of allergies with glioma has been independently replicated in three large well-conducted studies (Schlehofer et al. 1999; Brenner et al. 2002; Wiemels et al. 2002) that used a variety of study designs for ascertaining subjects. Further work to understand the basis of this observed relationship is warranted and might reveal a role for immunologic factors in gliomagenesis. The possible role of allergy medications, if any, might also deserve further study.

Head Trauma and Seizures. Head injuries have long been of interest in the etiology of brain tumors, with generally mixed results from case–control studies (reviewed in Preston-Martin and Mack 1996; Inskip et al. 1998).

Example 14–4 A recent large Danish cohort study found no important association between head injuries requiring hospitalization and risk of either glioma or meningioma occurring more than 1 year after injury (Inskip et al. 1998). The authors attributed a large increased risk within the first year after head injury to increased detection from procedures related to the injury, but they did not see a corresponding deficit of cases in subsequent years. Seven studies of meningioma and head trauma reviewed by Preston-Martin and Mack (1996) gave a median 90% increased risk of meningioma among persons with head trauma. Six of eight case–control studies reported elevated odds ratios of 1.1–1.6 for primary malignant brain tumors in adults (reviewed in Wrensch et al. 1993, 2000a) and one study reported an odds ratio for serious head injury of 10.6 among men with glioblastoma or anaplastic astrocytoma versus friend controls ($p = 0.004$) (Hochberg et al. 1984). Because Wrensch et al. (2000a) noted differential study participation by controls based on prior head injury, it seems possible that some bias in selection of friend controls might have explained the very high odds ratio for head injury reported by Hochberg et al. Preferential recall of injuries by those with a brain tumor further complicates interpretation. This example illustrates methodologic issues of recall bias, bias selection among controls, ascertainment issues, and the difficulties of ruling out acute versus long-term effects of head injury.

In most but not all studies, mothers of children with brain tumors have reported increased birth trauma or other head injury to the child compared to that reported by mothers of control children. Critics suggest that the magnitude of risk is compatible with preferential recall of head injuries by those whose children have had brain tumors. Most recent studies have tried to minimize this bias by asking only for severe injuries that most people would not forget (Gurney et al. 1996).

Because of the large size of the Danish cohort study of head injuries, Inskip et al. (1998) were able to examine risk of glioma among those with head injury stratified by gender, age at injury, type of injury (fractured skull, concussion, laceration, or contusion), type or location of accident (traffic, home, workplace, sports, or other), and presence of epilepsy. With one exception, none of these subgroups had marked or significantly elevated risk of glioma 1 or more years after head injury. Only people with epilepsy

listed as one of the discharge diagnoses for the injury hospitalization continued to have elevated glioma risk 1 or more years after head injury (standardized incidence ratio = 7.6, 95% confidence interval [CI] 2.4–17.7).

Histories of seizures or epilepsy have been fairly consistently linked with brain tumors in cohort studies of epileptics (Wrensch et al. 1993; reviewed in Inskip et al. 1998) and in case–control studies of adult glioma (Ryan et al. 1992; Wrensch et al. 1997b). Deciding whether the tumors or the seizures came first is problematic, however. For meningioma, one study found cases to be five times as likely as controls to report seizures even 10 years or more prior to diagnosis and adult glioma studies have reported elevated odds ratios associated with seizures occurring 3 or more years prior to diagnosis. Because epilepsy is relatively rare, head injuries are more common in people with seizures, and head injuries can cause seizures, only very large studies that could obtain information on timing of both seizures and head injuries relative to brain tumor diagnosis are likely to clarify this problem. Use of seizure medications also needs to be considered in interpreting these findings.

Drugs and Medications. Very few studies have examined medications and drugs in relation to either child or adult brain tumors (reviewed in Preston-Martin and Mack 1996). Methodologic difficulties in such studies include validity and reliability of drug recall, and pertinent time periods of exposure assessments (issues include documenting pre- and postnatal exposures for childhood tumors and latency of exposure to diagnosis for adult-onset tumors). Despite these problems, because nonsteroidal anti-inflammatory drugs may be protective against colorectal and certain other cancers, it would be worth investigating these drugs in relation to brain tumor risk.

Diet, Vitamins, Alcohol, Tobacco, and Residential Chemicals

Several mechanisms involving DNA damage through which N-nitroso compounds might operate to cause brain tumors are discussed in detail in other reviews (Berleur and Cordier 1995; Preston-Martin and Mack 1996). N-nitroso compounds have been identified as neurocarcinogens in experimental animal studies, where these compounds may initiate carcinogenesis either pre- or postnatally, although fetal exposures result in more tumors than postnatal exposures. Adult tumors may be a result of prenatal or early postnatal exposures, as the delay to tumor formation following pre- or postnatal exposure in animal models can be substantial. The induction of brain tumors by these compounds is species-sensitive, though a wide variety of primate and other mammalian species have been shown to be susceptible to chemically induced brain tumors (Berleur and Cordier 1995; Preston-Martin and Mack 1996). Furthermore, some of the tumors induced are histologically similar to prevalent human types.

Because N-nitroso compounds are virtually ubiquitous in the environment, epidemiologic evaluation of their role in human brain tumors has been extremely problematic. Humans may be exposed to N-nitroso compounds from endogenous and exogenous sources (Preston-Martin and Mack 1996). Some sources (such as vegetables) are high in nitrates, which can be converted to nitrites, but are also high in vitamins that block formation of N-nitroso compounds. Despite these assessment problems, many studies have attempted to examine major dietary sources of these chemicals and to assess the inhibition of nitrosourea formation that may come from certain vitamins.

The possible roles of oxidants and antioxidants in cancers and other degenerative diseases of aging also are being extensively evaluated (Ames et al. 1993). Oxidants are thought to damage DNA and this damage accumulates, and/or is more difficult to repair, with age. In contrast, antioxidants may directly block the effects of oxidative DNA damage by removing or lowering the concentration of oxidants and may further minimize DNA or cellular damage or enhance repair through other mechanisms. Oxidants and antioxidants derive from a variety of endogenous and exogenous sources including enzymes and foods. That increased consumption of vegetables and fruits is associated with decreased cancer risk, for most cancer sites studied, provides epidemiologic support for the hypothesis that antioxidants protect against cancer formation or progression (Patterson et al. 1997). Distinguishing the role of oxidants or antioxidants versus nitroso-compounds in epidemiologic studies is complex, as many foods that are high in nitroso compounds or protect against nitrosation are also oxidants or antioxidants.

Not surprisingly, given inherent methodologic difficulties in retrospective dietary assessment, compounded by problems in categorizing foods correctly for pertinent factors, epidemiologic studies of diet and vitamin supplementation provide mixed support for the hypothesis that dietary N-nitroso compounds or other nutrients might influence the risk of both childhood and adult brain tumors (Wrensch et al. 1993; reviewed in Berleur and Cordier 1995; Preston-Martin and Mack 1996; Kaplan et al. 1997; Lee et al. 1997; Blot et al. 1999; Cantor et al. 1999; Hu et al. 1999; Lubin et al. 2000; Mueller et al. 2001; Pogoda and Preston-Martin 2001; Tedeschi et al. 2001). Interpretation of dietary associations is also complicated by potential selection bias of controls, which might favor participation by those who consume "healthier" diets; such a bias would tend to falsely accentuate differences in the observed direction. Some interesting studies that have examined micronutrients and trace minerals (e.g., folate compounds [Bunin et al. 1993, 1994] and calcium [Tedeschi et al. 2001]) show the importance of considering alternatives to the N-nitroso compound and antioxidant hypotheses.

Many studies have considered the potential role of active, passive, and/or prenatal cigarette smoke exposures, known environmental sources of numerous carcinogens, in the development of brain tumors (Norman et al. 1996; Preston-Martin and Mack 1996; reviewed in Lee et al. 1997; Zheng et al. 2001a), with most evidence showing no effect from any source except personal smoking of unfiltered cigarettes. The blood–brain barrier may pose an obstacle to large polycyclic aromatic hydrocarbons and may explain why ordinary cigarette smoking does not seem to be a risk factor for brain tumors, but it is unclear why unfiltered cigarettes would be a risk factor when filtered cigarettes are not.

Neither childhood nor adult brain tumors have been convincingly linked with alcohol exposures, though some studies have shown positive associations (Wrensch et al. 1993; reviewed in Preston-Martin and Mack 1996; Wrensch et al. 2002).

Pre- and postnatal pesticide exposures in childhood brain tumors have been the focus of many studies of residential chemical exposures (Preston-Martin and Mack 1996). Although results have not been entirely consistent, a large population-based study found significantly increased risk of pediatric brain tumors with prenatal exposures to flea and tick pesticides (Pogoda and Preston-Martin 1997). Given that the finding was specific to these and not other types of pesticide exposures, the authors thought that the observed association was unlikely to be due to recall bias by mothers of affected children.

Industry and Occupation

No comprehensive review of occupational risk factors for brain tumors has been published since 1986 (Thomas and Waxweiler 1986), but the same issues discussed then are still relevant today. Workers in many jobs may be exposed to neurotoxic or carcinogenic substances or both, in the form of lubricating oils, organic solvents, formaldehyde, acrylonitrile, phenols and phenolic compounds, and polycyclic aromatic hydrocarbons. Some of these chemicals induce brain tumors in experimental animals. However, strain, gestational age, fetal versus adult status at time of exposure, and exposure route significantly influence tumor susceptibility in animals, and such factors usually cannot be accounted for or generalized to occupational cohort exposure studies.

Example 14–5 Some compounds, such as polycyclic aromatic hydrocarbons, induce brain tumors through direct implantation or transplacentally but not though inhalation or transdermally, the exposure routes that would be relevant to occupational groups. Moreover, workers are seldom exposed only to one chemical, and chemicals may well interact with other chemicals to increase or reduce risk. Even in the largest occupational cohort studies, the number of brain tumor cases is often too small to permit meaningful subgroup analyses to detect damaging chemicals, physical agents, work processes, or interactions. Random exposure misclassification in many types of jobs might bias results toward the null. For these reasons, no definitive associations of brain tumors with specific chemicals have been established, even for known or putative carcinogens.

Industries or occupations for which the available evidence has not ruled out the possibility of an association with brain tumors but for which doubt about a consistent or causal relationship exists include (1) occupations or industries involving exposures to pesticides and other agricultural chemicals (Bohnen and Kurland 1995; Khuder et al. 1998; Schreinemachers 2000); (2) production and processing of synthetic rubber (Thomas and Waxweiler 1986; Weiland et al. 1996); (3) polyvinyl chloride production (Thomas and Waxweiler 1986; Wu et al. 1989; Hagmar et al. 1990; Simonato et al. 1991; Wong et al. 1991; McLaughlin and Lipworth 1999; Mundt et al. 2000; Rice and Wilbourn 2000; Lewis 2001); (4) petrochemical, petroleum, and oil production industry workers (Wrensch et al. 1993; Preston-Martin and Mack 1996; Cooper et al. 1997; Delzell et al. 1999; Divine et al. 1999; Carozza et al. 2000; Divine and Hartman 2000; Beall et al. 2001a, 2001b; Rodu et al. 2001; Sathiakumar et al. 2001); (5) scientists and biomedical professionals (Burnett et al. 1999; Santana et al. 1999; Wennborg et al. 1999; Carozza et al. 2000; Rachet et al. 2000); and (6) firefighters (Vena and Fiedler

1987; Demers et al. 1991, 1992, 1994; Aronson et al. 1994; Tornling et al. 1994; Deschamps et al. 1995; Golden et al. 1995; Guidotti 1995; Firth et al. 1996; Moen and Ovrebo 1997; Ma et al. 1998). Two recent population-based studies identified a variety of occupations that would be reasonable candidates for more detailed exposure assessment in future studies (Carozza et al. 2000; Zheng et al. 2001b). In a recent large international study, no associations were found for glioma or meningioma with occupational or residential contacts with a wide variety of animals (Menegoz et al. 2002).

Suspected brain tumor clusters in occupational or residential settings have often been reported, but investigations of such clusters rarely lead to conclusive results because of small numbers of cases, disease heterogeneity and unknown or inadequately characterized exposures, latency periods, and/or base populations. Thus, we will not review the evidence for or against clusters here; guidance for evaluating clusters can be found in studies by the Centers for Disease Control and Prevention (1990) and Davis et al. (1999a).

Parents' workplace exposures might increase the risk of cancer in their children. A father's exposures before conception might damage his DNA, and a mother's exposures might have a direct impact on the developing fetus. Parents could expose their children to infectious agents that they contracted at their workplace or to chemical carcinogens that remain on their skin or clothing. There is no definitive evidence of such exposures causing brain tumors due to methodologic limitations, including small sample sizes, multiple or rare exposures, confounding factors, and insufficient follow-up data. Interested readers are referred to Wrensch et al. (1993) for a review of 16 studies published before 1993. More recent studies of parental exposures related to childhood brain tumors include those by Holly et al. (1998), Kristensen et al. (1996), and Kerr et al. (2000).

Ionizing Radiation

Reasonable agreement exists that there is strong increased risk of intracranial tumors following therapeutic ionizing radiation (Wrensch et al. 1993; reviewed in Preston-Martin and Mack 1996; Wrensch et al. 2002). People with even relatively low-dose exposures for ring worm treatment averaging 1.5 Gy (Grey) have shown relative risks of 18, 10, and 3 for nerve sheath tumors, meningiomas, and gliomas, respectively. A very high rate (17%) of prior therapeutic radiation among patients with glioblastoma or glioma and increased risk of brain tumors in children after radiation treatment for leukemia and other childhood cancers (including previous brain tumors) have been reported (Neglia et al. 1991; Salvati et al. 1991; Hodges et al. 1992; Little et al. 1998; Salminen et al. 1999; Loning et al. 2000). Radiation treatments of the nasopharynx for adenoid hypertrophy and for pituitary tumors have also been linked to increased risk of brain tumors (Erfurth et al. 2001; Yeh et al. 2001).

Whether prenatal radiation exposures cause childhood brain tumors is unclear. Studies of Japanese atomic bomb survivors have not shown increased brain tumor incidence among those exposed in utero (reviewed in Preston-Martin and Mack 1996). Relative risks of 1.2 to 1.6 for childhood brain tumors have been reported for prenatal radiation exposure, but some studies had too small a sample size to achieve statistical significance. Relative risks of this low magnitude in conjunction with a comparatively uncommon exposure would not account for many childhood brain tumors. Parental exposure to ionizing radiation prior to conception has not been shown to be a risk factor for childhood brain tumors (Preston-Martin and Mack 1996).

Diagnostic radiation does not appear to play an important role in malignant brain tumor risk (Wrensch et al. 2000a), but might be important for meningioma (reviewed in Preston-Martin and Mack 1996). Three glioma case–control studies reported relative risks of 0.4, 1.2, and 3.0 for exposure to dental X-rays. The evidence is slightly stronger for meningioma in which twofold or greater relative risks were found in three of four studies.

Nuclear facility employees and nuclear materials production workers have exhibited a small but significantly elevated risk of 1.2 for brain tumors (Loomis and Wolf 1996), but confounding or effect modification by chemical exposures makes interpretation of causality difficult. Studies of brain tumors among airplane pilots exposed to cosmic radiation at high altitudes have produced mixed results (Band et al. 1990; Salisbury et al. 1991).

Electromagnetic Fields

Cell Phones and Radio Frequency Exposures. Concern over possible health effects of using cellular telephones has prompted studies looking at the relation between cell phone use or radiofrequency exposure and brain tumor risk. Although most reports do not support an association (Morgan et al. 2000; Hardell et al. 2001; Johansen et al. 2001; Krewski et al. 2001), continued study in this area may be important for several reasons: (1) cell phone usage is becoming increasingly common; (2) most studies were conducted when analog phones were the predominant type of cell phone, whereas digital phones are most common today; (3) duration of phone use has increased, as have the number of cell phone users; and (4) some brain tumors may take a long time to develop.

Power Frequency Electromagnetic Fields. The potential health effects of power frequency (50–60 Hz) electromagnetic fields (EMF) have received substantial public and scientific attention (reviewed in Kheifets 2001). The interest arose from residential studies showing increased risks of brain tumors and leukemia in children whose homes have high EMF exposures and occupational studies showing higher than expected brain tumor incidence and mortality among presumably exposed workers. Recent meta-analyses of occupational studies suggest a statistically significant increased risk of 10% to 20% for brain malignancy among electrical workers (Kheifets et al. 1995; NIEHS 1999). Four recent oc-

cupational studies supported an association of brain tumors with EMF exposure (Robinson et al. 1999; Savitz et al. 2000; Minder and Pfluger 2001; Villeneuve et al. 2002) and three others did not (Floderus et al. 1999; Johansen and Olsen 1999; Sorahan et al. 2001). Maternal EMF exposures have not been linked to brain tumors in their children (Sorahan et al. 1999; Feychting et al. 2000). A comprehensive assessment of childhood brain tumors in relation to residential EMF concluded that the evidence did not support an association (Kheifets et al. 1999) but some disagree with this conclusion (Meinert and Michaelis 1996). Although it may be plausible that EMF exposure influences the risk of brain tumors, no causal connection has been established. It is very difficult to prove the existence of no association between power-frequency EMF fields and brain tumors. A definitive resolution to the question of whether EMF exposure causes brain tumors remains elusive for this and a variety of other reasons, as discussed by several groups (Blettner and Schlehofer 1999; National Institute of Environmental Health Sciences 1999; Wrensch et al. 1999, 2000b; Kheifets 2001). The lack of convincing biologic plausibility is often a primary reason given against a causal relation between EMF exposures and brain tumors, but two recently published studies showed that residential EMF exposures might depress the normal levels of nocturnal melatonin production; melatonin is thought to have oncostatic effects (Davis et al. 2001; Levallois et al. 2001).

Future Directions and Conclusions

The descriptive and analytic epidemiology of primary brain tumors furnishes many provocative challenges for further research. Primary brain tumors represent a heterogeneous collection of diseases and even common subtypes such as glioblastoma multiforme are likely to have a multifactorial etiology. Improved registration, a consensus on classification, and increased use of molecular tumor markers are necessary to characterize more homogeneous subgroups of tumors. A major unaccomplished task in descriptive brain tumor epidemiology is the explanation of gender and ethnic differences for glioma and meningioma. Further analytic studies of environmental factors (viruses, radiation, and carcinogenic or protective chemical exposures through diet, workplace, or other sources) and potentially relevant polymorphisms are likely to improve understanding of this devastating collection of diseases. Since currently established or suggested risk factors do not account for most cases, novel concepts of neurocarcinogenesis may be required before a more comprehensive picture of the natural history and pathogenesis of brain tumors can be formed. Given these formidable challenges, future epidemiologic research on brain tumors is likely to be exciting.

References

Aldape K, Simmons ML, Davis RL, et al. Discrepancies in diagnoses of neuroepithelial neoplasms: the San Francisco Bay Area Adult Glioma Study. *Cancer* 2000;88:2342–2349.

Ames BN, Shigenaga MK, Hagen TM. Oxidants, antioxidants, and the degenerative diseases of aging. *Proc Natl Acad Sci USA* 1993;90:7915–7922.

Aronson KJ, Tomlinson GA, Smith L. Mortality among fire fighters in metropolitan Toronto. *Am J Ind Med* 1994;26:89–101.

Bailey P, Cushing HA. A classification of the tumors of the glioma group on a histogenetic basis with a correlated study of prognosis. Philadelphia, PA: JB Lippincott, 1926.

Band PR, Spinelli JJ, Ng VT, et al. Mortality and cancer incidence in a cohort of commercial airline pilots. *Aviat Space Environ Med* 1990;61:299–302.

Beall C, Delzell E, Rodu B, et al. Case–control study of intracranial tumors among employees at a petrochemical research facility. *J Occup Environ Med* 2001a;43:1103–1113.

Beall C, Delzell E, Rodu B, et al. Cancer and benign tumor incidence among employees in a polymers research complex. *J Occup Environ Med* 2001b;43:914–924.

Berleur MP, Cordier S. The role of chemical, physical, or viral exposures and health factors in neurocarcinogenesis: implications for epidemiologic studies of brain tumors. *Cancer Causes Control* 1995;6:240–256.

Blettner M, Schlehofer B. Is there an increased risk of leukemia, brain tumors or breast cancer after exposure to high-frequency radiation? Review of methods and results of epidemiologic studies [in German]. *Med Klin* 1999;94:150–158.

Blot WJ, Henderson BE, Boice JD. Childhood cancer in relation to cured meat intake: review of the epidemiological evidence. *Nutr Cancer* 1999;34:111–118.

Bohnen NI, Kurland LT. Brain tumor and exposure to pesticides in humans: a review of the epidemiologic data. *J Neurol Sci* 1995;132:110–121.

Bondy M, Ligon BL. Epidemiology and etiology of intracranial meningiomas: a review. *J Neurooncol* 1996;29:197–205.

Bondy M, Wiencke J, Wrensch M, Kyritsis AP. Genetics of primary brain tumors: a review. *J Neurooncol* 1994;18:69–81.

Bondy ML, Kyritsis AP, Gu J, et al. Mutagen sensitivity and risk of gliomas: a case–control analysis. *Cancer Res* 1996;56:1484–1486.

Bondy ML, Wang LE, El-Zein R, et al. Gamma-radiation sensitivity and risk of glioma. *J Natl Cancer Inst* 2001;93:1553–1557.

Brenner AV, Linet MS, Fine HA, et al. History of allergies and autoimmune diseases and risk of brain tumors in adults. *Int J Cancer* 2002;99:252–259.

Bruner JM, Inouye L, Fuller GN, Langford LA. Diagnostic discrepancies and their clinical impact in a neuropathology referral practice. *Cancer* 1997;79:796–803.

Bunin G. What causes childhood brain tumors? Limited knowledge, many clues. *Pediatr Neurosurg* 2000;32:321–326.

Bunin GR, Kuijten RR, Boesel CP, et al. Maternal diet and risk of astrocytic glioma in children: a report from the Childrens Cancer Group (United States and Canada). *Cancer Causes Control* 1994;5:177–187.

Bunin GR, Kuijten RR, Buckley JD, et al. Relation between maternal diet and subsequent primitive neuroectodermal brain tumors in young children. *N Engl J Med* 1993;329:536–541.

Burnett C, Robinson C, Walker J. Cancer mortality in health and science technicians. *Am J Ind Med* 1999;36:155–158.

Caggana M, Kilgallen J, Conroy JM, et al. Associations between *ERCC2* polymorphisms and gliomas. *Cancer Epidemiol Biomarkers Prev* 2001;10:355–360.

Cairncross JG, Ueki K, Zlatescu MC, et al. Specific genetic predictors of chemotherapeutic response and survival in patients with anaplastic oligodendrogliomas. *J Natl Cancer Inst* 1998;90:1473–1479.

Cantor KP, Lynch CF, Hildesheim ME, et al. Drinking water source and chlorination byproducts in Iowa. III. Risk of brain cancer. *Am J Epidemiol* 1999;150:552–560.

Carozza S, Wrensch M, Miike R, et al. Occupation and adult glioma. *Am J Epidemiol* 2000;152:838–846.

Centers for Disease Control and Prevention (CDC). Guidelines for Investigating Clusters of Health Events—Appendix. Summary of Methods for Statistically Assessing Clusters of Health Events, 1990.

Central Brain Tumor Registry of the United States (CBTRUS). 2002. Web Site: www.cbtrus.org

Connecticut Department of Public Health. Connecticut Tumor Registry Web site, 2002. www.dph.state.ct.us/OPPE/hptumor.htm.

Cooper SP, Labarthe D, Downs T, et al. Cancer mortality among petroleum refinery and chemical manufacturing workers in Texas. *J Environ Pathol Toxicol Oncol* 1997;16:1–14.

Cuomo L, Trivedi P, Cardillo MR, et al. Human herpesvirus 6 infection in neoplastic and normal brain tissue. *J Med Virol* 2001;63:45–51.

Curran WJ Jr, Scott CB, Horton J, et al. Recursive partitioning analysis of prognostic factors in three Radiation Therapy Oncology Group malignant glioma trials [see comments]. *J Natl Cancer Inst* 1993;85:704–710.

Daumas-Duport C, Scheithauer B, O'Fallon J, Kelly J. Grading of astrocytomas. A simple reproducible method. *Cancer* 1988;62:2152–2165.

Davis FG, Bruner JM, Surawicz TS. The rationale for standardized registration and reporting of brain and central nervous system tumors in population-based cancer registries. *Neuroepidemiology* 1997;16:308–316.

Davis FG, Freels S, Grutsch J, et al. Survival rates in patients with primary malignant brain tumors stratified by patient age and tumor histological type: an analysis based on Surveillance, Epidemiology, and End Results (SEER) data, 1973–1991. *J Neurosurg* 1998;88:1–10.

Davis FG, Malinski N, Haenszel W, et al. Primary brain tumor incidence rates in four United States regions, 1985–1989: a pilot study. *Neuroepidemiology* 1996;15:103–112.

Davis FG, McCarthy BJ. Epidemiology of brain tumors. *Curr Opin Neurol* 2000;13:635–640.

Davis FG, McCarthy BJ, Freels S, et al. The conditional probability of survival of patients with primary malignant brain tumors: surveillance, epidemiology, and end results (SEER) data. *Cancer* 1999b;85:485–491.

Davis FG, McCarthy B, Jukich P. The descriptive epidemiology of brain tumors. *Neuroimaging Clin North Am* 1999a;9:581–594.

Davis S, Kaune WT, Mirick DK, et al. Residential magnetic fields, light-at-night, and nocturnal urinary 6-sulfatoxymelatonin concentration in women. *Am J Epidemiol* 2001;154:591–600.

de Andrade M, Barnholtz JS, Amos CI, et al. Segregation analysis of cancer in families of glioma patients. *Genet Epidemiol* 2001;20:258–270.

Del Valle L, Gordon J, Assimakopoulou M, et al. Detection of JC virus DNA sequences and expression of the viral regulatory protein T-antigen in tumors of the central nervous system. *Cancer Res* 2001;61:4287–4293.

Delzell E, Beall C, Rodu B, et al. Case-series investigation of intracranial neoplasms at a petrochemical research facility. *Am J Ind Med* 1999;36:450–458.

Demers PA, Checkoway H, Vaughan TL, et al. Cancer incidence among firefighters in Seattle and Tacoma, Washington (United States). *Cancer Causes Control* 1994;5:129–135.

Demers PA, Heyer NJ, Rosenstock L. Mortality among firefighters from three northwestern United States cities. *Br J Ind Med* 1992;49:664–670.

Demers PA, Vaughan TL, Schommer RR. Occupation, socioeconomic status, and brain tumor mortality: a death certificate-based case–control study. *J Occup Med* 1991;33:1001–1006.

Deschamps S, Momas I, Festy B. Mortality amongst Paris fire-fighters. *Eur J Epidemiol* 1995;11:643–646.

Divine BJ, Hartman CM. Update of a study of crude oil production workers 1946–94. *Occup Environ Med* 2000;57:411–417.

Divine BJ, Hartman CM, Wendt JK. Update of the Texaco mortality study 1947–93: Part I. Analysis of overall patterns of mortality among refining, research, and petrochemical workers. *Occup Environ Med* 1999;56:167–173.

Elexpuru-Camiruaga J, Buxton N, Kandula V, et al. Susceptibility to astrocytoma and meningioma: influence of allelism at glutathione *S*-transferase (GSTT1 and GSTM1) and cytochrome P-450 (CYP2D6) loci. *Cancer Res* 1995;55:4237–4239.

El-Zein R, Bondy ML, Wang LE, et al. Increased chromosomal instability in peripheral lymphocytes and risk of human gliomas. *Carcinogenesis* 1999;20:811–815.

Erfurth EM, Bulow B, Mikoczy Z, et al. Is there an increase in second brain tumours after surgery and irradiation for a pituitary tumour? *Clin Endocrinol (Oxf)* 2001;55:613–616.

Feychting M, Floderus B, Ahlbom A. Parental occupational exposure to magnetic fields and childhood cancer (Sweden). *Cancer Causes Control* 2000;11:151–615.

Firth HM, Cooke KR, Herbison GP. Male cancer incidence by occupation: New Zealand, 1972–1984. *Int J Epidemiol* 1996;25:14–21.

Fisher JL, Schwartzbaum JA, Johnson CC. Cold/influenza infection, influenza vaccination, and risk of adult glioma (abstract 116). *Am J Epidemiol* 2000;151(Suppl):S29.

Floderus B, Stenlund C, Persson T. Occupational magnetic field exposure and site-specific cancer incidence: a Swedish cohort study. *Cancer Causes Control* 1999;10:323–332.

Fuller GN. Central nervous system tumors. In: Parham DM, ed. Pediatric Neoplasia: Morphology and Biology. Philadelphia: Lippincott-Raven, 1996, pp 153–204.

Golden AL, Markowitz SB, Landrigan PJ. The risk of cancer in firefighters. *Occup Med* 1995;10:803–820.

Grossman SA, Osman M, Hruban R, Piantadosi S. Central nervous system cancers in first-degree relatives and spouses. *Cancer Invest* 1999;17:299–308.

Grotzer MA, Geoerger B, Janss AJ, et al. Prognostic significance of Ki-67 (MIB-1) proliferation index in childhood primitive neuroectodermal tumors of the central nervous system. *Med Pediatr Oncol* 2001;36:268–273.

Grovas A, Fremgen A, Rauck A, et al. The National Cancer Data Base report on patterns of childhood cancers in the United States. *Cancer* 1997;80:2321–2332.

Guidotti TL. Occupational mortality among firefighters: assessing the association. *J Occup Environ Med* 1995;37:1348–1356.

Gurney JG, Kadan-Lottick N. Brain and other central nervous system tumors: rates, trends, and epidemiology. *Curr Opin Oncol* 2001; 13:160–166.

Gurney JG, Preston-Martin S, McDaniel AM, et al. Head injury as a risk factor for brain tumors in children: results from a multicenter case–control study. *Epidemiology* 1996;7:485–489.

Hagel C, Krog B, Laas R, Stavrou DK. Prognostic relevance of TP53 mutations, p53 protein, Ki-67 index and conventional histological grading in oligodendrogliomas. *J Exp Clin Cancer Res* 1999;18:305–309.

Hagmar L, Akesson B, Nielsen J, et al. Mortality and cancer morbidity in workers exposed to low levels of vinyl chloride monomer at a polyvinyl chloride processing plant *Am J Ind Med* 1990;17:553–565.

Hardell L, Mild KH, Pahlson A, Hallquist A. Ionizing radiation, cellular telephones and the risk for brain tumours. *Eur J Cancer Prev* 2001;10:523–529.

Hemminki K, Li X, Vaittinen P, Dong C. Cancers in the first-degree relatives of children with brain tumours. *Br J Cancer* 2000;83: 407–411.

Hochberg F, Toniolo P, Cole P. Head trauma and seizures as risk factors of glioblastoma. *Neurology* 1984;34:1511–1514.

Hodges LC, Smith JL, Garrett A, Tate S. Prevalence of glioblastoma multiforme in subjects with prior therapeutic radiation. *J Neurosci Nurs* 1992;24:79–83.

Holly EA, Bracci PM, Mueller BA, Preston-Martin S. Farm and animal exposures and pediatric brain tumors: results from the United States West Coast Childhood Brain Tumor Study. *Cancer Epidemiol Biomarkers Prev* 1998;7:797–802.

Horn B, Heideman R, Geyer R, et al. A multi-institutional retrospective study of intracranial ependymoma in children: identification of risk factors. *J Pediatr Hematol Oncol* 1999;21:203–211.

Hu J, La Vecchia C, Negri E, et al. Diet and brain cancer in adults: a case–control study in northeast China. *Int J Cancer* 1999; 81:20–23.

Huang H, Reis R, Yonekawa Y, et al. Identification in human brain tumors of DNA sequences specific for SV40 large T antigen. *Brain Pathol* 1999;9:33–42.

Huncharek M, Kupelnick B. Epidermal growth factor receptor gene amplification as a prognostic marker in glioblastoma multiforme: results of a meta-analysis. *Oncol Res* 2000; 12:107–112.

Inskip PD, Linet MS, Heineman EF. Etiology of brain tumors in adults. *Epidemiol Rev* 1995;17:382–414.

Inskip PD, Mellemkjaer L, Gridley G, Olsen JH. Incidence of intracranial tumors following hospitalization for head injuries (Denmark). *Cancer Causes Control* 1998;9:109–116.

James CD, Smith JS, Jenkins RB. Genetic and molecular basis of primary central nervous system tumors. In: Levin V, ed. Cancer in the Nervous System. New York: Oxford University Press, 2002, pp 239–252.

Johansen C, Boice JD, McLaughlin JK, Olsen JH. Cellular telephones and cancer—a nationwide cohort study in Denmark. *J Natl Cancer Inst* 2001;93:203–207.

Johansen C, Olsen JH. Risk of cancer among Danish electricity workers. A cohort study [in Danish]. *Ugeskr Laeger* 1999;161:2079–2085.

Kaplan S, Novikov I, Modan B. Nutritional factors in the etiology of brain tumors: potential role of nitrosamines, fat, and cholesterol. *Am J Epidemiol* 1997;146:832–841.

Kernohan JW, Maybon RF, Svien HJ, Adson AW. A simplified classification of the gliomas. *Proc Staff Meet Mayo Clin* 1949; 24:71–75.

Kerr MA, Nasca PC, Mundt KA, et al. Parental occupational exposures and risk of neuroblastoma: a case–control study (United States). *Cancer Causes Control* 2000;11: 635–643.

Kheifets LI. Electric and magnetic field exposure and brain cancer: a review. *Bioelectromagnetics* 2001;Suppl:S120–S131.

Kheifets LI, Afifi AA, Buffler PA, Zhang ZW. Occupational electric and magnetic field exposure and brain cancer: a meta-analysis. *J Occup Environ Med* 1995;37:1327–1341.

Kheifets LI, Sussman SS, Preston-Martin S. Childhood brain tumors and residential electromagnetic fields (EMF). *Rev Environ Contam Toxicol* 1999;159:111–129.

Khuder SA, Mutgi AB, Schaub EA. Meta-analyses of brain cancer and farming. *Am J Ind Med* 1998;34:252–260.

Kleihues P, Burger PC, Scheithauer BW. The new WHO classification of brain tumors. *Brain Pathol* 1993;3:255–268.

Kleihues P, Cavenee WK. Tumors of the Central Nervous System: Pathology and Genetics, 2nd edition. Lyon, France: International Agency for Research on Cancer, 2000.

Kreftregisteret. Cancer Registry of Norway Web Site, Institute of Population-Based Cancer Research, 2002: http://www.kreftregisteret.no.

Krewski D, Byus CV, Glickman BW, et al. Recent advances in research on radiofrequency fields and health. *J Toxicol Environ Health B Crit Rev* 2001;4:145–159.

Kristensen P, Andersen A, Irgens LM, et al. Cancer in offspring of parents engaged in agricultural activities in Norway: incidence and risk factors in the farm environment. *Int J Cancer* 1996;65:39–50.

Krynska B, Del Valle L, Croul S, et al. Detection of human neurotropic JC virus DNA sequence and expression of the viral oncogenic protein in pediatric medulloblastomas. *Proc Nal Acad Sci USA* 1999;96:11519–11524.

Kyritsis AP, Bondy ML, Xiao M, et al. Germline p53 gene mutations in subsets of glioma patients. *J Natl Cancer Inst* 1994;86:344–349.

Lee M, Wrensch M, Miike R. Dietary and tobacco risk factors for adult onset glioma in the San Francisco Bay Area (California, USA). *Cancer Causes Control* 1997;8: 13–24.

Legler JM, Ries LA, Smith MA, et al. Cancer surveillance series [corrected]: brain and other central nervous system cancers: recent trends in incidence and mortality. *J Natl Cancer Inst* 1999;91:1382–1390.

Levallois P, Dumont M, Touitou Y, et al. Effects of electric and magnetic fields from high-power lines on female urinary excretion of 6-sulfatoxymelatonin concentration in women. *Am J Epidemiol* 2001;154:601–609.

Lewis R. Use of rank-order analysis of ordinal exposure data: application to vinyl chloride exposure. *Appl Occup Environ Hyg* 2001; 16:188–191.

Li Y, Millikan RC, Carozza S, et al. p53 mutations in malignant gliomas. *Cancer Epidemiol Biomarkers Prev* 1998;7:303–308.

Linos A, Kardara M, Kosmidis H, et al. Reported influenza in pregnancy and childhood tumour. *Eur J Epidemiol* 1998;14:471–475.

Little MP, de Vathaire F, Shamsaldin A, et al. Risks of brain tumour following treatment for cancer in childhood: modification by genetic factors, radiotherapy and chemotherapy. *Int J Cancer* 1998;78:269–275.

Loning L, Zimmermann M, Reiter A, et al. Secondary neoplasms subsequent to Berlin-Frankfurt-Munster therapy of acute lymphoblastic leukemia in childhood: significantly lower risk without cranial radiotherapy. *Blood* 2000;95:2770–2775.

Loomis DP, Wolf SH. Mortality of workers at a nuclear materials production plant at Oak Ridge, Tennessee, 1947–1990. *Am J Ind Med* 1996;29:131–141.

Lopez-Gonzalez MA, Sotelo J. Brain tumors in Mexico: characteristics and prognosis of glioblastoma. *Surg Neurol* 2000;53:157–162.

Lubin F, Farbstein H, Chetrit A, et al. The role of nutritional habits during gestation and child life in pediatric brain tumor etiology. *Int J Cancer* 2000;86:139–143.

Ma F, Lee DJ, Fleming LE, Dosemeci M. Race-specific cancer mortality in US firefighters: 1984–1993. *J Occup Environ Med* 1998; 40:1134–1138.

Malmer B, Gronberg H, Bergenheim AT, et al. Familial aggregation of astrocytoma in northern Sweden: an epidemiological cohort study. *Int J Cancer* 1999;81:366–370.

McKinley BP, Michalek AM, Fenstermaker RA, Plunkett RJ. The impact of age and sex on the incidence of glial tumors in New York state from 1976 to 1995. *J Neurosurg* 2000; 93:932–939.

McLaughlin JK, Lipworth L. A critical review of the epidemiologic literature on health effects of occupational exposure to vinyl chloride. *J Epidemiol Biostat* 1999;4:253–275.

McNally RJ, Cairns DP, Eden OB, et al. An infectious aetiology for childhood brain tumours? Evidence from space-time clustering and seasonality analyses. *Br J Cancer* 2002; 86:1070–1077.

Meinert R and Michaelis J. Meta-analyses of studies on the association between electromagnetic fields and childhood cancer. *Radiat Environ Biophys* 1996;35:11–18.

Menegoz F, Little J, Colonna M, et al. Contacts with animals and humans as risk factors for adult brain tumours. An international case–control study. *Eur J Cancer* 2002;38: 696–704.

Minder CE, Pfluger DH. Leukemia, brain tumors, and exposure to extremely low frequency electromagnetic fields in Swiss railway employees. *Am J Epidemiol* 2001;153: 825–835.

Mizumatsu S, Tamiya T, Ono Y, et al. Expression of cell cycle regulator p27Kip1 is correlated with survival of patients with astrocytoma. *Clin Cancer Res* 1999;5:551–557.

Moen BE, Ovrebo S. Assessment of exposure to polycyclic aromatic hydrocarbons during firefighting by measurement of urinary 1-hydroxypyrene. *J Occup Environ Med* 1997; 39:515–519.

Morgan RW, Kelsh MA, Zhao K, et al. Radiofrequency exposure and mortality from cancer of the brain and lymphatic/hematopoietic systems. *Epidemiology* 2000;11:118–127.

Mueller BA, Newton K, Holly EA, Preston-Martin S. Residential water source and the risk of childhood brain tumors. *Environ Health Perspect* 2001;109:551–556.

Mundt KA, Dell LD, Austin RP, et al. Historical cohort study of 10,109 men in the North American vinyl chloride industry, 1942–72: update of cancer mortality to 31 December 1995. *Occup Environ Med* 2000;57:774–781.

Nakamura M, Konishi N, Tsunoda S, et al. Analysis of prognostic and survival factors related to treatment of low-grade astrocytomas in adults. *Oncology* 2000;58:108–116.

Narod SA, Stiller C, Lenoir GM. An estimate of the heritable fraction of childhood cancer. *Br J Cancer* 1991;63:993–999.

National Institute of Environmental Health Sciences. NIEHS Health Effects from Exposure to Power-Line Frequency Electric and Magnetic Fields. Triangle Park, NC: 1999, Publication No. 99–4493.

Neglia JP, Meadows AT, Robison LL, et al. Second neoplasms after acute lymphoblastic leukemia in childhood. *N Engl J Med* 1991; 325:1330–1336.

Norman MA, Holly EA, Preston-Martin S. Childhood brain tumors and exposure to tobacco smoke. *Cancer Epidemiol Biomarkers Prev* 1996;5:85–91.

Patterson RE, White E, Kristal AR, et al. Vitamin supplements and cancer risk: the epidemiologic evidence. *Cancer Causes Control* 1997;8:786–802.

Paunu N, Pukkala E, Laippala P, Sankila R, Isola J, Miettinen H, Simola KO, Helen P, Helin H, Haapasalo H. Cancer incidence in families with multiple glioma patients. *Int J Cancer* 2002;97:819–822.

Peters ES, Kelsey KT, Wiencke JK, et al. *NAT2* and *NQO1* polymorphisms are not associated with adult glioma. *Cancer Epidemiol Biomarkers Prev* 2001;10:151–152.

Pobereskin LH, Sneyd JR. Incidence of hospital admission does not equal incidence of disease. Conclusions drawn from data are incorrect. *BMJ* 2000;320:1277.

Pogoda JM, Preston-Martin S. Household pesticides and risk of pediatric brain tumors. *Environ Health Perspect* 1997;105:1214–1220.

Pogoda JM, Preston-Martin S. Maternal cured meat consumption during pregnancy and risk of paediatric brain tumour in offspring: potentially harmful levels of intake. *Public Health Nutr* 2001;4:183–189.

Preston-Martin S, Mack W. Neoplasms of the nervous system. In: Scottenfeld DFJ, ed. Cancer Epidemiology and Prevention, Vol. 2. New York: Oxford University Press, 1996, pp 1231–1281.

Rachet B, Partanen T, Kauppinen T, Sasco AJ. Cancer risk in laboratory workers: an emphasis on biological research. *Am J Ind Med* 2000;38:651–665.

Rice JM, Wilbourn JD. Tumors of the nervous system in carcinogenic hazard identification. *Toxicol Pathol* 2000;28:202–214.

Ringertz N. Grading gliomas. *Acta Pathol Microbiol Scand* 1950;27:51–64.

Robinson CF, Petersen M, Palu S. Mortality patterns among electrical workers employed in the U.S. construction industry, 1982–1987. *Am J Ind Med* 1999;36:630–637.

Rodu B, Delzell E, Beall C, Sathiakumar N. Mortality among employees at a petrochemical research facility. *Am J Ind Med* 2001;39:29–41.

Ryan P, Hurley SF, Johnson AM, et al. Tumours of the brain and presence of antibodies to *Toxoplasma gondii*. *Int J Epidemiol* 1993; 22:412–419.

Ryan P, Lee MW, North B, McMichael AJ. Risk factors for tumors of the brain and meninges: results from the Adelaide Adult Brain Tumor Study. *Int J Cancer* 1992;51:20–27.

Salisbury DA, Band PR, Threlfall WJ, Gallagher RP. Mortality among British Columbia pilots. *Aviat Space Environ Med* 1991;62:351–352.

Salminen E, Pukkala E, Teppo L. Second cancers in patients with brain tumours—impact of treatment. *Eur J Cancer* 1999;35:102–105.

Salvati M, Artico M, Caruso R, et al. A report on radiation-induced gliomas. *Cancer* 1991; 67:392–397.

Santana VS, Silva M, Loomis D. Brain neoplasms among naval military men. *Int J Occup Environ Health* 1999;5:88–94.

Sathiakumar N, Delzell E, Rodu B, et al. Cancer incidence among employees at a petrochemical research facility. *J Occup Environ Med* 2001;43:166–174.

Savitz DA, Cai J, van Wijngaarden E, et al. Case–cohort analysis of brain cancer and leukemia in electric utility workers using a refined magnetic field job-exposure matrix. *Am J Ind Med* 2000;38:417–425.

Schlehofer B, Blettner M, Preston-Martin S, et al. Role of medical history in brain tumour development. Results from the international adult brain tumour study. *Int J Cancer* 1999; 82:155–160.

Schreinemachers DM. Cancer mortality in four northern wheat-producing states. *Environ Health Perspect* 2000;108:873–881.

Shadan FF, Koziol J. Induced genome instability as a potential screening test for cancer susceptibility? *Med Hypotheses* 2000;55: 69–72.

Simmons ML, Lamborn KR, Takahashi M, et al. Analysis of complex relationships between age, p53, epidermal growth factor receptor, and survival in glioblastoma patients. *Cancer Res* 2001;61:1122–1128.

Simonato L, L'Abbé KA, Andersen A, Belli S, Comba P, Engholm G, Ferro G, Hagmar L, LangÜrd S, Lundberg I, et al. A collaborative study of cancer incidence and mortality among vinyl chloride workers. *Scand J Work Environ Health* 1991;17:159–169.

Smith MA, Freidlin B, Ries LA, Simon R. Trends in reported incidence of primary malignant brain tumors in children in the United States. *J Natl Cancer Inst* 1998;90: 1269–1277.

Sorahan T, Hamilton L, Gardiner K, et al. Maternal occupational exposure to electromagnetic fields before, during, and after pregnancy in relation to risks of childhood cancers: findings from the Oxford Survey of Childhood Cancers, 1953–1981 deaths. *Am J Ind Med* 1999;35:348–357.

Sorahan T, Nichols L, van Tongeren M, Harrington JM. Occupational exposure to magnetic fields relative to mortality from brain tumours: updated and revised findings from a study of United Kingdom electricity generation and transmission workers, 1973–97. *Occup Environ Med* 2001;58:626–630.

Strojnik T, Kos J, Zidanik B, et al. Cathepsin B immunohistochemical staining in tumor and endothelial cells is a new prognostic factor for survival in patients with brain tumors. *Clin Cancer Res* 1999;5:559–567.

Surawicz TS, McCarthy BJ, Kupelian V, et al. Descriptive epidemiology of primary brain and CNS tumors: results from the Central Brain Tumor Registry of the United States, 1990–1994. *Neurooncology* 1999;1:14–25.

Surveillance, Epidemiology, and End Results (SEER). 2002a. Web site: www.seer.cancer.gov.

Surveillance Epidemiology and End Results (SEER). Surveillance, Epidemiology, and End Results Cancer Statistics Review (1973–1999), 2002b. http://seer.cancer.gov/csr/1973_1999/sections.html.

Tedeschi N, Schwartzbaum JA, Lee M, Wrensch M. Dietary calcium and adult glioma. *Nutr Cancer* 2001;39:196–203.

Thomas TL, Waxweiler RJ. Brain tumors and occupational risk factors. *Scand J Work Environ Health* 1986;12:1–15.

Tornling G, Gustavsson P, Hogstedt C. Mortality and cancer incidence in Stockholm fire fighters. *Am J Ind Med* 1994;25:219–228.

Vena JE, Fiedler RC. Mortality of a municipal-worker cohort: IV. Fire fighters. *Am J Ind Med* 1987;11:671–684.

Villeneuve PJ, Agnew DA, Johnson KC, Mao Y. Brain cancer and occupational exposure to magnetic fields among men: results from a Canadian population-based case–control study. *Int J Epidemiol* 2002;31:210–217.

Weiland SK, Mundt KA, Keil U, et al. Cancer mortality among workers in the German rubber industry: 1981–91. *Occup Environ Med* 1996;53:289–298.

Wennborg H, Yuen J, Axelsson G, et al. Mortality and cancer incidence in biomedical laboratory personnel in Sweden. *Am J Ind Med* 1999;35:382–389.

Wiemels JL, Wiencke JK, Sison JD, et al. History of allergies among adults with glioma and controls. *Int J Cancer* 2002;98:609–615.

Wiencke JK, Wrensch MR, Miike R, et al. Population-based study of glutathione S-transferase mu gene deletion in adult glioma cases and controls. *Carcinogenesis* 1997;18:1431–1433.

Wong O, Whorton MD, Foliart DE, Ragland D. An industry-wide epidemiologic study of vinyl chloride workers, 1942–1982. *Am J Ind Med* 1991;20:317–334.

Wrensch M, Bondy ML, Wiencke J, Yost M. Environmental risk factors for primary malignant brain tumors: a review. *J Neurooncol* 1993;17:47–64.

Wrensch M, Lee M, Miike R, et al. Familial and personal medical history of cancer and nervous system conditions among adults with glioma and controls. *Am J Epidemiol* 1997a; 145:581–593.

Wrensch M, Miike R, Lee M, Neuhaus J. Are prior head injuries or diagnostic X-rays associated with glioma in adults? The effects of control selection bias. *Neuroepidemiology* 2000a;19:234–244.

Wrensch MR, Minn Y, Bondy M. Epidemiology. In: Bernstein M, Berger M, eds. Neuro-Oncology: The Essentials. New York: Thieme, 2000b, pp 2–17.

Wrensch M, Minn Y, Chew TC, et al. Epidemiology of primary brain tumors: current concepts and review of the literature. *Neurooncology* 2002;4:278–299.

Wrensch M, Weinberg A, Wiencke J, et al. Does prior infection with varicella-zoster virus influence risk of adult glioma? *Am J Epidemiol* 1997b;145:594–597.

Wrensch M, Weinberg A, Wiencke J, et al. Prevalence of antibodies to four herpesviruses among adults with glioma and controls. *Am J Epidemiol* 2001;154:161–165.

Wrensch M, Yost M, Miike R, et al. Adult glioma in relation to residential power frequency electromagnetic field exposures in the San Francisco Bay area. *Epidemiology* 1999;10:523–527.

Wu W, Steenland K, Brown D, et al. Cohort and case–control analyses of workers exposed to vinyl chloride: an update. *J Occup Med* 1989;31:518–523.

Yeh H, Matanoski GM, Wang N, et al. Cancer incidence after childhood nasopharyngeal radium irradiation: a follow-up study in Washington County, Maryland. *Am J Epidemiol* 2001;153:749–756.

Zhen HN, Zhang X, Bu XY, et al. Expression of the simian virus 40 large tumor antigen (Tag) and formation of Tag-p53 and Tag-pRb complexes in human brain tumors. *Cancer* 1999;86:2124–2132.

Zheng T, Cantor KP, Zhang Y, et al. Risk of brain glioma not associated with cigarette smoking or use of other tobacco products in Iowa. *Cancer Epidemiol Biomarkers Prev* 2001a;10:413–414.

Zheng T, Cantor KP, Zhang Y, et al. Occupational risk factors for brain cancer: a population-based case–control study in Iowa. *J Occup Environ Med* 2001b;43: 317–324.

15

Neurodevelopmental Disabilities

COLEEN A. BOYLE AND CATHERINE C. MURPHY

Neurodevelopmental disorders comprise physical, cognitive, psychological, sensory, speech, and language impairments that result from neurologic damage or dysfunction and are identified between birth and age 18 years. Seventeen percent of children were reported to have a neurodevelopmental disorder on the National Health Interview Survey (Boyle et al. 1994). About 2% of children have a serious neurodevelopmental disorder that requires lifelong care and special services (Boyle et al. 1996). Table 15–1 shows the major neurodevelopmental disorders, including less common ones such as mental retardation, cerebral palsy, and autism, and more pervasive disorders such as attention deficit hyperactivity disorder and learning disabilities. Other disorders involving prenatal brain insults, such as schizophrenia, are sometimes included under the rubric of neurodevelopmental disorders (Susser et al. 1998).

The cause of most neurodevelopmental disorders is considered to be prenatal in origin, and impairments from the resulting brain damage may be manifest at birth. About 10% of mental retardation has known prenatal causes (e.g., genetic disorders, birth defects, and congenital infections), 5%–10% results from adverse perinatal conditions (birth asphyxia, neonatal infections), 5%–10% results from postnatal causes; the remainder are thought to arise from unknown prenatal or genetic factors (Yeargin-Allsopp et al. 1997).

Although most neurodevelopmental disorders are present at birth, parental and clinical recognition is usually delayed until an affected child misses major developmental milestones in the second or third year of life. The confirmatory diagnosis may not come until the child is even older. Some neurodevelopmental disabilities, such as mild mental retardation and attention deficit hyperactivity disorder, may not be diagnosed until the child faces the challenges of school at age 5 or 6 years. This delay in recognition and diagnosis presents methodologic challenges for epidemiologic studies. First, the lag makes it difficult to

Table 15–1 Major Neurodevelopmental Disorders

Disorder	Prevalence per 1000	References
Cerebral palsy	2–3	Kuban and Leviton 1994; Nelson and Grether 1999; Stanley et al. 2000
Mental retardation	10	Fryers 1984; Kiely 1987; Murphy et al. 1995a
Autism	1–3	Wing 1993; Fombonne 1999; Gillberg and Wing 1999
Epilepsy	6	Engel and Pedley 1990
Speech and language disorders	20–40	Tomblin et al. 1997; Shames et al. 2002
Behavior disorders	3–15	Cohen et al. 1993b; Shaffer et al. 1996
Sensory disorders	1	Davidson et al. 1989; Gilbert et al. 1999; Van Naarden et al. 1999; Steinkuller et al. 1999; Mervis et al. 2000

rely on available records to diagnose these conditions, especially at an early age. Second, the relatively long time period between exposure (pregnancy) and diagnosis of the condition at age 2–3 years or school age makes it difficult to develop sensitive measures of exposure for etiologic studies.

Neurodevelopmental disorders tend to co-occur (Table 15–2). About a fifth of children with mental retardation also have another neurodevelopmental disorder, primarily cerebral palsy; about three-quarters of children with autism also have mental retardation; and children with vision impairment are more likely to have multiple disabilities than children with hearing loss (Boyle et al. 1996; Gillberg and Wing 1999). Children with multiple neurodevelopmental disorders tend to have a distinct epidemiologic pattern compared with children who have only one neurodevelopmental disorder; however, most epidemiologic research on neurodevelopmental disorders has focused on each one separately.

Table 15–2 Coexisting Neurodevelopmental Disorders in Children

Disorder	Percent of children with any coexisting disorder
Mental retardation	22
Cerebral palsy	66
Autism	80
Vision impairment	73
Hearing impairment	23

Source: Boyle et al. (1996); Fombonne (1999).

Example 15–1 Among children with mental retardation and at least one other neurodevelopmental disorders, there is little if any association with maternal education and other socioeconomic factors (regardless of the level of the mental retardation), while among children with mental retardation without other neurodevelopmental disorders, maternal education is an extremely important risk factor (Decoufle and Boyle 1995). This phenomenon of co-occurrence may be related to the timing of exposure in pregnancy and in the early postnatal period. The same exposure during different windows of susceptibility may produce very different effects. Examples include the maternal exposures of thalidomide and alcohol, which cause various structural and neurodevelopmental outcomes, depending on the time of exposure in pregnancy (Coles et al. 1991; Stromland et al. 1994).

This chapter will concentrate on mental retardation, autism, and cerebral palsy. These three are highlighted because epidemiologic knowledge of them is more advanced; however, many of the important methodologic issues apply to other neurodevelopmental disorders as well.

Mental Retardation

Disease Description and Classification

Mental retardation (MR) is a heterogeneous group of disorders. The key feature of MR is cognitive impairment with onset up to age 18 years. Cognitive impairment is measured as a standard intelligence quotient (IQ) from individually administered psychometric tests (American Association of Mental Retardation 1992). Standardized tests of intelligence have a mean of 100 and a standard deviation of 15 or 16. An IQ score of 70 or below is usually considered mental retardation. An IQ score reflects an individual's verbal communication, reasoning, and motor and spatial capabilities; however, these do not describe the full range of a person's abilities. The American Association of Mental Retardation (AAMR) recommends that adaptive skills related to daily living and social functioning be taken into consideration when determining the level of MR in an individual (American Association of Mental Retardation 1992).

The level of cognitive or intellectual functioning, as measured by the *Diagnostic and Statistical Manual*–Fourth Edition and the *International Classification of Diseases— Clinical Modification,* Ninth Edition (1992), provide the following classifications: an IQ of 50–70 is mild MR; an IQ of 35–49 is moderate MR; an IQ of 20–34 is severe MR; and an IQ of less than 20 is profound MR (American Psychiatric Association 1994). Each level of intellectual impairment, as measured by IQ score, has a range of functional abilities associated with it (American Psychiatric Association 1994). Adaptive skills are also measured by standardized tests, including the Vineland Adaptive Behavior Scales and the Adaptive Behavior Scale, AAMR (American Association of Mental Retardation 1992).

Criteria for diagnosing MR have long been controversial, especially in the milder ranges of the disability. Underdiagnosis of the milder forms of MR can occur at younger ages, before the academic pressures of school make this disability apparent (Mercer 1973; Murphy et al. 1995a). Culturally inappropriate IQ tests may result in overdiagnosis in ethnically diverse populations.

Descriptive Studies

Period prevalence is used to describe the frequency of MR; *period prevalence* is the number of cases of MR at a specified time in a specified population. The incidence of MR is generally not reported, since the disorder is not usually diagnosed close to the time of occurrence (e.g., prenatal, birth). Accurately enumerating the population from which the incident cases would occur is difficult because of such factors as mortality and migration (Murphy et al. 1995a). In addition, since many genetic causes of MR also result in fetal loss, it would be difficult to estimate the true incidence of MR.

The expected prevalence of MR, if IQ is normally distributed in a population with a mean of 100, is 2.5%, with mild MR representing the majority of cases (75%–80%) (Roeleveld et al. 1997). However, prevalence rates of MR from numerous studies span a wide range, 1–97 per 1000 children 0 to 14 years of age (Kiely 1987; MacLaren and Bryson 1987; Murphy et al. 1995a; Roeleveld et al. 1997).

Example 15–2 As shown in Figure 15–1, the prevalence rates for mild MR show the greatest variation, whereas the rate for children with IQs below 50–55 (Fig. 15–2) is more stable at 2–4 per 1000 (Fryers 1984; Kiely 1987; Roeleveld et al. 1997; Leonard and Wen 2002). Review articles that have compiled rates from prevalence studies across populations and over time (Fryers 1984, Kiely 1987; MacLaren and Bryson 1987; Roeleveld et al. 1997; Leonard and Wen 2002) have shown that secular variations, particularly for mild MR, often reflect differences in case definitions, study designs, and case ascertainment procedures (i.e., registries, service provision, educational placement, and screening). In addition, population characteristics, such as age distribution, birth cohorts observed, race/ethnicity, availability of health and education services, and possibly migration patterns, will also influence rates. Because the rate of mild MR is so dependent on the method of case finding, i.e., population screening versus administrative prevalence, more consideration should be given to a more comprehensive enumeration of the population in epidemiologic studies.

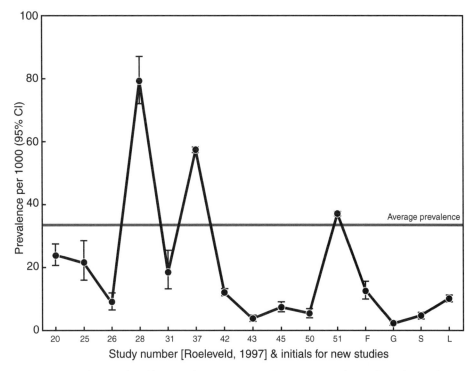

Figure 15–1 Prevalence of mild mental retardation in children of school age in 1960–2000. See Roeleveld et al. (1997) for studies listed by number. (Reprinted with permission from Leonard H, Wen X. The epidemiology of mental retardation: challenges and opportunities in the new millenium. *Ment Retard Disabil Res Rev* 2002; 8:117–134.)

The occurrence and number of coexisting neurosensory conditions increase as the severity of the MR increases. The prevalence of epilepsy is 4%–7% among children with mild MR and 20%–30% among children with severe MR; the prevalence of cerebral palsy is 6%–8% for mild MR and 30% for severe MR; and the prevalence of sensory deficits is 2% for mild MR and 11% for severe MR (Kiely 1987; Murphy et al. 1995b). Autism has been found in 9%–20% of children with MR and occurs more frequently in children with severe MR (Rapin, 1997).

Some investigators have postulated that MR is composed of two types of disorders, roughly corresponding to those with IQs in the mild range (50–70) and those with IQs below 50. The first group could have familial MR due to socioeconomic and/or inheritance patterns (Fryers 1984). These with IQs below 50 could have a more random biologic cause of MR (i.e., spontaneous mutations or trisomies) rather than a cause that segregates within families. However, this two-group definition of MR is not supported by the data, which show considerable overlap between the two groups (Zigler 1967; Fryers 1984; Drews et al. 1995).

Although children with severe MR are diagnosed at earlier ages, on average, the prevalence of severe MR peaks at 10–14 years and doesn't decrease until 20–29 years (Murphy et al. 1995a; Roeleveld et al. 1997). More males than females are found to have MR, primarily mild MR, with a prevalence odds ratio of about 1.4:1; the differences by gender decrease as the level of severity of MR increases (Kiely 1987;

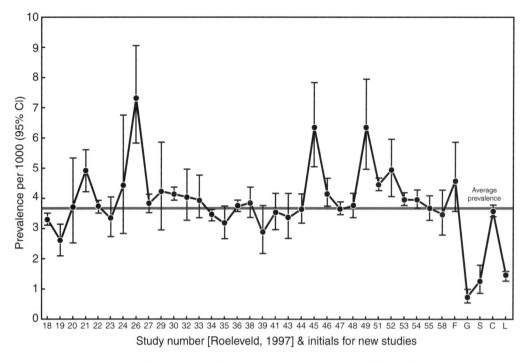

Figure 15–2 Prevalence of severe mental retardation in children of school age in 1960–2000. See Roeleveld et al. (1997) for studies listed by number. (Reprinted with permission from Leonard H, Wen X. The epidemiology of mental rerardation: challenge and opportunities in the new millennium. *Ment Retard Disabil Res Rev* 2002;8:117–134.)

Murphy et al. 1995a). The gender difference in mild MR may be due to social expectations of behavior that put boys at greater risk of being identified for testing procedures that subsequently diagnose mild MR (Mercer 1973). In addition, as discussed below, X chromosome—linked syndromes are expressed more often in males. Among some U.S. populations non-white children have a higher reported prevalence of MR than do white children (see Murphy et al. 1995a for summary). The causes of increased MR in some racial or ethnic groups are often difficult to separate from other prevailing sociodemographic factors. Unmeasured confounders, particularly factors related to social and economic disadvantage, are believed by many researchers to contribute to these findings; accurate measurement and control for these factors is particularly challenging (Leonard and Wen 2002).

Analytic Studies

Mental retardation results from many different types of disease processes and can have quite variable expression even for a single given cause (e.g., Down syndrome, fetal alcohol syndrome). The percentage of people with MR with a known cause is quite variable, depending on the number and types of factors that are considered causal. A known cause has been identified in 20%–24% of mild MR and in approximately 43%–70% of children with severe MR (Murphy et al. 1995a, 1999; Flint and Wilkie 1996; Yeargin-Allsopp et al. 1997). In case series of children seen in genetics clinics, known causes have been found in 10% to 80% of children (Curry et al. 1997; Hunter 2000).

When deciding on a cause or associated risk factors for MR, the use of a temporal sequence for hierarchal decision making is recommended (Table 15–3). Population studies report that the origin of severe and mild MR is prenatal in 25%–55% and 7%–23% of severe and mild MR, respectively; perinatal/neonatal in 10%–15% and 4%–18%, respectively; and postnatal in 7%–10% and 2%–4%, respectively (Hagberg and Kyllerman 1983; MacLaren and Bryson 1987; Yeargin-Allsopp et al. 1997).

Genetics of Mental Retardation

Recurrence risks for MR vary widely within families even when the severity of MR and gender of the index case are taken into consideration (Crow and Tolmie 1998). Among

Table 15–3 Nongenetic Causes or Risk Factors for Mental Retardation in Children

I. Prenatal
  A. Teratogens
    1. Congenital infections—TORCH
    2. Chemical agents
      Alcohol
  B. CNS birth defects
    1. Isolated CNS anomalies
      Hydrocephaly
      Spina bifida
      Cortical atrophy
      Holoprosencephaly
      Microcephaly
      Craniosynostosis
    2. Multiple CNS anomalies
II. Perinatal
  A. Intrauterine/intrapartum asphyxia
  B. Neonatal
    1. Meningitis, bacterial
    2. Neonatal hemorrhage
    3. Low birth weight, prematurity, multiple gestation
    4. Other
      Encephalitis (viral)
      Brain neoplasm
      Multiple congenital anomalies
III. Postneonatal events
  Meningitis (bacterial)
  Cerebrovascular accident (stroke)
  Head trauma
  Brain neoplasm
  Anoxia
IV. Sociocultural

CNS, central nervous system; TORCH, toxoplasmosis, rubella, cytomegalovirus, and herpes simplex.
Source: Adapted from Yeargin-Allsopp et al. (1997) and American Association of Mental Retardation (1992).

studies of siblings of males with severe MR, the recurrence risks for male and female siblings ranged from about 2% to 14%. When the severe MR index case was female, the recurrence risks for male and female siblings were similar but lower than those for the siblings of a male severe MR index case. Regardless of whether the index case was a male or female with mild MR, the recurrences risks were quite similar, ranging from 3% to 20% (Crow and Tolmie 1998).

Genetic conditions are responsible for approximately 7%–15% of all MR and 30%–40% of MR from known causes (Czeizel et al. 1990; Schaefer and Bodensteiner 1992; Yeargin-Allsopp et al. 1997). Chromosomal abnormalities account for up to 30% of severe MR and 4%–8% of mild MR with identifiable causes (Schaefer and Bodensteiner 1992; Crow and Tolmie 1998).

More than 500 genetic diseases are associated with MR (Flint and Wilkie 1996). Thapar et al. (1994) reported that approximately 210 single gene disorders, though rare, have been associated with MR. Several population-based studies have described some of the most widely recognized genetic causes of MR (Buyse 1990; American Association of Mental Retardation 1992; Cohen et al. 1993a; Thapar et al. 1994; Warren and Nelson 1994; Yeargin-Allsopp et al. 1997). Down syndrome (trisomy 21), with a prevalence of 0.8–1.0 per 1000 live births, is the most frequent cause of MR associated with chromosomal abnormalities, accounting for approximately 4%–12% of all MR cases and up to 22% of those cases of MR with a known etiology (Schaefer and Bodensteiner 1992; Yeargin-Allsopp et al. 1997).

New advances and refinements of genetic molecular techniques provide further definition of genetic causes of MR (Thapar et al. 1994; Trembath 1994; Flint and Wilkie 1996). Specialized culture media procedures and molecular cloning techniques have been used to detect "fragile" sites on chromosomes. Among these, fragile X syndrome, FRAXA (fragile site Xq27.3) is one of the best defined conditions and may be the most common single gene disorder that causes inherited MR. The syndrome has a prevalence of 1 per 4000 males and 1 per 8000 females (Turner 1998; Crawford et al. 1999) and accounts for 1%–6% of cases of MR with a known cause (Schaefer and Bodensteiner 1992). As much as 27% of all nonspecific MR in males is due to some sort of X-linked genetic defect (Herbst and Miller 1980; Crow and Tolmie 1998). Approximately 178 XLMR conditions have been identified, with 109 of these being mapped to a specific chromosomal region (Lubs et al. 1999).

Differential expression of genes according to paternal or maternal origin (genomic imprinting and uniparental disomy) is responsible for two genetic types of MR involving the same gene locus, Prader-Willi and Angelman syndromes (Cohen et al. 1993a). Genomic imprinting also has implications for other genetic causes of MR (e.g., myotonic dystrophy, fragile X syndrome, and neurofibromatosis types 1 and 2) (Chatkupt et al. 1995).

Since the mid-1970s, neonates in the United States and in other developed countries have been screened for several metabolic disorders, including phenylketonuria, hypothyrodism, and galactosemia, which, if left untreated, can result in severe neurologic disability as well as MR (Thapar et al. 1994).

There has been increased emphasis on risk factors for some of these genetic disorders (primarily Down syndrome) that result in MR. Potential risk factors include cigarette smoking, oral contraception use, and maternal folate metabolism (Yang et al. 1999; Hobbs et al. 2000; Martinez-Frias et al. 2001). The role that some of these factors play in the etiology of Down syndrome is controversial, however. Do they directly influence the risk of Down syndrome or, alternatively, do they increase the risk of fetal loss in affected pregnancies (Torfs and Christianson 2000)? Many of

the genetic factors described above may be viewed as the proximal cause.

Nongenetic Factors

Maternal Behaviors and Exposures During Pregnancy. Maternal smoking has been linked to MR in exposed children in several studies (Rantakallio and Koiranen 1987; Roeleveld et al. 1992; Drews et al. 1996). Fetal alcohol syndrome (FAS) from prolonged prenatal exposure to alcohol is characterized by a number of central nervous system (CNS) impairments, including MR (Abel 1995). Studies of case series of children with FAS have shown that 23% to 58% have IQs below 70 (Streissguth et al. 1991; Autti-Rämö et al. 1992; Spohr et al. 1993; Habbick et al. 1996). The level of cognitive deficit appears to be proportional to the severity and extent of the physical features of FAS. This suggests a dose effect of prenatal alcohol exposure on physical and cognitive outcomes (Streissguth et al. 1991; Spohr et al. 1993).

Example 15–3 Several environmental contaminants (i.e., lead, methyl-mercury, polychlorinated biphenols [PCBs]) in high doses can produce serious neurologic damage, including MR. Prospective cohort studies of school-age children have found a decrease of 2–6 points in mean IQ with previous lead exposures of >20 to >30 µg/dl relative to exposures <10 µg/dl (Bellinger et al. 1992; Dietrich et al. 1993; Shilu et al. 1996). These findings suggest that pervasive exposure to lead or other environmental toxins would shift the IQ distribution of children in the population and greatly increase the percentage with MR. Alternate explanations for the observed association between lead exposure and IQ include inadequate control of socioeconomic covariates of lead exposure and the possibility that children with initially low IQs are more likely to behave in ways that increase their exposure (i.e., pica) (Silva and Christophers 1997).

Of the two prospective cohort studies of the adverse effects of in utero and postnatal exposure to PCBs (Gladen and Rogan 1991; Jacobson and Jacobson 1996), only the second study reported persistent adverse cognitive effects at ages 4 and 11 years.

As discussed below, maternal infection may be an important factor in preterm labor and possibly in cerebral palsy. Such infection, either through direct infection of the mother or the fetus itself, may also play an important role for other neurodevelopmental outcomes, such as MR.

The role of congenital infections, known as TORCH infections in the etiology of MR, has decreased over the last several decades. The decreasing prevalence of congenital rubella syndrome, coupled with the relatively low prevalence of MR in such children, has made it a minor contributor to MR (Centers for Disease Control and Prevention 1994, 1998). Human cytomegalovirus (CMV), the most common congenital infection, occurs in approximately 3% of births. Whereas only about 5% of infected infants have symptoms at birth, 80%–90% of infants with *symptomatic* CMV infection will have serious neurologically based disabilities by age 2 years (Buyse 1990; Adler 1992; Fowler et al. 1992).

The prevalence of congenital syphilis (CS) was approximately 0.39 per 1000 live births in 1995, decreasing from a high of 1.1 per 1000 live births in 1991 (Dunn et al. 1993; Centers for Disease Control and Prevention, 1996a). Severe neurologic damage, including MR, occurs in about one-third of children with CS (Roizen and Johnson 1996).

Neonatal herpes simplex virus (HSV) infection (onset less than 7 days after birth) occurs in 1.3 per 1000 live births and is a potentially fatal disease (Roizen and Johnson 1996). Among 2-year survivors with HSV, however up to 50% will have permanent neurologic impairment that includes MR (Roizen and Johnson 1996).

Severe, prolonged perinatal asphyxia can result in mental handicap, but this appears to be responsible for only about 5% of all MR in children (Paneth and Stark 1983;

Yeargin-Allsopp et al. 1997). Low birth weight (<2500 grams), a marker of preterm delivery, has been associated with an increased risk for MR. Approximately 21%–28% of children with MR born since the mid-1970s were of low birth weight, compared to 7% of all births (Scottish Low Birthweight Study Group 1992; Cooke 1994; Hack et al. 1994; Mervis et al. 1995; Centers for Disease Control and Prevention 1999). Children from twin gestations have twice the risk for MR as children from singleton gestations (Rydhstroem 1995; Boyle et al. 1997). While most of this increase in risk is due to the higher proportion of preterm births among twins relative to singleton births, there is a substantial increase in the risk of MR in twins with a fetal or infant death of the co-twin (Boyle et al. 1997).

Postnatal insults (injury, infection, stroke) are the cause of MR in approximately 3%–15% of children with MR (MacLaren and Bryson 1987; Centers for Disease Control and Prevention 1996b). The Centers for Disease Control and Prevention (CDC) found that 68% of children with MR due to postnatal causes were more likely to suffer from multiple disabilities (including cerebral palsy, vision, and hearing impairments) than were children with MR due to all other causes (20%). Preventable causes such as head trauma from child battering, motor vehicle injuries, and falls accounted for 52% of MR due to postnatal causes, (Centers for Disease Control and Prevention 1996b).

The percentage of children with MR after contracting postnatal bacterial meningitis infection is 2.1% for *Neisseria meningitides*, 6.1% for *Haemophilus influenzae* (Hib), and 17% for *Streptococcus pneumoniae* (Baraff et al. 1993). Consequently, although the Hib vaccine has resulted in a substantial decrease in the incidence of Hib from 1989 to 1991, the decrease in all meningitis-associated MR may not be substantial. Currently, there are two vaccines for *Streptococcus pneumoniae*, one of which is recommended for children as young as 2 months of age (Centers for Disease Control and Prevention 2000).

Landmark studies from Scotland, England, and the United States on the social risks for MR reported that low socioeconomic status—however measured—is positively correlated with the prevalence of MR, in particular mild MR (Stein and Susser 1963; Birch et al. 1970; Rutter et al. 1970; Mercer 1973; Broman et al. 1987). Recent reports assessing individual, family, and community contributions to children's cognitive development have shown the negative impact of economic depression on the prevalence of MR in developing countries (Islam et al. 1993; Yi et al. 1993; Yaqoob et al. 1995) as well as in the United States (Yeargin-Allsopp et al. 1992, 1995; Decouflé and Boyle 1995; Drews et al. 1995).

Summary

Continued refinement of the classification scheme for defining homogeneous groups of people with MR is necessary to advance knowledge of risk factors and causes. Promising classification schemes include combining levels of severity of MR with the presence of other neurologic conditions. Discovery of additional genetic factors and their causal link to MR will continue to diminish the large percentage of children with MR of unknown cause. An additional challenge that remains in researching the relation between socioeconomic factors and MR is to adequately control for confounding from other risk factors.

Autism

Disease Description and Classification

Leo Kanner (1943) first described autism in the 1940s. He saw autistic children as having functional impairments in three areas: social interactions, communication, and restrictive or repetitive patterns of behaviors. While the field of autism has advanced considerably, these features remain the defining characteristics of the disorder. But the level of impairment necessary to diagnose autism has changed. The children initially described by Kanner (1943) had severe impairments in each of the three areas of functioning. We now have a better appreciation that autism varies widely in its presentation and severity (Rapin 1997; Gillberg and Wing 1999). This variation presents methodologic challenges in conducting epidemiologic studies of the disease. As with mental retardation, it is a challenge for researchers to develop a phenotypic grouping of autism that will facilitate the epidemiologic study of this (these) condition(s).

The age at parental recognition of symptoms of autism varies. Rogers and DiLalla (1990) reported that only 38% of parents recognize abnormalities in development in the first year of life, while 40% recognize a delay in the second year, and 21% notice one at age 2 or later. In the same study, the mean age at diagnosis was considerably later, 45.3 months, and did not vary significantly by age at parental recognition. Despite this late age at diagnosis, recent studies suggest that autism can be reliably diagnosed by 2 years of age (Cox et al. 1999; Stone et al. 1999).

Unlike some of the other neurodevelopmental disorders there are no objective tests for the diagnosis of autism. Instead the diagnosis is based on clinical observations of behaviors that are consistent with the diagnostic criteria for autism (Filipek et al. 1999), such as the criteria of the American Psychiatric Association's *Diagnostic and Statistical Manual, Fourth Edition* (DSM-IV) (1994) and the World Health Organization's (WHO) *International Classification for Diseases, 10th Edition* (ICD-10) (1992). These classification systems include criteria for autistic disorder, Asperger's disorder, and pervasive developmental disorder not otherwise specified (PDD-NOS); the latter two are considered lesser variants of autistic disorder (see Table 15–4). Under Asperger's disorder are included children with higher intellectual functioning who have the features of autism without the communication impairments; PDD-NOS is a default

Table 15–4 Diagnostic Criteria for Autism from ICD-10 and DSM-IV

Autistic Disorder (299.0)

Qualitative impairments in social interactions

Qualitative impairments in communication

Restricted repetitive and stereotyped patterns of behavior

Abnormal functioning in at least one of the above areas prior to age 3 years.

Pervasive Developmental Disorder Not Otherwise Specified (299.80)

Severe impairments in social interactions, communication or stereotyped behaviors, interests, and activities but criteria for autism are not fully met

Asperger Disorder (299.80)

Qualitative impairments in social interactions

No significant delay in language or cognitive development

Restrictive repetitive and stereotyped patterns of behaviors, interests, and activities

Disturbance causes clinically significant impairments in social, occupational, or other important areas of functioning

---

category for children who don't quite meet the criteria for autism. Autism is classified similarly between the two systems, DSM and ICD. Thus comparisons can be made between studies.

Structured diagnostic instruments, such as the Autism Diagnostic Schedule-Generic (ADOS-G) and the Autism Diagnostic Interview (ADI), have been developed for clinicians to diagnose autism (Lord et al. 1994, 2000). Extensive training and ongoing monitoring of the clinical reliability are necessary for the proper use of these instruments. The ADOS-G is used to guide the clinical observation and assessment of children while the ADI is a parent interview of the child's developmental history. While these instruments have improved the validity and reliability of the diagnosis of autism, they also have limitations. The ADOS is based on the current functioning of the child as observed in the clinical session; thus previous behaviors or those not observed during the session are not included. The ADI is a parent interview and is de-

pendent on accurate historical descriptions of a child's behaviors. Ideally these two instruments should be used together, but this may be too costly and burdensome for participating families (Lord and Risi 1998). The use of these state-of-the-art instruments in epidemiologic studies should be encouraged to ensure more reliable case definitions.

Descriptive Studies

The bulk of the epidemiologic studies of autism have been descriptive studies of the prevalence and characteristics of autism. The approach has generally been a process of case finding followed by confirmation of case status (Fombonne 1999; Bertrand et al. 2001). There have been a number of methods used in case finding, the most comprehensive one involving total population screening in which schools or pediatric well-child care visits are used as the vehicle for screening. The advantage of this method is that children who have not yet been diagnosed with autism will come to attention. However, the process is labor-intensive and has only been done in relatively small populations, limiting the number of children identified with autism (Gillberg and Wing, 1999). Other methods used in case finding have targeted *at risk* populations, including those in special education programs, specialty diagnostic clinics, and other service programs for children with neurodevelopmental disorders. Methods to identify children at such sources have varied from asking providers to identify children with possible autism to a comprehensive review of all service provider records. An advantage of this method is that large populations can be targeted, but the success of the method is dependent on the quality and comprehensiveness of diagnostic and treatment services in the community as well as the completeness of the medical records.

Methods used in the second phase, case confirmation, have also varied (Fombonne 1999, Wing and Potter 2002). The most comprehensive method has been a clinical evaluation of the child using standardized instruments to assess the presence of various behaviors of autism and the intellectual and other capabilities of the child. As with the case-finding techniques, the complexity and costs of this approach have generally limited its use in larger epidemiologic studies. A second approach has been to conduct an expert review based on the available diagnostic record information on the child. While this approach has resource advantages and potentially allows for a developmental perspective of the child's behavior, it is dependent on the quality of the records. A third approach is to use the diagnosis as provided by the record source. Because the diagnosis of autism varies widely, this approach needs to be used with caution, keeping in mind methodologic factors that might explain specific trends in the data. An example of this approach would be the use of the classification of autism from education records. Because this classification is based on the need for special education services, children with higher-functioning autism who may be less likely to require special education may be underrepresented in education records. In all these approaches, the case definition, while usually based on the DSM or ICD criteria, has been variably applied. Most studies rely on a clinical expert to either review records or examine the children directly. A few recent studies have used standardized instruments (such as the ADOS or ADI discussed above) for assessing the presence of the criteria when children are examined (Baird et al. 2000; Bertrand et al. 2001). A similar type of rigor to identify affected children is needed for studies based on record review. Studies that assess the validity of these various approaches for ascertaining prevalence should be conducted.

Prevalence. As with MR, most epidemiologic studies of autism have examined the period prevalence (Fombonne 1999). This frequency measure is influenced by in- and out-migrations to populations, so examining trends in prevalence over time may be influenced by changes in the underlying population. A few studies have examined the birth cohort prevalence—the number of cases of autism in a cohort of children who were born during a specified time period and population (Honda et al. 1996; Baird et al. 2000). This measure is more closely tied to changes in etiologic factors in the population. The challenge with birth cohort prevalence is to follow all children who were born into the birth cohort but move out of the geographical area. For example, in the Baird et al. study, which was conducted in the United Kingdom, 78.7% of the cohort of children initially assessed at 18 months was followed at age 3 years and 47.8% was followed at $5^1/_2$ years.

There has been an upward secular trend in the prevalence of autism. Early studies found prevalences of 4–6 per 10,000. More recent studies have found prevalences that are several-fold higher. Two recent reviews (Fombonne 1999; Gilberg and Wing 1999) of the prevalence of autism from studies published in the 1990s calculated average prevalences of 7.2 and 9.6 per 10,000 children. These reviews, however, did not include some of the very recent studies that have found prevalences as high as 2–6 per 1000 (Kadesjo et al. 1999; Baird et al. 2000; Bertrand et al. 2001; Chakrabarti and Fombonne 2001).

It is unclear why the rate of autism is higher than that previously found, although some factors have been identified. One is the current broader definition of autism (Wing and Potter 2002). The early criteria used by Kanner included *severe* impairments in social interactions and communication, e.g., a child who was socially unresponsive and mute. More recent criteria recognize that the behaviors of autism have varied manifestations and severities. Greater awareness of the condition among educators, clinicians, and parents may also contribute to higher prevalence rates. Along with the higher prevalence of autism, there have also been reports of increasing numbers of children receiving services for autism (California Department of Developmental Services 1999; U.S. Department of Education 1999). These service providers have often served in the case-finding aspects of prevalence studies; thus it is sometimes unclear which factor came first. A number of communities have been concerned that they may have an unusually high rate of autism. A recent study in one such community found a prevalence for autism of 4.0 per 1000 children (Bertrand et al. 2001). Whether this prevalence is unusual, however, is difficult to address given the uncertainty about the background prevalence of autism.

While rates of autism in older studies were somewhat higher in elementary school-age children than in preschool or teenage children (Fombonne 1999), more recent data suggest higher rates in preschool-age children (Bertrand et al. 2001). This may be related to the introduction of more early intervention services targeting children with autism. Other explanations include the introduction of causal factors into the environment (Wing and Potter 2002). Most studies have found more boys than girls with autism, with sex ratios ranging from 2:1 to 4:1, with a few exceptions (Fombonne 1999; Gillberg and Wing 1999). While it is likely that gender difference is due to a genetic susceptibility, some authors speculate that boys may be more likely to come to diagnostic attention than girls (Volkmar et al. 1993). This suggestion seems more likely when considering the sex ratio by IQ level—the sex ratio is close to 1:1 for children with IQ <50, while for higher functioning children (IQs >50) it is 3–4:1 (Fombonne 1999).

Little is known about variations in the prevalence of autism in various racial/ethnic groups. Most studies have been conducted in northern Europe or Japan. A number of the studies showing higher autism rates are from Japan (Ishii and Takahashi 1983; Matsuishi et al. 1987; Tanoue et al. 1988; Sugiyama and Abe 1989; Honda et al. 1996). However, these studies were of small populations and used well-child visits to screen the entire population. A few studies have suggested higher rates in immigrant populations (Gillberg and Gillberg 1996).

Analytic Studies

There are a limited number of analytic epidemiologic studies of autism. This is probably because autism was considered a rare disorder and it was too difficult to achieve adequate sample sizes for such studies. In addition, the emphasis of early studies was in understanding the prevalence and descriptive epidemiology of autism.

Family Aggregation/Genetic Studies

Family studies support the idea that there is a strong genetic basis for autism (Szatmari et al. 1998; Spiker 1999; Cook 2001). Siblings of children with autism have a higher than background risk of autism. Szatmari et al. (1998) reported a sibling risk of autism of 2.2%, based on a review of 12 family studies. If PDD-NOS (the lesser variant of autism) was included, the sibling risk increased to 5%. The prevalence among siblings is 5- to 10-fold higher than that in the general population, depending on the population used. Twin studies, which are used to help define the contribution of genetic and environmental factors, suggest that genetics may account for much of the family aggregation in autism. Concordance rates have ranged from 36% to 95% for monozygotic twins, but 0% to 23% for dyzygotic twins (Szatmari et al. 1998). The differences between the monozygotic and dizygotic concordances have been used to estimate the heritability of autism at greater than 90% and to suggest that the mode of transmission is non-Mendelian and most likely involves several genes (Szatmari et al. 1998). Because most genetic studies have been clinic based, issues such as ascertainment bias—i.e., the phenomenon of more families with twins/siblings concordant for the disorder coming to the attention of geneticists—may have biased these estimates.

Coexisting Disorders

Autism is likely to co-occur with MR. Previous studies have found that between 50%

and 90% of individuals with autism also had MR (Wing 1993; Fombonne 1999; Gillberg and Wing 1999). It is unclear whether autism and MR are independent conditions with a single genetic or environmental cause or whether combined gene susceptibility and environmental factors result in a single condition that manifests as impaired cognition (MR) and impaired sociability (autism). Such dilemmas make etiologic studies difficult.

Other disorders found to occur with greater frequency in persons with autism include epilepsy, fragile X syndrome, and tuberous sclerosis (Gillberg and Coleman 1996; Fombonne 1999).

Other Factors

A few exposures during pregnancy have been associated with an increased risk of autism. Chess (1977) found a high rate of autism in a cohort of children exposed in utero to the measles virus; however, in a number of the children, symptoms of the disorder improved with age. In another exposure cohort, individuals exposed in utero to thalidomide also experienced an unusually high rate of autism (Stromland et al. 1994). Because of detailed knowledge of the timing of exposure to thalidomide, it was estimated that exposure to thalidomide very early in pregnancy (day 20–24) most likely resulted in autism.

Example 15–4 A number of studies have examined prenatal and perinatal risk factors for autism, with varied results (Finegan and Quarrington 1979; Deykin and MacMahon 1980; Gillberg and Gillberg 1983; Bryson et al. 1988; Bolton et al 1997). These studies have a number of limitations that may explain their disparate findings, including narrow definitions of autism, incomplete methods for case finding, small sample sizes with low study power to examine all but common risk factors, and the lack of multivariate analyses to examine the independence of the many interrelated prenatal and intrapartum factors (Nelson 1991). Nevertheless, a few possible risk factors were identified that warrant further study: bleeding during pregnancy (especially mid-pregnancy); meconium aspiration syndrome, and high pregnancy optimality score (which reflects the total number of adverse prenatal and perinatal factors experienced during the pregnancy) (Torrey et al. 1975; Gillberg and Gillberg 1983; Matsuishi et al. 1999). Advanced maternal age was implicated in some but not all studies (Gillberg 1980; Tsai and Stewart 1983). Matsuishi et al. (1999) reported a higher prevalence of autism in neonatal intensive care survivors; however, the rate of 3.4 per 1000 children is within the range of prevalences reported in very recent studies.

Summary

Small samples sizes and incomplete case finding have hampered previous epidemiologic studies of autism. Significant advances have been made in the diagnosis of autism, which has important implications for epidemiologic research. Important studies have begun to examine the descriptive epidemiology of autism, including the prevalence and changes in the characteristics of the population over time. Future analytic epidemiologic studies need to be multicentered so that adequate sample size is achieved to examine the genetic and environmental risk factors for autism.

Cerebral Palsy

Disease Description and Classification

Cerebral palsy is an "umbrella term covering a group of non-progressive, but often changing, motor impairment syndromes secondary to lesions or anomalies of the brain arising in the early stages of development" (Mutch et al. 1992). This definition recognizes the clinical and etiological heterogeneity of the cerebral palsy diagnosis, which is based exclusively on the clinical signs and symptoms of motor impairment. Cerebral palsy is analogous to mental retardation in that both are the overt signs of CNS dysfunction (Nelson and Grether 1999). Clinical classification of cerebral palsy is generally by the type of motor disability, the extent of involvement of the limbs, and the severity of the motor disability (see Table 15–5). The prominent type of motor impairment is spasticity, which represents about 80% of cerebral palsy. Among those with spastic cerebral palsy, about a third are hemiplegia, another third are diplegic, and the remaining third are quadriplegic, although some registries have found lower proportions of children with quadriplegic cerebral palsy (Stanley et al. 2000). Because the classification of cerebral palsy is based on clinical findings, the reliability of clinical subtype may be questionable, especially for less common subtypes (Blair and Stanley 1985). This may explain some of the variation in subtype of cerebral palsy across studies. However, this variation in diagnosis does not appear to greatly affect the overall prevalence rate of cerebral palsy (discussed below). Attempts to examine the severity of cerebral palsy have used more objective indices, such as use of assistive devices, receipt of physical therapy, and motor scores on standardized developmental tests (Pinto-Martin et al. 1995)

A diagnosis of cerebral palsy is generally not given until the child reaches at least age 2 years, because motor disability in young children may be transient. Many registry programs for cerebral palsy actually use a later age (i.e., 3–5 years) for reporting. As Nelson and Ellenberg (1982) showed in their analysis of the U.S. Collaborative Perinatal Project data, 52% of children who were diagnosed with motor impairment at

age 1 no longer had signs of such impairment at age 7.

Descriptive Studies

Because cerebral palsy represents a heterogeneous condition, it is important to estimate the prevalence of cerebral palsy in specific subgroups, particularly those defined by type and birth weight. Case-finding methods in epidemiologic studies of cerebral palsy have primarily used service provider records, i.e. records of specialists who diagnosis or provide services to children with cerebral palsy and other neurodevelopmental disorders. Multiple sources may be necessary to capture all children, depending on the age of the child and the level of services in the community within a defined population (Yeargin-Allsopp et al. 1992). Some studies have used clinical examinations of the child to confirm the diagnosis and determine the specific type of cerebral palsy (Cummins et al. 1993), while others have relied on medical records, including physical and occupational therapy reports to confirm the type of cerebral palsy (Murphy et al. 1993). It is important to report age-specific prevalence rates for comparison across studies, especially when examining type of cerebral palsy, which continues to evolve as the child grows older.

Prevalence. Because most of cerebral palsy is considered to be prenatal in origin, with the resulting motor disability manifesting itself as the child fails to reach developmental motor milestones, epidemiologic studies have traditionally used a birth cohort prevalence measure. The numerator is the number of cases at a defined age and the denominator includes all live births or all neonatal/infant survivors from the birth cohort that gave rise to the case children. Prevalences based on live births will tend to be lower than those based on neonatal or infant survivors; this is especially true for children born with low birth weight or very preterm, when mortality in the first

Table 15–5 Classification of Cerebral Palsy by Type of Movement Disorder and Location of Impairment

Type of cerebral palsy	Percent of cases
Spastic	76–86
Hemiplegia	27–37
Diplegia	18–45
Quadriplegia	8–32
Dyskinesia	4–10
Athetoid	4

Adapted from Stanley et al. (2000), with permission.

year of life is considerable (Blair and Stanley 1997). Period prevalence, in which the denominator is the number of children defined by the same age and calendar time as the case children, has been used to describe the burden of cerebral palsy in the population (Murphy et al. 1993). While the period prevalence is considered useful for planning service provision, depending on the changes in the population over time—due to both in- and out-migration—it might be reflective of etiologic differences as well.

Despite the methodologic differences that can influence rates, the prevalence of cerebral palsy from recent studies is remarkably similar, ranging from 1.2 to 2.8, with the majority of studies at about 2.0 per 1000 live births (Stanley et al. 2000, table on pp 208–9). Similar to studies of autism and mental retardation, most of the cerebral palsy studies are from northern European countries (e.g., Hagberg et al. 1996; Topp et al. 1997; Pharoah et al. 1998), although there are also long-standing surveillance programs for cerebral palsy in Western Australia and the United States. The U.S. Centers for Disease Control and Prevention has an ongoing monitoring program for cerebral palsy in Atlanta, Georgia (Boyle et al. 1996; Stanley et al 2000).

The prevalence of cerebral palsy tends to increase with age up to early elementary school age; as with autism and mental retardation, this pattern reflects children going undiagnosed until they need special education services at school entry (Boyle et al. 1996). In addition, a small fraction of this increase stems from incidence of postnatal cerebral palsy—i.e., motor disability due to brain damage from such causes as postnatal infections and trauma (Centers for Disease Control and Prevention 1996b).

Among children with cerebral palsy, more males are found than females. The sex ratios range from 1.1 to 1.5:1, although there may be some variation by birth weight (Stanley et al. 2000). In the CDC data, children of African American descent had lower rates of cerebral palsy relative to white children if their birth weight was <2500 grams, but had higher rates if their birth weight was ≥2500 grams (Winter et al. 2002).

Very low birth weight (i.e., <1500 grams) is the most significant risk *indicator* for cerebral palsy (Nelson and Grether 1997). Extreme prematurity is perhaps the more important risk factor, but birth weight is used instead of gestational age because it is more accurately available for all children (Stanley et al. 2000). Because the descriptive and analytic epidemiology of cerebral palsy has been shown to vary by birth weight, epidemiologic studies of cerebral palsy should always present birth weight–specific findings (Mutch et al. 1992). To illustrate this remarkable association with birth weight, the birth weight distribution of case children relative to all live births in California for 1983–1987 is shown in Figure 15-3. Among children with cerebral palsy, there is a bimodal distribution of birth weights, which peaks at about 1200 grams and then parallels the distribution for all live-born children. About one-quarter of children with cerebral palsy are born at <1500 grams and about half are born at <2500 grams (Cummins et al. 1993), compared with about 1% and 7%, respectively, of births in the general population. Children from multiple births have a higher risk of cerebral palsy, which seems to be mostly attributable to being born prematurely (Grether et al. 1993; Petterson et al. 1993)

In examining trends over 30 years (1958–1989) from five different registry systems, Blair and Stanley (1997) did not find consistent trends in the overall birth prevalence of cerebral palsy, even though there have been remarkable improvements in obstetric and neonatal care during that time period. However, trends over time in neonatal survivors with birth weights <1500 grams suggest an increase in the rate of cerebral palsy from the mid-1960s to the late 1980s (Stanley et al. 2000). Two recent studies indicate a possible downward trend in the rate of cerebral palsy in very low–birth weight survivors in the most recent follow-up period

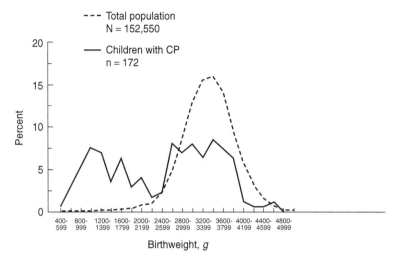

Figure 15–3 Birth weight distribution of singleton children with cerebral palsy (CP) and of total singleton population. Birth weight, in 200 gram intervals, is on the horizontal axis; the percentage of singleton children with CP and in the total surviving 3-year-old singleton population within each birth weight is plotted on the vertical axis. Thirty-five children in the total population with missing birth weight information were excluded. (Reprinted with permission from Cummins SK, Nelson KB, Grether JK, Velie EM. Cerebral palsy in four northern California counties, births 1983 through 1985. *J Pediatr* 1993; 123:230–237.)

(1990–1994) (O'Shea et al. 1998; Grether and Nelson 2000).

Analytic Studies

Because cerebral palsy has a relatively low prevalence, most population-based studies of children with cerebral palsy have relied on referral sources to identify case children. In analytic epidemiologic studies that focus on high-risk subgroups of the population where the prevalence of cerebral palsy and other neurodevelopmental disabilities is considerably higher (e.g., those born very preterm), clinical exams on all children in the cohort are possible.

Example 15–5 One methodologic issue that is more important for cerebral palsy than for the other neurodevelopmental disorders is the fact that cerebral palsy is so strongly associated with prematurity, and preterm infants have a high mortality rate. Hence, many preterm infants don't survive long enough to exhibit disease. If these children had survived, it is likely that a substantial proportion of them would have developed cerebral palsy. In studies of cerebral palsy in infant survivors, it has generally been assumed that the risk and protective factors are similar among the survivors with serious neurologic disability and their counterparts who die in the first year of life. Brain imaging techniques are currently being used to try to identify early markers of motor impairment (Leviton and Gilles, 1999). Periventricular echolucency as measured by ultrasound is evidence of white matter damage and is strongly linked to later motor disability (Pinto-Martin et al. 1995). Comparison of epidemiologic characteristics of children with early signs of brain damage with those who survive and develop cerebral palsy will determine if there are differences in risk or protective factors between these groups.

Family Aggregation

There is some family aggregation in cerebral palsy, but it tends to occur in association with unusual circumstances, such as populations with high rates of consanguinous marriages (Bundy, 1997). One interesting observation is that women who have given birth to a child with cerebral palsy are at increased risk for other adverse reproductive outcomes, such as prematurity or intrauterine growth retardation, but this may be a result of maternal rather than genetic factors (Palmer et al. 1994). Several studies have shown a higher proportion of birth defects in children with cerebral palsy relative to the general population, suggesting a common prenatal and perhaps genetic etiology (Nelson and Ellenberg 1986; Cronin et al. 2001).

Nongenetic Risk Factors

Among very-low–birth-weight infants, pre-eclampsia is associated with a reduced risk of cerebral palsy; however, there is a modest increase in risk of cerebral palsy associated with preeclampsia in normal–birth-weight infants (Collins and Paneth 1998). It is unclear why preeclampsia would be a protective factor in preterm infants, given that preeclampsia results in infants who have lower birth weight for gestational age, a risk factor for cerebral palsy. One group has suggested that this is an artifact of selection due to higher mortality in infants born very preterm to preeclamptic mothers (Murphy et al. 1996). Congenital infections, primarily rubella and CMV, are known to cause various neurologic impairments including cerebral palsy, primarily in term infants (Gilbert 1996). A number of markers of maternal infection in pregnancy, such as clinical chorioamnionitis, maternal fever and antibiotic use, uterine tenderness, and neonatal sepsis, have been linked to cerebral palsy in preterm infants in some (Murphy et al. 1995b; O'Shea et al. 1998) but not all studies (Grether and Nelson 1996). While it is unclear whether the link between maternal infection and cerebral palsy is independent of factors associated with preterm birth, these same markers of maternal infection, including biomarkers of neonatal inflammatory response, have been associated with cerebral palsy in term infants (Grether and Nelson 1996; Nelson et al. 1998). A variety of abnormalities in coagulation, including antiphospholipid anti-

bodies and factor V Leiden, have been linked to neonatal strokes and cerebral palsy in term infants (Nelson et al. 1998; Harum et al. 1999).

In preterm infants, intrapartum indications of fetal distress and factors that may reflect a compromised oxygen supply were not associated with cerebral palsy (Murphy et al. 1995b; Grether and Nelson 1996). In term infants, a recent study that examined obstetric complications that may have resulted in birth asphyxia found only one factor, tight nuchal cord, to be strongly associated with cerebral palsy. This factor explains only 6% of spastic cerebral palsy (Nelson and Grether 1998).

Studies have found that between 10% and 15% of cerebral palsy is due to postnatal causes (Stanley et al. 2000, pp 126–127). There is a fluctuating upper age limit for what is included as cerebral palsy, which may account for some of the variation in proportion of cerebral palsy due to a postnatal cause. The major causes of postnatal cerebral palsy include infection, stroke, and cerebral vascular accidents (Centers for Disease Control and Prevention 1996b).

Summary

Despite advances in prenatal and obstetric care, the prevalence of cerebral palsy has not declined in the past 30 years. In fact, there are some indications that the prevalence of cerebral palsy in very preterm infants who survive the neonatal period has increased, although we must await more data to confirm this finding. Promising advances have been made in identifying precursors of cerebral palsy, including the possible roles of maternal infection and coagulation abnormalities, which may offer prevention opportunities. Future studies must have sufficient statistical power to examine risk factors specific to birth weight and subtype of cerebral palsy.

Future Directions and Conclusions

Systematic disease monitoring and tracking programs exist for some childhood health problems, such as birth defects and childhood cancers, but no systematic programs exist for monitoring the occurrence of neurodevelopmental disorders, even though these conditions affect a sizable percentage of children. While there are selective registries worldwide for cerebral palsy, which have been monitoring rates since the 1970s (most notably, in Australia and Sweden), there is only one ongoing population-based study of autism in Sweden, which is limited by small sample size. Such programs are critical to understanding the descriptive epidemiology of neurodevelopmental disorders and to monitoring changes in prevalence over time, and as a resource for case children for analytic studies. Current questions as to whether the prevalence of some neurodevelopmental disabilities has changed over time (Wing and Potter 2002) are impossible to address because of the lack of such monitoring programs.

Valid and reliable case definitions of neurodevelopmental disorders need to be developed and applied in a standardized fashion in epidemiolgic studies. In monitoring trends, it is important to include all manifestations of the disorder even if the cause is known; in analytic studies, such case children can be excluded when appropriate.

The descriptive epidemiology of neurodevelopmental disorders needs to be better characterized. Determining how the prevalence of these conditions varies among various ethnic and racial population groups may provide useful insight into underlying etiology; however, to date, most research has focused on northern European populations. Because the neurodevelopmental disabilities are relatively uncommon and analytic studies often examine specific subtypes, large multicenter collaborative studies should be encouraged. Subtypes based on the presence or absence of other neurodevelopmental disorders should be considered. Establishing biomarkers of exposure and precursors of early disease during the relevant time periods (pregnancy and early postnatal period) is challenging in the study of neurodevelopmental disabilities. One promising area is the use of biologic materials collected and stored for other purposes in pregnancy and at birth, such a samples collected for alpha fetal protein screening, newborn blood spot screening, and placental pathologic evaluations. Genetics plays an important role in some of the neurodevelopmental disabilities, especially autism and mental retardation. We need to use genetic epidemiology techniques that include epidemiologic approaches to family studies (Khoury 1998) to aid in the search for gene markers to better understand the role of gene–environment interactions.

References

Abel EL. An update on incidence of FAS: FAS is not an equal opportunity birth defect. *Neurotoxicol Teratol* 1995;17:437–443.

American Association of Mental Retardation. Mental Retardation: Definitions, Classification, and Systems of Supports. Washington DC: American Association on Mental Retardation, 1992.

American Psychiatric Association. Diagnostic and Statistical Manual of Mental Disorders, Fourth Edition (DSM-IV). Washington, DC: American Psychiatric Association, 1994.

Autti-Rämö I, Korkman M, Hilakivi-Clarke L, et al. Mental development of 2-year-old children exposed to alcohol in utero. *J Pediatr* 1992;120:740–746.

Baird G, Charman T, Baron-Cohen S, Cox A, et al. A screening instrument for autism at 18 months: a 6-year follow-up study. *J Am Acad Child Adolesc Psychiatry* 2000;39:694–702.

Baraff LJ, Lee SI, Schriger DL. Outcomes of bacterial meningitis in children: a meta-analysis. *Pediatr Infect Dis J* 1993;12:389–394.

Bellinger DC, Stiles KM, Needleman HL. Low-level lead exposure, intelligence, and academic achievement: a long-term follow-up study. *Pediatrics* 1992;90:855–861.

Bertrand J, Mars A, Boyle C et al. Prevalence of autism in a United States population: the Brick Township, New Jersey, investigation. *Pediatrics* 2001;108:1155–1161.

Birch HG, Richardson SA, Baird D, et al. Mental Subnormality in the Community. Baltimore, MD: Williams and Wilkins, 1970.

Blair C, Stanley FJ. Issues in the classification and epidemiology of cerebral palsy. *Ment Retard Dev Disabil Res Rev* 1997;3:184–193.

Blair E, Stanley F. Interobserver agreement in the classification of cerebral palsy. *Dev Med Child Neurol* 1985;27:615–622.

Bolton P, Murphy M, MacDonald H, et al. Obstetric complications in autism: consequences or causes of the condition. *J Am Acad Child Adolesc Psychiatry* 1997;36: 272–281.

Boyle CA, Decoufle P, Yeargin-Allsopp M. Prevalence and health impact of developmental disabilities in U.S. children. *Pediatrics* 1994;93:399–403.

Boyle CA, Keddie A, Holmgreen P. The risk of mental retardation in twins. *Paediatr Perinat Epidemiol* 1997;11:A10.

Boyle CA, Yeargin-Allsopp M, Doernberg NS, et al. Prevalence and selected developmental disabilities in children 3–10 years of age: the Metropolitan Atlanta Developmental Disabilities Surveillance Program, 1991. *MMWR CDC Surveill Summ* 1996;45:1–14.

Broman S, Nichols PL, Shaughnessy P, et al. Retardation in Young Children. A Developmental Study of Cognitive Deficit. Hillsdate, NJ: Lawrence Erlbaum Associates, 1987.

Bundy S. Prevalence and type of cerebral palsy. *Dev Med Child Neurol* 1997;39:568.

Buyse ML, ed. Birth Defects Encyclopedia. Cambridge, MA: Blackwell Scientific Publications, 1990.

California Department of Developmental Services. Changes in the population of persons with autism and pervasive developmental disorders in California's Developmental Services System: 1987 through 1998. A report to the Legislature. Sacramento, CA: California Department of Developmental Services, 1999.

Centers for Disease Control and Prevention. Rubella and congenital rubella syndrome—United States, January 1, 1991—May 7, 1994. *MMWR Morb Mortal Wkly Rep* 1994; 43(21):391–401.

Centers for Disease Control and Prevention. Summary of notifiable diseases, United States 1995. *MMWR Morb Mortal Wkly Rep* 1996a;44:1–87.

Centers for Disease Control and Prevention. Postnatal causes of developmental disabilities in children aged 3–10 years—Atlanta, Georgia, 1991. *MMWR Morb Mortal Wkly Rep* 1996b;45:130–134.

Centers for Disease Control and Prevention. Measles, mumps, and rubella—vaccine use and strategies for elimination of measles, rubella,and congenital rubella syndrome and control of mumps: Recommendations of the advisory committee on immunization practices (ACIP). *MMWR* 1998;47(RR-8):1–57.

Centers for Disease Control and Prevention. Prevention and control of meningococcal disease. Recommendations of the advisory committee on immunization practices (ACIP). *MMWR* 1999;49(RR-7):1–10.

Centers for Disease Control and Prevention. Preventing pneumococcal disease among infants and young children: recommendations of the Advisory Committee on Immunization Practices (ACIP). *MMWR Recomm Rep* 2000; 49:1–35.

Chakrabarti S Frombonne E. Pervasive developmental disorder in preschool children. *JAMA* 2001;285:3093–3099.

Chatkupt S, Antonowicz M, Johnson WG. Parents do matter: genomic imprinting and parental sex effects in neurological disorders. *J Neurol Sci* 1995;130:1–10.

Chess S. Follow-up report on autism in congenital rubella. *J Autism Child Schizophr* 1977;7:69–81.

Cohen MM, Rosenblum LS, Prabhaker C. Human cytogenetics: a current overview. *Am J Dis Child* 1993a;147:1159–1166.

Cohen P, Cohen J, Kasen S, Velex CN. An epidemiological study of disorders in late childhood and adolescence I. Age- and gender-specific prevalence. *J Child Psychol Psychiatry* 1993b;34:851–867.

Coles CD, Brown RT, Smith IE, et al. Effects of prenatal alcohol exposure at school age. I. Physical and cognitive development. *Neurotoxicol Teratol* 1991;13:357–367.

Collins M, Paneth N. Pre-eclampsia and cerebral palsy: are they related? *Dev Med Child Neurol* 1998;40:207–211.

Cook EH Jr. Genetics of autism. *Child Adolesc Psychiatr Clin North Am* 2001;10:333–350.

Cooke RWI. Factors affecting survival and outcome at 3 years in extremely preterm infants. *Arch Dis Child Fetal Neonatal Ed* 1994; 71:F28–F31.

Cox A, Klein K, Charman T, et al. Autism spectrum disorders at 20 and 42 months of age: stability of clinical and ADI-R diagnosis. *J Child Psychol Psychiatry* 1999;40:719–732.

Crawford DC, Meadows KL, Newman JL, et al. Prevalence and phenotype consequence of *FRAXA* and *FRAXE* alleles in a large, ethnically diverse, special education-needs population. *Am J Hum Genet* 1999;64: 495–507.

Cronin LA, Grether JK, Curry CJ, Nelson KB. Congenital abnormalities among children with cerebral palsy: more evidence for prenatal antecedents. *J Pediatr* 2001;138:804–810.

Crow Y, Tolmie JL. Recurrence risks in mental retardation. *J Med Genet* 1998;35:177–182.

Cummins SK, Nelson KB, Grether JK, Velie EM. Cerebral palsy in four northern California counties, births 1983 through 1985. *J Pediatr* 1993;123:230–237.

Curry CJ, Stevenson RE, Aughton D, et al. Evaluation of mental retardation: recommendations of a Consensus Conference: American College of Medical Genetics. *Am J Med Genet* 1997;72:468–477.

Czeizel A, Sankaranarayanan K, Szondy M. The load of genetic and partially genetic diseases in man. *Mutat Res* 1990;232:291–303.

Davidson J, Hyde ML, Alberti PW. Epidemiologic patterns in childhood hearing loss: a review. *Int J Pediatr Otorhinolaryngol* 1989; 17:239–266.

Decouflé P, Boyle CA. The relationship between maternal education and mental retardation in 10-year-old children. *Ann Epidemiol* 1995;5:347–353.

Deykin EY, MacMahon B. Pregnancy, delivery, and neonatal complications among autistic children. *Am J Dis Child* 1980;134:860–864.

Dietrich KN, Berger OG, Succop PA, et al. The developmental consequences of low to moderate prenatal and postnatal lead exposure: intellectual attainment in the Cincinnati Lead Study Cohort following school entry. *Neurotoxicol Teratol* 1993;15:37–44.

Drews CD, Murphy CC, Yeargin-Allsopp M, Decouflé P. The relationship between idiopathic mental retardation and maternal smoking during pregnancy. *Pediatrics* 1996; 97:547–53.

Drews CD, Yeargin-Allsopp M, Decouflé P, Murphy, CC. Variation in the influence of selected sociodemographic risk factors for mental retardation. *Am J Public Health* 1995;85:329–334.

Dunn RA, Webster LA, Nakashima AK, Sylvester G. Surveillance for geographic and secular trends in congenital syphilis—United States, 1983–1991. *MMWR CDC Surveill Summ* 1993;4259–4271.

Engel J, Pedley TA, eds. Epilepsy: A Comprehensive Text Book, Vol. 1. Philadelphia: Lippincott-Raven, 1990.

Filipek PA, Accardo PJ, Baranek GT, et al. The screening and diagnosis of autistic spectrum disorders. *J Autism Dev Disord* 1999;29: 439–484.

Finegan J, Quarrington B. Pre-, peri-, and neonatal factors and infantile autism. *J Child Psychol Psychiatry* 1979;20:119–128.

Flint J, Wilkie AOM. The genetics of mental retardation. *Br Med Bull* 1996;52:453–464.

Fombonne E. Is the prevalence of autism increasing? *J Autism Dev Disord* 1996;26: 673–676.

Fombonne E. The epidemiology of autism: a review. *Psychol Med* 1999;29:769–786.

Fowler KB, Stagno S, Pass RF, et al. The outcome of congenital cytomegalovirus infection in relation to maternal antibody status. *N Engl J Med* 1992;326:663–667.

Fryers T. The Epidemiology of Severe Intellectual Impairment: The Dynamics of Prevalence. London: Academic Press, 1984, pp 32–59.

Gilbert CE, Anderton L, Dandona L, Foster A. Prevalence of visual impairment in children: a review of available data. *Ophthalm Epidemiol* 1999;6:73–82.

Gilbert GL. Congenital fetal infections. *Semin Neonatol* 1996;1:91–105.

Gillberg C. Maternal age and infantile autism. *J Autism Dev Disord* 1980;10:293–297.

Gillberg C, Coleman M. Autism and medical disorders: a review of the literature. *Dev Med Child Neurol* 1996;38:191–202.

Gillberg C, Gillberg IC. Infantile autism: a total population study of reduced optimality in the pre-, peri-, and neonatal period. *J Autism Dev Disord* 1983;13:153–166.

Gillberg C, Wing L. Autism: not an extremely rare disorder. *Acta Psychiatr Scand* 1999;99: 399–406.

Gillberg IC, Gillberg C. Autism in immigrants: a population-based study from Swedish rural and urban areas. *J Intellect Disabil Res* 1996;40:24–31.

Gladen BC, Rogan WJ. Effects of perinatal polychlorinated biphenlys and dichlorodiphenyl dichloroethene on later development. *J Pediatr* 1991;119:58–63.

Grether JK, Nelson KB. Prenatal and perinatal factors and cerebral palsy in very low birth weight infants. *J Pediatr* 1996;128:407–414.

Grether JK, Nelson KB. Possible decrease in prevalence of cerebral palsy in premature infants. *J Pediatr* 2000;136:133.

Grether JK, Nelson KB, Cummins SK. Twinning and cerebral palsy: experience in four northern California counties, births 1983 through 1985. *Pediatrics* 1993;92:854–858.

Habbick BF, Nanson JL, Snyder RE, et al. Foetal alcohol syndrome in Saskatchewan: unchanged incidence in a 20-year period. *Can J Public Health* 1996;87:204–207.

Hack M, Taylor HG, Klein N, et al. School-age outcomes in children with birth weights under 750 g. *N Engl J Med* 1994;331:753–759.

Hagberg B, Hagberg G, Olow I, von Wendt L. The changing panorama of cerebral palsy in Sweden VII. Prevalence and origin in the birth year period 1987–90. *Acta Paediatr* 1996;85:954–960.

Hagberg B, Kyllerman M. Epidemiology of mental retardation—a Swedish survey. *Brain Dev* 1983;5:441–449.

Harum KH, Hoon AH, Kato GJ, et al. Homozygous factor-V mutation as a genetic cause of perinatal thrombosis and cerebral palsy. *Dev Med Child Neurol* 1999;41:777–780.

Herbst DS, Miller JR. Nonspecific X-linked mental retardation II: the frequency in British Columbia. *Am J Med Genet* 1980;7:461–469.

Hobbs CA, Sherman SL, Yi P, Hopkins SE, Torfs CP, Hine RJ, Pogribna M, Rozen R, James SJ. Polymorphins in genes involved in folate metabolism as maternal risk factors for Down syndrome. *Am J Hum Genet* 2000;67:623–630.

Honda H, Shimizu Y, Misumi K, et al. Cumulative incidence and prevalence of childhood autism in children in Japan. *Br J Psychiatry* 1996;169:228–235.

Hunter A. Outcome of routine assessment of patients with mental retardation in a genetics clinic. *Am J Med Genet* 2000;90:60–68.

International Classification of Diseases, 9th Revision, Clinical Modification (ICD-9cm). Reno, NV: Channel Pub Ltd, 1993.

Ishii T, Takahashi I. The epidemiology of autistic children in Toyota, Japan: prevalence. *Jpn J Child Adolesc Psychiatry* 1983;24:311–321.

Islam S, Durkin MS, Zaman SS. Socioeconomic status and the prevalence of mental retardation in Bangladesh. *Ment Retard* 1993:31:412–417.

Jacobson JL, Jacobson SW. Intellectual impairment in children exposed to polychorinated biphenyls in utero. *N Engl J Med* 1996;335:783–789.

Kadesjo B, Gillberg C, Hagberg B. Brief report: autism and Asperger syndorme in seven-year-old children: a total population study. *J Autism Dev Disord* 1999;29:327–331.

Kanner L. Autistic disturbances of affective contact. *Nervous Child* 1943;2:217–250.

Khoury MJ. Genetic epidemiology. In: Rothman KJ, Greenland S, eds. Modern Epidemiology. Philadelphia: Lipponcott-Raven, 1998, pp 609–622.

Kiely M. The prevalence of mental retardation. *Epidemiol Rev* 1987;9:194–218.

Kuban KCK, Leviton A. Cerebral palsy. *N Engl J Med* 1994;330:188–195.

Leonard H, Wen X. The epidemiology of mental retardation: challenges and opportunities in the new millennium. *Ment Retard Dev Disabil Res Rev* 2002;8:117–134.

Leviton A, Gilles F. Ventriculomegaly, delayed myelination, white matter hypoplasia, and "perventricular" leudomalacia: how are they related? *Pediatr Neurol* 1999;15:127–136.

Lord C, Risi S. Frameworks and methods in diagnosing autism spectrum disorders. *Men Retard Dev Disabil* 1998;4:90–96.

Lord C, Risi S, Lambrecht L, et al. The Autism Diagnostic Observation Schedule–Generic: a standard measure of social and communication deficits associated with the spectrum of autism. *J Autism Dev Disord* 2000;30:205–223.

Lord C, Rutter M, Le Couteur A. Autism Diagnostic Interview–Revised: a revised version of a diagnostic interview for caregivers of individuals with possible pervasive developmental disabilities. *J Autism Dev Disord* 1994;24:659–657.

Lubs H, Chiurazzi P, Arena J, et al. *XLMR* genes: update 1998. *Am J Med Genet* 1999;83:237–247.

MacLaren J, Bryson SE. Review of recent epidemiological studies of mental retardation: prevalence, associated disorders, and etiology. *Am J Ment Retard* 1987;92:243–254.

Martinez-Frias M, Bermejo E, Rodriguea-Pinilla E, Preito L. Periconceptional exposure to contraceptive pills and risk for Down syndrome. *J Perinatol* 2001;21:288–292.

Matsuishi T, Shiotsuki Y, Yoshimura K, et al. High prevalence of infantile autism in Kurume City, Japan. *J Child Neurol* 1987;2:268–271.

Matsuishi T, Yamashita Y, Ohtani Y, et al. Brief report: incidence of and risk factors for autistic disorder in neonatal intensive care unit survivors. *J Autism Dev Disord* 1999;29:161–166.

Mercer JR. Labeling the Mentally Retarded. Berkeley, CA: University of California Press, 1973.

Mervis CA, Decouflé P, Murphy CC, Yeargin-Allsopp M. Low birthweight and the risk for mental retardation later in childhood. *Paediatr Perinat Epidemiol* 1995;9:455–468.

Mervis CA, Yeargin-Allsopp M, Winter S, Boyle C. Aetiology of childhood vision impairment, metropolitan Atlanta, 1991–93. *Paediatr Perinat Epidemiol* 2000;14:70–77.

Murphy CC, Yeargin-Allsopp M, Decoufle P, Drews CD. Prevalence of cerebral palsy among ten-year-old children in metropolitan Atlanta, 1985 through 1987. *J Pediatr* 1993;123:S13–S20.

Murphy CC, Yeargin-Allsopp M, Decoufle P, Drews C. The administrative prevalence of mental retardation in 10-year-old children in metropolitan Atlanta, 1985 through 1987. *Am J Public Health* 1995a;85:319–323.

Murphy DJ, Sellers S, MacKenzie IA, et al. Case–control study of antenatal and intrapartum risk factors for cerebral palsy in preterm singleton babies. *Lancet* 1995b;346:1449–1454.

Murphy DJ, Squier MV, Hope PL, et al. Clinical associations and term of onset of cerebral white matter damage in very preterm babies. *Arch Dis Child Fetal Neonatal Ed* 1996;75:F27–F32.

Mutch L, Alberman E, Hagberg B, et al. Cerebral palsy epidemiology epidemiology: where are we now and where are we going? *Dev Med Child Neurol* 1992;34:547–551.

Nelson KB. Prenatal and perinatal factors in the etiology of autism. *Pediatrics* 1991:87:761–766.

Nelson KB, Dambrosia JM, Grether JK, Phillips TM. Neonatal cytokines and coagulation factors in children with cerebral palsy. *Ann Neurol* 1998;44:665–675.

Nelson KB, Ellenberg JH. Children who 'outgrew' cerebral palsy. *Pediatrics* 1982;69:529–536.

Nelson KB, Ellenberg JH. Antecedents of cerebral palsy: multivariate analysis of risk. *N Engl J Med* 1986;315:81–86.

Nelson KB, Grether JK. Cerebral palsy in low-birthweight infants: etiology and strategies for prevention. *Ment Retard Dev Disabil Res Rev* 1997;3:112–117.

Nelson KB, Grether JK. Potentially asphyxiating conditions and spastic cerebral palsy in infants of normal birthweight. *Am J Obstet Gynecol* 1998;179:507–513.

Nelson KB, Grether JK. Causes of cerebral palsy. *Curr Opin Pediatr* 1999;11:487–491.

O'Shea TM, Preisser JS, Klinepeter KL, Dillard RG. Trends in mortality and cerebral palsy in a geographically based cohort of very low birth weight neonates born between 1982 and 1994. *Pediatrics* 1998;101:624–627.

Palmer L, Petterson B, Blair E, Burton P. Family patterns of gestational age at delivery and growth in utero in moderate and severe cerebral palsy. *Dev Med Child Neurol* 1994; 36:1108–1119.

Paneth N, Stark RI. Cerebral palsy and mental retardation in relation to indicators of perinatal asphyxia. *Am J Obstet Gynecol* 1983; 147:960–966.

Petterson B, Nelson KB, Watson L, Stanley F. Twins, triplets, and cerebral palsy in births in Western Australia in the 1980s. *BMJ* 1993;307:1239–1243.

Pharoah PO, Cooke T, Johnson MA, et al. Epidemiology of cerebral palsy in England and Scotland 1984–9. *Arch Dis Child Fetal Neonatal Ed* 1998;79:F21–F25.

Pinto-Martin JA, Riolo S, Cnaan A, et al. Cranial ultrasound prediction of disabling and nondisabling cerebral palsy at age two in a low birth weight population. *Pediatrics* 1995;95:249–254.

Rantakallio P, Koiranen M. Neurologic handicaps among children whose mothers smoked during pregnancy. *Prev Med* 1987;16:597–606.

Rapin I. Autism. *New Engl J Med* 1997;337: 97–104.

Roeleveld N, Vingerhoets E, Zielhuis G, Gabreels F. Mental retardation associated with parental smoking and alcohol consumption before, during, and after pregnancy. *Prev Med* 1992;21:110–119.

Roeleveld N, Zielhuis GA, Gabreels F. The prevalence of mental retardation: a critical review of recent literature. *Dev Med Child Neurol* 1997;39:125–132.

Rogers SJ, DiLalla DL. Age of symptom onset in young children with pervasive developmental disorders. *J Am Acad Child Adolesc Psychiatry* 1990;29:863–872.

Roizen NJ, Johnson D. Congenital Infections. Developmental Disabilities in Infancy and Childhood, 2nd ed. Vol I: Neurodevelopmental Diagnosis and Treatment. Baltimore, MD: Paul H. Brookes, 1996, pp 175–193.

Rousseau F, Heitz D, Tarleton J, et al. A multicenter study of genotype–phenotype correlations in the fragile X syndrome, using direct diagnosis with probe StB12.3: the first 2,253 cases. *Am J Hum Genet* 1994;55:225–237.

Rutter M, Tizard J, Whitmore K. Education, Health and Behavior; Psychological and Medical Study of Childhood Development. New York: John Wiley, 1970.

Rydhstroem H. The relationship of birth weight and birth weight discordance to cerebral palsy or mental retardation later in life for twins weighing less than 2500 grams. *Am J Obstet Gynecol* 1995;173:680–686.

Schaefer GB, Bodensteiner JB. Evaluation of the child with idiopathic mental retardation. *Pediatr Clin North Am* 1992;39:929–943.

Scottish Low Birthweight Study Group. The Scottish Low Birthweight Study: II. Language attainment, cognitive status, and behavioural problems. *Arch Dis Child* 1992; 67:682–686.

Shaffer D, Fisher P, Dulcan MK, et al. The NIMH Diagnostic Interview Schedule for Children Version 2.3 (DISC-2.3): description, acceptability, prevalence rates, and performance in the MECA study. Methods for the Epidemiology of Child and Adolescent Mental Disorders Study. *J Am Acad Child Adolesc Psychiatry* 1996;35:865–877.

Shames, GH, Anderson NB. Human Communication Disorders: An Introduction, 6th ed. Boston: Allyn and Bacon/Longman, 2002.

Shilu T, Baghurst P, McMichael A, et al. Lifetime exposure to environmental lead and children's intelligence at 11–13 years: the Port Pirie cohort study. *BMJ* 1996;312: 1569–1575.

Silva PD, Christophers AJ. Lead exposure and children's intelligence: do low levels of lead in blood cause mental deficit? *J Pediatr Child Health* 1997;33:12–17.

Spiker D. The role of genetics in autism. *Infant Young Child* 1999;12:55–63.

Spohr HL, Willms J, Steinhausen HC. Prenatal alcohol exposure and long-term developmental consequences. *Lancet* 1993;341: 907–910.

Stanley F, Blair E, Alberman E. Cerebral Palsies: Epidemiology and Causal Pathways. London: Mac Keith Press, 2000.

Stein Z, Susser M. The social distribution of mental retardation. *Am J Ment Defic* 1963; 67:811–821.

Steinkuller PG, Du L, Gilbert C, Foster A, Collins ML, Coats DK. Childhood blindness. *J AAPOS* 1999;3:26–32.

Stone WL, Lee EB, Ashford L, et al. Can autism be diagnosed accurately in children under 3 years? *J Child Psychol Psychiatry* 1999;40: 219–226.

Streissguth AP, Aase JM, Clarren SK, et al. Fetal alcohol syndrome in adolescents and adults. *JAMA* 1991;265:1961–1967.

Stromland K, Nordin V, Miller M, et al. Autism in thalidomide embryopathy: a population study. *Dev Med Child Neurol* 1994;36:351–356.

Sugiyama T, Abe T. The prevalence of autism in Nagoya, Japan: a total population study. *J Autism Dev Disord* 1989;19:87–96.

Susser E, Hoek HW, Brown A. Neurodevelopmental disorders after prenatal famine. The story of the Dutch Famine Study. *Am J Epidemiol* 1998;147:213–216.

Szatmari P, Jones MB, Zwaigenbaum L, MacLean JE. Genetic of autism: overview and new directions. *J Autism Dev Disord* 1998;28:351–368.

Tanoue Y, Oda S, Asano F, Kawashima K. Epidemiology of infantile autism in southern Ibaraki, Japan: differences in prevalence in birth cohorts. *J Autism Dev Dis* 1988;18: 155–166.

Thapar A, Gottesmann II, Owen MJ, O'Donovan C. The genetics of mental retardation. *Br J Psychiatry* 1994;164:747–758.

Tomblin JB, Smith E, Zhang X. Epidemiology of specific language impairment: prenatal and perinatal risk factors. *J Commun Disord* 1997;30:325–344.

Topp M, Uldall P, Langhoff-Roos J. Trend in cerebral palsy birth prevalence in eastern Denmark: birth year period 1979–86. *Paediatr Perinat Epidemiol* 1997;11:451–460.

Torfs CP, Christianson RE. Effect of maternal smoking and coffee consumption on the risk of having a recognized Down syndrome pregnancy. *Am J Epidemiol* 2000;152:1185–1191.

Torrey EF, Hersh SP, McCabe KD. Early childhood psychosis and bleeding during pregnancy. A prospective study of gravid women and their offspring. *J Autism Child Schizophr* 1975:5:287–297.

Trembath RC. Genetic mechanisms and mental retardation. *J R Coll Phys Lond* 1994;28: 121–125.

Tsai LY, Stewart MA. Etiological implications of maternal age and birth order in infantile autism. *J Autism Dev Dis* 1983;13:57–65.

Turner G, Webb T, Wake S, Robinson H. Prevalence of fragile X syndrome. *Am J Med Genet* 1998;64:196–197.

U.S. Department of Education. To assure the free appropriate public education of all children with disabilities. Twenty-first annual report to Congress on the implementation of the Individuals with Disabilities Education Act. Washington, DC: U.S. Department of Education, 1999, p A–30.

Van Naarden K, Decoufle P, Caldwell K. Prevalence and characteristics of children with serious hearing impairment in metropolitan Atlanta, 1991–1993. *Pediatrics* 1999;103: 570–575.

Volkmar FR, Szatmari P, Sparrow SS. Sex differences in pervasive developmental disabilities. *J Autism Dev Disord* 1993;23:579–591.

Warren ST, Nelson DL. Advances in molecular analysis of fragile X syndrome. *JAMA* 1994;217:536–542.

Wing L. The definition and prevalence of autism: a review. *Eur Child Adolesc Psychiatry* 1993;2:61–74.

Wing L, Potter D. The epidemiology of autistic spectrum disorders: is the prevalence rising? *Ment Retard Dev Disabil Res Rev* 2002; 8:151–161.

Winter S, Autry A, Boyle C, Yeargin-Allsopp M. Trends in the prevalence of congenital cerebral palsy in Atlanta, Georgia. *Pediatrics* 2002;110:1220–1225.

World Health Organization. The ICD-10 Classification of Mental and Behavioral Disorders: Clinical Descriptions and Diagnostic Guidelines. World Health Organization, Geneva: 1992.

Yang Q, Sherman SL, Hassold TJ, et al. Risk factors for trisomy 21: maternal cigarette smoking and oral contraceptive use in a population-based case–control study. *Genet Med* 1999;1:80–88.

Yaqoob M, Bashir A, Tareen K, et al. Severe mental retardation in 2- to 24-month-old children in Lahore, Pakistan: a prospective cohort study. *Acta Paediatr* 1995;84: 267–272.

Yeargin-Allsopp M, Drews CD, Decouflé P, Murphy CC. Mild mental retardation in black and white children in metropolitan Atlanta: a case–control study. *Am J Public Health* 1995;85:324–328.

Yeargin-Allsopp M, Murphy CC, Cordero JF, et al. Reported biomedical causes and associated medical conditions for mental retardation among 10-year-old children , metropolitan Atlanta, 1985 to 1987. *Dev Med Child Neurol* 1997;39:142–149.

Yeargin-Allsopp M, Murphy CC, Oakley GP, Sikes RK. A multiple-source method for studying the prevalence of developmental disabilities in children: the Metropolotan Atlanta Development Disabilitities Study. *Pediatrics* 1992;89:624–630.

Yi S, Luo X, Wan G, et al. Epidemiological investigation in a village with high prevalence of mental retardation. *Chin Mental Health J* 1993;7:270–272.

Zigler E. Familial mental retardation: a continuing dilemma. *Science* 1967;155:292–298.

16

Prognosis of Neurologic Diseases

W. T. LONGSTRETH JR. AND VALERIE McGUIRE

This chapter returns to the methodological principles of the first section of the book and reviews how they can be applied to clinical questions, specifically questions of prognosis. Although the methodological approaches are similar, the questions posed in classic epidemiology and clinical epidemiology differ (Fig 16–1). In classic epidemiology, epidemiologists pose a question about the etiology of a disease and identify causal factors that can be manipulated or modified to prevent the disease in a population of people. In clinical epidemiology, clinicians pose a question about the prognosis of a disease in a population of patients. Prognosis can be regarded as a set of outcomes and their associated probabilities following the occurrence of some defining event or diagnosis that can be a symptom, sign, test result, or disease (Longstreth et al. 1987b). If the efforts of classic epidemiology are successful, a disease is prevented, and clinical epidemiology is no longer pertinent. Though the distinction between classic and clinical epidemiology is not always as clear-cut as suggested

by Figure 16–1, it plays an important part in convincing clinicians of the relevance of these methodological principles to the care they provide their patients (Sackett et al. 1991; Fletcher et al. 1996).

Prognosis is the keystone of clinical neurology (Longstreth et al. 1992). Clinical epidemiology also includes important issues about diagnosis, including reliability and validity (Longstreth et al. 1987a; Sackett et al. 1991; Fletcher et al. 1996). Classic epidemiologic studies may begin with populations of healthy people, but they end with the occurrence of a disease, and an accurate diagnosis is essential. A similar need exists in clinical epidemiologic studies that begin with a population of patients with a particular diagnosis. However, issues of diagnosis will not be addressed in this chapter. Prognosis links a diagnosis to an outcome; without such a link, a diagnosis is little more than a descriptive term that lacks implications for the patient's future. A numb hand could be explained by carpal tunnel syndrome or multiple sclerosis; prognosis is what makes these conditions,

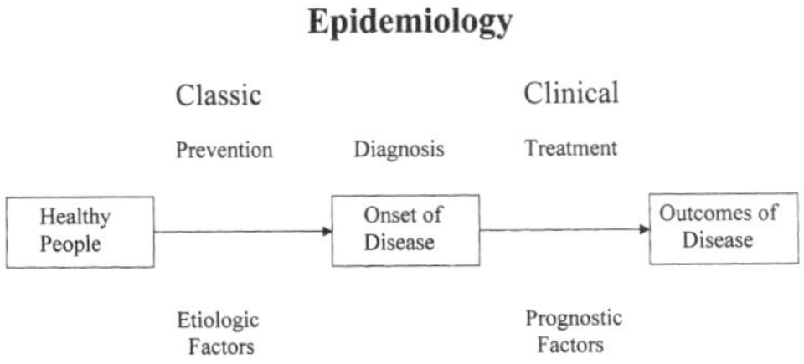

Epidemiology

Figure 16–1 Contrast of classic and clinical epidemiology. (Modified from previous work [reprinted with permission from Longstreth WT Jr, Koepsell TD, van Belle G. Neuroepidemiology as it applies to occupational neurology. In: Bleecker ML, Hanson JA, eds. Occupational Neurology and Clinical Neurotoxicology. Baltimore: Williams and Wilkins, 1994, pp 1–21].)

which can start in an identical fashion, so different.

This chapter will cover study design, analytic considerations, and genetics, while highlighting the challenges presented by studies of prognosis. Observational studies are needed to study prognosis because many of the prognostic factors being evaluated are not easily modified, for example, age at onset, coma on presentation, or histologic pattern. Modifiable prognostic factors, such as medications, diet, or exercise, may also be identified through observational studies and further studied by randomized controlled clinical trials (experimental studies). Randomized controlled trials are our most powerful tool for establishing whether or not a modifiable prognostic factor is causally related to an outcome. Clinical trials are the focus of Chapter 17. Once we recognize the importance of prognostic factors that go beyond the specific patient and once we broaden our view of what constitute the important outcomes from a disease, we have a better understanding of what is meant by health services research and outcomes research—the topics of Chapter 18. Finally, the lessons of clinical epidemiology are not meant to be limited to academic physician-epidemiologists, who sometimes have more interest in analyzing data than caring for patients, but also to provide clinicians with the tools to improve their patients' outcomes. Evidence-based medicine teaches clinicians

the practical application of clinical epidemiology, which includes how to find the best evidence relevant to a specific problem, how to assess the quality of that evidence, and how to decide if it applies to a specific patient. Evidence-based medicine will be discussed in Chapter 19.

Study Designs

Getting Started

The first step in designing a study of prognosis is to ask an important clinical question. A thorough clinical understanding of the condition to be studied is an asset in devising a relevant question. A review of the literature allows the investigator to decide if the question is unanswered and, if so, which study design has the greatest likelihood of answering the question. Altman and Lyman (1998) describe several types of studies of prognosis that depend on how well the question is formulated. They define phase I prognostic studies as those with the least well-defined hypotheses. These studies are exploratory and serve to generate hypotheses to be examined further in phase II prognostic studies. Phase III studies serve to confirm and validate prognostic factors that appear promising in the phase II studies. Unfortunately, most studies of prognosis in neurology and other fields are of the first two types, which explains the sometimes inconclusive results (Kernan et al. 1991).

The focus of studies of prognosis may differ. Some studies try to demonstrate a robust association of a prognostic factor or marker with an outcome. Control for other factors in this setting may be important, not to identify confounding, but to explore whether the new prognostic factor adds anything to established factors. For example, clinicians should not use an expensive new laboratory test to clarify prognosis if it does no better than knowing the patient's demographics and conducting a neurologic examination. Other studies aim to predict outcome from the information available rather than to identify new prognostic factors. Prediction is based on multivariate models, e.g., how well these models classify the outcome of patients with the condition in question. Still other studies focus on establishing a causal association between a prognostic factor and outcome, with confounding of prime concern. Understanding that a prognostic factor causes an outcome may lead to a better understanding of pathophysiology, treatment, or both. Often studies with observational designs cannot resolve causal issues, so experimental studies are needed.

As described in Chapter 2 and summarized in Table 16–1, several designs are available to address questions of etiology in classic epidemiology. These have parallels in designs to address questions of prognosis in clinical epidemiology. The simplest studies are descriptive. Outcomes are described in a population of patients with a specified condition. Once hypotheses are generated, analytic designs are needed to explore what factors are related to outcomes. The best approach would be an experimental design whereby the factor of interest would be randomly assigned to patients with the condition of interest to determine whether or not outcomes differed by some modifiable prognostic factor. Such an approach is taken in randomized controlled clinical trials, although it is often not practical or feasible because many prognostic factors of interest may not be easily modified or randomized. In such situations, we turn to observational study designs. In addition, unlike classic epidemiology, in which etiologic associations are important, in studies of prognosis, strong associations are important regardless of whether or not they imply a causal link.

Example 16–1 In a study of diffusion-weighted magnetic resonance imaging (DWI) of patients with an acute ischemic stroke, DWI was related to the long-term outcome (van Everdingen et al. 1998). The correlations between lesion size on early DWI and follow-up of the patients' clinical status using the National Institutes of Health Stroke Scale and the Modified Rankin Scale were 0.62 ($p < 0.001$) for both measures. The imaging result may be a useful clinical marker for outcome. Note that the investigators did not address whether or not the imaging results add clinically meaningful prognostic information to what is already available from demographics information and the early neurological examination.

Observational studies come in several varieties, as discussed in Chapter 2, the most common being the case–control study and the cohort study. In classic epidemiology, the case–control study is efficient when the disease is relatively rare. If the outcome of interest is rare, with prevalence of 10% or less, the case–control design can still be employed in studies of prognosis. Most often in studies of prognosis, however, the outcomes of interest are not rare and the

Table 16–1 Types of Designs and Purpose of Prognostic Studies

Type of design	Purpose
Observational Studies Cohort studies Case–control studies Cross-sectional studies Nonrandomized trials	• Identify clinical and other factors (genetic, lifestyle, demographic) associated with a poor outcome • Develop prognostic models to enable better classification of individuals into distinct prognostic subgroups, e.g., patients at high or low risk of disease progression or death
Randomized Clinical Trials	• Guide clinical decision making to identify subsets of patients likely to benefit from therapy • Use nontreated subjects (placebo group) to identify factors associated with outcome (a natural history study)

case–control design provides little, if any, advantage over the cohort design. In the cohort design, a group of patients with the same condition are identified, followed over time, and have their outcomes documented.

Example 16–2 Investigators wanted to know what factors were associated with long-term survival in patients with glioblastoma multiforme (Scott et al. 1999). In their population-based study of 689 patients with histologically verified glioblastoma multiforme, 15 (2.2%) patients survived at least 3 years—a rare outcome in this population. Each long-term survivor was matched to three patients from among the remaining patients according to age, gender, and year of diagnosis. The investigators reviewed medical records on these 60 patients rather than the entire cohort of 689 patients. They identified several factors associated with long-term survival, such as better neurologic function at diagnosis as assessed by the Karnofsky Performance Status, gross total surgical resection (40% for long-term survivors compared with 14% for controls), adjuvant chemotherapy (40% of long-term survivors underwent this compared with 0% for controls), and certain features of the tumor histology.

Cohort designs can be either prospective or retrospective. In prospective cohort studies, the investigators assemble the cohort and follow it forward in time. The Framingham Study is an example of an ongoing prospective cohort study (Wolf et al. 1978). In a retrospective cohort study, information on prognostic factors and outcomes were collected at some time in the past, and the investigator uses these retrospective data. Many examples of retrospective cohort studies come from the Mayo Clinic because of the excellent medical records linkage system used there (Kurland and Brian 1978).

Ideally, a cohort study of prognosis would emulate a randomized trial. Several authors have suggested the essential features for valid studies of prognosis (Sackett et al. 1991; Longstreth et al. 1992; Lau-pacis et al. 1994; Simon and Altman 1994; Altman and Lyman 1998), and some of these considerations are summarized in Table 16–2. The condition, prognostic factors, and outcomes must be defined explicitly and assessed similarly in all study subjects. Defining and assessing the neurologic condition requires a thorough understanding of diagnosis. Lack of precision in diagnosis may result in a heterogeneous rather than homogeneous cohort. For example, when examining prognostic factors for hemorrhagic stroke, patients with intraparenchymal hemorrhage and subarachnoid hemorrhage should be considered separately. Statistical power may be eroded, making the investigators less likely to identify associations that in fact exist (type II error). Many of the methodological issues about measurement discussed in Chapter 3 apply equally well to defining and assessing prognostic factors and outcomes. Imprecision in measurements may also erode statistical power or, even worse, introduce bias if prognostic factors and outcomes are not determined independently or blindly.

Table 16–2 Considerations for Design of Prognostic Studies

Develop and define prognostic research question
• Concrete issue that advances understanding of prognosis

Define and assess similarly in all study subjects:
• Neurologic diagnosis
• Prognostic factors
• Outcomes, such as disease severity, disability, death

Choose and define cohort of study subjects
• Describe the source of patients and the inclusion/exclusion criteria
• Assemble newly diagnosed patients
• Minimize losses to follow-up over time

Identify prognostic factors based on the following:
• Literature review of previous studies
• Single best prognostic factor or marker
• Best model with multiple factors that predicts outcome
• Biological reasoning about disease pathogenesis
• Relevance to the clinical setting

Given all these potential problems that can weaken studies, the fact that associations are ever found is remarkable.

Investigators strive to design internally valid studies, but the clinician must also consider external validity. Unfortunately, a high level of internal validity is no guarantee of external validity, which is how well the results of an internally valid study can be applied to other populations. Studies that lack internal validity do not warrant such a consideration. Clinicians need the critical reading skills to judge the internal and external validity of the study. The greater challenge is often with external validity and deciding if the results of a valid study apply to a particular patient (Justice et al. 1999). Clinicians are faced with the same task in interpreting and applying results of randomized trials.

Prognostic Factors and Outcomes

Prognostic factors come in many varieties, such as clinical signs, symptoms, test results, medications, demographic factors, and lifestyle behaviors (e.g., exercise, smoking). The literature abounds with examples of clinical features as prognostic indicators; for example, numbness as the first symptom of multiple sclerosis is associated with a benign course (Hawkins and McDonnell 1999). For patients admitted to the hospital after onset of subarachnoid hemorrhage, survival of patients was significantly related to Hunt and Hess grade (Longstreth et al. 1993) (Fig. 16–2). Low mean distal compound muscle action potential on electromyography is associated with delayed or incomplete recovery from Guillain-Barré syndrome (Cornblath et al. 1988). Seizures as the presenting manifestation of a brain tumor are associated with a favorable survival (Gehan and Walker 1977). Investigators often collect information on several clinical factors with plans to adjust for other factors or to find the best predictive model. Information based on the history and physical examination may have irreducible imprecision, so clinicians often seek more reliable information from imaging studies and laboratory tests. A reliable and

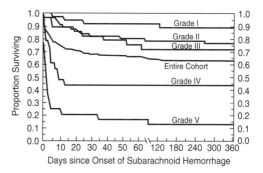

Figure 16–2   Survival after onset of subarachnoid hemorrhage for the entire cohort ($n = 171$) and for those admitted according to Hunt and Hess grade (Hunt and Hess, 1968) on admission ($n = 166$). (Reprinted with permission from Longstreth WT Jr, Nelson LM, Koepsell TD, van Belle G. Clinical course of spontaneous subarachnoid hemorrhage in population-based study in King County, Washington. *Neurology* 1993;43:712–718.)

reproducible prognostic factor is necessary but not sufficient to assure its accuracy. Accuracy of a prognostic factor is often assessed using approaches developed for diagnostic tests, such as sensitivity, specificity, and predictive values. An important difference between diagnosis and prognosis is that time is not as important in diagnosis as it is in prognosis. Concepts such as sensitivity, specificity, and predictive values lack a time dimension. When applied to assessment of prognostic factors, investigators must eliminate time, for example, considering not the time of death but the proportion dead at some specified time.

Just as prognostic factors come in many varieties, so do outcomes. Fletcher and colleagues (1996) describe six categories of outcome: disease, death, disability, discomfort, dissatisfaction, and destitution. Outcomes will be discussed in greater depth in a subsequent chapter, especially those that move beyond death and disability. Sometimes the easiest outcomes to measure may not be appropriate, such as death as an assessment of outcome after idiopathic facial nerve dysfunction due to Bell's palsy. Often the outcomes that patients and clinicians find the most relevant are the most difficult to measure. The number of years lived may be viewed as less important than the quality of life during those years, for example. Whatever the outcome that the investigators define, it should be determined similarly in all study subjects, and the outcome and prognostic factors should be determined separately to avoid having information about one influence decisions about the other.

The Cohort

Care is required in assembling the cohort of patients with the condition of interest. An inception cohort is best, with all the patients being at a similar and early stage of their disease. As the cohort becomes more heterogeneous, with its members at different stages of the disease upon entry into the study, the greater is the threat to the study's internal validity. When an inception cohort is not used, a characteristic of the disease, such as severity, may influence which patients are included in the cohort and thus what sort of outcomes are experienced. Both bias due to the use of prevalent patients and referral bias demonstrate this point. Enrolling at some point in time all the patients with malignant brain tumors (prevalent patients) will select out preferentially those patients with longer survival, a design flaw that can be avoided by enrolling all patients with newly diagnosed malignant brain tumors over some time period (incident patients). The source of the patients comprising the cohort may also bias the study (referral bias). If the sample from which the subjects are drawn is not representative of the general population, the results will be skewed (Fig. 16–3).

Example 16–3 A classic example is a study of febrile seizures (Ellenberg and Nelson 1980). The authors compared the frequency of febrile seizures from referral centers and from population-based studies. The prevalence of febrile seizures among clinic-based studies varied widely compared to that among population-based studies. In this example, referral center patients were more severely affected than the general population of patients, but the outcome may also be more favorable among patients seen at referral centers. For instance, patients

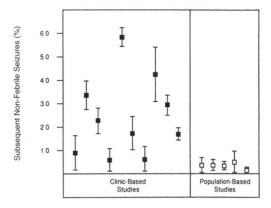

Figure 16–3 Rate of nonfebrile seizures following febrile convulsion. Closed squares represent studies form referral centers and open squares those from population-based surveys. Rates and their 95% confidence intervals are shown. (Modified from Ellenberg and Nelson [1980]; Sackett et al. [1991]; reprinted with permission from Longstreth WT Jr, Koepsel TD, van Belle G. Clinical Neuroepidemiology. II. Outcomes. *Arch Neurol* 1987b;44:1196–1202.)

with subarachnoid hemorrhage identified from referral centers have better survival than those from the general population (Whisnant et al. 1993). Selection bias may have played a role in improved survival for referral patients. Referral patients showed better early survival rates than community patients because patients who died or were in poor clinical condition could not be referred to the clinic.

Many other biases can compromise a study's internal validity, as reviewed in the earlier chapters. A major concern in cohort studies of prognosis is that patients are lost to follow-up. If a factor related to outcome is also related to the likelihood of being lost to follow-up, this may bias the study. Often, the potential for this bias is known, but the direction of the effect is not. Is the patient whose seizures are poorly controlled likely to continue to seek care from the study investigator, to seek care elsewhere, or to die suddenly? Investigators can perform sensitivity analyses, thus setting bounds on the effect of patients having been lost to follow-up. Nonetheless, as the numbers lost to follow-up rise, the internal validity of the study is compromised, along with any useful clinical information that can be derived from it.

Statistical Analyses

A first step in analyses is to summarize the outcome of interest in the group of patients under study. The analyses used are determined in part by the form of the outcome variable. Dichotomous outcomes are appealing because of their simplicity: the stroke patient survived or not; the patient stopping antiseizure medications had a recurrent seizure or not; or the patient with multiple sclerosis experienced a benign course or not. In these situations, time is ignored altogether. Sometimes a time interval is implied but not specified and unlikely to be the same for all patients, such as the status of some outcome measure by the time of hospital discharge. Such shortcomings can be avoided by using a fixed time interval, such as the proportion with the dichotomous outcome at 3 months or 5 years, or whatever interval is deemed appropriate by the investigators for the condition being studied.

> *Example 16–4* Although summaries such as the 5-year survival for patients with oligodendrogliomas are simple and easily understood, much information can be lost. For example, the 2-year survival may be identical for two groups of patients. In one group, most of the deaths occur early in their clinical course, such as with subarachnoid hemorrhage. In the other group, deaths accumulate over time, such as with amyotrophic lateral sclerosis. The clinician would be wrong to conclude that the prognosis of these two conditions is similar because the 2-year survival is similar. A richer summary of the outcome is possible by allowing the outcome to be a function of time: a dichotomous outcome still occurs but now at a specific time. Such information is summarized in a powerful technique called *survival analysis* (Peto et al. 1977).

In its purest form, a survival analysis includes all patients followed over the same time interval and provides the proportion with a certain dichotomous outcome as a function of time. Problems arise when patients are lost to follow-up or are followed for variable periods of time. The solution to these problems involves assumptions that are demonstrable in examples of the technique (Longstreth et al. 1992; Fletcher et al. 1996). An important assumption is typically made concerning the prognosis of patients who are not known to experience the outcome but who are also not followed to the end of the study. These patients are censored from the analyses and their prognosis is assumed to be the same as the prognosis of those who continue under observation. Review of a survival curve should always call to mind this hidden assumption and prompt an attempt to judge the impact of those no longer followed at a particular point in time. As time goes on and the number of patients observed decreases, results become unstable and require caution in interpretation.

> *Example 16–5* A community-based study in Perth, Australia examined prognostic factors for death within 5 years of incident stroke among 362 patients (Hankey et al. 2000). Only 2% of patients were lost to follow-up. This study also compared the observed survival after incident stroke with expected survival in the age- and gender-matched general population in Western Australia. Using this technique, the authors were able to obtain estimates of the absolute and relative risks of dying. Patients with incident stroke had a 10-fold increase of dying in the first year and a 4-fold increase of dying over 5 years compared with the individuals of the same age and gender in the general population.

Survival analyses serve an important descriptive role by summarizing a dichotomous outcome in a group of patients. Despite the name, survival analysis can be applied to any time-dependent dichotomous outcome, not just survival. It can also be used to address specific hypotheses about the effect of a prognostic factor on survival, for instance, comparing survival in men and women. Although the summary is simple, is easily understood, and can be illustrated graphically, it is limited to a single dichotomous outcome variable. Because of the need to examine more than one variable and continuous outcomes, investigators often turn to multivariate techniques.

Multivariate techniques assess which predictors are independently associated with the outcome after adjusting or controlling for the other variables in the model. The analyses provide coefficients for each predictor variable in the model. Many multivariate techniques are available and choosing the appropriate test depends largely on the form of the outcome variable. A popular technique in epidemiologic studies is logistic regression (Hall and Round 1994). Coefficients from logistic regression can be converted to odds ratios. Logistic regression is often used in etiologic studies of disease because the odds ratio is a reasonable estimate for the relative risk when the disease (or outcome) is rare. This rare disease assumption is not satisfied in many studies of prognosis because clinically important outcomes are usually not rare. In situations where the outcome is more common among the diseased cohort, say, more than 10%–15%, the odds ratio is still an acceptable measure of association but should not be presented as a relative risk with the corresponding interpretation. If the outcome of interest has more than two categories, logistic regression is no longer appropriate. Polytomous and ordinal logistic regression are available for prognostic measures that are ordinal or continuous, but these analyses can be complex (Bender and Grouven 1997). Alternatives include log-linear modeling and discriminant analysis. If the outcome of interest is continuous, multiple linear regression can be used.

None of these models allows the investigator to consider the timing of the outcome. To include time in the analyses, the Cox proportional hazard model is needed (Cox 1972). Cox regression allows for both the outcome and predictor variables to be time-dependent. The coefficients for the predictor variables can be used to obtain adjusted estimates of the relative risk. This powerful and sophisticated analytic tool for studies of prognosis is demanding and requires that certain assumptions be met, most importantly that of proportional hazards.

Other statistical techniques are suited to the analysis of studies of prognosis but are used less frequently than the multivariate techniques described above. Two examples include recursive partitioning and artificial neural networks. Recursive partitioning yields a classification tree with a series of binary branches (Breiman et al. 1984). The form of the outcome variable and the means by which associations are assessed are flexible. All predictor variables must be made dichotomous; for non-dichotomous predictors, all potential cut-points are examined to identify the best split. The process is repeated at each branch point and a tree is grown. Procedures are available that allow trimming of the tree and assessment of validity. Despite the appeal of the resulting trees to clinicians, relatively few examples are found in the neurological literature; the best known example concerns outcome from nontraumatic coma (Levy et al. 1981, 1985). The technique of artificial neural networks provides a computationally intense alternative to linear statistical approaches (Baxt 1995; Wyatt 1995). It uses computerized artificial intelligence processes to predict outcomes; however, few examples are found in the neurological literature (Edwards et al. 1999).

Statistical Modeling for Prognostic Studies

Although many of these modeling techniques are readily available to investigators through standard statistical packages, performing the analyses and testing for assumptions are challenging and should only be done with the guidance of an epidemiologist or biostatistician experienced in multivariate analyses (Harrell et al. 1985, 1996). Some of the key steps in multivariate modeling are outlined in Table 16–3.

Table 16–3 Steps to Multivariate Modeling for Prognostic Studies

Formulate hypotheses about associations and interactions

Prepare data set
- Examine for selection bias by determining if patients with missing outcome variables are different from patients who have outcome data
- Apply methods for dealing with missing values
- Include at least 10 outcomes of interest for each prognostic variable

Develop model
- Check model assumptions (linearity, additivity, and proportional hazards)
- Seek and evaluate overly influential observations
- Limit use of stepwise selection in favor of using all hypothesized predictors

Validate model
- Data-splitting, cross-validation, bootstrapping

Present results

Source: Harrell et al. (1996)

The more predictor variables and the fewer outcomes experienced by the patients being studied, the greater the risk that the results will simply reflect some quirk of the particular data set or, if basic assumptions of the technique are violated, will be uninterpretable and misleading. To avoid these problems, at least 10 outcomes of interest should be included for each prognostic variable in a multivariate model (Peduzzi et al. 1996). For example, if investigators want to evaluate five variables to predict death after subarachnoid hemorrhage, they will need a group of patients in which 50 or more have died. Altman and Lyman (1998) have suggested that influential studies of prognosis should probably include 250 to 500 end points, although accumulating that many subjects with the outcome of interest can be challenging for many neurological conditions.

Attention must also be paid to the predictor variables. Missing values can be especially problematic in retrospective studies. A patient with a missing value on any of the variables being considered in a multivariate model will automatically be excluded from the model. If many variables are being considered, the number of patients excluded from the analyses may be great, and the validity of the results threatened. Faced with such difficulties, investigators may estimate the missing values by a number of methods, such as using surrogate variables to improve the prediction of missing values or investigating a missing-at-random assumption so that the multivariate models can include as many patients as possible (Vach 1997). Nonetheless, the best protection for the study's validity is provided not by estimating missing values but by minimizing, as much as possible, missing values.

Dichotomous predictors are the easiest to understand, but often the underlying variable is continuous. Dichotomizing a continuous variable assumes that the patients in the two resulting groups are homogeneous. If the assumption is incorrect, statistical power may suffer. Leaving a predictor variable continuous may preserve statistical power if the basic assumptions of the model are met. The continuous variable may need to be transformed or divided into categories, such as into quartiles or quintiles, to meet the model assumptions. To the extent that such decisions about predictor variables are made after the data begin to be analyzed rather than before (a priori), the model may fit the data well, but the model may not be believable. For example, using results of analyses to decide the best cut-point increases the risk through multiple comparisons of concluding that an association is true when in fact it is not (type I error).

Once investigators have decided on the outcome variable and candidate predictor variables and have chosen a multivariate technique, they must decide how to build the model. In epidemiologic applications, because investigators have clearly delineated a priori hypotheses about etiologic factors based on their understanding of the underlying biology, they are often very deliberate about multivariate modeling strategies in terms of variable selection, confounders to adjust for, and so on. For prognostic applications, however, the investigator may have an interest in a number of closely related or correlated prognostic factors (e.g., clinical features, demographic features) and a multivariate technique is needed to select the best predictors among a number of similar (correlated) predictors. Often an approach such as stepwise selection is used; in stepwise selection, the strength of the association of a predictor variable and the outcome determines which variable enters the model. For example, in the Perth Community Stroke study, the investigators screened 26 independent prognostic variables for their association with the outcome variable (Hankey et al. 2002). The variables with a significance level of 0.05 were included in the initial multivariate model. Using the stepwise regression technique, the significant prognostic factors associated with the outcomes death or institutionalization 5 years after first stroke included age, prestroke functional status, history of current smoking, a history of intermittent claudication, severe hemiparesis, and recurrent stroke during follow-up. The stronger the association required, the more conservative the model. The resulting model is not necessarily the best model. If predictor variables are correlated among themselves, the entry of one variable into the model may preclude the entry of any of the other variables, even variables with similar associations with the outcome variable. Although the approach yields a single model, other models containing some of these other variables may perform overall as well or better than the model produced by the stepwise selection. Techniques are available to examine all the possible models and to choose the best among them. Also, techniques such as data-splitting, cross-validation, and bootstrapping can validate multivariate models, increasing the likelihood that the final model is the best summary of the data (Harrell et al. 1996; Schumacher et al.

1997). Such procedures do not address the external validity of the model. Assessment of external validity requires the model to be applied to a data set different from the one from which it was derived. Data sets may differ in historical, geographic, and methodologic aspects, in spectrum of disease, and in follow-up interval (Justice et al. 1999). Predictive performance falls as such differences increase. Nowhere is the contrast of internal and external validity more apparent than with these multivariate models.

How multivariate modeling is performed and interpreted depends on the original goals of the analyses. If the focus was on identifying a new predictor, the results may be used to show the multivariate-adjusted association (or lack of association) of a predictor with an outcome. If the focus was on developing a model that best predicts outcome, the results may be used to identify the group of variables that do so in that data set. The coefficients from the model can be used to generate weights for the predictor variables, and simple equations can be generated. If the focus was on identifying causal relations between a predictor variable and the outcome, special attention is needed in constructing and interpreting the model.

Confounding and Effect Modification

When the question is whether a prognostic factor causes an outcome, confounding and effect modification must be carefully considered. Confounding can occur when a factor is related to both the prognostic factor and the outcome, resulting in a change in the strength of association between the prognostic factor and the outcome when the confounding factor is considered.

Example 16–6 An example may help to clarify these concepts. Say investigators wanted to explore predictors of death after an ischemic stroke. Two candidate predictors are both related to outcome in univariate analyses: being 75 years or older (yes or no) and the ischemic stroke subtype being cardioembolic (yes or no). The investigators wonder if the association for cardioembolic stroke is due to age because most cardioembolic strokes are in the setting of atrial fibrillation and most patients with atrial fibrillation are 75 years or older. Thus age, not cardioembolic stroke, may be the predictor of a fatal outcome following a stroke—or, stated differently, the relation between cardioembolic stroke and death may be confounded by age.

Several approaches are available to examine the possibility of confounding and to control for its effects. The measure of association between cardioembolic stroke and death overall may differ from the association seen when controlling for age. In the context of multivariable models, such as the Cox proportional hazards model, the relative risk derived from the model may change after age is added to the model. The relative risk for cardioembolic stroke is thus controlled or adjusted for age. If the adjusted and unadjusted relative risks differ substantively, confounding is present.

Example 16–7 For many clinical uses of prognosis, confounding may not be an issue. A clinician will be correct in concluding that a patient with a cardioembolic stroke is more likely to die of a cardioembolic stroke than a patient without one, even if age is a confounder. The most clinically useful prognostic markers may not be those that are causally related to the outcome but those that are readily available, reliably determined, and inexpensive. On the other hand, if causality is the issue, confounding is important but may be difficult to eliminate in an observational study. For example, blood glucose levels are related to outcomes after ischemic brain injuries—both focal injuries such as after ischemic stroke and global injuries such as after cardiac arrest (Li et al. 1997). Does the elevated glucose worsen ischemic brain damage and thus outcome, as suggested by experimental studies, or is glucose simply a marker for the severity of the insult? Note that if the association is causal, it suggests the pos-

sibility of a treatment, namely lowering the blood glucose level to improve outcome. Controlling for severity may be appropriate if it is considered to be confounding the relation between glucose and outcome but may be inappropriate if it is in the causal pathway between glucose and outcome. Such conflicting hypotheses may not be resolved in studies with observational designs, in which case studies with experimental designs are needed.

Controlling for other variables may be inappropriate for many other reasons. In the example with cardioembolic stroke, we have assumed that the association between cardioembolic stroke and death is the same for those less than 75 years old and those 75 years or older. If the relative risk is similar in these two groups or strata, then combining the two risks into one is appropriate. If the risks differ substantially in these two strata, combining the two risks would be inappropriate, and the question of confounding would be superseded by the presence of effect modification. The effect of cardioembolic stroke on outcome would be modified by age. Besides examining the size of associations in the different strata, effect modification can be sought by adding an interaction term to the multivariate model containing the two variables in question. Some of the best examples of effect modification come from experimental studies of prognosis, namely clinical trials. Subgroups that benefit either more or less from a particular treatment are defined by variables that modify the effects of treatment. For example, hippocampal sclerosis defined by magnetic resonance imaging identifies a subgroup of patients with intractable temporal lobe epilepsy who are more likely to benefit from surgical approaches than those lacking this finding (Bronen et al. 1997). The effect of surgery is modified by the results of the imaging. We probably underestimate the occurrence of effect modification in studies of prognosis because, for a given study, the power to address interactions is limited and less than for the study overall.

Genetics

The genetic aspect of a disease has several potential roles in studies of prognosis, both in defining the condition whose prognosis is sought and as a prognostic factor. Susceptibility genes may be associated with prognosis, alone or in combination with other factors. For example, one study examined the association of the ε4 allele *APOE* and survival in men and women with Alzheimer's disease (Dal Forno et al. 2002). After adjusting for age at onset, the relative risk of death in men was significantly increased compared with women carriers of the ε4 allele *APOE*. Consider also the normal person with expanded CAG trinucleotide repeats on chromosome 4 of a number known to be associated with the development of Huntington's disease (Huntington's Disease Collaborative Research Group 1993). What is the prognosis for the person or patient with this genetic profile? The search for factors that determine the onset of cognitive deficits or chorea is the same as in other studies of prognosis. Evaluating a single prognostic factor or seeking a multivariate prognostic rule may be of interest, but identifying a causal association may advance the understanding of the pathophysiology and may suggest treatments. What are the determinants of the onset of symptoms of Huntington's disease? Some may be genetic factors, such as the number of CAG repeats (Ranen et al. 1995), which at this time cannot be easily modified, but some may be nongenetic factors. If a modifiable prognostic factor were found to explain the remaining variability, the possibility would exist to treat patients with expansion of trinucleotide repeats so as to delay or avoid the onset of symptoms. Similar arguments could be forwarded for other genetic diseases, namely that the expression of or outcome from the disease may be determined in part by prognostic risk factors.

Besides genetic factors defining the disease for which prognostic factors and outcomes are sought, genetic factors can act as prognostic factors for both genetic and nongenetic diseases. For example, continuing with Huntington's disease, a TAA repeat polymorphism in close linkage to the kainate receptor on chromosome 6 is associated with age of onset, even after controlling for the number of CAG repeats on chromosome 4 (MacDonald et al. 1999). Perhaps the variability in age of onset is explained entirely by genetic factors without a contribution from environmental factors. Consider another example of a disorder that is not genetic, such as head trauma. Many prognostic factors that are associated with outcome after head trauma have been identified.

Example 16–8 Investigators hypothesized that apolipoprotein E, usually considered in the context of Alzheimer's disease, has an important role in the response of the nervous system to a variety of injuries. They found that having the apolipoprotein E4 isoform of the protein was associated with a poor outcome after head injury, even after controlling for the effects of more traditional prognostic factors such as age, Glasgow Coma Scale results, and findings on computed tomography of the head (Teasdale et al. 1997). Thus given comparable patients with head injury, the one with the E4 isoform will have a worse outcome than the one without it.

As more is learned about the genetics of certain diseases, the genetic profile may come to define the disease. If normal people with the genetic profiles to define porphyria or phenylketonuria are considered to be disease-free, the environmental exposures that trigger the expression of the disease are etiologic risk factors and the genetic profile, a potent effect modifier. The environmental exposures trigger disease in those with the genetic profiles for porphyria or phenylketonuria, but not among those without such profiles. Alternatively, if normal people with such profiles are considered to have a disease, the environmental exposures that trigger the outcome of the disease can be considered causal prognostic factors. Avoidance of the prognostic factor results in a good outcome from the disease. As with any genetically defined disease, consideration of genetic aspects of an individual serves to blur the distinction between classic epidemiology and clinical epidemiology, between studies of etiology and studies of prognosis.

Future Directions and Conclusions

For the clinician and the patient for whom a diagnosis is established, no study is more salient than a valid study of prognosis. Accurate information on prognosis is what patients demand and what clinicians must supply. As expressed by Fletcher and colleagues (1996), "[t]he object is to avoid expressing prognosis with vagueness when it is unnecessary, and with certainty when it is misleading." Prognostic studies are often the starting point for understanding the pathophysiology of disease and for formulating treatments. Prognostic studies should be used to help investigators design clinical trials by suggesting important strata or subgroups to consider in the randomization or in the analyses. For investigators, these studies pose many challenges, some of which have been addressed in this chapter and elsewhere in this book.

Unfortunately, financial support is scarce to perform studies of prognosis, despite their clinical importance. Most studies of prognosis do not have the necessary resources to achieve the elements listed in Table 16–2. Studies of prognosis are based in tertiary referral centers and are comprised of descriptive characteristics of patients with a particular condition, which probably explains why so many studies of prognosis are methodologically flawed. Because they have been based in referral centers, any prognostic studies of neurologic conditions have included only demographic and clinical features as they relate to prognosis. When case–control studies obtain lifestyle information on patients newly diagnosed with a neurologic disorder, these

data provide the investigator with an opportunity to evaluate any potentially modifiable lifestyle behaviors that may independently and significantly affect the risk of disability or death. Therefore, many case–control studies of newly diagnosed patients are ideally suited for extension into prognostic studies, and much could be gained by conducting follow-up studies of these incident cohorts. Using randomized trials as a source of prognostic information has its advantages, especially with respect to standard definitions and assessments of the condition, the prognostic factors and the outcomes. Unfortunately, clinical trials have their shortcomings as prognostic studies because a select population of patients defined by inclusion and exclusion criteria are studied. Population-based randomized trials are the exception. When an etiologic case–control study is employed to investigate a question of etiology, the investigator may have a unique opportunity to investigate prognosis, if the case group is population based and consists of newly diagnosed patients. Although outcomes may be determined prospectively, information on prognostic factors typically comes from review of medical records with a lack of standard definitions and assessments and with all but the most basic information often missing.

Given the many designs and variable quality of studies of prognosis, the difficulty in combining information from such studies, such as in a meta-analysis, is not unexpected (Altman and Lyman 1998). Conducting multicenter studies would allow data to be combined in the analysis. Some useful meta-analyses do exist but typically for narrowly defined prognostic factors. For example, investigators performed a systematic review of early predictors of poor outcome from coma after cardiac arrest (Zandbergen et al. 1998). Death or survival in a vegetative state was predicted in numerous studies by certain physical examination features, certain findings on electroencephalogram, and bilateral absence of the N20 response on somatosensory evoked potentials. The best predictor was the somatosensory evoked potentials. Combining results from 11 studies yielded 563 patients with the testing. None of the 187 patients with bilateral absence of the N20 response had a good outcome, yielding 100% specificity with a 95% confidence interval of 98% to 100%. Although each of the 11 studies had a specificity of 100%, the 95% confidence interval for any individual study was broad. The result of this systematic review of prognosis allows clinicians to be more confident about their predictions of a poor outcome based on this test.

Studies of prognosis are the core of clinical neurology and clinical epidemiology and are central to the work of clinicians and clinician investigators. Only with prognostic information can patients and clinicians decide if a diagnosis should prompt such disparate actions as initiation of aggressive treatment or withdrawal of all but comfort measures. Subsequent chapters will detail specialized studies of prognosis. First will be studies where the focus is on modifiable prognostic factors, namely treatments that are evaluated in clinical trials (Chapter 17). Next will come studies with an expanded view of prognostic factors and outcomes, namely health services research and outcomes research (Chapter 18). The final chapter will be on evidence-based medicine (Chapter 19), namely an attempt to show clinicians how to use the accumulating wealth of clinical epidemiologic studies in caring for patients.

References

Altman DG, Lyman GH. Methodological challenges in the evaluation of prognostic factors in breast cancer. *Breast Cancer Res Treat* 1998;52:289–303.

Baxt WG. Application of artificial neural networks to clinical medicine. *Lancet* 1995;346:1135–1138.

Bender R, Grouven U. Ordinal logistic regression in medical research. *J R Coll Physicians Lond* 1997;31:546–551.

Breiman L, Friedman J, Olshen R, Stone C. Classification and Regression Trees. Belmont, CA: Wadsworth International Group, 1984.

Bronen RA, Fulbright RK, King D, et al. Qualitative MR imaging of refractory temporal lobe epilepsy requiring surgery: correlation with pathology and seizure outcome after surgery. *AJR Am J Roentgenol* 1997;169:875–882.

Cornblath DR, Mellits ED, Griffin JW, et al. Motor conduction studies in Guillain-Barre syndrome: description and prognostic value. *Ann Neurol* 1988;23:354–359.

Cox DR. Regression models and life tables. *J R Stat Soc B* 1972;34:187–220.

Dal Forno G, Carson KA, Brookmeyer R, et al. *APOE* genotype and survival in men and women with Alzheimer's disease. *Neurology* 2002;58:1045–1050.

Edwards DF, Hollingsworth H, Zazulia AR, Diringer MN. Artificial neural networks improve the prediction of mortality in intracerebral hemorrhage. *Neurology* 1999;53:351–357.

Ellenberg JH, Nelson KB. Sample selection and the natural history of disease. *JAMA* 1980;243:1337–1340.

Fletcher RH, Fletcher SW, Wagner EH. Clinical Epidemiology: The Essentials, 3rd ed. Baltimore, MD: Williams & Wilkins, 1996.

Gehan EA, Walker MD. Prognostic factors for patients with brain tumors. *Natl Cancer Inst Monogr* 1977;46:189–195.

Hall GH, Round AP. Logistic regression—explanation and use. *J R Coll Physicians Lond* 1994;28:242–246.

Hankey G, Jamrozik K, Broadhurst RJ, et al. Five-year survival after first-ever stroke and related prognostic factors in the Perth Community Stroke Study. *Stroke* 2000;31:2080–2086.

Hankey G, Jamrozik K, Broadhurst RJ, et al. Long-term disability after first-ever stroke and related prognostic factors in the Perth Community Stroke Study, 1989–1990. *Stroke* 2002;33:1034–1040.

Harrell FE Jr, Lee KL, Mark DB. Multivariable prognostic models: issues in developing models, evaluating assumptions and adequacy, and measuring and reducing errors. *Stat Med* 1996;15:361–387.

Harrell FE Jr, Lee KL, Matchar DB, Reichert TA. Regression models for prognostic prediction: advantages, problems, and suggested solutions. *Cancer Treat Rep* 1985;69:1071–1077.

Hawkins SA, McDonnell GV. Benign multiple sclerosis? Clinical course, long-term follow up, and assessment of prognostic factors. *J Neurol Neurosurg Psychiatry* 1999;67:148–152.

Hunt WE, Hess RM. Surgical risk as relates to time of intervention in the repair of intracranial aneurysms. *J Neurosurg* 1968;28:14–20.

Huntington's Disease Collaborative Research Group. A novel gene containing a trinucleotide repeat that is expanded and unstable on Huntington's disease chromosomes. *Cell* 1993;72:971–983.

Justice AC, Covinsky KE, Berlin JA. Assessing the generalizability of prognostic information. *Ann Intern Med* 1999;130:515–524.

Kernan WN, Feinstein AR, Brass LM. A methodological appraisal of research on prognosis after transient ischemic attacks. *Stroke* 1991;22:1108–1116.

Kurland LT, Brian DD. Contributions to neurology from records linkage in Olmsted County, Minnesota. *Adv Neurol* 1978;19:93–105.

Laupacis A, Wells G, Richardson WS, Tugwell P. Users' guides to the medical literature. V. How to use an article about prognosis. Evidence-Based Medicine Working Group. *JAMA* 1994;272:234–237.

Levy DE, Bates D, Caronna JJ, et al. Prognosis in nontraumatic coma. *Ann Intern Med* 1981;94:293–301.

Levy DE, Caronna JJ, Singer BH, et al. Predicting outcome from hypoxic-ischemic coma. *JAMA* 1985;253:1420–1426.

Li PA, Siesjo BK. Role of hyperglycemia-related acidosis in ischemic brain damage. *Acta Physiol Scand* 1997;161:567–580.

Longstreth WT Jr, Koepsell TD, Nelson LM, van Belle G. Prognosis: keystone of clinical neurology. In: Evans RW, Baskin DS, Yatsu FM, eds. Prognosis in Neurological Disease. New York: Oxford University Press, 1992, pp 29–44.

Longstreth WT Jr, Koepsell TD, van Belle G. Clinical neuroepidemiology. I. Diagnosis. *Arch Neurol* 1987a;44:1091–1099.

Longstreth WT Jr, Koepsell TD, van Belle G. Clinical neuroepidemiology. II. Outcomes. *Arch Neurol* 1987b;44:1196–1202.

Longstreth WT Jr, Koepsell TD, van Belle G. Neuroepidemiology as it applies to occupational neurology. In: Bleecker ML, Hansen JA, eds. Occupational Neurology and Clinical Neurotoxicology. Baltimore: Williams & Wilkins, 1994, pp 1–21.

Longstreth WT Jr, Nelson LM, Koepsell TD, van Belle G. Clinical course of spontaneous subarachnoid hemorrhage: a population-based study in King County, Washington. *Neurology* 1993;43:712–718.

MacDonald ME, Vonsattel JP, Shrinidhi J, et al. Evidence for the GluR6 gene associated with

younger onset age of Huntington's disease. *Neurology* 1999;53:1330–1332.

Peduzzi P, Concato J, Kemper E, et al. A simulation study of the number of events per variable in logistic regression analysis. *J Clin Epidemiol* 1996;49:1373–1379.

Peto R, Pike MC, Armitage P, et al. Design and analysis of randomized clinical trials requiring prolonged observation of each patient. II. Analysis and examples. *Br J Cancer* 1977;35:1–39.

Ranen NG, Stine OC, Abbott MH, et al. Anticipation and instability of IT-15 (CAG)n repeats in parent–offspring pairs with Huntington disease. *Am J Hum Genet* 1995;57:593–602.

Sackett DL, Haynes RB, Guyatt GH, Tugwell P. Clinical Epidemiology: A Basic Science for Clinical Medicine, 2nd ed. Boston: Little, Brown and Company, 1991.

Schumacher M, Hollander N, Sauerbrei W. Resampling and cross-validation techniques: a tool to reduce bias caused by model building? *Stat Med* 1997;16:2813–2827.

Scott JN, Rewcastle NB, Brasher PM, et al. Which glioblastoma multiforme patient will become a long-term survivor? A population-based study. *Ann Neurol* 1999;46:183–188.

Simon R, Altman DG. Statistical aspects of prognostic factor studies in oncology. *Br J Cancer* 1994;69:979–985.

Teasdale GM, Nicoll JA, Murray G, Fiddes M. Association of apolipoprotein E polymorphism with outcome after head injury. *Lancet* 1997;350:1069–1071.

Vach W. Some issues in estimating the effect of prognostic factors from incomplete covariate data. *Stat Med* 1997;16:57–72.

van Everdingen KJ, van der Grond J, Kappelle LJ, et al. Diffusion-weighted magnetic resonance imaging in acute stroke. *Stroke* 1998;29:1783–1790.

Whisnant JP, Sacco SE, O'Fallon WM, et al. Referral bias in aneurysmal subarachnoid hemorrhage. *J Neurosurg* 1993;78:726–732.

Wolf PA, Kannel WB, Dawber TR. Prospective investigations: the Framingham Study and the epidemiology of stroke. *Adv Neurol* 1978;19:107–120.

Wyatt J. Nervous about artificial neural networks? *Lancet* 1995;346:1175–1177.

Zandbergen EG, de Haan RJ, Stoutenbeek CP, et al. Systematic review of early prediction of poor outcome in anoxic-ischaemic coma. *Lancet* 1998;352:1808–1812.

17

Clinical Trials in Neurology

CONNIE MARRAS, STEVEN R. SCHWID, AND KARL KIEBURTZ

Observational studies have made important contributions to our understanding of the natural history and etiology of many diseases, but they afford limited ability to assess treatments. Retrospective studies of interventions are limited by the potential for recall bias (differential recall of outcomes related to the subject's perception of the effectiveness of treatment) and the lack of systematic data collection. Both prospective and retrospective observational studies can be affected by selection bias, whereby treatment assignment is influenced by characteristics of the subject that are related to outcome, some of which may be unknown.

A randomized, controlled clinical trial is an experiment in which investigators randomly assign a group of patients to an experimental or control treatment and observe them prospectively to compare treatment effects. Randomly assigned controls aid the detection of changes in outcome that are unrelated to the experimental treatment, such as placebo response and any effects related to the increased scrutiny and

medical attention inherent in participating in a clinical trial. By assuming that the only important difference between the treatment and control patients is whether or not they received the experimental treatment, any differences in the outcome may be reasonably ascribed to the treatment. A randomized, controlled clinical trial is therefore often an ideal way of demonstrating the benefits and risks of a treatment.

Certain circumstances may render controlled clinical trials too difficult or expensive to conduct. As is often the case for rare neurological diseases, clinical trials of interventions may be prohibitively expensive because of the difficulties of recruiting sufficient numbers of patients. Rarity of outcomes or small incremental benefits over the current treatment can also prohibit study by clinical trial, because of the large sample size required. Clinical trials may also be impractical if the duration of follow-up required to observe outcomes is very long. In these situations, observational studies can be helpful.

Clinical trials may also be difficult to carry out when expert opinion is polarized between the two treatments to be compared because individual investigators may be reluctant to randomize patients to one treatment option or the other. Focusing on the existing evidence that supports each position will generally determine whether enough uncertainty exists to justify a randomized trial, although enlisting support from individual physicians may still be difficult.

Example 17–1 Levodopa is the cornerstone of treatment for Parkinson's disease; however, there are concerns that it may be toxic to dopaminergic neurons and may thus promote neurodegeneration despite its symptomatic benefits. The ELLDOPA (Earlier vs. Later L-DOPA) study was designed to help understand the long-term effects of early levodopa therapy. Patients with mild symptoms were randomized to receive levodopa, the most potent symptomatic therapy for Parkinson's disease, or placebo (Fahn 1999). Given the concerns about possible toxicity, some clinicians and patients were reluctant to participate, despite the importance of the research question.

Occasionally, it may appear that a treatment has such an obvious biological rationale or significant clinical benefit that a controlled clinical trial is not necessary. Such assumptions should be made with great caution, however. Apparently rational and effective therapies, adopted as standard of practice, have subsequently proved to be of no value or even harmful when studied in a controlled fashion.

Example 17–2 Extracranial-to-intracranial (EC-IC) bypass was adopted as a preventive treatment for stroke in patients with carotid stenosis. Many clinicians believed that this procedure was effective, and for years patients underwent it. Once studied in a randomized, controlled trial, however, it became evident that patients operated on had worse outcomes than those not undergoing the procedure (EC/IC Bypass Study Group 1985).

In general, the controlled clinical trial remains the preferred method for demonstrating treatment efficacy and safety. In this chapter we describe the main issues in clinical trial design, conduct, and analysis, illustrated with examples from neurological research.

Planning a Clinical Trial

The Research Question

The first and probably most critical step in planning a clinical trial is defining the research question. There should be a biological or economic rationale for the treatment under investigation that might come from basic research. Pathological and animal studies, for example, indicate that inflammation may play a role in the development of plaques and tangles in Alzheimer's disease, and that specific prostaglandins may be involved (Fiebich et al. 1998), suggesting that inhibitors of inflammation, such as nonsteroidal anti-inflammatory drugs, might slow the progression of Alzheimer's disease. Many different research questions could arise from this hypothesis. For example, in patients with mild to moderate Alzheimer's disease, does treatment with 325 mg per day of ASA reduce deterioration on the Alzheimer's Disease Assessment Scale–Cognitive subscale, measured at 6 months, compared to placebo?

A fully developed research question should precisely describe the patient population to be studied, the experimental and control interventions, and the primary outcome of interest, and should suggest the relevance and ethical nature of the proposed research.

A good research question must be relevant to current clinical practice. This implies proposing an alternative to a currently acceptable treatment that may have benefits in efficacy, cost, or safety. The question must be important, having either the potential to benefit a large number of patients, as in a treatment for stroke prevention, or the potential to make a dramatic impact on a smaller group of patients, as with deep-brain stimulation for tremor. For a research question to be considered ethical, there must be uncertainty in the professional community about the relative benefits of the interventions to be compared. The question must also be answerable, and the knowledge gained must be likely to benefit the population being studied to justify the risk and/or inconvenience to the subjects.

Phases of Clinical Trials

When testing new drug therapies, the investigation customarily progresses through multiple stages of experimental trials, designated phases I through IV (Table 17–1). Phase I trials are small studies designed to study pharmacokinetics and pharmacodynamics, as well as to provide initial evidence of safety. These trials are usually uncontrolled and include only a small number of subjects. Early phase II trials are designed to provide evidence that the treatment will have the desired effect and establish dosing ranges and tolerability. These "proof-of-concept" studies often focus on biological rather than clinical outcomes. Later phase II trials are designed to gather more information about optimal dosage regimens, patient selection, and end points to ensure that the definitive trial will be informative. Phase III trials are randomized controlled trials designed to show efficacy and safety with clinical outcomes. These are often large, multicenter trials. Phase IV trials are supplemental studies of

the new treatment on large numbers of patients after a drug has been approved for widespread use. Phase IV studies can help to identify uncommon adverse effects which may not have occurred (or have rarely occurred) during the phase I–III trials. They may also focus on different patient groups or end points than those of the phase III studies.

Clinical Trial Designs

Parallel Group Designs

The most common and straightforward clinical trial design is a parallel-group design (Table 17–2 and Fig. 17–1). In this approach, subjects are randomly assigned to receive the experimental or control treatment at the time of enrollment and this treatment assignment is maintained throughout the trial unless safety issues arise. Subjects may be randomized to any number of trial arms, limited only by sample size and practicality. As assignment to groups is in random order, there will likely be subjects in either group being followed concurrently, and there will not be a tendency for subjects receiving any particular treatment assignment to be enrolled earlier or later. This avoids confounding by changes in clinical practice over time. Alternative designs generally attempt to reduce the required sample size for the amount of information obtained. Such designs include factorial, crossover, and N-of-1 designs.

Factorial Designs

A factorial design allows investigators to efficiently test more than one treatment in a single trial (Table 17–2 and Fig. 17–1). In a 2×2 factorial design, two treatments are investigated and participants are randomly assigned to one of four treatment arms, with the possibility of receiving neither, either, or both new treatments. This design is particularly useful when large numbers of patients or a long treatment duration will be required, as the sample size required is half that of performing separate trials for

Table 17–1 Study Phases

Phase	Goals
I	Gather pharmacodynamic/kinetic data
	Initial safety
II	Establish effectiveness
	Establish dose range
	Gather additional safety data
III	Establish efficacy
	Gather additional safety data
IV	Refine understanding of efficacy (e.g., in subgroups)
	Gather additional safety data

Table 17–2 Study Designs: Advantages and Disadvantages

Design	Major advantages	Major disadvantages
Simple parallel group	Concurrent enrollment Straightforward interpretation	Single treatment per group: larger sample size to compare multiple treatments
Factorial	Assess combined effects of treatments Sample size reduced compared with two separate trials or parallel group	Interactions between treatments may distort apparent treatment effects
Crossover	Reduced sample size requirement compared with parallel group design Reduced possibility for confounding due to unrecognized factors	Longer duration than parallel group Carryover effects may distort apparent treatment effects May not be suitable in short-duration or rapidly progressing diseases
N-of-1 trials	Feasible in very rare diseases	Questionable generalizability Carryover effects may distort apparent treatment effects

each intervention and also less than that of performing a four-arm parallel group randomized-controlled trial.

Example 17–3 In trials of selegiline and α-tocopherol use in Parkinson's disease (Parkinson Study Group 1989) and Alzheimer's disease (Sano et al. 1997),

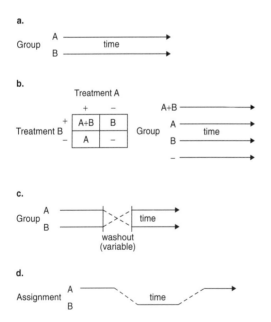

Figure 17–1 Study designs: (**a**) two-arm parallel-group design; (**b**) 2 × 2 factorial design; (**c**) two-phase crossover design; (**d**) three-phase N-of-1 design.

participants were randomized to one of four groups: tocopherol, selegiline, both treatments, or placebo. All participants on selegiline were compared to all those not on selegiline; participant on or not on tocopherol were similarly compared. Both of these trials attempted to assess the influence of each treatment on rate of progression of slowly progressive diseases, thus it was necessary to allow for a long trial duration (2 years for each trial). Although the studies were primarily designed to assess the individual effects of each treatment, the combined effects of both treatments were also of interest, making the factorial design particularly attractive. Patients on each treatment alone could be compared to those on both treatments together.

While factorial designs offer efficiency in administration for interventions requiring the same outcome assessments, any interaction between the two treatments with respect to a single outcome may confound the results. For example, if the effect of selegiline and tocopherol together were greater than the effect of each individually, then the apparent effect of each drug individually would be inflated. Similarly, if one treatment reduces the effect of the other, then the estimate of each treatment's effect will be reduced. Ideally, the effects of the two treatments are additive on the outcome of interest.

Crossover Designs

In a crossover trial, participants receive both the treatment under investigation and the control treatment in random order (Table 17–2 and Fig. 17–1). Outcomes are assessed at the end of each phase of treatment. Since all participants receive each treatment, the duration of a crossover trial is longer than that of a parallel-group trial. A crossover design has more power than a parallel-group design, however, because there is less variability in the outcome measure. Since each subject serves as his or her own control, the treatment and control "groups" are automatically balanced for potentially important variables such as age, gender, and any other unknown confounding factors. As the study is twice as long as an equivalent parallel-group trial, however, retention of subjects is a greater challenge in crossover trials.

Carryover effects—the influence of the first treatment on the outcomes of the second phase—may confound the analysis of a crossover trial and may negate the advantages of this design. Scheduled washout periods, where time is allowed to elapse between treatment phases, attempt to minimize these effects; however, the potential duration of treatment effects is not always known. Data can be analyzed for carryover effects, but no analysis can salvage a negative result due to carryover effects.

Crossover designs are most useful when a treatment is unlikely to have effects on the outcome measure after a few weeks of stopping treatment, when the effects of treatment are rapid and subjects are scarce. Rapidly progressive diseases make poor candidates for crossover designs because the outcomes may change significantly during the trial simply from the natural history of the disease. Even when the disorder appears stable and carryover effects are not apparent, the patient's condition at the start of the first period may not be the same at the start of the second period. Thus, even the most rigorously performed crossover trial is less convincing than the equivalent parallel-group trial (Pocock 1983).

Crossover designs have been used to study migraine, epilepsy, tic disorders, and excessive daytime sleepiness, which are nonprogressive disorders that have outcomes that can be rapidly assessed (Schapel et al. 1993; Shukla et al. 1995; Broughton et al. 1997; Marras et al. 2001).

N-of-1 Trials

A trial of $N = 1$ consists of sequential trials of a treatment and its comparator in a single patient, where outcomes are systematically assessed at the beginning and end of each treatment phase (Table 17–2 and Fig. 17–1). Ideally, investigators and the patient are blinded to treatment status. Several N-of-1 trials can be combined and the results analyzed statistically. This can be a useful approach when the condition of interest is particularly rare, such that assembling a group of patients to answer the research question is not possible. The criteria for feasibility are the same as those of a crossover trial: prompt treatment response and lack of carryover effects. The results of N-of-1 trials are of questionable generalizability to other patients, however, given that they were generated on only one subject.

Single versus Multicenter Trials

Multicenter designs should be considered when sample size needs are large and recruiting subjects from a single center would prolong the trial beyond the planned time frame. This may be the case when studying a rare disease or when a large sample is required to detect small treatment effects. The results of multicenter studies are more likely to be generalizable, but they require considerably greater resources in staff and time than single-center trials. Central mechanisms are often required to ensure that randomization is coordinated across centers. Monitors from the coordinating center must regularly visit each center to ensure that treatments are being provided in a uniform fashion and that data are being collected properly and completely. Each center's progress in recruitment must be monitored to ensure that the center's continued participation is cost-effective.

Selecting the Trial Participants

Goals of internal validity, generalizability, and feasibility, which often compete, must be weighed to determine inclusion and exclusion criteria for a clinical trial. As the inclusion criteria are narrowed, the internal validity of the study increases; groups are more likely to be similar with respect to factors that influence the outcomes. At the same time, generalizability of the study is reduced; the applicability of the results to patients unlike those participating in the trial is not certain. Loosening the inclusion criteria can increase generalizability and lead to broad treatment recommendations, but the results may not apply uniformly to all subgroups within a population.

Excluding some groups of patients is necessary for reasons of feasibility. In trials of neurological diseases it is often necessary to consider excluding patients with cognitive impairment, significant physical impairment, or poor prognosis; such patients may have difficulty attending scheduled visits or participating appropriately in outcome measurement. It also may be necessary to restrict the inclusion criteria to those with a sufficiently high rate of the outcome events to keep sample size requirements manageable. For example, trials of antiplatelet agents for the prevention of vascular events have generally enrolled patients with previous vascular events because of their greater likelihood of benefit. These trials have clearly shown the benefit of antiplatelet agents in secondary prevention (Antiplatelet Trialists' Collaboration 1994). Primary prevention trials have attempted to increase the likelihood of demonstrating benefit by including only patients with known risk factors for vascular events (Hart et al. 2000).

Ethical considerations also influence the inclusion criteria for a clinical trial. Principles of beneficence and nonmaleficence support the exclusion of those with little or no chance of benefiting from an intervention, as well as those with a high likelihood of adverse effects. Considerations of justice have resulted in an emphasis on providing equal access to research across age groups, races, and genders. Groups should not be excluded unless that trial would be compromised in internal validity or feasibility to the extent that it could not be performed. Equal representation policies have led to the inclusion of more elderly subjects in clinical research, for example, increasing the generalizability of results.

Participants in a trial are not only determined by the inclusion and exclusion criteria but also by the methods of sampling. For convenience, subjects are often recruited from tertiary care clinics, where eligible subjects are concentrated and enrollment is efficient. Patients attending tertiary care clinics may not be representative of all patients with the disease, however, unless the disease is rare. Tertiary care centers see a higher proportion of difficult cases with poor prognosis. Such selective sampling can introduce biases, possibly limiting the generalizability of the results. The lack of an observed treatment effect in severely affected patients at tertiary care centers might not apply to more mildly affected patients from primary care practices, for example.

The Ethics of Controlled Clinical Trials

Once the design of a trial has been finalized, ethical approval is required before implementation. Research ethics boards (institutional review boards) are in place to ensure that research on human subjects is conducted with due respect for persons, in particular that research subjects are not exposed to undue risk. Clinical trial design is guided by the same ethical principles as observational studies; however, more difficult ethical issues are likely to arise in clinical trials because an intervention is being applied. In this section we will discuss ethical issues relevant to controlled clinical trials, and refer the reader to Chapter 1 for a more general discussion of ethical issues in clinical research.

Reducing risk or ensuring that the risk involved is justified can be accomplished in the following ways:

1. Ensuring that the proposed treatment has been demonstrated to be safe or at least that common adverse effects are known such that an accurate assessment of the risk/benefit ratio can be made.
2. Excluding from the trial subjects unlikely to benefit or likely to experience toxicity.
3. Providing the current standard of care to the control group. Exceptions may include nondisabling conditions.
4. Ensuring that there is sufficient uncertainty regarding the benefits of the new treatment compared to the current standard of care to justify random allocation to one or the other strategy. There is debate over the ethical grounds on which an individual physician can justify offering participation in a randomized trial to his or her patients. Some feel that uncertainty must be present at the level of the individual investigator or physician (referred to as the *uncertainty principle*); others feel that collective uncertainty (clinical equipoise) is sufficient (Weijer et al. 2000). It is important to periodically review the level of uncertainty regarding the relative benefits of the treatments being compared during the trials, as results from other ongoing research and interim results from the trial in question may provide evidence that one treatment is clearly superior to the other. In this situation it is appropriate to stop the trial.
5. Providing a mechanism for stopping the trial if the treatment is clearly shown to be effective before all patients finish the protocol, or if adverse events are excessively severe or frequent, or if enrollment or retention of subjects is too poor to provide useful results to answer the research question. This may involve setting up a committee (Data Safety Monitoring Board [DSMB]) whose members are external to the study and have no vested interest in seeing the trial completed or stopped early. Scheduled review of the data at intervals after predetermined numbers of subjects have finished the protocol or a certain number of outcomes have occurred provides interim analysis of results to assess efficacy relative to control, and the trial is continued or stopped according to preset criteria. Continuous review of adverse events serves to monitor safety of the new treatment. Such procedures are common in large, multicenter trials but are not often undertaken for small trials. Interim analyses are discussed under Data Analysis, below.
6. Providing a 24-hour mechanism for unblinding should medical emergencies arise for individuals within the trial. This may or may not be necessary depending on the known toxicities of the treatment being tested.
7. Not placing the control group at undue risk for the sake of blinding (see Blinding, below). Sham procedures, such as burr holes in the skull or sham plasma exchange, subject the subjects to discomfort and risk of physical injury. The perceived benefits of the trial and the adverse consequences of unblinding on the validity of the trial must be sufficient to justify such risks.

The requirement of informed consent is common to most research involving human subjects, not just clinical trials. Two aspects of informed consent are particularly relevant to clinical trials, however. First, subjects may erroneously perceive participation as the only way to obtain proper treatment for their disorder, and this must be put into proper perspective by explaining the range of options for treatment outside the trial. Also, risks and benefits of both the treatment and control procedures must be presented. An exhaustive list of the possible risks of each treatment is impractical and probably inappropriate, but it is important to inform subjects of common adverse effects and severe adverse effects, even if they are rare.

Ethical considerations influence the selection criteria for a clinical trial. The principle of justice supports the inclusion of all populations that may benefit from the treatment under study (e.g., the very elderly, children, those with comorbid illness) as long as the risks do not outweigh the benefits. It is important, however, to also consider the ability to enroll subjects without coercion and with properly informed consent. Certain socially disadvantaged populations (those without access to health insurance and prisoners, for example) may perceive participating in the trial as a way to obtain benefits other than the potential to receive the experimental treatment. Offering participation to such individuals may under some circumstances be considered coercive. The inclusion of cognitively impaired individuals must also be carefully considered. Consent cannot be considered "informed" unless subjects or those providing consent for them can fully understand the risks and benefits of participating and the alternatives presented to them. Although ethical considerations support the inclusion of all those who can potentially benefit from an intervention, researchers have an obligation to protect vulnerable persons from the emotional and physical risks of research participation.

Choosing Measures of Treatment Response

Clinical and Nonclinical Outcomes

The desire to use a clinically important outcome measure must be balanced against the practical issues of trial duration and sample size. Surrogates for the clinical outcome measure of choice may be more easily measured and more responsive to the intervention but are less likely to change treatment policy. The choice of measurement perspective, therefore, depends on the phase of hypothesis testing.

Initially, laboratory or radiologic measurements that are plausibly associated with clinical outcomes of interest may be most appropriate. New treatments for multiple sclerosis are often screened in this way, using the incidence of active magnetic resonance imaging (MRI) lesions as the primary outcome measure. These studies may detect statistically significant treatment effects with as few as 30 patients studied for 6 months (Andersen et al. 1996), whereas a trial using clinical measures of disease activity, such as relapse rates, would generally require several hundred patients being followed for 2 to 3 years. Studies based on such sensitive nonclinical outcome measures may demonstrate an appropriate physiologic effect of treatment using small numbers of patients, providing "proof of concept" to justify the resources required for larger clinical trials with clinically relevant outcome measures. An accepted risk of this strategy, though, is that treatments which result in positive changes in nonclinical outcomes may not meaningfully improve clinical outcomes.

Choosing the Specific Outcome Measure

In addition to being clinically important, measures of treatment effect should be reproducible, responsive, and valid (Table 17–3). A measure is reproducible when it can give the same or similar results over time. A responsive measure reflects changes in the outcome when they occur, and must at least be sensitive to changes that are clinically important. Validity implies that a measurement tool is measuring what it is intended to measure. Each of these attributes must be considered with the disease and patient population of interest in mind.

Table 17–3 Desirable Characteristics in Outcome Measures

Valid—measuring what is intended
Reproducible
Responsive to change in disease status
Objective
Easily measured
Clinically meaningful

Reproducibility avoids spurious changes in outcome related to random measurement error rather than to true change in disease status. Although random measurement error may not bias the outcome if enough observations are taken, the power of the study to show a treatment effect will be reduced. For example, the Expanded Disability Status Scale (EDSS) is commonly used to summarize disability in patients with multiple sclerosis. Because it is based on subjective ratings of neurologic signs, the scale tends to have relatively poor intra- and interrater reliability. Training investigators before starting the study in order to standardize assessment has been shown to improve reliability substantially (Noseworthy et al. 1990; Goodkin et al. 1992).

The responsiveness of a rating scale may change across the full range of disease severity, and this must be considered in the context of the inclusion criteria for the clinical trial.

> *Example 17–4* In describing the course of multiple sclerosis, most studies report changes in the EDSS. The most rigorously performed population-based studies indicate that the disease worsens slowly through milder levels of disability, much more rapidly as patients develop significant ambulatory impairment, and more slowly again after patients become wheelchair bound (Weinshenker et al. 1991). It is unclear whether these observations truly reflect changes in the disease process or are an artifact of the EDSS, which is heavily weighted to report impairment in ambulation. The EDSS would be more sensitive to change when subjects are developing ambulatory difficulties, and relatively unresponsive in patients with mild or severe disease.

Demonstrating validity is important for rating scales that attempt to measure a construct that cannot be measured directly but must be inferred; examples are the EDSS for multiple sclerosis severity, the Unified Parkinson's Disease Rating Scale (UPDRS) for Parkinson's disease severity, and the Alzheimer's Disease Assessment Scale–Cognitive Subscale (ADAS-Cog) for cognitive impairment. Validity can be supported by showing that scores on a measurement tool correlate with a biological measure of disease activity or with other scales attempting to measure the same construct (convergent validity). It is also helpful to demonstrate that the scores behave as one would expect, when interventions are applied that would be expected to worsen or improve disease (construct validity).

The scale chosen should be appropriate for the population under study. A self-administered quality of life rating scale may not be appropriate for the cognitively impaired in a trial of therapy for Alzheimer's disease. An instrument designed for use by the caregiver and validated for this use may be more appropriate.

The assessment of outcome should be standardized as much as possible to reduce subjectivity. This will minimize random error in measurement due to differing criteria between investigators for determining end point status and systematic error due to investigators altering their assessment depending on their suspicion of the patient's treatment allocation (measurement bias).

> *Example 17–5* If the proportion of patients responding to a new chemotherapy for brain tumours is the outcome measure of interest, then the determination of "response to treatment" should not be left as a global judgement by investigators. Instead, a "complete response" is often defined as total disappearance of all enhancing disease on MRI, a "partial response" as greater than 50% reduction in the area of enhancing disease, and "progressive disease" as greater than 25% increase in the area of enhancing disease or any new area of enhancement or worsening clinical status. Although they don't remove all measurement error, such definitions increase uniformity of measurement and give a more objective indication of the clinical significance of the results.

Usually, subjectivity cannot be removed completely from the chosen outcome measure(s). If an outcome can be assessed in the absence of the subject (such as radiographic findings), an independent adjudication committee may be helpful. The adjudication committee is a group of experts who are blinded to treatment allocation and are not involved in the assessment of individual patients within the trial protocol. The members decide by consensus whether or not the outcome had occurred. This strategy is often employed in large, multicenter trials and helps to maintain uniformity of outcome assessment across participating centers. Centralized rating of videotaped examinations may have similar advantages in cases where evaluations of outcome involve physical examination findings.

Choosing the Form of the Outcome Measure

The clinical, laboratory, or radiologic outcome measure of interest is generally expressed in one of three forms: categorical (usually dichotomous), continuous, or time to event. Events such as death are dichotomous, but two treatment groups may also be compared using the proportion of deaths (continuous) or the time to death (time to event). The choice of form depends largely on what makes sense clinically; if the treatment is expected to delay a negative outcome, then a time-to-event analysis may be most appropriate, but if the treatment is expected to prevent an outcome altogether, a proportion-of-events comparison may be more useful.

Outcomes based on rating scales (such as a visual analogue scale for the assessment of pain or a multi-item scale such as the ADAS-Cog for cognitive impairment) can be used as continuous measures. On the other hand, if there is an established clinically significant change on the scale of interest, or if there is a threshold, which marks a functionally or physiologically relevant event (such as independence in activities of daily living or an abnormal level of a laboratory measurement), then it may make sense to dichotomize the outcome. For example, if functional disability after

stroke is the outcome feature of interest, then the specific outcome measure might be the score on the Modified Rankin Scale (MRS, rated 0, absence of symptoms, to 5, severe disability) at 90 days. Alternatively, since scores of 0 or 1 represent nondisabling outcomes and scores above this threshold indicate some level of disability due to stroke, the outcome measure could be dichotomized to compare the proportion of patients in each group achieving a "favorable outcome," defined as a MRS score of 0 or 1. Such dichotomous transformations of stroke disability scales (MRS, Barthel Index, NIH Stroke Scale) have been used in several large trials (Hacke et al. 1995; National Institute for Neurologic Disorders and Stroke rt-PA Stroke Study Group 1995). The transformation of a multilevel interval or continuous scale to a dichotomous outcome may make outcomes easier to interpret clinically but may reduce statistical power. Eliminating the distinction between a score of 0 and 1 or between a score of 3 and 5 necessitates larger treatment effects, and thus larger sample sizes, to show a statistically significant difference. It may be meaningful to use a prespecified change in score as an outcome event if that amount of change has been shown to have clinical significance across a relevant range of the outcome scale. For example, most investigators agree that a 1-point worsening on the EDSS is a clinically significant change (Goodkin et al. 1998) and the time to a 1-point worsening on the EDSS has been used as an outcome in clinical trials of treatment for multiple sclerosis. In such a case, it is desirable for 1-point worsening to have similar clinical significance across the entire range of the scale that is relevant to the population eligible for the trial.

Disease-specific versus Generic Outcome Scales

Given the diverse and often unique manifestations of neurological disease, disease-specific outcome scales can be very useful and are becoming increasingly available. Investigators must often choose between a disease-specific scale and a generic scale. Disease-specific outcome scales are likely to be more responsive to change as all items within the scale are relevant to the disease of interest and the most important aspects of the disease are emphasized. Irrelevant items introduce random noise into the data and make treatment effects more difficult to detect. However, clinicians who are not experts on the disease being studied are usually unfamiliar with the content of disease-specific scales and are thus often unequipped to judge the clinical significance of changes on these scales. Generic instruments are often widely used and well validated. Demonstrating favorable outcomes on these scales is likely to be accepted as important.

Disease-specific and generic instruments are often available to measure health-related quality of life, for example. For the measurement of quality of life in Parkinson's disease the PDQ-39 (Peto et al. 1995) and the PDQL (de Boer et al. 1996) are disease-specific instruments; alternatively the SF-36 or the EuroQol are generic health-related quality of life instruments which could be used. In addition to rating general difficulties with mobility, self-care, discomfort, and emotional functioning, the PDQ-39 inquires about avoidance of eating or drinking in public and ability to communicate, and the PDQL is even more specific, inquiring about "on/off" periods, shaking of the hands, and difficulty turning while walking. The only physical impairment specifically referred to in the EuroQol, by contrast, is difficulty walking. This does not necessarily make it less valid, but it may be less responsive. As generic and disease-specific measures each have advantages and disadvantages, one of each is often used.

Measures of Neurological Functioning

The World Health Organization has recommended that disease impact be divided into impairment (altered function in a system, e.g., strength), disability (altered function in an activity, e.g., walking), and handicap (altered function in a societal role, e.g., working). Most neurological conditions have an impact on patients at each level, but outcome measures tend to focus on a particular level. Measures based on the neurologic exam, such as the UPDRS motor section, are primarily measures of impairment. Functional measures, such as timed gait tests, are primarily measures of disability. Finally, quality of life scales are primarily measures of handicap. Measures of handicap may have greater relevance to patients than measures of impairment or disability, but measures of impairment and disability tend to have better reproducibility and responsiveness than handicap measures. As a result, the most informative studies evaluate all of these features.

Primary and Secondary Outcomes

Clinical trials often consider multiple outcome measures to capture several dimensions of response to treatment (survival, quality of life, adverse events etc.). Usually, a single primary outcome is assigned to allow for planning of sample size and to indicate the most important analysis. Specifying the primary analysis helps to avoid compromising the confidence in the result of the most important analysis when several analyses of less important outcomes are also being performed. Occasionally, two or three primary outcomes will be specified if they seem to be complementary or equally important. Otherwise, less important outcomes are designated as secondary outcomes. Secondary outcomes can help to increase confidence in the primary analysis by demonstrating consistency of effect across different outcomes. For example, phase III studies in multiple sclerosis may choose a change in EDSS or relapse rate as a primary outcome, supplemented by a change in MRI-documented activity of disease as a secondary outcome.

Randomization

Randomization between treatment and control groups allows unbiased allocation of subjects. This generally ensures that treatment and control groups will be similar, aside from chance variation, for the characteristics that could affect treatment response. If this is the case, then any difference between groups should be attributable to the intervention under study. To ensure adherence to proper randomization procedures, every effort must be taken to avoid disclosing the randomization scheme or schedule to the investigators enrolling subjects. Allocating treatment by subject characteristics (such as even or odd year of birth) or the time of randomization (such as even or odd date) do not guarantee that every subject has an equal probability of being allocated to each intervention and are susceptible to selection bias due to prior knowledge of the study arm to which the subject would be allocated. Such methods are sometimes referred to as "pseudo-randomization." Methods such as allocation by random number tables or other truly random computer program methods are preferred. The major types of randomization strategies are outlined in Table 17–4.

In small trials, groups resulting from random allocation may differ with respect to important variables associated with the outcome just by chance. To guard against this, randomization can be blocked and/or stratified. *Blocked* randomization divides allocation into small groups of subjects (such as four or six) and ensures that within groups of this size equal numbers of subjects will be allocated to each study arm. The order of treatment allocation within the block is random, and the size of the blocks can also be varied randomly to prevent investigators from predicting treatment allocation. *Stratified* randomization, by contrast, ensures that study groups are similar with respect to important variables (usually one, two, or at most three) that may be associated with the outcome. This strategy can increase the power of a study by decreasing the variation in outcome between groups that will be due to variables other than the intervention under study.

Stratified randomization has also been used to allow an informative analysis of treatment effect on interesting subgroups of subjects. For example, there is concern that patients with primary and secondary progressive multiple sclerosis may not respond equally to course-modifying therapies (Thompson et al. 1997). To maintain a relatively uniform study population, some studies have limited inclusion to one group or the other (PRISMS Study Group 1998). A recent trial of methotrexate for progressive multiple sclerosis, by contrast, chose to include both groups, stratifying the randomization to provide similar numbers of patients with primary and secondary progressive multiple sclerosis in each group (Goodkin et al. 1995). This not only helped to balance the treatment groups with regard to a potentially important prognostic factor but also ensured that there were adequate numbers of patients in each treatment group to perform separate analyses of treatment effects in the primary and secondary progressive subgroups.

Occasionally it may be desirable to allocate unequal numbers of subjects to the treatment and control arms of the trial. This can be done to increase the proportion of subjects exposed to the new intervention if

Table 17–4 Randomization

- *Strategy:* allocate subjects to treatments so that both measured and unmeasured factors are comparable between the treatment and control groups.
- *Simple randomization:* randomly assign patients to either treatment or control group.
- *Blocked randomization:* randomization is set up within "blocks." For example, there are 6 patients in each block: 3 treatment and 3 placebo.
- *Stratified randomization:* randomization is done within subgroups defined by prognostic factors. For example, subgroups are mild, moderate, or severe at outset.
- *Adaptive randomization:* randomization changes as the trial proceeds to achieve balance on one or more factors throughout the trial.

it is particularly promising. To some, this may make the trial more ethically acceptable, though equal randomization is more consistent with the ethical requirement of uncertainty about the relative benefits of the treatments being compared. As an additional benefit, this strategy also provides more safety data on the new treatment.

Adaptive randomization methods alter the probability of being allocated to treatment or control groups over the course of the trial. Adaptation may be in response to imbalances in the number of subjects assigned to each arm of the study. To ensure equal numbers of subjects in each study arm, the proportion of subjects already assigned to each group can be calculated. If there is an unacceptable imbalance in the size of the groups, then the randomization scheme adjusts the probability of allocation to each group such that the imbalance is gradually corrected. This is called *biased coin randomization*. This method can also be extended to important prognostic factors. For example, the probability that males and females are allocated to treatment or control groups can be selectively altered according to imbalances that arise.

Adaptive randomization may also be in response to outcomes of previous subjects. This allows subjects to have a higher probability of being assigned to the more successful intervention, and such strategies are referred to as *playing the winner*. Playing the winner requires that the outcome be assessed relatively quickly, to allow allocation probabilities be adjusted after each subject or at intervals throughout the study. Therefore, more subjects will receive the more effective intervention, and thus there are fewer ethical concerns about randomization. Despite the potential advantages, adaptive randomization strategies are complex and not commonly used.

Blinding

The Importance of Blinding

Concealing treatment allocation is an important mechanism for minimizing differences in outcome not due to treatment effects. In the absence of blinding, bias can arise from various sources. Study personnel may alter the likelihood of enrolling individual subjects according to their own opinion of what would serve the best interest of the subject or the study. Patients who have opinions about the relative efficacy of the treatments being compared may also introduce bias. They may be more compliant if they perceive that they are receiving the beneficial treatment. They may undertake additional out-of-study treatments (co-interventions) in an attempt to compensate for receiving what they perceive to be the less effective treatment. Patients' perception and reporting of outcome are also likely to differ according to whether or not they received the "better" treatment. Investigators interacting with subjects at their visits may encourage co-intervention to varying degrees, depending on treatment allocation. For example, in a trial of a lipid-lowering agent versus placebo, investigators who believe that lipid-lowering agents are an important intervention for a particular subject may be more likely to emphasize dietary change or exercise as an alternate treatment if they suspect that a subject is receiving placebo. Lastly, the investigators assessing outcomes may be biased by knowledge of treatment status and alter their measurements accordingly. Even if there is no intention to influence study results, bias may be active at a subconscious level.

Example 17–6 The potential consequences of unblinding were demonstrated in a sham treatment-controlled trial of plasmapheresis and chemotherapy for progressive multiple sclerosis (Noseworthy et al. 1994). Patients were evaluated by both blinded "evaluating" physicians and unblinded "treating" physicians. The unblinded evaluations indicated that treated patients did better than controls, but the blinded evaluations did not demonstrate a difference. Further analysis showed that the unblinded raters perceived more rapid worsening in the placebo group and more rapid improvement in the treated group, showing that the "placebo effect" may have both positive and negative aspects. Although the additional attention to investigator blinding complicated the study design, it prevented drawing a false-positive conclusion from the study.

Because of the bias that may be introduced, unblinded studies are not as convincing as their blinded counterparts. As a result, investigators have gone to great lengths to enhance blinding. A particularly striking example is the use of sham surgery. Burr holes were drilled into the skulls of all subjects enrolled in a clinical trial of fetal cell transplantation for Parkinson's disease, regardless of treatment or control group allocation (Freed et al. 2001). This study and other similar designs have prompted a spirited debate over the ethical implications of sham procedures (Macklin 1999).

Example 17–7 The usefulness of sham surgery was demonstrated in a randomized, controlled trial of endolymphatic sac decompression for Menière's disease. Subjects received either an endolymphatic shunt or a placebo (mastoidectomy) procedure. While small differences in outcome between the active and placebo-treated groups were found, far greater differences were found between the pre- and postoperative symptom scores in both groups. Had it not been for the presence of a control group, the apparent effect of treatment would have been much greater in magnitude. While this does not establish that less invasive control procedures would not also provide a valuable control group, a nonsurgical control would not have permitted blinding of the subjects (Thomsen et al. 1981).

In some studies, blinding of patients and all study personnel is not possible. This may be because of side effects of treatment such as a distinctive taste from the active medication, bleeding from venipuncture sites after anticoagulant administration, or characteristic alterations in laboratory values due to the active treatment. Therefore it

may be helpful to ask patients and investigators at the end of a study protocol to guess what treatment was received. If they are correct more often than would be expected by chance, then it is possible that unblinding may have biased the results.

Minimizing Bias due to Unblinding

When blinding is not possible or unlikely to be successfully maintained, several strategies can be undertaken to minimize biases that result. First, the outcome measures can be made as objective as possible. Death and laboratory values are less susceptible to measurement bias than outcomes such as a global clinical assessment of change or even a radiologic assessment. Second, personnel assessing the outcome can be different from those seeing the patients at study visits or allocating treatment. Some studies have used a two-investigator paradigm (Jacobs et al. 1996). The treating physician monitors the subject's clinical status, including any adverse events that may reveal treatment allocation. The examining physician is not permitted to discuss any of these issues, and only reports observations from the neurological examination. This reduces the possibility that the examining physician's perceptions will be biased, regardless of whether the patient was unblinded. Sometimes this may be taken even further, using outcome measures that may be analyzed by someone who has no contact with the patient at all. Thus some studies have used videotaped examinations evaluated by blinded neurologists (Lozano et al. 1995) or MRI outcome measures evaluated by blinded radiologists (Paty and Li 1993). Third, a strategy for minimizing alterations in behavior that may result from unblinding of patients is to provide explicit instructions about allowable co-interventions that may influence an outcome. Subjects may be requested, for example, to avoid any prescription or over-the-counter medications or foods that may alter lipid profiles if lipid levels are the outcome of interest. In addition, all subjects can be provided with general recommendations for diet and exercise to help reduce differences in co-interventions between groups of patients.

Pilot Studies

Once the study protocol has been created, it may be useful to conduct a small pilot study. Pilot studies help identify problems in data-recording forms, questionnaires, and all study procedures. The necessary contents of an operations manual become clear as the procedures are implemented. As subjects are recruited for the pilot study, a sense of the willingness of patients to participate is obtained. Barriers to participation may be revealed and plans can be made to overcome them. Recruitment strategies can be tested and modified. Any procedures within the study that subjects find to be a negative experience may also be revealed and addressed. Pilot studies can also help to determine the sample size required for the definitive trial by providing an estimate of the standard deviation of the outcome variable in the population of interest, if this is not available from the literature.

The disadvantage of pilot studies is that they require subjects who may then be ineligible for the formal trial. If substantive changes are made to a protocol after the pilot study, or if the pilot study is carried out in an unblinded way, then data from pilot subjects cannot be used for the subsequent trial. For this reason, pilot studies are often conducted with patients similar to the target population but who would not be eligible on the basis of inclusion and exclusion criteria. In general, pilot studies are an important means of ensuring smooth running of the study protocol.

Clinical Trial Conduct

The amount of work involved in running a clinical trial is often underestimated. Recruitment of subjects, randomization, blinding, treatment delivery, outcome measurement, and adverse event recording must not only be performed in a timely manner but also be continuously reviewed throughout the study to ensure efficiency and adherence to proper protocol and that subjects are not being exposed to excessive risks. In multicenter trials, periodic investigator meetings may be necessary to ensure standardization across participating centers. This section will review the main tasks of conducting clinical trials.

Recruitment and Retention of Subjects

Successful recruitment of subjects is fundamental to the success of the clinical trial. The rate of patient enrollment is almost always less than anticipated, and reviews have been devoted to exploring barriers to recruitment (Ross et al. 1999). Recruitment of both patients and physicians can be a challenge.

Participating physicians are often recruited to provide access to their patient population or to actually participate in the conduct of the trial. The time commitment required may be a barrier, particularly in studies that do not provide reimbursement. More difficult to address is the ethical barrier imposed when a physician has a definite opinion about the superiority of one study treatment over another. When studies are dependent upon physician support, a survey of the range of opinions surrounding the treatment and control procedures may be helpful to ensure feasibility of the trial.

From the patient's point of view, a number of barriers to participation may arise. First, they may be unable to make the time and travel commitments required. They may also be unwilling to be assigned to a placebo group if the study treatment is available outside the trial setting. Some may be unwilling to undergo treatments that they see as unproven or "experimental." Regardless of treatment choices available, some patients are simply averse to having their treatment allocated by chance. Emphasizing to potential subjects the importance of the study's aims and the uncertainty concerning the preferred treatment can overcome many of these barriers.

Because of the tendency for recruitment to be slower than projected, the pace of subject enrollment must be continuously reviewed. Reasons for not attaining target numbers must be assessed and strategies developed to improve recruitment. To increase awareness of the trial, it may be necessary to place advertisements in disease-specific society newsletters or send personal mailings to society members. Sending information about the trial to physicians treating potential subjects and encouraging them to refer patients can boost recruitment. One of the most important determinants of patient willingness to participate is the opinion of their personal physician (Ross et al. 1999). Thus, securing the support of community physicians can be very important. Depending on how broad the inclusion criteria for the study are, it may be cost-effective to place advertisements on the radio or on television.

The likelihood of patient participation and retention in the trial can be increased by minimizing the time and travel commitments required and by minimizing costs to the patient. Reimbursement for travel costs, meals purchased, and parking is quite acceptable and reinforces the appreciation felt by the investigators toward the participants. Extra honoraria beyond reimbursement for costs incurred are sometimes given. If promised during the recruitment process they can be seen as inducements and their appropriateness is controversial. This is probably not a significant issue for a minimal honorarium but larger sums should be presented or promised after consent is given.

Crossover trials may be better received by patients than parallel-group trials. Participants can be assured that they will receive the active treatment at some point in the trial, and this certainty may be more acceptable to them than the possibility of receiving only placebo. Of course, crossover trials are only feasible in certain settings (see Trial Designs, above).

Continued contact with the subjects throughout trials can maintain interest and encourage completion of the trial protocol. Sending newsletters with research updates and organizing group activities can help to make the subjects feel that their work is important and that they are part of a valued group of people. Such strategies are most useful for trials of long duration when months may go by without contact between subjects and investigators. Establishing a personal relationship with the subject is also very helpful—by personalizing all communications, sending birthday or holiday cards, and maintaining continuity of contact between specific research personnel and specific subjects. Obviously, rapidly addressing questions or concerns from subjects is necessary to maintain good will and participation.

Follow-up and Compliance

Inevitably, there will be subjects who do not adhere to the study protocol, either by missing follow-up visits or not complying with the study intervention. If sufficient numbers do not attend follow-up visits, the study may become underpowered to demonstrate a significant difference between treatment and control, or bias may result if subjects lost to follow-up are systematically different from those who finish the study protocol. Subjects lost to follow-up may be those who die or become too ill to attend visits before the study is over and thus represent patients with particularly poor prognoses. They may be those who suffer adverse effects and failure to obtain this information would produce biased safety data. They may be those not perceiving benefit from the study intervention, leaving in the trial only those who are doing particularly well.

To minimize bias due to loss to follow-up, it is important to attempt to obtain outcome data on missing subjects, both for efficacy and adverse effects. This can be attempted by telephone or mail if the subject is unwilling to return to the study center. If the subject is deceased, proxy information may be obtainable from a family member. Tracking services may be useful if no alternate contact can provide information on the subject's whereabouts. If none of these methods is successful, then many studies will use the last observation available as a surrogate for the final outcome (last observation carried forward [LOCF] analysis) and a relatively unbiased method of imputing missing data.

It is important to obtain information on compliance so that failure to take the study medication can be explored as a possible reason if efficacy is not demonstrated. Compliance can be assessed through directly asking the subject or by counting pills, but is most accurately assessed by testing for levels of the medication or its metabolites in blood or urine. Pill bottles that count the number of times medication is dispensed can be used, but there are no methods for ensuring that the subject is taking the medication other than by direct observation. If subjects have indicated that they are not willing to comply with the study intervention, then they should still be encouraged to continue to attend follow-up visits. The primary analysis usually includes outcomes from noncompliant patients in the group to which they were assigned, to avoid selection bias (see Intention to Treat and Explanatory Analyses, below).

Monitoring Adverse Events

It is imperative when testing a new treatment that mechanisms are in place to recognize and react to adverse events. Not only is it necessary to advise individual subjects as to whether or not they should continue the study medication, but, when adverse events are occurring more often than is acceptable, the trial may need to be stopped or modified. A clear understanding of the natural history of the condition being studied is invaluable in these situations, since one of the tasks is to determine whether any of the groups is experiencing "unexpected" adverse events or outcomes. When reviewing individual adverse events or comparing adverse event rates between treatment groups before the end of the trial,

it is necessary to reveal data related to treatment assignment. Since this process has the potential to unblind investigators or provide outcome data that can affect subsequent trial conduct, an external Data and Safety Monitoring Board (DSMB), or Data Monitoring Committee (DMC) is often set up to review these data throughout the course of the trial.

The decision to stop a trial because of adverse events must take into account the probability that differences in adverse event frequency in the treatment and control groups has occurred by chance, and must weigh the seriousness of the adverse events against the potential benefits of the treatment under investigation. For some anticipated adverse events predetermined stopping rules can be made for both individual subjects and the study as a whole. This may set out a threshold of adverse event frequency (or difference compared to control) above which the trial should be stopped. Inevitably, unexpected adverse event will occur, requiring review without preset stopping rules. Such decisions require considerable judgment and are best performed by a committee without conflicts of interest. Practical issues of interim analyses are discussed below, under Data Analysis.

Data Monitoring Committees

A data monitoring committee (DMC) is a group of individuals who have the responsibility of reviewing outcome and adverse event data that become available as the trial is ongoing. Their charge is to ensure that the subjects are not exposed to excessive risk of adverse outcomes and that there continues to be a sound scientific rationale for continuing the trial. Data monitoring committee members should ideally be independent experts who can make unbiased decisions about the need to stop or alter the trial. The DMC members should not be involved in the ongoing conduct of the trial, so that knowledge of interim data will not affect subsequent enrollment, intervention, or outcome assessment beyond any changes in trial design recommended by the DMC.

They should also be free of any conflicts of interest between their monitoring responsibility and any financial or professional ties to the sponsor and other investigators.

The DMC must provide expertise in biostatistics and experimental therapeutics, as well as clinical expertise with the disease and anticipated adverse events of the interventions being studied. Medical ethics expertise is also desirable.

Typically, the DMC will meet several times during the course of the trial to review safety and efficacy data. In most cases, data can be summarized by treatment group without unblinding DMC members about the intervention each group is receiving. If disparities in adverse event frequency or clinical outcomes between groups are noted and are large enough to raise concern, it may be necessary to reveal treatment allocation as well. The DMC may recommend stopping the trial in response to a high frequency of treatment-related adverse events. Alternatively, a decision may be made to modify the trial design to reduce the risk of adverse events. For example, a subgroup of the population that appears to be at particularly high risk may be excluded from further participation and enrollment, or the range of dosages being administered may change. Differences in efficacy outcomes between groups that clearly indicate the efficacy or futility of the intervention may also be grounds to stop the trial. Guidelines for the frequency and timing of interim analyses and criteria for stopping or altering the trial may be specified in advance by the study protocol. These guidelines should not, however, unduly interfere with DMC independence.

Some clinical trials—namely shorter or smaller trials or those evaluating interventions with well-characterized safety profiles—may not have formal DMCs, but they should all have a plan for monitoring safety during the course of the study.

Data Management

Data management refers to the process of recording data from subjects and transfer-

ring it into a database suitable for statistical analysis. This includes quality assurance of entered data. We will highlight some of the more important aspects of this process.

Data should be entered into a database as soon as possible after collection. The sooner data are entered and missing or ambiguous data on the case report forms identified, the greater the chance of successful clarification. Clarification may require checking source documents, contacting the data collector, or even repeating the measurement. Subject responses may be time-sensitive, such that after a delay subjects may not be able to provide a response that accurately reflects their status on the day of original data collection.

To minimize the frequency of missing data or ambiguous responses, personnel (study monitors) with the specific task of quality assurance may be assigned to periodically review data and procedures at study sites. Forms will be reviewed for completeness, and adherence to aspects of the protocol such as entry criteria can be reviewed. Monitors are usually employed in multicenter trials where methods and quality of data collection cannot be directly overseen by the principal investigator or his/her coworkers.

Data entry may be done from paper forms or directly into a computer as the data are collected. Direct data entry avoids transcription errors, but does not provide any written source documents to check for accuracy of data entry. Machine-readable forms can help to minimize data entry errors, but the computer's interpretation of written information must still be verified between the original form and the database. In a multicenter trial, data entry may be centralized or performed by each center collecting the data. The latter method may allow for more prompt data entry as well as faster resolution of ambiguities and missing values.

Data entry errors can be minimized in various ways. Double data entry involves re-entering all or a proportion of the data at a separate session, ideally by different study personnel who are less likely to make the same errors. The two versions can then be compared and discrepancies flagged for resolution. If only a portion of the data is to be double entered, then an acceptable limit of errors (e.g., 1/1000 entries) is set. If the number of errors exceeds the limit, then a second random sample of the data is double entered and so on until the proportion of erroneous entries falls within the acceptable limit.

Other ways of checking the database for errors include range checks and logic checks. Range checks flag data points that fall outside a specified range of acceptable values. Such ranges must be set narrowly enough to catch most errors, but widely enough to avoid flagging too many correct entries. Through logic checks, the compatibility of data for the same subject across fields can be verified. For example, the number of pregnancies should be 0 for any male subject.

Data Analysis

Intention-to-Treat and Explanatory Analyses

Intention-to-treat analyses compare outcomes according to the groups to which subjects were initially assigned, regardless of which intervention they actually received. Subjects may not receive the assigned treatment because of noncompliance or development of circumstances that necessitate alternative treatment. For example, in a trial of carotid endarterectomy for asymptomatic carotid stenosis, a subject with a high-grade stenosis who experienced a transient ischemic attack (TIA) or stroke during the trial would have to be offered an endarterectomy as standard of care regardless of initial allocation to treatment or control group. Most clinical trials use an intention-to-treat analysis as the primary analysis, as it is felt to give the most unbiased assessment of the benefits of treatment.

An alternative analysis approach is an *on-treatment analysis*, which compares outcomes according to the treatment actually received. Subjects may become difficult to classify if the intervention is a medical one, where a subject may be compliant for part of the observation time and then stop the study drug. In this case a subject can be dropped from the analysis at the time of stopping the assigned treatment and the observations recorded at last visit prior to discontinuation can be used as the outcome for that subject. This is called a *censored analysis*. In trials being analyzed by survival analysis, subjects in the control group who cross over to the treatment group may contribute to the denominator for the control group until they cross over and then contribute to the denominator for the treatment group. This is called a *transition analysis*.

A *per-protocol analysis* restricts analysis to those following important aspects of the protocol, including receiving the assigned intervention (compliant with study drug, undergoing the surgical procedure), completing the final visit, and meeting all of the inclusion criteria. Per-protocol and on-treatment analyses are often referred to as *explanatory analyses,* because they can help provide insight into the results obtained from the primary, intention-to-treat analysis.

Intention-to-treat analyses tend to underestimate treatment effects by including in the treated group those not receiving the intervention and retaining in the control group those subjects "crossing over" to receive the treatment. However, those who adhere to the protocol tend to be systematically different in ways that relate to outcome (for example, better prognosis, not suffering adverse effects or complications of therapy, and doing generally well on treatment). Therefore, an on-treatment or per protocol analysis can produce biased results. The intention-to-treat analysis usually provides a result that more closely approximates the effects of treatment that would be achieved in regular practice. Thus intention-to-treat analysis helps to determine whether or not an intervention is *effective*, and can be thought of as a test of treatment policy rather than treatment efficacy (performance under ideal circumstances).

Per-protocol and on-treatment analyses can be useful to explore whether or not an intervention might be of value under ideal circumstances. They can therefore be considered *efficacy* analyses, and may help to determine if it is reasonable to pursue treatment with those individuals who are likely to be particularly compliant or meet strict inclusion criteria, for example. The results should be interpreted with caution, however, as it is rarely possible to know with certainty who these patients are before making a treatment decision. All non–intention-to-treat analyses lose the benefits of randomization, as the groups may no longer be balanced with regard to factors that influence the outcome. All of the factors that determine compliance and adverse event development are not known.

Example 17–8 The European Cooperative Acute Stroke Study (ECASS) study (Hacke et al. 1995) of intravenous recombinant tissue plasminogen activator (rtPA) for acute stroke provides an example of how explanatory analysis approaches can be useful for guiding future investigation. Two analyses were performed: an intention-to-treat analysis and a per-protocol analysis. Of 620 subjects, 109 were excluded from the per-protocol analysis, because they had major protocol violations, such as having signs of early infarct on CT scan, being randomized but not treated, being unavailable for follow-up, or receiving prohibited concomitant therapy such as heparin. There was no difference in the primary end points on the intention-to-treat analysis, but the per-protocol analyses showed significantly better recovery at 90 days for the treatment group. As most of the protocol violations were due to the presence of early infarct signs on CT, a second trial was launched (ECASS-II) with particular attention to enforcing strict CT inclusion criteria (Hacke et al. 1998). Rt-PA was not demonstrated to be effective in the ECASS, however, it may be efficacious when used under strict conditions.

The complementary role of per-protocol analysis is particularly evident in trials designed to show equivalence. Because intention-to-treat analyses make it difficult to find a significant difference due to dilution of treatment effect, it is more likely to draw a false conclusion of a lack of difference between treatment and controls. If per-protocol and on-treatment analyses also show no difference between groups, then a conclusion of equivalence is more convincing. Table 17–5 contrasts intention-to-treat and per-protocol analyses.

Subgroup Analysis

Analysis of outcomes in a subset of the study subjects defined by interesting prerandomization factors can be a useful way to learn more about the effects of an intervention. However, such analyses do not carry the same weight as the primary analysis, because of the tendency for investigators to carry out many subgroup analyses. The likelihood of finding positive results due to chance alone can become too high to allow conclusions to be based on these results.

The results of subgroup analyses can be made legitimate by specifying one or a few

Table 17–5 Characteristics of Intention-to-Treat versus Per-Protocol Analyses

Intention-to-treat analysis	Per-protocol analysis
Measures effectiveness (treatment performance under usual clinical circumstances)	Measures efficacy (treatment performance under ideal circumstances of compliance and tolerance)
Preserves randomized assignment; there is less opportunity for bias because original treatment assignments are retained.	Groups no longer randomized; there is greater potential for bias because treatment crossovers and dropouts are not included.
May underestimate treatment effect or toxicity	More accurate estimate of treatment effect and toxicity in compliant and tolerant patients
More generalizable results	Less generalizable results

select subgroup analyses before the trial begins. Also, the hypothesis to be tested by the subgroup analysis should be biologically plausible, and the sample size should be large enough to ensure adequate observations within each subgroup to provide sufficient power to find the minimally clinically significant difference. Randomization stratified by the variable(s) that determine the subgroup(s) of interest can help to ensure maximum power for a given overall sample size.

Evaluating the Placebo Response

The purpose of having a control group in a clinical trial is to permit estimation of the response that is solely due to the intervention, subtracting effects due to spontaneous improvement, the beneficial effects (psychological and practical) of increased medical attention inherent in a clinical trial, and the beneficial psychological effects of knowing that one might be taking an active medicine. It is usually assumed that the difference between the response in the active treatment group and the control group represents the effects attributable to active treatment, but this is not necessarily true. For example, if subjects in the placebo group undertake effective co-interventions (treatments other than the study intervention) more frequently because they are not perceiving a benefit, then the difference between the responses in the active treatment and control groups will underestimate the effect of the treatment.

The extent of differences in behavior between groups that may influence the outcome in the control group is difficult to estimate accurately. It can be useful, therefore, to compare the outcome in the control group to that which was expected from previous experience (natural history studies, placebo or similarly treated control groups in other studies). When outcomes in control groups are better than expected, based on experience with historical controls, it may indicate that by chance patients allocated to the control group may have had a better prognosis or been destined to have a marked placebo response.

In such a case, it would be more difficult to show a beneficial effect of the treatment under investigation. Conversely, poor outcomes in the control group make a treatment effect easier to demonstrate. Therefore, outcomes in the control arm better or worse than expected are sometimes cited as reasons for a negative trial, or diminish confidence in a positive result.

The applicability of historical control experience to the current trial is questionable. Differences in standards of supportive care, baseline severity of disease, co-interventions, and the success of blinding between trials may account for differences in outcome in similarly treated control groups between trials. Also, greater than expected improvement in the control group may occur because patients doing particularly poorly are preferentially selected to participate in the trial. Patients doing poorly may be preferentially selected by study entry criteria or simply because those doing poorly are looking for alternative treatments. Such patients will, on average, tend to improve spontaneously toward the average course of disease. This phenomenon is referred to as *regression to the mean*. When patients with frequent relapses are chosen for multiple sclerosis clinical trials, for example, the rate of relapses during the study is usually less than half the rate before the study (Johnson et al. 1995). Without a control group, there would be no way to differentiate this tendency to "regress" to the mean relapse frequency from true treatment effects. The influence of regression to the mean on the apparent treatment effect is likely to apply equally to the treatment and control groups. Therefore, differences in outcome in the control group compared to expected outcomes based on experience with historical controls do not necessarily indicate that a treatment effect was underestimated. Thus for many reasons, concurrent control groups are preferred over historical controls.

Interim Analyses

The main purpose of interim analysis of data is to ensure that patients are not receiving a clearly inferior or more toxic treatment, whether they are in the treatment or the control group. Once the study questions have been answered by demonstrating clinically and statistically significant treatment differences, it is usually unethical to continue the trial. Interim analysis may also serve to assess whether or not the trial, as designed, still has a chance of demonstrating a meaningful effect of treatment (futility analysis). For example, if the interim data suggest that no difference between treatment and control can be demonstrated within the time frame of the trial, it may be unethical to continue to expose subjects to risk, as well as a waste of resources. It may be reasonable to continue, however, if the trial design is altered in response to interim analysis.

Interim analysis should also be restricted to a few major variables to minimize issues with multiple comparisons, and the outcome variable(s) for interim analysis may not be the same as those used for the final analysis of the trial results.

Rules for stopping the trial according to the results of interim analyses should take into account both statistical and clinical significance of the differences between treatment and control groups. If statistical significance alone leads to stopping a trial, this may provide results that are insufficiently convincing to guide practice. In this case it would be important to continue until more precise estimates of treatment differences could be obtained. This is particularly important when a treatment poses significant risks of toxicity, and toxicity is not the reason for stopping the trial. In such situations, imprecise estimates of treatment effect may provide insufficient information to weigh the risks and benefits of the treatment. Toxicity rates outside the trial setting may not be the same as those in the trial as subjects are often selected for their likelihood of tolerating the treatment.

Example 17–9 Several clinical trials of warfarin as preventive therapy for stroke in nonrheumatic atrial fibrillation have been stopped early because of the finding of a statistically significant positive effect of treatment. This has led to the widespread recommendation of warfarin prophylaxis, but the confidence intervals on the absolute risk reduction were wide. The Boston Area Anticoagulation Trial for Atrial Fibrillation (Boston Area Anticoagulation Trial for Atrial Fibrillation Investigators 1990) was terminated prematurely because of a clear beneficial effect of warfarin for stroke prophylaxis. The 95% confidence interval for the relative risk reduction of stroke was 51% to 96%. These results may leave uncertainty regarding the risk/benefit ratio for patients at higher risk of bleeding. Continuing the trials to obtain more precise estimates could have reduced uncertainty. This presents an ethical dilemma, however, denying a clearly beneficial therapy for the duration of the trial to some for the sake of a subgroup with a higher risk of toxicity. In such a situation, a trial can be continued by refining the entry criteria to include only those for whom the balance of risks and benefits is still uncertain.

A more stringent level of statistical significance than $\alpha = 0.05$ is often set for interim analyses to account for the fact that more than one analysis of the data will be performed. Otherwise, the chance of finding an effect of treatment, positive or negative, due to chance alone can become unacceptably high. The appropriate level of significance is determined at the beginning of the trial, based on the projected number of interim analyses (O'Brien and Fleming 1979; Pocock 1983).

Interim analyses should be conducted at predetermined intervals. Selective analyses in response to "interesting" trends greatly increases the chances of significant results, either true or false. The frequency of interim analysis depends on recruitment rates and the time between subject enrollment and informative interpretation of the interim outcome variables. Interim analyses may be planned after a given number of patients are enrolled for an outcome that can be measured at a fixed, short time interval after patient enrollment. Alternatively, if an outcome is an event that may occur at an uncertain interval after enrollment (such as death or tumor recurrence), then it may be more appropriate to wait until a given number of outcomes have been observed.

If an interim analysis does not lead to stopping a trial but is suggestive of a difference in outcome due to the treatment, this knowledge may become a significant barrier to retention and further recruitment of patients, compromising the validity of the study. For this reason, interim analyses are conducted by data monitoring committees external to the trial and data from interim analyses are often suppressed when they do not lead to termination of the study.

Other Types of Analyses

Assessing Bias from Loss to Follow-up. Analyzing the baseline characteristics of those enrolled but lost to follow-up is an important way to assess bias in the results of a clinical trial. Those completing the trial and those lost to follow-up can be compared according to baseline characteristics, which are known to be associated with outcome. This gives insight into the likelihood that the effectiveness of a medication was over- or underestimated by selective loss to follow-up. Listing the reasons for discontinuation (if known) for those lost to follow-up is also useful information. For example, it may provide a more complete picture of the adverse event profile of the active treatment.

Comparing Adverse Event Rates between Groups. The active treatment and control groups need to be compared for the frequency of adverse events. Each type of adverse event is compared for both the magnitude and the statistical significance of the difference in frequency between the treatment and control groups. A greater magnitude of difference in frequency would be acceptable for less serious adverse events.

Future Directions and Conclusions

Clinical trials are often the culmination of a long history of investigation that began in the laboratory or in observational epidemiologic studies. Knowledge of disease prevalence and the health-care burdens associated with disease helps to put the potential impact of a clinical trial's results into perspective, and helps to guide the size of treatment effect that is worthwhile pursuing. When a disease is highly prevalent and leads to significant morbidity, smaller treatment effects are seen as worthwhile. Knowledge of the natural history of a disease is essential for guiding clinical trial design. Rates of occurrence of the outcome of interest help determine study duration and sample size, and suggest appropriate design. They also help in the interpretation of results by giving an estimate of the expected outcomes in a placebo arm, although caution must be taken in such extrapolation, as described above. Observational studies help to characterize the patients who are experiencing the target problem. Ways to identify prognostic subgroups may be discovered in epidemiologic studies, and this allows those most likely to benefit and most likely to experience the outcome of interest to be targeted through the inclusion criteria. An accurate knowledge of prognosis from observational studies also allows appropriate limits to be set on what would be considered acceptable therapy (Longstreth et al. 1987). For example, as more is learned about progressive accumulation of MRI lesions, brain atrophy, axonal damage, and cognitive impairment in multiple sclerosis patients who were thought to have relatively benign disease, more aggressive interventions are being considered at an earlier stage of the disease (Rudick et al. 1997).

Neuroepidemiologic studies may provide clues to potential treatments or preventive strategies by identifying factors that are related to the incidence or prognosis of the disease. Observational studies suggested, for example, that estrogen replacement can significantly reduce the risk for the development of Alzheimer's disease in postmenopausal women (Henderson et al. 1994; Tang et al. 1996). These observations led to randomized trials that demonstrated that estrogen replacement led to improvements in cognitive function in postmenopausal women with Alzheimer's disease (Asthana et al. 2001).

Thus, clinical trial design and interpretation should be based on the knowledge of disease and outcome frequency, natural history, and prognostic factors that comes from observational research.

Clinical trials is a relatively young and rapidly developing field of research in many areas of neurology. Much work remains to be done to develop improved methods for conducting clinical trials of many neurologic diseases, for example, developing accurate measures of disease progression. In diseases for which treatment remains inadequate, methods for efficiently screening potential treatments must be developed. This is particularly challenging when choosing targets for trials of preventive therapy in slowly progressive diseases. In areas with well-developed treatments, work may still be necessary to expand the population studied beyond tertiary-care referral centers to community-based samples for a better understanding of the effectiveness of current treatments. Given the rarity of many neurologic diseases, collaborative efforts of investigators from many centers will be necessary to ensure rapid progress toward achieving these important goals.

References

Andersen O, Lycke J, Tollesson PO, et al. Linomide reduces the rate of active lesions in relapsing-remitting multiple sclerosis. *Mult Scler* 1996;1:348.

Antiplatelet Trialists' Collaboration. Collaborative overview of randomised trials of antiplatelet therapy—I: Prevention of death, myocardial infarction, and stroke by prolonged antiplatelet therapy in various categories of patients. *BMJ* 1994;308:81–106.

Asthana S, Baker L D, Craft S, et al. High-dose estradiol improves cognition for women with AD: results of a randomized study. *Neurology* 2001;57:605–612.

Boston Area Anticoagulation Trial for Atrial Fibrillation Investigators. The effect of low-dose warfarin on the risk of stroke in patients with nonrheumatic atrial fibrillation. *N Engl J Med* 1990;323:1505–1511.

Broughton RJ, Fleming JA, George CF, et al. Randomized, double-blind, placebo-controlled crossover trial of modafinil in the treatment of excessive daytime sleepiness in narcolepsy. *Neurology* 1997;47:445–451.

de Boer AG, Wokler W, Speelman JD, de Haes JC. Quality of life in patients with Parkinson's disease: development of a questionaire. *J Neurol Neurosurg Psychiatry* 1996;61:70–74.

EC/IC Bypass Study Group. Failure of extracranial-intracranial arterial bypass to reduce the risk of ischemic stroke. Results of an international randomized trial. *N Engl J Med* 1985;313:1191–1200.

Fahn S. Parkinson disease, the effect of levodopa, and the ELLDOPA trial. Earlier vs later L-DOPA. *Arch Neurol* 1999;56:529–535.

Fiebich BL, Hull M, Lieb K, et al. Potential link between interleukin-6 and arachidonic acid metabolism in Alzheimer's disease. *J Neural Transm Suppl* 1998;54:268–278.

Freed CR, Greene PE, Breeze RE, et al. Transplantation of embryonic dopamine neurons for severe Parkinson's disease. *N Engl J Med* 2001;344:710–719.

Goodkin DE, Cookfair D, Wende K, et al. Inter- and intrarater scoring agreement using grades 1.0 to 3.5 of the Kurtzke Expanded Disability Status Scale (EDSS). Multiple Sclerosis Collaborative Research Group. *Neurology* 1992;42:859–863.

Goodkin DE, Priore R L, Wende KE, et al. Comparing the ability of various compositive outcomes to discriminate treatment effects in MS clinical trials. The Multiple Sclerosis Collaborative Research Group (MSCRG). *Mult Scler* 1998;4:480–486.

Goodkin DE, Rudick RA, VanderBrug Medendorp S, et al. Low-dose (7.5 mg) oral methotrexate reduces the rate of progression in chronic progressive multiple sclerosis. *Ann Neurol* 1995;37:30–40.

Hacke W, Kaste M, Fieschi C, et al. Intravenous thrombolysis with recombinant tissue plasminogen activator for acute hemispheric stroke. *JAMA* 1995;274:1017–1025.

Hacke W, Kaste M, Fieschi C, et al. Randomised double-blind placebo-controlled trial of thrombolytic therapy with intravenous alteplase in acute ischaemic stroke (ECASS II).

Second European-Australasian Acute Stroke Study Investigators. *Lancet* 1998;352:1245–1251.

Hart RG, Halperin JL, McBride R, et al. Aspirin for the primary prevention of stroke and other major vascular events: meta-analysis and hypotheses. *Arch Neurol* 2000;57:326–332.

Henderson VW, Paganini-Hill A, Emanuel CK, et al. Estrogen replacement therapy in older women. Comparisons between Alzheimer's disease cases and nondemented control subjects. *Arch Neurol* 1994;51:896–900.

Jacobs LD, Cookfair DL, Rudick RA, et al. Intramuscular interferon β-1a for disease progression in relapsing multiple sclerosis. The Multiple Sclerosis Collaborative Research Group (MSCRG). *Ann Neurol* 1996;39:285–294.

Johnson KP, Brooks BR, Cohen JA, et al. Copolymer 1 reduces relapse rate and improves disability in relapsing-remitting multiple sclerosis: results of a phase III multicenter, double-blind placebo-controlled trial. The Copolymer 1 Multiple Sclerosis Study Group. *Neurology* 1995;45:1268–1276.

Longstreth WT Jr, Koepsell TD, van Belle G. Clinical neuroepidemiology. II. Outcomes. *Arch Neurol* 1987;44:1196–1202.

Lozano AM, Lang AE, Galvez-Jimenez N, et al. Effect of GPi pallidotomy on motor function in Parkinson's disease. *Lancet* 1995;346:1383–1387.

Macklin R. The ethical problems with sham surgery in clinical research. *N Engl J Med* 1999;341:992–996.

Marras C, Andrews D, Sime E, Lang AE. Botulinum toxin for simple motor tics: a randomized, double-blind, controlled clinical trial. *Neurology* 2001;56:605–610.

National Institute of Neurological Disorders and Stroke rt-PA Stroke Study Group. Tissue plasminogen activator for acute ischemic stroke. *N Engl J Med* 1995;333:1581–1587.

Noseworthy JH, Ebers GC, Vandervoot MK, et al. The impact of blinding on the results of a randomized, placebo-controlled multiple sclerosis clinical trial. *Neurology* 1994;44:16–20.

Noseworthy JH, Vandervoort MK, Wong CJ, Ebers GC. Interrater variability with the Expanded Disability Status Scale (EDSS) and Functional Systems (FS) in a multiple sclerosis clinical trial. The Canadian Cooperation MS Study Group. *Neurology* 1990;40:971–975.

O'Brien PC, Fleming TR. A multiple testing procedure for clinical trials. *Biometrics* 1979;35:549–556.

Parkinson Study Group. DATATOP: a multicenter controlled clinical trial in early Parkinson's disease. *Arch Neurol* 1989;46:1052–1060.

Paty DW, Li DK. Interferon β-1b is effective in relapsing-remitting multiple sclerosis. II. MRI analysis results of a multicenter, randomized, double-blind, placebo-controlled trial. UBC MS/MRI Study Group and the IFNB Multiple Sclerosis Study Group. *Neurology* 1993;43:662–667.

Peto V, Jenkinson C, Fitzpatrick R, Greenhall R. The development and validation of a short measure of functioning and well being for individuals with Parkinson's disease. *Qual Life Res* 1995;4:241–248.

Pocock SJ. Monitoring trial progress. In: Clinical Trials: A Practical Approach. New York: John Wiley, 1983, pp 143–155.

PRISMS (Prevention of Relapses and Disability by Interferon β-1a Subcutaneously in Multiple Sclerosis) Study Group. Randomised double-blind placebo-controlled study of interferon β-1a in relapsing/remitting multiple sclerosis. *Lancet* 1998;352:1498–1504.

Ross S, Grant A, Counsell C, et al. Barriers to participation in randomised controlled trials: a systematic review. *J Clin Epidemiol* 1999;52:1143–1156.

Rudick RA, Cohen JA, Weinstock-Guttman B, et al. Management of multiple sclerosis. *N Engl J Med* 1997;337:1604–1611.

Sano M, Ernesto C, Thomas RG, et al. A controlled trial of selegiline, α-tocopherol, or both as treatment for Alzheimer's disease. The Alzheimer's Disease Cooperative Study. *N Engl J Med* 1997;336:1216–1222.

Schapel GJ, Beran RG, Vajda FJ, et al. Double-blind, placebo controlled, crossover study of lamotrigine in treatment resistant partial seizures. *J Neurol Neurosurg Psychiatry* 1993;56:448–453.

Shukla R, Garg RK, Nag D, Ahuja RC. Nifedipine in migraine and tension headache: a randomised double blind crossover study. *J Assoc Physicians India* 1995;43:770–772.

Tang MX, Jacobs D, Stern Y, et al. Effect of oestrogen during menopause on risk and age at onset of Alzheimer's disease. *Lancet* 1996;348:429–432.

Thompson AJ, Polman CH, Miller DH, et al. Primary progressive multiple sclerosis. *Brain* 1997;120(Pt 6):1085–1096.

Thomsen J, Bretlau P, Tos M, Johnsen NJ. Meniere's disease: endolymphatic sac decompression compared with sham (placebo) decompression. *Ann N Y Acad Sci* 1981;374:820–830.

Weijer C, Shapiro SH, Cranley Glass K. For and against: clinical equipoise and not the uncertainty principle is the moral underpinning of the randomised controlled trial. *BMJ* 2000;321:756–758.

Weinshenker BG, Rice GP, Noseworthy JH, et al. The natural history of multiple sclerosis: a geographically based study. 3. Multivariate analysis of predictive factors and models of outcome. *Brain* 1991;114(pt 2):1045–1056.

18

Health Services Research in Neurology

BARBARA G. VICKREY AND ROBERT G. HOLLOWAY

Health services research in neurology is the study of neurologic care and its consequences. This research encompasses the design and execution of studies of access to care, quality of care and outcomes, effectiveness, and cost-effectiveness. The goal of neurologic health services research is to create a scientific basis for measurably improving the care provided to patients with both chronic and acute neurological conditions. It is multidisciplinary research that draws on the expertise of neurologists with training in clinical research methods, economists, biostatisticians, epidemiologists, sociologists, and other social scientists. Most health services researchers employ a combination of quantitative and qualitative research methods, and they work in collaboration with administrators and organizations that provide health care. Typical sources of data for health services research studies are surveys and interviews, medical records, and administrative data sets. Figure 18–1 shows the relationship of health services research to traditional biomedical research. A list of common health services research terms is provided at the end of the chapter in Appendix 18–1.

Health services research is critical to achieving the ultimate goal of traditional biomedical research, which is to understand and reduce the population's burden of disease (Holloway and Ringel 1998). Basic neuroscience research seeks to identify mechanisms of disease; clinical trials tell us whether a treatment has potential value in humans under ideal conditions. There is ample evidence, however, that without observational and intervention studies to evaluate the translation of these innovations into actual care delivery to populations, these treatments may be delayed or varied in their application, or both (Rogers 1995). For example, studies of the introduction of thrombolytic therapy for acute myocardial infarction into clinical practice have shown delays of over a decade between the time when randomized clinical trial evidence showed a strongly positive benefit, and when textbooks and review articles recom-

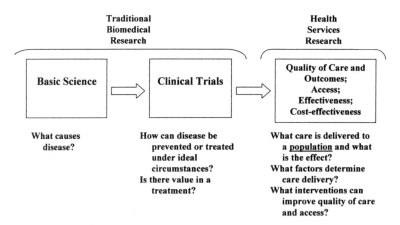

Figure 18–1 The continuum of and the relationships between basic science, clinical trials, and health services research. (Adapted from Holloway RG, Ringel SP. Narrowing the evidence-practice gap. Strengthening the link between research and clinical practice. *Neurology* 1998;50:319–321, reprinted with permission.)

mended its routine use in clinical care (Antman et al. 1992).

The introduction of new therapies can have unanticipated impacts on health in populations receiving care in nonclinical trial or "real-world" settings by typical care providers. Health services research is needed to answer questions about patterns of care in populations, such as a managed care population, and about factors that determine what care is delivered and how, and what interventions can improve quality of and access to care. While health services research for conditions like diabetes and asthma has received considerable attention and funding, there is growing recognition of the need for studies of neurologic care.

Access to Care

The U.S. health-care system has traditionally been a multitiered system in which access varies according to socioeconomic status, availability or type of insurance, race/ethnicity, and place of residence. It is well established that for certain non-neurological conditions, the uninsured, underserved minorities, and people with lower socioeconomic status have lower access to care. There has been a paucity of research on the extent to which subgroups of people

with neurologic conditions have limited access to care. This research is important because many neurologic diseases, like other chronic non-neurological diseases, require care in the context of close supervision by a qualified practitioner, the ability to obtain additional expert input when appropriate, and a system of care that does not place either logistical or financial barriers in the way of obtaining care. Managed care plans in the 1990s promoted the use of gatekeepers, potentially limiting access to specialists such as neurologists, but the effect of this trend on neurologic conditions has not been well studied. One national survey of primary care physicians and of neurologists found large differences in their preferences for referral to a specialist of cases (presented in vignette form) having dementia, Parkinson's disease, and cerebrovascular disease (Swarztrauber et al. 2002). Primary care physicians reported much less referral of these cases to a specialist than what the neurologists reported would be their preference for primary care providers' referral. Clearly, additional research is needed in the area of access to care for people with acute and chronic neurologic conditions and in developing, refining, and measuring outcomes of different models of generalist–specialty care coordination.

Example 18–1 One study found that of 930 adults with multiple sclerosis (MS) who were receiving care in one of two managed care settings or in a fee-for-service setting, only two-thirds of those needing to contact a neurologist for an MS-related problem in the prior 6 months had done so (Vickrey et al. 1999). The proportion of patients with unmet need was similar in the three different systems of care. One of the managed care plans had a policy of open access to specialists, and the other had no financial disincentives for referral to specialists within the health maintenance organization (HMO). Greater unmet need was observed among the MS patients for accessing other kinds of services than for accessing neurologists. For example, less than half of those needing mental health care or counseling, rehabilitation services, or home health care accessed those services in the prior 6 months (Vickrey et al. 1999).

Quality of Care and Outcomes Research

Quality of care research has four distinct phases: (*1*) establishing measures of quality and quality care standards or goals, (*2*) measuring current care patterns and identifying variations in actual care relative to those care standards or goals, (*3*) developing interventions to improve quality of care and conducting studies to evaluate these interventions, and (*4*) disseminating successful interventions to other settings and institutions.

The Institute of Medicine has defined quality of care as "the degree to which health services for individuals and populations increase the likelihood of desired health outcomes and are consistent with current professional knowledge" (Lohr 1990). Substantial progress has been made, particularly over the last decade, in developing reliable and valid instruments to measure quality of care for neurological disorders. In the United States, these efforts have been fueled by concerns about whether the major changes in health care reimbursement mechanisms, such as the introduction of the prospective payment system by the Health Care Financing Administration and the rise of managed care, would adversely affect quality of care. The most prominent model for conceptualizing quality of care defines quality of care as a multidimensional construct that includes structural elements, process of care, and outcomes (Donabedian 1980) (Fig. 18–2).

Structural elements of a health system that may affect quality of care include its facilities, the characteristics of its service providers, and the characteristics of the community it serves. Facilities influence care through such factors as the physical safety of hospitals and the availability of stroke units. Provider characteristics that shape quality of neurological care include whether or not doctors are board certified, how long doctors have been in practice, the quality of doctors' training, the availability

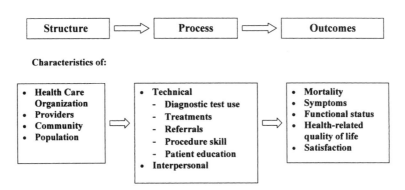

Figure 18–2 Conceptual framework for quality of care. (Source: American Academy of Neurology syllabus, Clinical Research Methods 3FC.003 [2000]).

and staffing of nurse specialists in neurology wards, and the availability of case managers for patients with chronic neurological diseases such as dementia. Community characteristics include the prevalence of neurological diseases in the population, the ratio of neurologists to the general population, the proportion of uninsured members of the population, and the socioeconomic profile of the population.

The process dimension of quality has two main features: technical aspects and interpersonal aspects. Technical aspects of quality of care pertain to actions that occur in the delivery of neurologic services, for example, whether or not a swallowing evaluation is performed in a stroke patient or whether a patient with transient ischemic attacks (TIAs) and atrial fibrillation receives treatment with coumadin. Technical aspects can refer to how skillfully a procedure or test is performed, or simply to whether or not a particular procedure or test is performed at all. Interpersonal aspects concern the extent to which care is provided in a humane fashion and the quality of doctor–patient communication. An example is whether or not patients receive understandable information about possible side effects of an antiepileptic medication. Structural and process aspects of quality of care are important ultimately because they influence health outcomes, and the goal of

the health services researcher is to study and evaluate ways to modify these aspects, such as to maximize health outcomes.

Example 18–2   A study of cerebrovascular disease care showed racial variation in a process-of-care measure, use of noninvasive cerebrovascular testing. Data were analyzed from a representative, national sample of over 17,000 Medicare beneficiaries hospitalized in 1991 with a discharge diagnosis of TIA (Mitchell et al. 2000). The proportion of African Americans who received a carotid duplex or Doppler study was significantly lower than the proportion of whites (40% vs. 48%). In addition to this racial variation, it is notable that the proportion receiving this test was under 50% in both groups, well below target recommendations for noninvasive testing, which are to noninvasively evaluate the carotid arteries of all patients with suspected cerebral ischemia in the anterior circulation.

Outcomes are the third key dimension of quality and the ultimate goal of health care delivery efforts. Relevant outcomes include both traditional clinical outcomes, such as disease symptoms and mortality, and "patient-centered" outcomes, such as health-related quality of life (HRQOL) and satisfaction with care (Guyatt et al. 1993; Vickrey 1999) (Table 18–1). The measure-

Table 18–1   Outcomes Relevant to Quality of Care Assessment

Dimension	Example
Traditional Clinical Outcomes	
Symptoms	Number of seizures
Signs	Degree of weakness in a limb
Labs	Phenobarbital level
Mortality	Case fatality rate at 30 days post-stroke
Patient-Centered Outcomes	
Physical function	Ability to climb stairs or walk up and down ramps
Social health	Ability to participate in recreational activities
Mental health	Time individual has felt discouraged or depressed
Satisfaction	
Satisfaction with explanations of care received	
Satisfaction with physician's willingness to listen and respond to patient's concerns and questions	

ments of HRQOL for neurologic conditions have advanced substantially over the last decade. Challenges remain, however, particularly in the areas of assessing HRQOL among the cognitively impaired and improving the ability of HRQOL measures to detect clinically meaningful changes over time. Measurement of HRQOL in cognitively impaired populations, such as those with dementia, may require proxy respondents such as spouses or caregivers to evaluate the patient's experience; yet, this may not reflect the patient's perceptions of their HRQOL (Stewart et al. 1996). Alternatively, some research has been conducted to develop HRQOL measures that are reliable and appear valid in patients with dementia having mild or even moderate cognitive impairment (Brod et al. 1999). Development of reliable and valid measures of patient-centered outcomes such as HRQOL and functional status has been an important focus of health services research. Notably, while these outcome measures were developed for studies of health care delivery, they have also enjoyed growing popularity and application in epidemiologic studies and clinical trials (Sacco et al. 1995a, 1995b).

Once quality of care is conceptualized and measures for assessing quality are constructed, the next step of outcomes research is to evaluate the extent to which existing care patterns deviate from quality of care goals. Blumenthal (1994) contends that the goal of outcomes research is to associate variations in patterns of care with differences in outcome so that patterns associated with better outcomes can be encouraged and those associated with poorer outcomes can be modified.

Example 18–3 A neurologic process of care that has been the subject of a series of research studies is carotid endarterectomy. A review of Medicare administrative data from 1981 revealed a fourfold variation in rates of use of carotid endarterectomy in 13 sites across the United States among Medicare beneficiaries. Age-

and gender-adjusted procedure rates varied approximately fourfold, from 6 per 10,000 to 23 per 10,000, with a mean of 14 per 10,000 (Chassin et al. 1986). Such geographic variation cannot be accounted for by differences in the clinical characteristics of subjects across these large regions, but likely reflects differences in physician training, knowledge, and preferences regarding the procedure, availability of surgeons, and other structural elements of the health-care delivery system. Findings of such variation highlight the need for additional studies to determine whether or not this observed geographic variation in use of carotid endarterectomy is associated with differences in outcomes.

With the exceptions of stroke and dementia, studies of quality of care for neurologic conditions have been lacking. There is a great need for research to identify combinations of structural and process elements that give the best possible health outcomes for neurologic diseases across a variety of settings. One such study is the Veterans Health Administration's Quality Enhancement Research Initiative (QUERI; Feussner et al. 2000), which seeks to translate findings from clinical research into improved patient outcomes and includes cerebrovascular disease and spinal cord injury among its target diseases (Oddone et al. 2000; Weaver et al. 2000).

Effectiveness Research

Efficacy studies provide information about the potential value of a therapy under ideal conditions and in highly selected samples of patients. Large, well-controlled randomized trials of new therapies are desirable for assessing efficacy. *Effectiveness* refers to evaluation of the impact of these therapies in "real-world" settings—i.e., as provided by typical practitioners to typical patients. These patients may be quite dissimilar to participants in efficacy studies, either in measurable characteristics (e.g., age and co-morbidities) or in unmeasured ways (Wells 1999). An example of the difficulty of introducing new treatments into practice without conducting effectiveness studies is use of recombinant tissue plasminogen activator (rtPA) for stroke. While overall health benefits have been shown from use of rtPA under ideal conditions, its impact may be less when used in community hospitals by non-stroke specialists or among older patients or patients with comorbidities (Katzan et al. 2000). Use in these settings warrants further rigorous study.

Example 18–4 An example of effectiveness research is a study of the use of carotid endarterectomy across one region of Canada (Wong et al. 1997). In the last decade, a number of large, well-conducted randomized controlled trials have demonstrated the benefits of carotid endarterectomy in appropriately selected candidates evaluated under strict protocol at centers with low surgical complication rates. To assess the appropriateness of carotid endarterectomy, a retrospective medical record review of all 291 consecutive carotid endarterectomies performed in this region was conducted. The indications for the procedure were abstracted from the medical record and coded into categories previously defined as "appropriate," "equivocal," or "inappropriate." Angiographic studies were obtained and remeasured using criteria applied in the randomized controlled trials. Outcomes were assessed as 30-day stroke or mortality rates. The study found that over 40% of the carotid endarterectomies were performed in asymptomatic individuals (Table 18–2). Nearly one-fifth of all the procedures performed were categorized as "inappropriate," with the most common reason being that, on re-analyzing the angiograms, individuals previously classified as having high-grade stenosis and who were asymptomatic were determined to have less than 60% stenosis according to the method for measuring stenosis used in one of the clinical trials. In addition, 30-day combined stroke and mortality rates were 5%, exceeding those of the clinical trials. This study exemplifies the value of effectiveness research, as it was used to identify specific areas where treatment could be changed to improve cerebrovascular disease care in the region.

Effectiveness studies can inform the design, implementation, and evaluation of healthcare interventions to address identified deficiencies in the quality of treatment (Grimshaw 2001). The ultimate goal of such research is to identify strategies for improving quality of care that can be generalized to many settings. In the case of the above example of carotid endarterectomy, a subsequent quality improvement intervention was indeed undertaken. This included education of surgeons at hospital rounds, distribution of clinical practice guidelines for carotid endarterectomy, and dissemination of the findings of the preintervention study. Improvements in health-care quality were subsequently documented (Wong et al. 1999).

Table 18–2 Appropriateness of Carotid Endarterectomy

Level of appropriateness	Subcategories	No. of cases*	% Total	95% CI
Appropriate	Symptomatic stenoses ≥70%	92	33	27–38
Uncertain	Symptomatic stenoses <70% *or*	63	22	18–27
	asymptomatic stenoses ≥60%	75	27	22–32
Inappropriate	Asymptomatic stenoses <60% or	37	13	9–17
	Neurologically unstable[†] or	8	3	1–6
	Medically unstable[‡]	6	2	1–5

*A total of 281 angiograms were available for review.

[†]Preoperative neurological instability was defined per selected criteria (Sundt et al. 1975; McCrory et al. 1993): progressing neurological deficit or neurological deficit within 1 day before carotid endarterectomy.

[‡]High-risk preoperative medical conditions included unstable angina, myocardial infarction within 3 months before carotid endarterectomy, or uncontrolled heart failure.

Reprinted with permission from Wong JH, Findlay JM, Suarez-Almazor ME. Regional performance of carotid endarterectomy. Appropriatenees, outcomes, and risk factors for complications. *Stroke* 1997;28:891–898.

Cost-effectiveness

The goal of cost-effectiveness evaluations is to systematically assess the costs (i.e., inputs) and the consequences (i.e., outputs) of a treatment or health-care program (Drummond et al. 1987; Gold et al. 1996). No health-care system has unlimited resources. The goal of cost-effectiveness research is to assign explicit values to new and existing technologies and health-care programs and to improve resource allocation.

A cost-effectiveness analysis can be defined as "a comparative analysis of alternative courses of action in terms of both their costs and consequences" (Eisenberg 1989). An example of a cost-effectiveness analysis would be a study to determine the incremental cost and benefit of a new medication, such as a dopamine agonist for early Parkinson's disease, compared with the current standard of practice (e.g., levodopa). This comparison can be interpreted as an "incremental cost-effectiveness ratio" (e.g., $20,000 to achieve a unit of health effect by using the new therapy compared with the old one).

An activity closely related to cost-effectiveness analysis is estimating the economic impact of an illness in terms of annual costs associated with diagnosing and treating the illness (i.e., direct costs) and the economic costs associated with patients' lost wages and reduced productivity while at work (i.e., indirect costs). This approach differs from cost-effectiveness analysis in that it estimates the economic burden of an illness at a population level. Chapter 13, "Migraine and Tension Type Headache," provides an excellent summary of the direct and indirect economic costs of migraine and tension headache.

An increasing number of cost-effectiveness studies on drugs and surgeries for patients with neurological conditions have been published recently (Lee et al. 1997; Hoerger et al. 1998; Neuman et al. 1999). Cost-effectiveness analyses, however, should not be limited to drugs or surgeries, but should include new models for delivering neurologic care—for example, the development and implementation of stroke units at hospitals (Grieve et al. 2000). With the advent of new therapeutics for neurologic disease as well as the development of new programs for delivering health care to people with acute or chronic neurologic conditions, cost-effectiveness analyses will be increasingly critical.

Many health services research studies rely on nonexperimental study designs, either because of the nature of the research question or external constraints on study design. For example, a new policy on coverage or financing may be introduced into a health-care system without a researcher's ability to control or influence which parts of the system (if any) are left unaffected. Thus, an evaluation of the policy's impact must rely on a nonexperimental study design and must address the potential for bias in the aspects of the design that the researcher can control in the analysis stage. Many health services researchers train in epidemiologic methods so that they can better design studies that minimize bias.

Future Directions and Conclusions

A remarkable body of basic neuroscience research in recent years has already yielded many new therapies for treating neurologic diseases. Health services research can help apply these advances in the effort to achieve measurable gains in health for persons afflicted with neurologic diseases. The methodology used by health services researchers is at a relatively early stage of development and will require researchers with training and understanding of epidemiologic methods to lead multidisciplinary teams in this vital research agenda.

References

American Academy of Neurology. AAN syllabus, Clinical Research Methods 3FC.003, 2000, 3FC.003-87.

Antman EM, Lau J, Kupelnick B, et al. A comparison of results of meta-analyses of randomized control trials and recommendations of clinical experts. Treatments for myocardial infarction. *JAMA* 1992;268:240–248.

Blumberg MS. Risk adjusting health care outcomes: a methodologic review. *Med Care Rev* 1986;43:351–393.

Blumenthal D. The variation phenomenon in 1994. *N Engl J Med* 1994;331:1017–1018.

Blumenthal D. Quality of health care. Part 1. Quality of care—what is it? *N Engl Med J* 1996;335:891–894.

Brod M, Stewart AL, Sands L, Walton P. Conceptualization and measurement of quality of life in dementia: The Dementia Quality of Life Instrument (DQoL). *Gerontologist* 1999; 39:25–35.

Brook RH, Park RE, Chassin MR, et al. Predicting the appropriate use of carotid endarterectomy, upper gastrointestinal endoscopy, and coronary angiography. *N Engl J Med* 1990;323:1173.

Chassin MR, Brook RH, Park RE, et al. Variations in the use of medical and surgical services by the Medicare population. *N Engl J Med* 1986;314:285–290.

Donabedian A. The Definition of Quality and Approaches to its Assessment. Ann Arbor, MI: Health Administration Press, 1980.

Drummond MF, Stoddart GL, Torrance GW. Methods for the Economic Evaluation of Health Care Programmes. Oxford, UK: Oxford University Press, 1987.

Eisenberg JM. Clinical economics: a guide to the economic analysis of clinical practices. *JAMA* 1989;262:2879–2886.

Feussner JR, Kizer KW, Demakis JG. The Quality Enhancement Research Initiative (QUERI): from evidence to action. *Med Care* 2000; 38:I1–I6.

Gold MR, Siegel JE, Russell LB, Weinstein MC, eds. Cost-effectiveness in Health and Medicine. New York: Oxford University Press, 1996.

Grieve R, Porsdal V, Hutton J, Wolfe C. A comparison of the cost-effectiveness of stroke care provided in London and Copenhagen. *Int J Technol Assess Health Care* 2000;16: 684–695.

Grimshaw JM, Shirran L, Thomas R, et al. Changing provider behaviour: an overview of systematic reviews of interventions. *Med Care* 2001;39 (Suppl 2):II2–45.

Guyatt GH, Feeny EH, Patrick DL. Measuring health-related quality of life. *Ann Intern Med* 1993;118:622–629.

Hoerger TJ, Bala MV, Rowland C, et al. Cost-effectiveness of pramipexole in Parkinson's disease in the US. *Pharmacoeconomics* 1998;15:541–557.

Holloway RG, Ringel SP. Narrowing the evidence-practice gap. Strengthening the link between research and clinical practice. *Neurology* 1998;50:319–321.

Katzan IL, Furlan AJ, Lloyd LE, et al. Use of tissue-type plasminogen activator for acute ischemic stroke: the Cleveland area experience. *JAMA* 2000;283:1151–1158.

Lee TT, Solomon NA, Heidenreich PA, et al. Cost-effectiveness of screening for carotid stenosis in asymptomatic patients. *Ann Intern Med* 1997;126:337–346.

Lohr KN, ed. Medicare: A Strategy for Quality Assurance, Vol. 1. Washington, DC: National Academy Press, 1990.

McCrory DC, Goldstein LB, Samsa GP, et al. Predicting complications of carotid endarterectomy. *Stroke* 1993;24:1285–1291.

McLaughlin CP, Kaluzny AD. Defining total quality management/continuous quality improvement. In: McLaughlin CP, Kaluzny AD, eds. Continuous Quality Improvement in Health Care: Theory, Implementation, and Applications. Gaithersburg, MD: Aspen Publishers Inc, 1994, pp 3–10.

Mitchell JB, Ballard DJ, Matchar DB, et al. Racial variation in treatment for transient ischemic attacks: impact of participation by neurologists. *Health Serv Res* 2000;34: 1413–1428.

Neumann PJ, Hermann RC, Kuntz KM, et al. Cost-effectiveness of donepezil in the treatment of mild or moderate Alzheimer's disease. *Neurology* 1999;52:1138–1145.

Oddone E, Brass LM, Booss J, et al. Quality Enhancement Research Initiative in stroke: prevention, treatment, and rehabilitation. *Med Care* 2000;38:I92–I104.

Rogers EM. Diffusion of Innovations, 4th edition. New York: The Free Press, 1995.

Sacco R, Boden-Albala B, Kargman D, et al. Quality of life after ischemic stroke: the Northern Manhattan Stroke Study. *Ann Neurol* 1995b;38:322.

Sacco RL, Kargman DE, Gu Q, Zamanillo MC. Race-ethnicity and determinants of intracranial atherosclerotic cerebral infarction. The Northern Manhattan Stroke Study. *Stroke* 1995a;26:14–20.

Stewart AL, Sherbourne CD, Brod M. Measuring health-related quality of life in older and demented populations. In: Spilker B, ed. Quality of Life and Pharmacoecnomics in Clinical Trials, Second Edition. Philadelphia: Lippincott-Raven, 1996, pp 58–67.

Sundt TM, Sandok BA, Whisnant JP. Carotid endarterectomy complications and preoperative assessment of risk. *Mayo Clin Proc* 1975;50:301–306.

Swarztrauber K, Vickrey BG, Mittman BS. Physicians' preferences for specialty involvement in the care of patients with neurological conditions. *Med Care* 2002;40:1196–1209.

Vickrey BG. Getting oriented to patient-oriented outcomes. *Neurology* 1999;53:662–663.

Vickrey BG, Wolf S, Shatin D, et al. Comparison of care for persons with multiple sclerosis in fee-for-service and managed care systems. Presented at Association for Health Services Research 16th Annual Meeting, 1999, Chicago, IL. http://www.ahsr.org/1999/abstracts/vickrey.htm.

Weaver FM. Hammond MC, Guihan M, Hendricks RD. Department of Veterans Affairs Quality Enhancement Research Initiative for spinal cord injury. *Med Care* 2000;38:I82–I91.

Wells KB. Treatment research at the crossroads: the scientific interface of clinical trials and effectiveness research. *Am J Psychiatry* 1999;156:5–10.

Wong JH, Findlay JM, Suarez-Almazor ME. Regional performance of carotid endarterectomy. Appropriateness, outcomes, and risk factors for complications. *Stroke* 1997;28:891–898.

Wong JH, Lubkey TB, Suarez-Almazor ME, Findlay JM. Improving the appropriateness of carotid endarterectomy: results of a prospective city-wide study. *Stroke* 1999;30:12–15.

Appendix 18–1　Common Health Services Research Terms

Access to care The opportunity to attain adequate and effective medical care. Dimensions of access include (1) *potential access,* which is related to the availability of providers and health-care resources and to the organization and financing of medical care, and (2) *actual (or realized) access,* which is actual utilization of care.

Appropriateness A method for assessing quality of care, often applied to use of procedures. A procedure is considered appropriate if "its health benefit exceeds its health risk by a sufficiently wide margin that the service or procedure is worth performing." (Brook et al. 1990). Indications for appropriate care are typically developed using a structured methodology involving expert panels and a systematic review of the scientific literature.

Continuous quality improvement in health care "A structured organizational process for involving personnel in planning and executing a continuous stream of improvements in systems in order to provide quality health care that meets or exceeds expectations" (McLaughlin and Kaluzny 1994).

Cost/benefit analysis A comparison of the cost (usually in dollars or other monetary units) of an intervention to the expected benefit (measured in the same units).

Cost-effectiveness analysis An estimate of the cost required to produce a desired outcome—for example, the cost of screening and treatment for carotid artery stenosis to prevent one stroke.

Cost-utility analysis An estimate of the cost per unit of a measure of patient utility such as quality-adjusted life years (QALYs)—for example, the cost of thrombolysis in acute stroke to achieve one QALY.

Effectiveness A scientific evaluation of the impact of a treatment in average or "real-world" settings, i.e., as provided by typical practitioners to typical patients. This is in contrast to efficacy studies, which are usually large, well-controlled randomized trials of the therapy when applied under ideal conditions and in highly selected (often homogeneous) research samples.

Health-related quality of life A patient-oriented health outcome; health-related quality of life is multidimensional and can be conceptualized as including physical, mental, and social health.

Quality of care "The degree to which health services for individuals and populations increase the likelihood of desired health outcomes and are consistent with current professional knowledge" (Lohr 1990).

Risk adjustment "A way to remove or reduce the effects of confounding factors in studies where the cases are not randomly assigned to different treatment. The key confounding factors are those aspects of health status that are causally related to the outcome under study" (Blumberg 1986). Risk adjustment is a necessity for most outcomes research studies because the objective is to adjust for key patient characteristics prior to drawing conclusions about effectiveness of alternative health-care strategies.

Variation "The observation of differences in the way apparently similar patients are treated from one health care setting to another. . . . Differences in patterns of care [that] cannot be explained away by confounding factors or technical errors such as undetected variation in the case mix of patients or inadequacies in data or methods of analysis" (Blumenthal 1994).

19

Evidence-Based Medicine in Neurology

ROBERT G. HOLLOWAY, BARBARA G. VICKREY,
AND DAVID H. THOM

Evidence-based medicine (EBM) provides a systematic approach to integrating the best research evidence with the expertise of the clinician and the values and preferences of the patient with the goal of improving patient care. In EBM, concepts from epidemiology, health services research, and information technology are combined to reach this goal. It differs from these disciplines primarily by focusing on decisions that affect the clinical care of individual patients. In applying research results to patient care, EBM practitioners have adapted and combined existing concepts and created new approaches for summarizing and interpreting research data. While disease-oriented outcomes have an important role in research and related activities, in EBM patient-oriented outcomes are emphasized as more relevant to most clinical decisions. This shift in focus has in turn affected the design of studies, the type of studies done, and the ways in which results are reported in the literature. Principles of EBM have been incorporated into advances in infor-

mation access for busy neurologists, from commercial and public access Web sites providing EBM-oriented reviews of clinical questions, literature review services, textbooks, and clinical guidelines (see Appendix 19–1). Since clinicians and researchers at McMaster University in Canada described the principles of EBM in 1992 (Evidence-Based Medicine Working Group 1992), there has been an explosion of published articles and textbooks. A literature search using PubMed found over 700 articles with "evidence-based" in the title in the year 2001, compared to just 9 such articles in 1993.

Evidence-based medicine embodies a skill set to improve a practitioner's ability to find and appraise the best available evidence and apply it to the patients they are seeing. There are several reasons why such a skill set is important for both physicians and patients (Table 19–1). First, it is impossible for clinicians to keep up with the medical literature, which is voluminous and poorly organized. More than 9 million ci-

Table 19–1 Reasons for Practicing Evidence-Based Medicine in Neurology

- Medical literature is voluminous
- Medical literature is poorly organized
- Advances in evidence processing
- Wide clinical practice variations and evidence that practice often falls short of the ideal
- Traditional continuing medical education offerings are not evidence based
- Traditional modes of continuing medical education employ few techniques to effectively change physician behavior
- Time constraints

tations from over 4000 journals have been indexed in MEDLINE since 1966 and research is being published at an unprecedented pace. Second, most of the peer-reviewed neurological literature is geared toward scientist-to-scientist communication, rather than targeted toward physicians for clinical application. Third, there have been advances in evidence-processing techniques such as systematic reviews, clinical guidelines, prediction rules, and journals of secondary publications that can facilitate the practice of EBM. Fourth, there is also evidence that practice often falls short of the ideal and that many processes of care may be underused, overused, or misused (Schuster et al. 1998). One explanation for this evidence–practice discord is that the best evidence often fails to reach its intended audience (i.e., clinicians). Fifth, traditional modes of continuing medical education (CME) do little to bridge this gap since most CME offerings are neither evidence based nor employ methods of education to change clinical practice (Davis 1998). Finally, ever-increasing time constraints limit one's ability to systematically keep up with the literature, even if it is only to review selected journals on a monthly basis.

The primary goal of EBM is better utilization of information technology to provide high-quality information to neurologists in an efficient manner that maximizes the opportunity for applying this information in daily clinical practice. Examples of

information technology include PubMed and other search engines to locate published articles of interest, Web sites that provide high-quality EBM information, information stored on compact discs, programs for PDAs (personal data assistants), and information incorporated into electronic medical records. Evidence-based information can range from primary research reports to well-developed guidelines or algorithms. The goal of EBM in neurology, to provide information that can potentially change the course of care of a patient in real time, can only be widely realized when such information can be rapidly located by busy neurologists. This ideal has not yet been achieved, although the advances in computer hardware, PDAs and other portable devices, faster search engines, and better synthesis of existing data bring us ever closer to this goal.

Neuroepidemiological Contributions to Evidence-Based Medicine

Data from neuroepidemiological investigations are used in the practice of EBM. Table 19–2 lists the publication types addressed in the *Journal of American Medical Association (JAMA)* series, Users' Guide to the Medical Literature (also see Appendix 19–1C *Journal of American Medical Association* Series on Evaluation of the Medical Literature). The table shows article types that rely on neuroepidemiological data. Articles that address issues of prognosis, harm, or variations in the outcomes of health services often rely on data obtained from primary neuroepidemiological investigations. The actual example used in the *JAMA* series article about how to use a prognosis article (Laupacis et al. 1994) dealt with survival outcomes in outpatients with Alzheimer's disease (Walsh et al. 1990). In addition, evidence from neuroepidemiological research is often used in integrative studies such as in review articles, clinical decision analysis, practice guidelines, and economic analysis. Therefore, data from neuroepidemiological research

Table 19–2 *Journal of American Medical Association* Series Users' Guides to the Medical Literature with Particular Relevance to Evidence-Based Medicine in Neurological Disorders*

Type of Article	Reference
Therapy or prevention	Guyatt et al. 1993, 1994
Diagnosis	Jaeschke et al. 1994a, 1994b
Harm[†]	Levine et al. 1994
Prognosis[†]	Laupacis et al. 1994
Overview/review[‡]	Oxman et al. 1994
Clinical decision analysis[‡]	Richardson et al. 1995a, 1995b
Clinical practice guidelines[‡]	Hayward et al. 1995
Variations in the outcomes of health services*	Naylor et al. 1996a
Clinical utilization review	Naylor et al. 1996b
Health-related quality of life	Guyatt et al. 1997
Economic analysis[†]	Drummond et al. 1997; O'Brien et al. 1997
Applicability of trial results to patients	Dans et al. 1998
How to use an article about disease probability for differential diagnosis	Richardson et al. 1999
How to use a treatment recommendation	Guyatt et al. 1999
Guidelines and recommendations about screening	Barratt et al. 1999

*Listed in Appendix 19–2.

[†]Indicates type of primary research article that relies heavily on neuroepidemiological research designs (cohort studies).

[‡]Indicates type of integrative research article that commonly incorporates research from neuroepidemiological investigations.

have far-reaching implications for the practicing neurologist attempting to answer patient-oriented questions about prognosis, harm, or variations in outcomes. In addition, data from neuroepidemiological research can be integrated into synthesis studies that answer broader clinical questions pertaining to optimal treatment strategies in the form of reviews, decision analysis, guidelines, or cost-effectiveness research.

Practice of Evidence-Based Medicine

In this section we will describe the principles and practice of EBM, using examples from the neurologic literature, and will discuss the limitations and future directions of EBM. A list of common EBM terms is provided at the end of the chapter in Appendix 19–2.

Recognizing an important gap in clinical knowledge, while not included as a formal step in EBM, is an obvious prerequisite for applying EBM. The importance of recognizing what one does not know is fundamental in medicine, as it is in most fields. Evidence-based medicine encourages both the student and practicing physician to

question the basis for and extent of their knowledge. While many gaps in knowledge have only minimal impact on practice, there are often situations where additional information is important for providing the best medical care. Being able to recognize which gaps are important—and therefore worth the effort to try to fill—requires experience.

The practice of EBM consists of five basic steps: (*1*) formulating a meaningful and potentially answerable question; (*2*) locating the best evidence available for answering the question; (*3*) critically appraising the evidence; (*4*) integrating the evidence with expert clinical opinion, clinical experience, and the patient's particular characteristics and preferences; and (*5*) evaluating and seeking ways to improve the efficiency of Steps 1 through 5 and their impact on patient care (Sackett 2000).

Step 1. Formulating a meaningful and potentially answerable question. This depends on a clear recognition of what is sought and knowledge of the likely types of information that can be located (Richardson 1995). The template recommended for formulating an appropriate EBM question is PICO, where the *P* is for patient and problem, *I* is the intervention (or exposure or prognostic factor), *C* is for the comparison intervention (or exposure or prognostic factor), and *O* is for the outcome. Patient and problem should be defined specifically enough so that the results can be applied to the patient, but not so narrowly as to preclude any reasonable chance of finding relevant evidence. Preferably, the outcome should be one that is clinically relevant to the patient, often termed "patient-oriented evidence that matters" (POEM), not simply disease-oriented evidence (DOE), such as a laboratory value or imaging findings. For example, a shorter time to resumption of usual work or role function after carpal tunnel syndrome is a patient-oriented outcome, while improvement of nerve conduction velocity would be a disease-oriented outcome. While this template does not work well for every question, it is surprisingly versatile and helps focus the search for and appraisal of information. An example of a question in the PICO format would be: "For an older man with atrial fibrillation, what is the incidence of fatal and nonfatal stroke with aspirin compared to warfarin therapy?".

Step 2. Locating the best evidence available for answering the question. This is often the most frustrating step for many clinicians. *Available* means able to be located within the constraints of the resources on hand, which includes the clinician's time and access to information technology. Sometime the best evidence available may be a textbook or even the opinion of a knowledgeable colleague. Evidence-based medicine, however, focuses on locating primary studies or secondary reviews that use EBM principles. Good secondary reviews often provide a more efficient answer to a clinical question, although to remain relevant, they need to be continually updated. Even so, most questions that arise in clinical practice have not been answered by an EBM-based secondary review.

Primary studies are most broadly accessed via PubMed, a publicly available search program that accesses the National Library of Medicine database (www.ncbi.nlm.nih.gov/pubmed). In practicing EBM one must be able to perform efficient searches in PubMed (Verhoeven et al. 2000, Alper et al. 2001), which includes articles from virtually every medical periodical as well as other sources, and thus does not limit its listings on the basis of scientific merit or clinical relevance. There are also several commercial sources that provide selected, searchable medical databases of primary and secondary publications in specific areas of medicine and neurology. These databases are selected for scientific merit and clinical importance.

Secondary sources of evidence include review articles, formal meta-analyses, systematic reviews, critically appraised topics, decision analyses, and evidence-based guidelines. Review articles and meta-analyses (which use statistical methods to combine results from two or more studies) are usually listed in PubMed. Systematic reviews (SRs) use explicit principals and procedures to locate, evaluate and synthesize research information on a focused clinical topic or question (Bero and Rennie 1995; Hunt and McKibbon 1997; McQuay and Moore 1997; Mulrow et al. 1997). Such reviews may be limited to randomized controlled trials but may also include well-designed observational studies. Often SRs include formal meta-analyses when sufficient data are available. The most widely cited source of systematic reviews is the Cochrane Library (Bero and Rennie 1995), which provides systematic reviews of health interventions (for example, the use of interferon in relapsing-remitting multiple sclerosis) (Rice et al. 2002). Systematic reviews are often available through EBM Internet sites and may be listed in PubMed. Critically appraised topics (CATs) are a less formal summary of the evidence to answer a particular clinical question, such as whether steroids reduce the time to recovery of motor function in patients with Bell's palsy. Critically appraised topics can refer to reviews posted on publicly or commercially available Web sites or to an informal one-page summary of the results of an EBM inquiry to answer a specific clinical question.

Clinical decision analysis is the application of quantitative methods to compare the likely consequences of two or more screening or treatment strategies (Richardson et al. 1995). In decision analysis the best evidence, ideally from well-designed studies, is used to estimate probabilities of all possible outcomes. The result is presented in a horizontal, branching tree-structure, with the final outcomes at the end of each "twig." Outcomes can be weighted by patient's stated preference ("utility") for that outcome. In some cases, quality-adjusted life years (QALYs) are calculated for each pathway. While it is usually not feasible to construct a decision analysis tree de novo for a given situation, published decision trees may provide a useful summary of outcome information.

Example 19–1 An example of decision analysis from the neurology literature is the decision to surgically treat asymptomatic intracranial saccular aneurysms (Koprowski et al. 1989). The decision tree is diagramed in Figure 19–1. An initial pathway is created for each decision option; in

this case there are two options (no surgery or surgery). Possible outcomes for each pathway are generated and assigned probabilities. In this example, initial outcomes from no surgery are bleeding from a ruptured aneurysm and no bleeding (A in Figure 19–1), with three possible secondary outcomes for patients with bleeding (death, morbidity, or remaining intact) (B in Figure 19–1). Probabilities are estimated for each outcome on the basis of studies. Similarly, outcomes and probabilities for death, morbidity, and remaining intact are generated for the option of surgery (C in Figure 19–1). Final outcomes are weighted by patient values. Note that lower values are assigned to morbidity and death associated with surgery, presumably reflecting the fact that these outcomes would occur on average sooner, being largely the result of surgical complications. The slightly lower value for remaining intact without surgery probably reflects, in part, loss of quality of life while living with the risk of future rupture or re-bleeding. The consequences of each decision can then be compared by multiplying the probability of each outcome by the value placed on that outcome and summing the products for all of the outcomes from a given decision, as shown at the bottom of the figure. Based on the numbers used in this decision analysis, the value of no surgery (0.925) out-

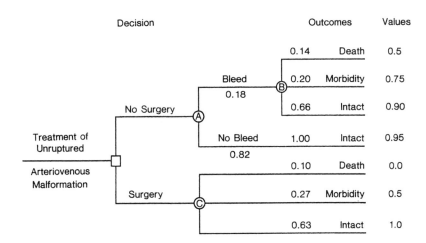

Figure 19–1 Decision analysis on treatment of unruptured arteriovenous malformations. See text for determination of values. (Adapted from Iansek et al. [1983]), reprinted with permission from Koprowski CD, Longstreth WT, Cebul RD. Clinical neuroepidemiology: III. Decisions. *Arch Neurol* 1989;46:223–229.)

weighs the value of surgery (0.765). Alternative decisions trees can be generated with different values to test the sensitivity of the result to changes in estimated probabilities or values.

Developing guidelines and recommendations requires reviewing the literature for the purpose of establishing recommendations for clinical actions such as screening, use of diagnostic tests, and treatment (Cook et al. 1997). Guidelines vary in the degree to which they use formal methods for comprehensively and critically evaluating the literature and the steps used to construct recommendations. Increasingly, guidelines are developed using the principles from the U.S. Preventive Services Task Force (U.S. Preventive Services Task Force 1996) and similar well-established groups. Such principles include explicit criteria for locating relevant information and ratings of the level of evidence for a recommendation.

The American Academy of Neurology (AAN) has published over 40 "Practice Parameters" since 1990, providing guidelines and recommendations for the evaluation and treatment of a wide range of neurologic conditions (Franklin and Zahn 2002), including the evaluation of children and adolescents with recurrent headache (Lewis et al. 2002), electrodiagnostic studies in carpal tunnel syndrome (Jablecki et al. 2002), and the diagnosis and management of dementia (Doody et al. 2001; Knopman et al. 2001).

Example 19–2 One example from the Quality Standards Subcommittee of the American Academy of Neurology is the updated practice parameter for initiation of treatment for Parkinson's disease (Miyasaki et al. 2002). In this review the authors searched the English literature published between 1966 and 2000 using MEDLINE and EMBASE (a commercially available database that indexes over 3600 journals published in 70 countries). The article provides a detailed description of the search strategy used as well as criteria for inclusion and exclusion of articles located. Articles were rated as to their level of evidence using the classification system shown in Table 19–3. The strength of the recommendations were rated A (established as effective, ineffective, or harmful), B (probably effective, ineffective, or harmful), or C (possibly effective, ineffective, or harmful). Table 19–4 provides a description of the criteria used for each rating.

While the above categories help us to understand the common types of information

Table 19–3   Levels of Evidence Quality, Class I (Best) to Class IV (Weakest)

Class I	Prospective, randomized, controlled clinical trial with masked outcome assessment, in a representative population that fulfills the following criteria: a. Primary outcome(s) is (are) clearly defined. b. Exclusion/inclusion criteria are clearly defined. c. There is adequate accounting for dropouts and crossovers with numbers sufficiently low to have minimal potential for bias. d. Relevant baseline characteristics are presented and are substantially equivalent among treatment groups or there is appropriate statistical adjustment of differences.
Class II	Prospective matched group cohort study in a representative population with masked outcome assessment that meets a–d above *or* a randomized controlled trial in a representative population that lacks one criterion from a–d above.
Class III	All other controlled trials (including well-defined natural history controls or patients serving as own controls) in a representative population where outcome assessment is independent of patient treatment
Class IV	Evidence from uncontrolled studies, case series, case reports, or expert opinion

Adapted from Miyasaki et al. (2002), reprinted with permission.

Table 19–4 Rating of Recommendations Based on Quality of Evidence

Rating of Recommendation	Translation of Evidence to Recommendations
A: Established as effective, ineffective, or harmful for the given condition in the specified population	Requires at least one convincing class I study or at least two consistent, convincing class II studies
B: Probably effective, ineffective, or harmful for the given condition in the specified population	Requires at least one convincing class II study or at least three convincing class III studies
C: Possibly effective, ineffective, or harmful for the given condition in the specified population	Requires at least two convincing and consistent class III studies

Adapted from Miyasaki et al. (2002), reprinted with permission.

sources relevant to EBM, types of information are commonly combined and distinctions may be blurred. Several commercial services provide structured, EBM-based reviews of topics as well as links to the primary studies and to guidelines. For example, a computer algorithm could provide an estimate of the utility of a CT scan in a patient with a minor head injury, based on the Canadian CT Head Rule (Stiell et al. 2001). Providing efficient access to the best evidence for answering clinical questions is an evolving process that depends on advances in hardware and information systems. Examples of sources for evidence are provided in Appendix 19–1.

Step 3. Critically appraising the evidence. This step can seem daunting, especially to clinicians with relatively little research training, but it can also be the most rewarding. Appraising the evidence is often broken down into three steps: (*1*) evaluating the internal validity of the study (are the results true for the subjects in the study?); (*2*) estimating the effect size, predictive value, or similar measure of the magnitude of the finding (are the results important?); and (*3*) the generalizability of the study (can I apply the results to my patients?). The evaluation of the internal validity of a study is based on the same principles and concepts taught in epidemiology (Chapters 1–3) and health services research and depends on the type of study. While most clinicians will not be as methodologically sophisticated as epidemiologists or health services researchers, basic concepts

such as confounding, intention-to-treat analysis, blinding, and confidence intervals are easily mastered. There are several excellent books and journal articles, including a widely respected series in the *Journal of the American Medical Association* (see Appendix 19–1C), that provide approaches for clinicians to use in evaluating common types of studies, such as screening and diagnostic testing, and prognosis and treatment studies, as well as meta-analyses, systematic reviews, decision analyses, and evidence-based guidelines. Reviewing these approaches is outside the scope of this chapter; however, a list of resources is provided in Appendix 19–1A.

Assessing the effect size reported for therapies has been facilitated by the increasingly common practice of reporting both absolute risk reduction and number needed to treat (NNT) (or number needed to screen) to achieve the desired outcome. The *NNT* is simply the inverse of the absolute risk reduction. For example, a randomized controlled trial of patients with migraine headache found that 56% of subjects taking L-acetylsalicylic acid (1620 mg) plus metoclopramide (10 mg) reported relief compared to 28% of those taking a placebo. The absolute risk reduction was 28% (i.e., 56% − 28%), yielding a NNT of 1/0.28, or approximately 4 (Chabriat et al. 2001). This indicates that, on average, one would need to treat four patients to prevent one headache.

Another measure, the likelihood ratio (LR), is helpful in assessing the usefulness of a test. The *likelihood ratio* is the likelihood that a given test result would be obtained in a patient with the condition, compared to the likelihood that it would occur in a patient without the condition. The LR for a positive test is equal to the sensitivity of the test divided by 1 minus the specificity (or the true-positive rate divided by the false-positive rate). Multiplying the pretest odds of a condition (i.e., that the patient has the condition of interest before the test is performed) by the LR for a positive test provides the post-test odds that the patient has the condition if the test is positive. Tests with LRs nearer to 1 are less useful than those with LRs much less or much more than 1.

Determining the applicability of the study to the patient in question requires clinical judgment. Demographic characteristics, comorbidities, severity of disease, type of symptoms, and practice environment of the study subjects are often different from those of the patients to whom the information is applied in practice. For example, the effectiveness of carotid endarterectomy in prevention of stroke depends on the patient's age, level of symptoms, and degree of stenosis and the complication rate of the surgeon performing the procedure (Cina et al. 1999).

Step 4. Integrating the evidence with expert clinical opinion. This step, which also entails integrating evidence with clinical experience and the patient's particular characteristics and preferences, is as much an art as a science. Evidence-based medicine does not provide a "cookbook" answer to a clinical question. Clinical expertise, the opinions of other physicians that are based on their experiences, and, most importantly, the preferences of the patient all must be integrated with the information provided by EBM. Eliciting patient preferences requires excellent communication and partnering skills between a physician and her or his patients.

Step 5. Evaluating and seeking ways to improve the efficiency of the EBM process.

This step requires reviewing steps 1 through 4 in light of the outcome achieved and the effort required. Was there a better way to formulate the question? Could the search have been performed more efficiently? With experience, it is possible to choose questions that are both clinically important and likely to be answered, at least partially, by evidence. Likewise, experience allows for more efficient searches and better evaluation and integration of evidence.

Applying Evidence-Based Medicine in Practice: A Case Vignette

Dr. Martin is seeing Mr. Thomas Newcomb, a 66-year-old man with a 3-year history of recurrent trigeminal neuralgia (TN) who is currently being treated with sustained-release carbamazepine at 400 mg, twice a day. The patient has continued to have significant pain (6/10) and when his primary care physician increased the dose of carbamazepine, he experienced nausea and an unsteady gait. Mr. Newcomb would like to try a different medication to relieve his pain. Dr. Martin knows that carbamazepine is considered the first-line treatment for TN, but the best alternative medication is less clear, so she decides to use EBM tools to locate evidence to help evaluate treatment options.

Dr. Martin first formulates a question using the principles of PICO: "In an older, healthy man with chronic pain from TN (Patient/Problem), what alternative to carbamazepine (Intervention and Comparison) is most effective for reducing pain (Outcome)?". Using the computer terminal in the examination room, she goes to her bookmarked Cochrane Library site and conducts a search for "trigeminal neuralgia". She is pleased to find two systematic reviews, one of which includes treatment of TN (Wiffen et al. 2000). From this review she finds that of the three drugs compared to carbamazepine in controlled studies, only pimozide, a dopamine receptor antagonist, was found to be more effective than carbamazepine (Lechin et al. 1989). In the table provided she sees that in this randomized, double-blind, crossover study, patients in the pimozide (12 mg per day) group reported a 78% improvement in their symptom score, compared to 56% improvement when taking carbamazepine (1200 mg per day) ($p < 0.05$). However, adverse events were also more common when taking pimozide (83% vs. 44%, $p < 0.05$). The quality of the study was rated 4 out of a possible 5. The mean age of the patients was 59 years, the median duration of TN was 13 years, and 50% of the patients were men. The review also reported a second double-blind crossover study of 14 patients with refractive TN (10 taking carbamazepine only and 4 taking phenytoin ± carbamazepine) that compared the addition of lamotrigine (400 mg per day) versus placebo (Zakrzewska et al. 1997). Global improvement was reported by 77% of patients when taking their usual medication plus lamotrigine, compared to 57% of those taking their usual medication plus the placebo (NNT = 5). The quality of this smaller study has also 4 out of 5, with patient characteristics similar to those of the first study. There was no difference in the incidence of side effects for patients taking lamotrigine or placebo.

While neither study reported the effects on pain alone, both were reasonably well designed but had limited follow-up (8 weeks and 2 weeks, respectively). Both reports enrolled patients similar in age to Mr. Newcomb, though with TN of longer duration. Dr. Martin summarizes the evidence for Mr. Newcomb and presents two possibilities: switching from carbamazepine to pimozide, which may be more effective than carbamazepine but appears to have more side effects, or adding lamotrigine, which appears to be effective and less likely to have side effects (a finding based on a smaller number of patients studied). Because Mr. Newcomb is concerned about side effects, he decides to try adding the lamotrigine carefully titrated as currently recommended to his current carbamazepine dose.

That evening, Dr. Martin reflects back on her EBM experience and wonders if she would have found more evidence if she had had more time. She notes that the Cochrane site was last updated 1 year earlier and was limited to evaluation of anticonvulsants, so she does a literature search on PubMed for the past 10 years, using the title/abstract words "trigeminal neuralgia" and "treatment". She limits the search to clinical trials and finds 22 articles, none of which seems to provide any important additional data. She decides that, while the evidence for the effectiveness of lamotrigine is limited, it was probably a reasonable choice for treatment, given Mr. Newcomb's preference for minimizing the chance of side effects.

Limitations of Evidence-Based Medicine

The most basic limitation of EBM is the lack of good-quality, relevant evidence for many of the clinically important questions neurologists encounter in practice. Many questions have not been addressed with studies, or have been inadequately addressed by observational studies or inadequately powered randomized trials. Even when good studies exist, they may not be relevant to a given patient. While additional evidence is being added daily, new questions are also being generated as additional treatments and diagnostic technologies become available. Thus it is unlikely that we will ever have the evidence we would like to answer all, or even most, of our clinical questions. Nonetheless, when good evidence is available, it can provide an essential part of decision making and patient care. Even determining a lack of evidence can be helpful, as it may free us from errors resulting from unsupported assumptions or beliefs.

A second limitation of EBM is clinician time. Typically, a clinician has only a few minutes or less to access, evaluate, and integrate evidence (Ely et al. 1999). To some extent, the impact of this limitation depends on the given technology for information access and the availability and quality of secondary review sources. Inevitably, however, there is an upfront time cost associated with searching for evidence to supplement clinical experience or opinion.

Another limitation of EBM is clinicians' relative lack of skills in critically and efficiently assessing the quality of evidence. Most clinicians do not have the formal training needed to be maximally effective in assessing evidence. To some extent this limitation can be addressed by books, tutorials, and courses on the practice of EBM. Appropriate skills can also be acquired through modeling of teachers, educators, and colleagues.

A fourth limitation of EBM is in implementing pertinent evidence in the care of the patient; certain diagnostic tests or treatments may not be available in a neurologist's practice setting. There is ample evidence, for example, that designated stroke units provide better care for stroke patients than does conventional care on medical wards (Stroke Unit Trialists' Collaboration 1997). To apply this evidence, however, would require organizational-level changes.

Finally, there is a lack of evidence for the utility of EBM. Little is known about the impact of EBM, compared to that of traditional practice patterns, on patient outcomes. We do not yet know in what circumstances an EBM approach is most likely to change patient care or if EBM is cost-effective.

Despite these limitations, EBM is growing. In the technological era, it is the logical extension of the principle espoused by William Osler 100 years ago of applying the best available scientific evidence to the practice of medicine (Osler 1932).

Future Directions and Conclusions

Evidence-based medicine is not cookbook medicine. Rather, is the conscientious, explicit, and judicious application of the best available evidence in making decisions about the care of individual patients. Neuroepidemiologic studies provide the groundwork for EBM by supplying research about patient risk, prognosis, and harm, as well as data to inform clinical decision analysis and practice guidelines. Evidence-based medicine provides a set of tools for formulating a clinically important question about a particular patient and efficiently accessing and critically evaluating relevant information. The neurologist can then integrate the evidence with clinical judgment and patient preferences to provide better patient care. The goal of EBM is to provide high-quality information in real time for neurologists to use in practice. Additional steps needed to achieve this goal include physician training in EBM principals and techniques, more and better patient-oriented research on important clinical questions, and improvements in information technology. In the mean time, EBM can provide a useful approach to maximizing the scientific basis for the practice of medicine in general and neurology in particular.

References

Alper BS, Stevermer JJ, White DS, Ewigman BG. Answering family physicians' clinical questions using electronic medical databases. *J Fam Pract* 2001;50:960–965.

Bero L, Rennie D. The Cochrane Collaboration. Preparing, maintaining, and disseminating systematic reviews of the effects of health care. *JAMA* 1995;274:1935–1938.

Chabriat H., Joire JE, Danchot J, et al. Combined oral lysine acetylsalicylate and metoclopramide in the acute treatment of migraine: a multicentre double-blind placebo-controlled trial. *Cephalagia* 1994;14:297–300.

Cina CS, Clase CM, Haynes BR. Redefining the indications for carotid endarterectomy in patients with symptomatic carotid stenosis. *J Vasc Surg* 1999;30:606–617.

Cook DJ, Greengold NL, Ellrodt AG, Weingarten SR. The relation between systematic reviews and practice guidelines. *Ann Intern Med* 1997;127:210–216.

Davis DA. Physician education, evidence and the coming to age of CME. *J Gen Intern Med* 1996;705–706.

Doody RS, Stevens JC, Beck C, et al. Practice parameter: management of dementia (an evidence-based review). Report of the Quality Standards Subcommittee of the American Academy of Neurology. *Neurology* 2001;56: 1154–1166.

Ely JW, Osheroff JA, Ebell MH, et al. Analysis of

questions asked by family doctors regarding patient care. *BMJ* 1999;319:358–361.

Evidence-Based Medicine Working Group. Evidence-based medicine. A new approach to teaching the practice of medicine. *JAMA* 1992;268:2420–2425.

Franklin GM, Zahn CA. American Academy of Neurology clinical practice guidelines: above the fray. *Neurology* 2002;59:975–976.

Hunt DL, McKibbon KA. Locating and appraising systematic reviews. *Ann Intern Med* 1997;126:532–538.

Iansek R, Elstein AS, Balla JI. Application of decision analysis to management of cerebral arteriovenous malformations. *Lancet* 1983; 1:1132–1135.

Jablecki CK, Andary MT, Floeter MK, et al. Practice parameter: Electrodiagnostic studies in carpal tunnel syndrome. Report of the American Association of Electrodiagnostic Medicine, American Academy of Neurology, and the American Academy of Physical Medicine and Rehabilitation. *Neurology* 2002; 58:1589–1592.

Knopman DS, DeKosky S, Cummings JL, et al. Practice parameter: diagnosis of dementia (an evidence-based review). Report of the Quality Standards Subcommittee of the American Academy of Neurology. *Neurology* 2001;56:1143–1153.

Koprowski CD, Longstreth WT, Cebul RD. Clinical neuroepidemiology: III. Decisions. *Arch Neurol* 1989;46:223–229.

Laupacis A, Wells G, Richardson WS, Tugwell P. Evidence-Based Medicine Working Group. User's guide to the medical literature: V. How to use an article about prognosis. *JAMA* 1994;272:234–237.

Lechin F, van der Dijs B, Lechin ME, et al. Pimozide therapy for trigeminal neuralgia. *Arch Neurol* 1989;46:960–963.

Lewis DW, Ashwal S, Dahl G, et al. Practice parameter: evaluation of children and adolescents with recurrent headaches: report of the Quality Standards Subcommittee of the American Academy of Neurology and the Practice Committee of the Child Neurology Society. *Neurology* 2002;59:490–498.

McQuay HJ, Moore RA. Using numerical results from systematic reviews in clinical practice. *Ann Intern Med* 1997;126:712–720.

Miyasaki JM, Martin W, Suchowersky O, et al. Practice parameter: initiation of treatment for Parkinson's disease: an evidence-based review: report of the Quality Standards Subcommittee of the American Academy of Neurology. *Neurology* 2002;58:11–17.

Mulrow CD, Cook DJ, Davidoff F. Systematic reviews: critical links in the great chain of evidence. *Ann Intern Med* 1997;126:389–391.

Osler W. Medicine in the nineteenth century. In: Aequanimitas with Other Address, 3rd edition. Philadelphia: The Blakiston Company, 1932, pp 219–262.

Rice GPA, Incorvaia B, Munari L, et al. Interferon in relapsing-remitting multiple sclerosis (Cochrane Review). In: *The Cochrane Library,* Issue 4, 2002, Oxford: Update Software.

Richardson WS, Wilson MC, Nishikawa J, Hayward RS. The well-built clinical question: a key to evidence-based decisions. *ACP Journal Club* 1995;Nov/Dec:A12–A13.

Richardson WS, Detsky AS, Evidence-Based Medicine Working Group. Users' guides to the medical literature: VII. How to use a clinical decision analysis. A. Are the results of the study valid? *JAMA* 1995;273:1292–1295.

Sackett DL, Strauss SE, Richardson WS, Rosenberg W, Haynes B. Evidence-Based Medicine: How to Practice and Teach EBM, 2nd edition. New York: Churchill Livingston, 2000.

Schuster MA, McGlynn EA, Brook RH. How good is the quality of health care in the United States? *Milbank Q* 1998;76:517–563.

Stiell IG, Wells GA, Vandemheen K, et al. The Canadian CT Head Rule for patients with minor head injury. *Lancet* 2001;1391–1396.

Stroke Unit Trialists' Collaboration. Collaborative systematic review of the randomised trials of organised inpatient (stroke unit) care after stroke. *BMJ* 1997;314:1151–1159.

U.S. Preventive Services Task Force. Guide to Clinical Preventive Services, second edition. Alexandria, VA: International Medical Publishing, 1996.

Verhoeven AAH, Boerma EJ, Meyboom-de Jung B. Which literature retrieval method is most effective for GPs? *Fam Pract* 2000;17:30–35.

Walsh JS, Welch HG, Larson EB. Survival of outpatients with Alzheimer-type dementia. *Ann Int Med* 1990;113:429–434.

Wiffen P, Collins S, McQuay H, et al. Anticonvulsant drugs for acute and chronic pain. In: *The Cochrane Library,* Issue 4, 2000. Oxford: Update Software.

Zakrzewska JM, Chaudhry Z, Nurmikko TJ, et al. Lamotrigine (Lamictal) in refractory trigeminal neuralgia: results from a double-blind placebo controlled crossover trial. *Pain* 1997;73:223–230.

Appendix 19–1 Evidence-Based Medicine Resources

A. Textbooks

General Evidence-Based Medicine Texts

Friedland DJ, Go AS, Davoren JB, Shlipak MG, Bent SW, Subak LL, Medelson T. Evidence-Based Medicine. Stamford CT: Appleton & Lange, 1998.

Geyman JP, Deyo RA, Ramsey SD. Evidence-Based Clinical Practice: Concepts and Approaches. Burlington, MA: Butterworth-Heinemann Medical, 2000.

Guyatt G, Rennie D. User's Guide to the Medical Literature: Essentials of Evidence-Based Clinical Practice. Chicago: American Medical Association, 2001.

McKibbon A. PDQ Evidence-Based Principles and Practices. Hamilton, IN: B.C. Deckers, Inc., 1999.

Muir Gray JA. Evidence-Based Healthcare: How to Make Health Policy and Management Decisions. Philadelphia: WB Saunders, 2001.

Sackett DL, Straus SE, Richardson WS, Rosenberg W, Haynes RB. Evidence-Based Medicine: How to Practice and Teach EBM, second edition. New York: Churchill Livingston, 2000.

Neurology Chapters in Evidence-Based Medicine Texts

McGee S. Neurologic examination. In Evidence-Based Physical Diagnosis. Philadelphia: WB Saunders, 2001, pp 671–828.

Salinas R, Neurological disorders. In Clinical Evidence. London: British Medical Journal Publishing Corporation, 2001, pp 961–1035.

B. Internet Sources for Evidence-Based Medicine

General Web Sites

Centre for Evidence-Based Medicine: http://www.cebm.jr2.ox.ac.uk

Michigan State University tutorial on evidence-based medicine: http://www.poems.msu.edu/infoMastery/

Netting the Evidence: http://www.sheffield.ac.uk/~scharr/ir/netting/

PubMed. Provides searches of contents of National Library of Medicine. http://www.ncbi.nlm.nih.gov/entrez/query.fcgi

Neurology-Specific Web Sites

ABN: Evidence-based Neurology. Provides links to multiple EBM sites. http://www.theabn.org/education/evidence.html

Cochrane Neurological Network. Part of the Cochrane Collaboration. http://www.cochraneneuronet.org/

Evidence-based Neurology. Provides EBM tools as well as critically appraised topics (CATs) in neurology. http://www.uwo.ca/clinns/ebn/

C. Journal of American Medical Association Series on Evaluation of the Medical Literature (in Chronological Order)

Oxman AD, Sackett DL, Guyatt GH, Evidence-Based Medicine Working Group. Users' guides to the medical literature: I. How to get started. *JAMA* 1993;270:2093–2097.

Guyatt GH, Sackett DL, Cook DJ, Evidence-Based Medicine Working Group. Users' guides to the medical literature: II. How to use an article about therapy or prevention. A. Are the results of the study valid? *JAMA* 1993;270:2598–2601.

Guyatt GH, Sackett DL, Cook DJ, Evidence-Based Medicine Working Group. Users' guides to the medical literature: II. How to use an article about therapy or prevention. B. What were the results and will they help me in caring for my patients? *JAMA* 1994;271:59–63.

Jaeschke R, Guyatt GH, Sackett DL, Evidence-Based Medicine Working Group. Users' guides to the medical literature: III. How to use an article about a diagnostic test. A. Are the results of the study valid? *JAMA* 1994a;271:389–391.

Jaeschke R, Guyatt GH, Sackett DL, Evidence-Based Medicine Working Group. Users' guides to the medical literature: III. How to use an article about a diagnostic test. B. What are the results and will they help me in caring for my patients? *JAMA* 1994b;271:703–707.

Levine M, Walter S, Lee H, Haines T, Holbrook A, Moyer V, Evidence-Based Medicine Working Group. Users' guides to the medical literature: IV. How to use an article about harm. *JAMA* 1994;271:1615–1619.

Laupacis A, Wells G, Richardson S, Tugwell P, Evidence-Based Medicine Working Group. Users' guides to the medical literature: V. How to use an article about prognosis. *JAMA* 1994;272:234–237.

Oxman AD, Cook DJ, Guyatt GH, Evidence-Based Medicine Working Group. Users' guides to the medical literature: VI. How to use an overview. *JAMA* 1994;272:1367–1371.

Richardson WS, Detsky AS, Evidence-Based Medicine Working Group. Users' guides to the medical literature: VII. How to use a clinical decision analysis. A. Are the results of the study valid? *JAMA* 1995a;273:1292–1295.

Richardson WS, Detsky AS, Evidence-Based Medicine Working Group. Users' guides to the medical literature: VII. How to use a clinical decision analysis. B. What are the results and will they help me in caring for my patients? *JAMA* 1995b;273:1610–1613.

Hayward RSA, Wilson MC, Tunis SR, Bass EB, Guyatt GH, Evidence-Based Medicine Working Group. Users' guides to the medical literature: VIII. How to use clinical practice guidelines A. Are the recommendations valid? *JAMA* 1995;274:570–574.

Guyatt GH, Sackett DL, Sinclair JC, et al. Users' Guides to the Medical Literature: IX. A method for grading health care recommendations. *JAMA* 1995;274:1800–1804.

Naylor CD, Guyatt GH, Evidence-Based Medicine Working Group. Users' guides to the medical literature: X. How to use an article reporting variations in the outcomes of health services. *JAMA* 1996a;275:554–558.

Naylor CD, Guyatt GH, Evidence-Based Medicine Working Group. Users' guide to the medical literature: XI. How to use an article about a clinical utilization review. *JAMA* 1996b;275:1435–1439.

Guyatt GH, Naylor CD, Juniper EF, Heyland KD, Jaeschke R, Cook DJ, Evidence-Based Medicine Working Group. Users' guides to the medical literature: XII. How to use articles about health-related quality of life. *JAMA* 1997;277:1232–1237.

Drummond MF, Richardson S, O'Brien BJ, Levine M, Heyland D, Evidence-Based Medicine Working Group. Users' guides to the medical literature: XIII. How to use an article on economic analysis of clinical practice. A. Are the results of the study valid? *JAMA* 1997;277:1552–1557.

O'Brien BJ, Heyland D, Richardson WS, Levine M, Drummond MF, Evidence-Based Medicine Working Group. Users' guides to the medical literature: XIII. How to use an article on economic analysis of clinical practice. B. What are the results and will they help me in caring for my patients? *JAMA* 1997;277:1802–1806.

Dans AL, Dans LF, Guyatt GH, Richardson S, Evidence-Based Medicine Working Group. Users' guides to the medical literature: XIV. How to decide on the applicability of clinical trial results to your patients. *JAMA* 1998;279:545–549.

Richardson WS, Wilson MC, Guyatt GH, Cook DJ, Nishikawa J, Evidence-Based Medicine Working Group. Users' guides to the medical literature: XV. How to use an article about disease probability for differential diagnosis. *JAMA* 1999;281:1214–1219.

Guyatt GH, Sinclair JC, Cook DJ, Glasziou PP, Evidence-Based Medicine Working Group. Users' guides to the medical literature: XVI. How to use a treatment recommendation. *JAMA* 1999;281:1836–1843.

Barratt A, Irwig L, Glasziou PP, Cummings RG, Raffle A, Hicks N, Muir Gray JA, Guyatt GH, Evidence-Based Medicine Working Group. Users' guides to the medical literature: XVII. How to use guidelines and recommendations about screening. *JAMA* 1999;281:2029–2034.

Randolph AG, Haynes RB, Wyatt JC, et al. Users' Guides to the Medical Literature: XVIII. How to use an article evaluating the clinical impact of a computer-based clinical decision support system. *JAMA* 1999;282:67–74.

Bucher HC, Guyatt GH, Holbrook A, McAlister FA. Users' Guides to the Medical Literature: XIX. Applying clinical trial results. A. How to use an article measuring the effect of an intervention on surrogate end points. *JAMA* 1999;282:771–778.

McAlister FA, Laupacis A, Wells GA, Sackett DL. Users' Guides to the Medical Literature: XIX. Applying clinical trial results. B. Guidelines for determining whether a drug is exerting (more than) a class effect. *JAMA* 1999;282:1371–1377.

McAlister FA, Straus SE, Guyatt GH, Haynes RB. Users' Guides to the Medical Literature: XX. Integrating research evidence with the care of the individual patient. *JAMA* 2000;283:2829–2836.

Hunt DL, Jaeschke R, McKibbon KA. Users' Guides to the Medical Literature: XXI. Using electronic health information resources in evidence-based practice. *JAMA* 2000;283:1875–1879.

McGinn TG, Guyatt GH, Naylor CD, et al. Users' Guides to the Medical Literature: XXII. How to use articles about clinical decision rules. *JAMA* 2000;284:79–84.

Giacomini MK, Cook DJ. Users' Guides to the Medical Literature: XXIII. Qualitative research in health care A. Are the results of the study valid? *JAMA* 2000;284:357–362.

Giacomini MK, Cook DJ. Users' Guides to the Medical Literature: XXIII. Qualitative research in health care B. What are the results and how do they help me care for my patients? *JAMA* 2000;284:478–482.

Richardson WS, Wilson MC, Williams JW Jr, et al. Users' Guides to the Medical Literature: XXIV. How to use an article on the clinical manifestations of disease. *JAMA* 2000;284:869–875.

Guyatt GH, Haynes RB, Jaeschke RZ, et al. Users' Guides to the Medical Literature: XXV. Evidence-based medicine: applying the Users' Guides to patient care. *JAMA* 2000;284:1290–1296.

Appendix 19–2 Common Evidence-Based Medicine Terms

Critically appraised topic (CAT) Evaluation of the evidence using EBM tools, to help answer a clinical question. Less comprehensive and formal than a systematic review.

Disease-oriented evidence (DOE) Evidence based on disease outcomes, usually a biologic or anatomic measure. Examples would be sedimentation rate in patients with intracerebral vasculitis or the number of white matter lesions on MRI in patients with multiple sclerosis.

Likelihood ratio negative (LR−) The ratio of the probability that a particular test will be negative in a patient with the condition of interest to the probability that the test will be negative in a patient without the condition. Equal to $(1 - \text{sensitivity})/\text{specificity}$. When a test is negative, the pretest odds of a condition multiplied by the LR− yields the post-test odds for the condition.

Likelihood ratio positive (LR+) The ratio of the probability that a particular test will be positive in a patient with the condition of interest to the probability that the test will be positive in a patient without the condition. Equal to $\text{sensitivity}/(1 - \text{specificity})$. When a test is positive, the pretest odds of a condition multiplied by the LR+ yields the post-test odds for the condition.

Negative predictive value (NPV) Probability that a patient with a negative test will not have the condition of interest.

Number needed to treat (NNT) The average number of patients that would need to receive the intervention for one patient to have the outcome of interest. Equal to the inverse of the absolute risk reduction. For example, if 56% of patients in the placebo group died, and only 22% in the treatment group died, then on average one would need to treat three patients to prevent one death $(1/(0.56 - 0.22) = 3)$.

Patient intervention comparison outcome (PICO) A mnemonic for structuring an evidence-based question. *Patient* refers to the key characteristics of the patient to whom the answer is to be applied, *intervention* can be a treatment or screening or other action, *comparison* refers to the alternative to the intervention (a different intervention or no intervention) and *outcome* refers to the clinically relevant results attributable to the intervention.

Patient-oriented evidence that matters (POEM) Evidence based on patient-centered outcomes, such as functional status, pain, or quality of life, as opposed to biological measures such as improvement in nerve conduction, normalization of laboratory values, or changes on imaging studies.

Positive predictive value (PPV) Probability that a patient with a positive test will have the condition of interest.

Post-test odds The odds that the patient has the condition of interest after the test is performed. Odds are calculated as probability/(1 − probability). Thus a probability of disease of 0.80 yields an odds of $0.8/(1 − 0.8) = 4$ (four patients with the disease for every patient without the diseases).

Post-test probability The probability that the patient has the condition of interest after the test is performed. Probability can be calculated as odds/(1 + odds). Thus if the odds of disease are 4 (four patients with the disease for every patient without the disease) the probability of disease would be $4/(1 + 4) = 0.8$.

Pre-test odds The odds that the patient has the condition of interest prior to the test. Odds are calculated as probability/(1 − probability). Thus a probability of disease of 0.25 yields an odds of 0.33 (one patient with the disease for every three patients without the disease).

Pre-test probability The probability that the patient has the condition of interest before the test is performed. Probability can be calculated as odds/(1 + odds). Thus if the odds of disease are 0.25 (one patient with the disease for every four patients without the disease) the probability of disease would be $0.25/(1 + 0.25) = 0.2$.

SnNout A mnemonic for remembering that for a test with high **S**e**n**sitivity, a **N**egative result effectively rules **out** a condition.

SpPin A mnemonic for remembering that for a test with high **S**pecificity, a **P**ositive result effectively rules **in** a condition.

Systematic review (SR) A comprehensive review of the literature that uses explicit principals and procedures to locate, evaluate, and synthesize research information on a topic or question.

Index